Handbook of Pulmonary Diseases

Handbook of Pulmonary Diseases

Editor: Beatrice Gunther

AMERICAN
MEDICAL PUBLISHERS
www.americanmedicalpublishers.com

AMERICAN
MEDICAL PUBLISHERS
www.americanmedicalpublishers.com

Cataloging-in-Publication Data

Handbook of pulmonary diseases / edited by Beatrice Gunther.
p. cm.
Includes bibliographical references and index.
ISBN 979-8-88740-567-4
1. Lungs--Diseases. 2. Lungs--Diseases, Fungal. 3. Lungs--Diseases, Obstructive.
4. Lungs—Blood-vessels--Diseases. 5. Pulmonary manifestations of general diseases.
6. Respiratory organs—Diseases. I. Gunther, Beatrice.
RC756 .P85 2023
616.24--dc23

American Medical Publishers,
41 Flatbush Avenue,
1st Floor, New York,
NY 11217, USA

ISBN 979-8-88740-567-4 (Hardback)

Contents

Preface

This book aims to highlight the current researches and provides a platform to further the scope of innovations in this area. This book is a product of the combined efforts of many researchers and scientists, after going through thorough studies and analysis from different parts of the world. The objective of this book is to provide the readers with the latest information of the field.

Pulmonary diseases are the disorders that inhibit the lungs and respiratory system from functioning properly. They can be classified into three main types, namely, airway diseases, lung tissue diseases and lung circulation diseases. Smoking is considered as the main cause of pulmonary diseases. Some other causes include infection, radon, asbestos, and other types of air pollution. The most common pulmonary diseases are asthma, chronic obstructive pulmonary disease (COPD), lung cancer pulmonary fibrosis, and pneumonia. Some major symptoms of pulmonary diseases are cough, chest pain, and shortness of breath, which can be diagnosed through chest X-ray, CT scan, bronchoscopy, pleural biopsies and pulmonary function tests. Treatments of pulmonary diseases include medications, oxygen therapy, pulmonary rehabilitation, and lung transplantation. Preventive measures like quitting smoking, proper nutrition and getting vaccinated can help reduce the progression of these diseases. This book unravels the recent studies on pulmonary diseases. It consists of contributions made by international experts. This book will serve as a valuable source of reference for graduate and post graduate students.

I would like to express my sincere thanks to the authors for their dedicated efforts in the completion of this book. I acknowledge the efforts of the publisher for providing constant support. Lastly, I would like to thank my family for their support in all academic endeavors.

Editor

1

Neutrophils in Tuberculosis-Associated Inflammation and Lung Pathology

Caleb N. Muefong* and Jayne S. Sutherland

Vaccines and Immunity Theme, Medical Research Council Unit, The Gambia at the London School of Hygiene and Tropical Medicine, Fajara, The Gambia

***Correspondence:**
Caleb N. Muefong
cmuefong@mrc.gm

Protective immunity to *Mycobacterium tuberculosis (Mtb)*—the causative agent of tuberculosis (TB)—is not fully understood but involves immune responses within the pulmonary airways which can lead to exacerbated inflammation and immune pathology. In humans, this inflammation results in lung damage; the extent of which depends on specific host pro-inflammatory processes. Neutrophils, though increasingly linked to the development of inflammatory disorders, have been less well studied in relation to TB-induced lung pathology. Neutrophils mode of action and their specialized functions can be directly linked to TB-specific lung tissue damage observed on patient chest X-rays at diagnosis and contribute to long-term pulmonary sequelae. This review discusses aspects of neutrophil activity associated with active TB, including the resulting inflammation and pulmonary impairment. It highlights the significance of neutrophil function on TB disease outcome and underlines the necessity of monitoring neutrophil function for better assessment of the immune response and severity of lung pathology associated with TB. Finally, we propose that some MMPs, ROS, MPO, S100A8/A9 and Glutathione are neutrophil-related inflammatory mediators with promising potential as targets for developing host-directed therapies for TB.

Keywords: tuberculosis, neutrophils, inflammatory mediators, lung damage, sequelae

INTRODUCTION

Tuberculosis (TB) is the single deadliest infectious disease known to man with 10 million new cases and 1.6 million deaths (including 300,000 HIV coinfected) in 2018 (1). This report does not account for health impairment nor deaths during and following TB treatment; which is suggested to be about three times higher than those observed in the general population or suitably matched controls (2). It is known today that despite being diagnosed as microbiologically cured from TB, about 50% of patients still suffer from some form of pulmonary impairment after tuberculosis (PIAT), irrespective of smoking habits (3). The definition of PIAT encompasses several clinical conditions; which in former TB patients is suggested to result from chronic inflammation, characterized by disrupted pulmonary structure and function (residual lung deficits) (4, 5); a state described as thoracic/TB sequelae (6). These include parenchymal, airway, vascular and mediastinal lesions manifested mainly through structural [cicatrization, calcification, fibrosis and reduction in cavity wall thickness (6)] and functional [deficit in forced expiratory volume (4)] damage; the establishment (7) and severity (8–10) of which, are associated to neutrophil abundance and (hyper-)activity.

As compelling as these effects of TB may be, PIAT is presently not included in global estimates of TB burden despite increasing scientific interest and evidence of associated morbidity and mortality (3–5, 11–14).

A recent cohort study showed that subjects with a history of fully treated active TB (ATB) lost 3.6 years on average of disability-adjusted life expectancy compared to subjects with latent TB infection (LTBI) who did not progress to the active state (12). Despite the lack of data to support disease burden resulting from long-term sequelae (11), the above reduced life expectancy is a direct result of TB sequelae and suggests that a considerable proportion of the TB disease burden is contributed by subjects who have successfully cleared Mtb. Indeed, a study in Texas, USA reported that the number of years lived with chronic TB disability accounts for 75% of non-fatal health effects of TB (11). This same study suggests that the most health and financial savings may be achieved by preventing rather than shortening therapeutic strategies. Additionally, a recent retrospective study reveals the negative effect of drug-resistance and disease recurrence on PIAT (15). Consequently, early detection of parameters which increase the likelihood of ATB complication into chronic inflammation and long-term sequelae would inform clinicians on the need for case-specific treatment measures and contribute to minimizing the global TB burden (13). Such parameters can be realistically linked to neutrophil function and/or interaction with other immune cell populations in the view of their specific activities described in subsequent sections below.

Generally, protective immunity to *Mycobacterium tuberculosis* (Mtb)—the causative agent of TB—is a combination of innate and adaptive immune responses within the pulmonary airways via which this pathogen gains entrance into the human host (16, 17). This immune response to TB is described as a chronic granulomatous inflammation; caused by close interaction between Mtb bacilli and host immune agents at the infection site (18). Indeed, the term "chronic granulomatous" draws from a condition, chronic granulomatous disease (CGD), with similar inflammatory outcomes; resulting from genetic mutations of reduced nicotinamide adenine dinucleotide phosphate ($NADPH_2$) oxidase-encoding genes (19, 20). Disruption in the production of this enzyme; which normally catalyzes the synthesis of reactive oxygen species (ROS) used by phagocytes to destroy bacteria during phagocytosis, leads to enhanced susceptibility to infectious pathogens and granuloma formation; particularly in the lungs (21). Despite several gaps in knowledge, the contribution of adaptive immune responses: particularly T-cells [reviewed in Jasenosky et al. (22)] and to a lesser extent B-cells [reviewed in Achkar et al. (23)] have been addressed. Furthermore Dyatlov et al. recently reviewed the role of B cells on reducing neutrophil influx to infection sites (24) and; these Mtb-specific immune responses having been studied extensively and will not form a focus of this review.

Recent studies have revealed that the innate arm of the immune system plays a bigger role in the onset and regulation of inflammatory processes during ATB than previously thought. ROS-generating cells are central to Mtb-induced inflammatory response; and that they are main actors of relevant cell death processes (i.e., apoptosis, necrosis, pyroptosis, necroptosis, pyronecrosis, NETosis, and autophagy) that influence TB disease progression [reviewed by Mohareer et al. (25)], suggests that their activity contributes considerably to destructive immunity to Mtb infection. The aim of this review is to provide an update on the importance of neutrophils during ATB and to identify related immune mediators associated with anti-TB treatment response and lung damage.

TB-INDUCED INFLAMMATORY RESPONSE

Innate immune responses play a central role in the pathology of infectious and inflammatory diseases including acute abdominal inflammation (26), cancers (27, 28) and respiratory tract disorders (29, 30). Phagocytic cells (i.e., neutrophils and macrophages) are the predominant components of this response in TB (17). In collaboration with inflammatory mediators like cytokines (31) and proteases, they are key contributors to the host interaction with Mtb, in a process which generally ends with the destruction of the pathogen and resolution of inflammation (32). In many cases, however, the inflammatory response is relatively ineffective and can lead to destruction of host tissues as reviewed by Fullerton and Gilroy (33). Such an unwanted scenario is characterized by a constant influx of inflammatory mediators and innate immune cells to the site of infection with progressive deterioration of the affected tissue. The end result is the formation of tuberculous granulomas whose structure, immune/pathogen cell balance (34), and intrinsic T-cell activity (35) ultimately determine the degree of formation of tissue lesions (36).

Defining and Assessing Lung Impairment

In order to understand the role of neutrophils in lung pathology, we need consensus on structural versus functional impairment. There are currently no international guidelines describing how to classify levels of structural impairment following TB as well as identifying TB sequelae in general (37). ATB is increasingly further classified with respect to disease severity into the extent of functional and/or structural lung damage, however, a decisive classification of TB patient pathology has not been reached at this time. Nonetheless, certain criteria have allowed the severity of active pulmonary TB to be determined following assessment of impaired pulmonary function via spirometry testing (38) and the observation of lesions and/or lung cavities through chest x-rays (CXR) and computed tomography (CT) (39).

Structural lung abnormalities determined by x-ray or computed topography (CT) scores have been observed to correlate to a degree with lung function in pulmonary TB (40). Reports also suggest that functional pulmonary impairment at diagnosis only begins to improve significantly several months after the end of successful TB therapy (4, 40). Saldana et al. observed that CXR abnormalities are inversely proportional to and more reliable than spirometry evaluations when assessing severity of lung impairment in cured ATB patients (41). An even earlier study by Plit et al. showed that the change in CXR score (pre- vs. post-treatment) is the most reliable predictor of the severity of functional lung impairment in ATB: here too, an inverse proportionality was observed between CXR

TABLE 1 | Clinical studies assessing TB sequelae.

References	Study site	Study type and design post-treatment commencement	ATB sample size, *n*	Nature of residual lung impairment	Associated inflammatory response
Ngahane et al. (46)	Cameroon	Cross-sectional Includes HIV+	269	Structural (CXR lesions) and Functional (dyspnoea and spirometry)	No
Ralph et al. (13)	Indonesia	Longitudinal [Baseline (BL), 6M & over 6M] Includes HIV+	200	Structural (CXR score of lesions and cavitation) and Functional (dyspnoea, SGRQ, spirometry)	No
Kumar et al. (47)	India	Longitudinal (BL & 6M) No HIV+ cases Part of larger study involving patients with co-morbidities	24	Structural (cavitation; no CXR-score)	Yes
Ravimohan et al. (48)	USA	Prospective (over 6M) All TB/HIV+	14	Functional (spirometry)	Yes (MMPs)
Pasipanodya et al. (11)	USA	Longitudinal (BL, 6M & over 6M) Includes HIV+	177	Functional (SGRQ and spirometry)	No
Plit et al. (42)	South Africa	Longitudinal (BL & 6M) Includes HIV+	76	Structural (CXR score of lung infiltrates) Functional (spirometry)	Yes (c-reactive protein (CRP) and serum α1-protease inhibitor (α1-PI)
Cole et al. (43)	South Africa	Cross-sectional Includes HIV+	55	Functional (SGRQ and spirometry)	No
Patil and Patil (44)	India	Longitudinal (6M, 9M, & 12M) No HIV+ cases	118	Functional (dyspnoea and spirometry)	No
Hnizdo et al. (4)	South Africa	Retrospective (BL-–375M) Includes HIV+	2,599	Functional (spirometry)	No
Maguire et al. (45)	Indonesia	Longitudinal (BL, 2M, & 6M) Includes HIV+	115	Functional (dyspnoea, SGRQ, spirometry)	No
Saldana et al. (41)	Mexico	Cross-sectional Includes HIV+	127	Functional (Spirometry) and Structural (CXR abnormalities)	No
Vecino et al. (14)	USA	Longitudinal (BL, 6M, & over 6M)	123	Functional (Spirometry)	No
Chushkin et al. (3)	Russia	Prospective (Over 12M) Undetermined HIV status	214	Functional (Spirometry)	No

scores and forced expiratory volume (FEV1; a spirometric parameter) (42). These suggest that monitoring variations in structural impairment during TB therapy is essential (or at least of significant added value) when attempting to determine the extent of TB sequelae. However, whilst most relevant clinical studies have generally attempted to monitor ATB-linked signs of TB sequelae via assessment of dyspnoea and disrupted lung function by spirometry (3, 4, 11, 14, 43–45), fewer cases have accounted for both structural and functional damage (13, 41, 42, 46), and none focussing on the former exclusively (see **Table 1**). Relevant follow-up parameters, where available (especially involving longitudinal cohort studies), appear to have relied on the researchers' study objective and understanding of TB sequelae—variably assessing different forms of pulmonary damage, lung rehabilitation and even treatment responses but not the potential inflammatory triggers of these events as the Ravimohan group's latest review hints (49). This is probably owing to absence of a referential guideline as mentioned above. At this time, a few studies: Ravimohan et al. (48) and Plit et al. (42) have assessed severity of lung impairment in ATB in relation to the expression of inflammatory mediators: matrix metalloproteinases (MMPs) in the former and; serum c-reactive protein (CRP), serum α1-protease inhibitor (α1-PI) and urine cotinine in the latter. To account for these limitations, a multisite trial is currently underway to monitor host-pathogen and socioeconomic factors that influence the development of pulmonary sequelae in ATB patients (50).

EVIDENCE OF NEUTROPHIL IMPACT ON DESTRUCTIVE TB INFLAMMATION

Neutrophilia and Hyperinflammation

Polymorphonuclear neutrophils are the most abundant type of white blood cells and play a central role in the immune response to bacterial pathogens (51). The protective activity of neutrophils in TB infection is observed during granuloma formation where mycobacteria are phagocytosed from infected macrophages by oxidative killing (52).

Previous work indicates that the levels of granulocytes (neutrophils and eosinophils) in circulation are higher in patients with ATB disease than those with latent TB infection (LTBI); with levels decreasing significantly following successful TB treatment (53). It has also been demonstrated that neutrophilia independently associates not only with increased risk of cavity formation and lung tissue damage (54), but also mortality in patients undergoing TB therapy (55), suggesting that the neutrophil count in tuberculosis positively correlates with bacillary load and disease outcome. Recently, Leem et al. (56) monitored inflammatory markers in TB patients and found that the neutrophil counts and neutrophil to lymphocyte ratios (NLR) were decreased following a 6-months anti-TB drug therapy compared to baseline. These results hint that inflammation might be resolved only following the 6-month treatment completion, suggesting that progress to chronic inflammation and development of pulmonary lesions is a silent process potentially mediated by secondary products of inflammatory response whose activity persist in tissue long after mycobacterial clearance.

Despite the lack of a consensus on neutrophil classification, varying attributes: granule content (cytotoxic species/enzyme concentration), density (low or normal density granulocytes), nuclear segmentation [banded or (hyper)-segmented], tumor suppressive/enhancing functions (N1/N2), to surface antigen expression [CD177 (7, 57, 58); CD16, CD62L and CD11b] and cytokine/chemokine secretion levels have been associated to disease and immunoregulation [reviewed in Hellebrekers et al. (59), Perobelli et al. (60), and Wang (61)]. It is therefore arguable that a combination of these attributes could constitute a neutrophil profile suggestive of disease severity at an early stage as well as anticipated development of sequalae if chronic conditions (in TB potentially) were to be established. However, given the vast discrepancies in markers, experimental conditions and disease models investigated by previous studies as described in the reviews cited above, these functional differences in neutrophil subsets will not constitute a focus here. Nevertheless, the severity of ATB is linked to neutrophilia as discussed above; but also a specific hyperactivated profile of the circulating neutrophils; which has predominantly been associated with immature banded (or non-segmented) neutrophils (8). Interestingly, the bulk of neutrophil cytotoxic (and antibacterial) molecules are concentrated in their granules. Hence, neutrophil degranulation and exocytosis: processes requiring phosphatidylinositol 3-kinase, (PI3-K) (62); are closely related to the severity of neutrophil-mediated inflammation. We therefore anticipate that a potential neutrophil bio-signature of ATB would encompass enhancement/inhibition of some specific chemokines and increased neutrophil-specific enzyme concentrations. In fact, a recent review by Leisching (7) exposes the regulatory role of PI3-K on enhanced neutrophil mobility and hyperactivity and; the effect on neutrophil-driven TB inflammation. This hyperactivity is equally suggested to be at play in chronic periodontis where it is associated with increased migratory capacity as well as pro-inflammatory cytokine (IL-8, TNF, and IL-1, notably) production by circulating neutrophils (63). Taken together, neutrophil relative abundance (in circulation and at infection sites) and cytokine/enzyme release are potentially major agents of hyperinflammatory conditions observed in ATB.

The mechanisms responsible for this inflammatory response mainly result from three neutrophil functions: oxidative burst, necrosis and NETosis.

Oxidative Burst Capacity

Although neutrophils have the capacity to protect against Mtb infection, if left uncontrolled their collective activity may produce pathogenic effects through different functions (64). One such phagocytic function is oxidative burst, which is the release of reactive oxygen species (ROS) mainly by neutrophils and to a lesser extent, macrophages during phagocytosis, a process which is mediated by nicotinamide adenine dinucleotide phosphate (NADP) oxidase (65). This antibacterial activity is performed by a myeloperoxidase system composed mainly of reduced NADP ($NADPH_2$), reduced glutathione (GSH), azide, cyanide, thiocyanate, Tapazole, thiourea, cysteine, ergothioneine, thiosulfate, reduced nicotinamide adenine dinucleotide ($NADH_2$), and tyrosine (66).

GSH levels have been shown to reduce significantly in PMBCs and red blood cells isolated from tuberculosis patients compared to healthy controls (67), while increased GSH levels are reported to enhance T-cell capacity to inhibit Mtb growth inside macrophages (68). Also, ROS produced by neutrophils during oxidative burst have been reported to drive Mtb-induced necrosis; which in turn promotes Mtb growth (69). It has also been suggested that rapid assessment of individual neutrophil oxidative burst capacity could distinguish patients at risk of excessive immune responses and thus could potentially guide therapy (70). Hence, correlating neutrophil oxidative burst capacity with GSH and/or $NADPH_2$ levels in TB patients may provide avenues for novel host-directed therapies.

Neutrophil Extracellular Traps (NETs)

In-vitro studies by Brinkmann (71) revealed that neutrophil activation with lipopolysaccharide (LPS), interleukin 8 or phorbol myristate acetate (PMA) led to the release of cell components, which form an extracellular fibril matrix called neutrophil extracellular traps (NETs). These components are proteins [namely neutrophil elastase (NE) and myeloperoxidase (MPO)], DNA and chromatin-derived fibers; which destroy bacteria extracellularly (71, 72). This process, NETosis, is a powerful neutrophil-mediated response to a range of infections but also acts as a double-edged sword during inflammatory diseases (73). Interestingly, neutrophils can sense pathogen size and can produce more NETs in presence of larger pathogens like *Mycobacterium bovis* (74). Although aggregated NETs are reported to degrade neutrophil-derived inflammatory mediators in an attempt to resolve inflammation (75), NETs also stimulate unwanted immune reactions and trigger tissue injury (73, 76).

In TB pathogenesis, Mtb is reported to induce the formation of NETs, which trap Mycobacteria *in vitro* but are unable to kill them (77). This may be partially explained by the fact that expression of enzyme systems such as those required in inflammatory pathways [i.e., to degrade proteins within the phagolysosome (e.g., MPO) and for the phagocytic burst, NADPH-oxidase complex and the generation of ROS] are suppressed (78). Furthermore, these Mtb-induced NETs are also associated with macrophage activation in humans (79) and could thus help elucidate specific inflammatory mechanisms of lung damage in TB pathogenesis. Indeed, a recent study by De Melo et al. revealed high levels of citrullinated H3—a common NET marker—in serum samples from TB patients with extensive pulmonary damage (54). Although this marker is usually measured in combination with others (i.e., MPO and NE) to specifically identify NETs, this study suggests that NET formation is centrally linked with severe lung tissue damage in TB patients and could be implicated in subsequent pulmonary pathology.

Neutrophil-mediated lung injury is not just restricted to Tuberculosis. For example, excessive neutrophil recruitment and NETosis was linked to acute lung injury in a mouse model of Influenza pneumonitis (80). Additionally, more recent studies reveal that reduced neutrophil recruitment into infected tissue promotes resolution of inflammation (81). Hence, monitoring NETosis and neutrophil-associated inflammatory mediators within inflamed tissue could be useful in developing therapeutic targets against chronic inflammatory conditions like TB (72).

Metalloproteinases in Destructive TB Immunity

A group of molecules increasingly associated with excessive lung inflammation is the matrix metalloproteinases (MMPs). In the case of cystic fibrosis, which results in loss of pulmonary architecture, Pardo et al. described in a review (82) the essential role played by MMPs in modifying the tissue microenvironment and modulating cell signaling through their ability to degrade constituents of the extracellular matrix. Although the origin of most MMPs cannot be directly linked to neutrophils, MMP-9 is known to be secreted rapidly by neutrophils in whole blood from healthy volunteers following proinflammatory stimulus (83) and is suggested to facilitate transmembrane neutrophil migration (84); also reviewed in Pardo et al. (82). Similar to MMP-9, MMP-8 synthesis in ATB patients is also suspected to be of neutrophil origin (85). In effect, Ravimohan et al. (48) assessed the role of MMPs on TB-immune reconstitution inflammatory syndrome and observed increased MMP-8; whilst MMP-2, -3 and -9 levels reduced (MMP-1 did not vary significantly) in patients with impaired lung function post-TB cure following antiretroviral therapy. MMP-1 and MMP-8 have previously been shown to correlate with pulmonary tissue damage (PTD) in patients with ATB (85, 86) while MMP-14 has been shown to play a central role in TB pathogenesis by provoking collagen degradation and regulating monocyte migration (87). Interestingly, a more recent study by De Melo et al. found lower levels of serum MMP-8 in TB patients with severe PTD showing no radiological improvement after 60 days of anti-TB treatment (54). Whether this change in trend is related to plasma vs serum or due to the presence/absence of HIV infection is unknown, however, the latter observation is inconsistent with that from the previous studies reported above and suggests that MMP regulation in TB patients might differ between the circulation and the lung as well as in the presence of coinfection. Nonetheless, de Melo et al. (54) did find higher MMP-1 levels in these patients compared to those with improved chest-x rays. Hence, whilst there is clearly a role for MMPs in TB-linked tissue damage, more detailed studies, with assessment of coinfections, are required to ascertain which MMPs are predominant mediators. This will help to determine potential host-directed therapeutic strategies.

Furthermore, a few clinical studies on major TB comorbidities have recently emerged. One shows that sputum levels of MMP-1, -2, -3 and -9 are higher in HIV negative TB patients than in TB healthy controls (HC) and HIV positive TB patients with a correlation found between the degree of chest x-ray inflammation and both MMP-1 and MMP-3 levels in HIV negative TB patients (88). Moreover, the clinical severity of TB is known to increase in TB patients with diabetes mellitus (DM). Kumar et al. have shown that circulatory levels of MMP-1, -2, -3, -8, and -13 in these patients decrease following successful TB treatment and that MMP-1 (in sputum) and MMP-1, -2, -3, -9, and -12 levels (in serum) were higher in patients with more severe structural lung damage at baseline (47) as determined from chest x-rays.

These findings suggest that MMPs (MMP-1, -2, -3, -8, and -9, particularly) may promote tissue injury following Mtb infection. Hence, monitoring the correlation of these particular MMPs together with the downregulation of other neutrophil-related inflammatory proteins and pro-inflammatory cytokines associated with intracellular killing pathways during TB infection would increase our understanding of the active inflammatory pathways which enhance susceptibility to development of PIAT and subsequent sequelae. Importantly, natural regulation of MMP activity is performed by tissue inhibitors of metalloproteinases (TIMPs). The levels of TIMPs have not yet been monitored in TB patients; an aspect of TB research which should be addressed for optimal understanding of inflammatory mechanisms involved in development and host control of TB-related PTD.

NEUTROPHIL-RELATED TB HDT

With increasing cases of co-infections, co-morbidities, drug resistance; as well as the cost associated with the relatively long standard antibiotic TB-treatment, new treatment regiments like host directed therapies (HDT) could complement existing Mtb-targeted approaches. Meanwhile biomarkers for efficiently identifying and treating TB disease progressors at an early stage are being actively researched (89), those that could single out individuals who develop unresolving inflammation-induced lung damage are still greatly under-investigated. This means that research on HDTs should ideally focus on diagnosis and prevention of the latter long-lasting condition as well. Recent reviews have highlighted various established as well as promising host directed adjuvant therapies against the development of TB disease (90), TB-linked inflammation (91, 92) and lung damage (93). Drugs that potentially inhibit pulmonary damage and/or promote lung repair range from steroids to nonsteroidal anti-inflammatory drugs, statins, metformin, dietary supplements,

TNF blockers etc. (10). Of these, we observe that those suppressing pro-inflammatory aspects of the disease appear to be potent targets in preclinical and clinical trials. In fact, Young et al. have recently reviewed current targets in TB HDT with some of the most advanced ATB-relevant in clinical trials being modulators of pro-inflammatory mediators which: dampen inflammatory responses, curb immunopathology and resolve lung damage (93). These include the phase 3 drugs: cox-2 inhibitor (Meloxicam) and corticosteroids (Prednisolone and Dexamethasone) amongst others. This HDT potential of inflammatory mediators has also been addressed with inhibitory effects on neutrophil recruitment (Ibuprofen) and neutrophil-derived inflammatory mediators such as ROS and MPO as reviewed by Dallenga et al. (94).

Also, a combination of the anti-inflammatory drug, zileuton (an inhibitor of the synthesis of pro-inflammatory eicosanoid; already approved against asthma) and prostaglandin E2 (95) is reported to reduce bacillary load and TB-induced lung damage in mice. Statins are also interesting HDT targets against destructive lung pathology following ATB (96); with a promising phase 2 trial using pravastatin being investigated in South Africa (ClinicalTrials.gov Identifier: NCT03456102). Moreover, a phase 2b trial testing the effect of atorvastatin against PIAT in patients with or without HIV is about to begin in South Africa (ClinicalTrials.gov Identifier: NCT04147286); underlining the potential of these agents.

Potentially, some mediators of neutrophil function (mentioned in previous sections) could provide suitable HDT targets. Amongst others, these involve: vitamin D which is reported to inhibit Mtb-induced expression of MMP-7 and−10 as well as MMP-9 gene expression, secretion and activity by peripheral blood mononuclear cells (PBMCs) (97). Although the authors reported that the latter inhibition occurs irrespective of infection, MMP-9 is reported to be of neutrophil origin and in-depth investigation may be warranted. Doxycycline is also a known MMP-inhibitor which in TB-HIV co-infection particularly, is shown to suppress the secretion of TNF, MMP-1 and−9 by primary human macrophages while reducing Mtb growth in the guinea pig model of TB (98). Also, Allen et al. reviewed the importance of considering GSH as HDT against TB and TB/HIV co-infection (99). Furthermore, it is important to note that N-acetylated proline glycine proline (ac-PGP) induces neutrophil chemotaxis and neutrophil production of MMP-9 and IL-8 (100, 101) which has led this molecule to be suggested as potential HDT-target against chronic neuroinflammatory diseases (102) and cystic fibrosis (103); which result in MMP activation and result in considerable tissue damage like TB.

Besides these, calprotectin, a hetero-dimer made up of proteins S100A8 and S100A9 is a mediator of inflammatory responses and a potent diagnostic and HDT target against inflammatory diseases (104). Actually, Gopal et al. (9) reported that S100A8/A9 accumulates in TB-induced granulomas. The authors showed that this accumulation was neutrophil-driven (in humans) and the animal models they employed suggested an association between S100A8/A9 and the degree of inflammation and lung pathology during ATB. Recently, it has been shown that these high levels of S100A8/A9 as well as an S100A8/A9-mediated enhanced accumulation of neutrophils in lungs of mice and macaques are associated with Mtb proliferation in chronic TB disease (105). Both studies reveal a close interaction between neutrophils and S100A8/A9 in ATB suggesting that neutrophils and S100A8/A9, particularly could be targeted in TB HDT.

CONCLUDING REMARKS AND FUTURE PERSPECTIVES

In conclusion, we believe that observation and monitoring of neutrophil subsets and related inflammatory mediators is important not only for studies aiming at developing novel therapeutic targets against TB (72) but also for improved estimation of host immuno-modulatory effects on the severity of TB sequalae. It is foreseeable that the extent of long-term pulmonary injury sustained and potentially resorbed following TB therapy (irrespective of HIV coinfection) could be correlated to a specific neutrophil function. It is also likely that ATB patients who express a specific form of neutrophil-mediated inflammatory response over the period from diagnosis through treatment are more susceptible to developing chronic PIAT than otherwise. A major challenge will be harmonizing the categorization of disease severity (structural and functional) to ease comparison between clinical studies. Moreover, we believe that prediction of treatment response and residual pulmonary impairment in future clinical studies would be made more effective and reproduceable by evaluating inflammatory responses as well as simultaneously monitoring variations in pulmonary structure and function during and months after treatment completion. Finally, prospective HDTs; which rely on inflammatory mediators of neutrophil activity particularly, should be investigated further.

AUTHOR CONTRIBUTIONS

CM was the primary author of the manuscript. JS provided substantial writing support, edits, and suggestions.

REFERENCES

WHO. *Global Tuberculosis Report 2018*. Geneva: World Health Organization (2018).

Romanowski K, Baumann B, Basham CA, Khan FA, Fox GJ, Johnston JC. Articles long-term all-cause mortality in people treated for tuberculosis: a systematic review and meta-analysis. *Lancet Infect Dis.* (2019) 3099:1–9. doi: 10.1016/S1473-3099(19)30309-3

Chushkin MI, Ots ON. Impaired pulmonary function after treatment for tuberculosis: the end of the disease? *J Bras Pneumol.* (2017) 43:38– 43. doi: 10.1590/s1806-37562016000000053

Hnizdo E, Singh T, Churchyard G. Chronic pulmonary function impairment caused by initial and recurrent pulmonary tuberculosis following treatment. *Thorax.* (2000) 55:32–8. doi: 10.1136/thorax.55.1.32

Chakaya J, Kirenga B, Getahun H. Long term complications after completion of pulmonary tuberculosis treatment: a quest for a public health approach. *J Clin Tuberc Other Mycobact Dis.* (2016) 3:10– 2. doi: 10.1016/j.jctube.2016.03.001

Kim HY, Song K.-S, Goo JM, Lee JS, Lee KS, Lim T.-H. Thoracic sequelae and complications of tuberculosis. *RadioGraphics.* (2001) 21:839– 58. doi: 10.1148/radiographics.21.4.g01jl06839

Leisching GR. Susceptibility to Tuberculosis is associated with PI3K- dependent increased mobilization of neutrophils. *Front Immunol.* (2018) 9:1669. doi: 10.3389/fimmu.2018.01669

Panteleev AV, Nikitina IY, Burmistrova IA, Kosmiadi GA, Radaeva TV, Amansahedov RB, et al. Severe tuberculosis in humans correlates best with neutrophil abundance and lymphocyte deficiency and does not correlate with antigen-specific CD4 T-cell response. *Front Immunol.* (2017) 8:963. doi: 10.3389/fimmu.2017.00963

Gopal R, Monin L, Torres D, Slight S, Mehra S, McKenna KC, et al. S100A8/A9 proteins mediate neutrophilic inflammation and lung pathology during tuberculosis. *Am. J Respir Crit Care Med.* (2013) 188:1137– 46. doi: 10.1164/rccm.201304-0803OC

Stek C, Allwood B, Walker NF, Wilkinson RJ, Lynen L, Meintjes G. The immune mechanisms of lung parenchymal damage in tuberculosis and the role of host-directed therapy. *Front Microbiol.* (2018) 9:2603. doi: 10.3389/fmicb.2018.02603

Pasipanodya JG, McNabb SJ, Hilsenrath P, Bae S, Lykens K, Vecino E, et al. Pulmonary impairment after tuberculosis and its contribution to TB burden. *BMC Public Health.* (2010) 10:259. doi: 10.1186/1471-2458-10-259

Hoger S, Lykens K, Beavers SF, Katz D, Miller TL. Longevity loss among cured tuberculosis patients and the potential value of prevention. *Int J Tuberc Lung Dis.* (2014) 18:1347–52. doi: 10.5588/ijtld.14.0242

Ralph AP, Kenangalem E, Waramori G, Pontororing GJ, Tjitra E, Maguire GP, et al. High morbidity during treatment and residual pulmonary disability in pulmonary tuberculosis: under-recognised phenomena. *PLoS ONE.* (2013) 8:1–11. doi: 10.1371/journal.pone.0080302

Vecino M, Pasipanodya JG, Slocum P, Bae S, Munguia G, Miller T, et al. Evidence for chronic lung impairment in patients treated for pulmonary tuberculosis. *J Infect Public Health.* (2011) 6:244–52. doi: 10.1016/j.jiph.2011.08.005

Vashakidze SA, Kempker JA, Jakobia NA, Gogishvili SG, Nikolaishvili KA, Goginashvili LM, et al. Pulmonary function and respiratory health after successful treatment of drug-resistant tuberculosis. *Int J Infect Dis.* (2019) 82:66–72. doi: 10.1016/j.ijid.2019.02.039

Scriba TJ, Coussens AK, Fletcher HA. Human immunology of tuberculosis. *Tuberc Tuber Bacillus..* (2016) 5:213–37. doi: 10.1128/9781555819569.ch11

O'Garra A, Redford PS, McNab FW, Bloom CI, Wilkinson RJ, Berry MPR. The immune response in tuberculosis. *Annu Rev Immunol.* (2013) 31:475– 527. doi: 10.1146/annurev-immunol-032712-095939

Kiran D, Podell BK, Chambers M, Basaraba RJ. Host-directed therapy targeting the Mycobacterium tuberculosis granuloma: a review. *Semin Immunopathol.* (2016) 38:167–83. doi: 10.1007/s00281-015-0537-x

Holland SM. Chronic granulomatous disease. *Hematol Oncol Clin North Am.* (2013) 27:89–99. doi: 10.1016/j.hoc.2012.11.002

Heyworth PG, Cross AR, Curnutte JT. Chronic granulomatous disease. *Curr Opin Immunol.* (2003). 15:578–584. doi: 10.1016/S0952-7915(03)00109-2

Roos D, de Boer M. Molecular diagnosis of chronic granulomatous disease. *Clin Exp Immunol.* (2014) 175:139–49. doi: 10.1111/cei.12202

Jasenosky LD, Scriba TJ, Hanekom WA, Goldfeld AE. T cells and adaptive immunity to *Mycobacterium tuberculosis* in humans. *Immunol Rev.* (2015) 264:74–87. doi: 10.1111/imr.12274

Achkar JM, Chan J, Casadevall A. B cells and antibodies in the defense against *Mycobacterium tuberculosis* infection. *Immunol Rev.* (2015) 264:167– 81. doi: 10.1111/imr.12276

Dyatlov V, Apt AS, Linge IA. B lymphocytes in anti-mycobacterial immune responses : Pathogenesis or protection? *Tuberculosis.* (2018) 114:1– 8. doi: 10.1016/j.tube.2018.10.011

Mohareer K, Asalla S, Banerjee S. Cell death at the cross roads of host-pathogen interaction in Mycobacterium tuberculosis infection. *Tuberculosis.* (2018) 113:99–121. doi: 10.1016/j.tube.2018.09.007

Bilyy R, Fedorov V, Vovk V, Leppkes M, Dumych T, Chopyak V, et al. Neutrophil extracellular traps form a barrier between necrotic and viable areas in acute abdominal inflammation. *Front Immunol.* (2016) 7:1– 7. doi: 10.3389/fimmu.2016.00424

Liu J, Geng X, Li Y. Milky spots: omental functional units and hotbeds for peritoneal cancer metastasis. *Tumor Biol.* (2016) 37:5715– 26. doi: 10.1007/s13277-016-4887-3

Clark R, Krishnan V, Schoof M, Rodriguez I, Theriault B, Chekmareva M, et al. Milky spots promote ovarian cancer metastatic colonization of peritoneal adipose in experimental models. *Am J Pathol.* (2013) 183:576– 91. doi: 10.1016/j.ajpath.2013.04.023

Robb CT, Regan KH, Dorward DA, Rossi AG. Key mechanisms governing resolution of lung inflammation. *Semin Immunopathol.* (2016) 38:425– 48. doi: 10.1007/s00281-016-0560-6

Porto BN, Stein RT. Neutrophil extracellular traps in pulmonary diseases: too much of a good thing? *Front Immunol.* (2016) 7:1– 13. doi: 10.3389/fimmu.2016.00311

Etna MP, Giacomini E, Severa M, Coccia EM. Pro-and anti-inflammatory cytokines in tuberculosis: A two-edged sword in TB pathogenesis. *Semin Immunol.* (2014) 26:543–51. doi: 10.1016/j.smim.2014.09.011

Newson J, Stables M, Karra E, Arce-Vargas F, Quezada S, Motwani M, et al. Resolution of acute in fl ammation bridges the gap between innate and adaptive immunity. *Blood.* (2015) 124:1748–65. doi: 10.1182/blood-2014-03-562710

Fullerton JN, Gilroy DW. Resolution of inflammation: a new therapeutic frontier. *Nat Rev.* (2016) 15:551–67. doi: 10.1038/nrd.2016.39

Marakalala MJ, Raju RM, Sharma K, Zhang YJ, Eugenin EA, Prideaux B, et al. Inflammatory signaling in human tuberculosis granulomas is spatially organized. *Nat Med.* (2016) 22:531–8. doi: 10.1038/nm.4073

Gideon HP, Phuah J, Myers AJ, Bryson BD, Rodgers MA, Coleman MT, et al. Variability in tuberculosis granuloma T cell responses exists, but a balance of pro- and anti-inflammatory cytokines is associated with sterilization. *PLoS Pathog.* (2015) 11:1–28. doi: 10.1371/journal.ppat.1004603

Lin PL, Ford CB, Coleman MT, Myers AJ, Gawande R, Ioerger T, et al. Sterilization of granulomas is common in active and latent tuberculosis despite within-host variability in bacterial killing. *Nat Med.* (2014) 20:75– 9. doi: 10.1038/nm.3412

van Kampen SC, Wanner A, Edwards M, Harries AD, Kirenga BJ, Chakaya J, et al. International research and guidelines on post-tuberculosis chronic lung disorders: a systematic scoping review. *BMJ Glob Heal.* (2018) 3:1– 8. doi: 10.1136/bmjgh-2018-000745

Pellegrino R, Viegi G, Brusasco V, Crapo RO, Burgos F, Casaburi RE, et al. Interpretative strategies for lung function tests. *Eur Respir J.* (2005) 26:948–68. doi: 10.1183/09031936.05.00035205

Yeh JJ. Predictors of initial smear-negative active pulmonary tuberculosis with acute early stage lung injury by high-resolution computed tomography and clinical manifestations: an auxiliary model in critical patients. *Sci Rep.* (2019) 9:1–13. doi: 10.1038/s41598-019-40799-w

Long R, Maycher B, Dhar A, Manfreda J, Hershfield E, Anthonisen N. Pulmonary tuberculosis treated with directly observed therapy: serial changes in lung structure and function. *Chest.* (1998) 113:933– 43. doi: 10.1378/chest.113.4.933

Báez-Saldaña R, López-Arteaga Y, Bizarrón-Muro A, Ferreira- Guerrero E, Ferreyra-Reyes L, Delgado-Sánchez G, et al. A novel scoring system to measure radiographic abnormalities and related spirometric values in cured pulmonary tuberculosis. *PLoS ONE.* (2013) 8:1–12. doi: 10.1371/journal.pone.0078926

Plit ML, Anderson R, Van Rensburg CE, Page-Shipp L, Blott JA, Fresen JL, et al. Influence of antimicrobial chemotherapy on spirometric parameters and pro-inflammatory indices in severe pulmonary tuberculosis. *Eur Respir J.* (1998) 12:351–6. doi: 10.1183/09031936.98.12020351

Cole G, Miller D, Ebrahim T, Dreyden T, Simpson R, Manie S. Pulmonary impairment after tuberculosis in a South African population. *South Afr J Physiother.* (2016) 72:1–6. doi: 10.4102/sajp.v72i1.307

Patil P, Patil S. A six-month follow-up study to evaluate changes of pulmonary function test in Category I pulmonary tuberculosis treatment completed patient. *Natl J Physiol Pharm Pharmacol.* (2017) 8:31– 6. doi: 10.5455/njppp.2018.8.0724121072017

Maguire GP, Anstey NM, Ardian M, Waramori G, Tjitra E, Kenangalem E, et al. Pulmonary tuberculosis, impaired lung function, disability and quality of life in a high-burden setting. *Int J Tuberc Lung Dis.* (2009) 13:1500–6.

Ngahane BH, Nouyep J, Motto MN, Njankouo YM, Wandji A, Endale M, et al. Post-tuberculous lung function impairment in a tuberculosis reference clinic in Cameroon. *Respir Med.* (2016) 114:67–71. doi: 10.1016/j.rmed.2016.03.007

Kumar NP, Moideen K, Viswanathan V, Shruthi BS, Sivakumar S, Menon PA, et al. Elevated levels of matrix metalloproteinases reflect severity and extent of disease in tuberculosis-diabetes co-morbidity and are predominantly reversed following standard anti-tuberculosis or metformin treatment. *BMC Infect Dis.* (2018) 18:1–10. doi: 10.1186/s12879-018-3246-y

Ravimohan S, Tamuhla N, Kung SJ, Nfanyana K, Steenhoff AP, Gross R, et al. Matrix metalloproteinases in tuberculosis-immune reconstitution inflammatory syndrome and impaired lung function among advanced HIV/TB co-infected patients initiating antiretroviral therapy. *EBioMedicine.* (2016) 3:100–7. doi: 10.1016/j.ebiom.2015.11.040

Ravimohan S, Kornfeld H, Weissman D, Bisson GP. Tuberculosis and lung damage: from epidemiology to pathophysiology. *Eur Respir Rev.* (2018) 27:170077. doi: 10.1183/16000617.0077-2017

Rachow A, Ivanova O, Wallis R, Charalambous S, Jani I, Bhatt N, et al. TB sequel: incidence, pathogenesis and risk factors of long-term medical and social sequelae of pulmonary TB - A study protocol 11 Medical and Health Sciences 1117 Public Health and Health Services. *BMC Pulm Med.* (2019) 19:1–9. doi: 10.1186/s12890-018-0777-3

Jenne CN, Wong CH, Zemp FJ, McDonald B, Rahman MM, Forsyth PA, et al. Neutrophils recruited to sites of infection protect from virus challenge by releasing neutrophil extracellular traps. *Cell Host Microbe.* (2013) 13:169– 80. doi: 10.1016/j.chom.2013.01.005

Yang CT, Cambier CJ, Davis JM, Hall CJ, Crosier PS, Ramakrishnan L. Neutrophils exert protection in the early tuberculous granuloma by oxidative killing of mycobacteria phagocytosed from infected macrophages. *Cell Host Microbe.* (2012) 12:301–12. doi: 10.1016/j.chom.2012. 07.009

Moideen K, Kumar NP, Nair D, Banurekha VV, Bethunaickan R, Babu S. Heightened systemic levels of neutrophil and eosinophil granular proteins in pulmonary tuberculosis and reversal following treatment. *Infect Immun.* (2018) 86:1–8. doi: 10.1128/IAI.00008-18

de Melo MG, Mesquita ED, Oliveira MM, Silva-Monteiro CD, Silveira AK, Malaquias TS, et al. Imbalance of NET and alpha- 1-antitrypsin in tuberculosis patients is related with hyper inflammation and severe lung tissue damage. *Front Immunol.* (2019) 9:1–17. doi: 10.3389/fimmu.2018.03147

Lowe DM, Bandara AK, Packe GE, Barker RD, Robert J. Europe PMC Funders Group Neutrophilia independently predicts death in tuberculosis. *Eur Respir J.* (2014) 42:1752–7. doi: 10.1183/09031936.00140913

Leem AY, Song JH, Lee EH, Lee H, Sim B, Kim SY, et al. Changes in cytokine responses to TB antigens ESAT-6, CFP-10 and TB 7.7 and inflammatory markers in peripheral blood during therapy. *Sci Rep.* (2018) 8:4–11. doi: 10.1038/s41598-018-19523-7

Zhou G, Yu L, Fang L, Yang W, Yu T, Miao Y, et al. CD177+ neutrophils as functionally activated neutrophils negatively regulate IBD. *Gut.* (2018) 67:1052–63. doi: 10.1136/gutjnl-2016-313535

Wang X, Qiu L, Li Z, Wang XY, Yi H. Understanding the multifaceted role of neutrophils in cancer and autoimmune diseases. *Front Immunol.* (2018) 9:1–10. doi: 10.3389/fimmu.2018.02456

Hellebrekers P, Vrisekoop N, Koenderman L. Neutrophil phenotypes in health and disease. *Eur J Clin Invest.* (2018) 48:e12943. doi: 10.1111/eci.12943

Perobelli SM, Galvani RG, Gonçalves-Silva T, Xavier CR, Nóbrega A, Bonomo A. Plasticity of neutrophils reveals modulatory capacity. *Braz J Med Biol Res.* (2015) 48:665–75. doi: 10.1590/1414-431x2015 4524

Wang J. Neutrophils in tissue injury and repair. *Cell Tissue Res.* (2018) 371:531–9. doi: 10.1007/s00441-017-2785-7

Lacy P. Mechanisms of degranulation in neutrophils. *Aller Asthma Clin Immunol.* (2006) 2:98–108. doi: 10.1186/1710-1492-2-3-98

Ling MR, Chapple ILC, Matthews JB. Peripheral blood neutrophil cytokine hyper-reactivity in chronic periodontitis. *Innate Immun.* (2015) 21:714– 25. doi: 10.1177/1753425915589387

Villanueva E, Yalavarthi S, Berthier CC, Hodgin JB, Khandpur R, Lin AM, et al. Netting Neutrophils Induce Endothelial Damage, Infiltrate Tissues, and Expose Immunostimulatory Molecules in Systemic Lupus Erythematosus. *J Immunol.* (2011) 187:538–552. doi: 10.4049/jimmunol.1100450

Babior BM. Oxidants from phagocytes: agents of defense and destruction. *Blood.* (1984) 64:959–66. doi: 10.1182/blood.V64.5.959.959

Klebanoff SJ. Myeloperoxidase-halide-hydrogen peroxide antibacterial system. *J Bacteriol.* (1968) 95:2131–8. doi: 10.1128/JB.95.6.2131-2138.1968

Venketaraman V, Millman A, Salman M, Swaminathan S, Goetz M, Lardizabal A, et al. Glutathione levels and immune responses in tuberculosis patients. *Microb Pathog.* (2008) 44:255–61. doi: 10.1016/j.micpath.2007.09.002

Guerra C, Morris D, Sipin A, Kung S, Franklin M, Gray D, et al. Glutathione and adaptive immune responses against mycobacterium tuberculosis infection in healthy and HIV infected individuals. *PLoS ONE.* (2011) 6:e28378. doi: 10.1371/journal.pone.0028378

Dallenga T, Repnik U, Corleis B, Eich J, Reimer R, Griffiths GW, et al. *M. tuberculosis*-induced necrosis of infected neutrophils promotes bacterial growth following phagocytosis by macrophages. *Cell Host Microbe.* (2017) 22:519–30. e3. doi: 10.1016/j.chom.2017.09.003

Vernon PJ, Schaub LJ, Dallelucca JJ, Pusateri AE, Sheppard FR. Rapid detection of neutrophil oxidative burst capacity is predictive of whole blood cytokine responses. *PLoS ONE.* (2015) 10:1–13. doi: 10.1371/journal.pone.0146105

Brinkmann V, Reichard U, Goosmann C, Fauler B, Uhlemann Y, Weiss DS, et al. Neutrophil extracellular traps kill bacteria. *Sciene.* (2004) 3033:1532– 5. doi: 10.1126/science.1092385

Gupta S, Kaplan MJ. The role of neutrophils and NETosis in autoimmune and renal diseases. *Nat Rev Nephrol.* (2016) 12:402–13. doi: 10.1038/nrneph.2016.71

Kaplan JM. Neutrophil extracelullar traps (NETs): double-edged swords of innate immunity 1. *J Immunol.* (2013) 189:2689– 95. doi: 10.4049/jimmunol.1201719

Branzk N, Lubojemska A, Hardison SE, Wang Q, Gutierrez MG, Brown GD, et al. Neutrophils sense microbe size and selectively release neutrophil extracellular traps in response to large pathogens. *Nat Immunol.* (2014) 15:1017–25. doi: 10.1038/ni.2987

Schauer C, Janko C, Munoz LE, Zhao Y, Kienhöfer D, Frey B, et al. Aggregated neutrophil extracellular traps limit inflammation by degrading cytokines and chemokines. *Nat Med.* (2014) 20:511–7. doi: 10.1038/nm.3547

Mayadas TN, Cullere X, Lowell CA. The multifaceted functions of neutrophils. *Annu Rev Pathol.* (2014) 9:181– 218. doi: 10.1146/annurev-pathol-020712-164023

Ramos-Kichik V, Mondragón-Flores R, Mondragón-Castelán M, Gonzalez- Pozos S, Muñiz-Hernandez S, Rojas-Espinosa O, et al. Neutrophil extracellular traps are induced by *Mycobacterium tuberculosis*. *Tuberculosis.* (2009) 89:29–37. doi: 10.1016/j.tube.2008.09.009

von Both U, Berk M, Agapow PM, Wright JD, Git A, Hamilton MS, et al. *Mycobacterium tuberculosis* exploits a molecular off switch of the immune system for intracellular survival. *Sci Rep.* (2018) 8:1– 17. doi: 10.1038/s41598-017-18528-y

Braian C, Hogea V, Stendahl O. *Mycobacterium tuberculosis*-induced neutrophil extracellular traps activate human macrophages. *J Innate Immun.* (2013) 5:591–602. doi: 10.1159/000348676

Narasaraju T, Yang E, Samy RP, Ng HH, Poh WP, Liew AA, et al. Excessive neutrophils and neutrophil extracellular traps contribute to acute lung injury of influenza pneumonitis. *Am J. Pathol.* (2011) 179:199– 210. doi: 10.1016/j.ajpath.2011.03.013

Sugimoto MA, Vago JP, Teixeira MM, Sousa LP. Annexin A1 and the resolution of inflammation: modulation of neutrophil recruitment, apoptosis, and clearance. *J Immunol Res.* (2016) 2016:8239258. doi: 10.1155/2016/8239258

Pardo A, Cabrera S, Maldonado M, Selman M. Role of matrix metalloproteinases in the pathogenesis of idiopathic pulmonary fibrosis. *Respir Res.* (2016) 17:23. doi: 10.1186/s12931-016-0343-6

Pugin J, Widmer MC, Kossodo S, Liang CM, Preas HL, Suffredini AF. Human neutrophils secrete gelatinase B *in vitro* and *in vivo* in response to endotoxin and proinflammatory mediators. *Am J Respir Cell Mol Biol.* (1999) 20:458–64. doi: 10.1165/ajrcmb.20.3.3311

Delclaux C, Delacourt C, D'Ortho MP, Boyer V, Lafuma C, Harf A. Role of gelatinase B and elastase in human polymorphonuclear neutrophil migration across basement membrane. *Am J Respir Cell Mol Biol.* (1996) 14:288– 95. doi: 10.1165/ajrcmb.14.3.8845180

Ong CW, Elkington PT, Brilha S, Ugarte-Gil C, Tome-Esteban MT, Tezera LB, et al. Neutrophil-derived MMP-8 drives AMPK-dependent matrix destruction in human pulmonary tuberculosis. *PLoS Pathog.* (2015) 11:1– 21. doi: 10.1371/journal.ppat.1004917

Elkington PTG, Friedland JS. Matrix metalloproteinases in destructive pulmonary pathology. *Thorax.* (2006) 61:259– 66. doi: 10.1136/thx.2005.051979

Sathyamoorthy T, Tezera LB, Walker NF, Brilha S, Saraiva L, Mauri FA, et al. Membrane type 1 matrix metalloproteinase regulates monocyte migration and collagen destruction in tuberculosis. *J Immunol.* (2015) 195:882– 91. doi: 10.4049/jimmunol.1403110

Walker NF, Wilkinson KA, Meintjes G, Tezera LB, Goliath R, Peyper JM, et al. Matrix degradation in human immunodeficiency virus type 1-associated tuberculosis and tuberculosis immune reconstitution inflammatory syndrome: a prospective observational study. *Clin Infect Dis.* (2017) 65:121–32. doi: 10.1093/cid/cix231

Sumner T, Scriba TJ, Penn-Nicholson A, Hatherill M, White RG. Potential population level impact on tuberculosis incidence of using an mRNA expression signature correlate-of-risk test to target tuberculosis preventive therapy. *Sci Rep.* (2019) 9:11126. doi: 10.1038/s41598-019-47645-z

Kolloli A, Subbian S. Host-directed therapeutic strategies for tuberculosis. *Front Med.* (2017) 4:171. doi: 10.3389/fmed.2017.00171

Ndlovu H, Marakalala MJ. Granulomas and inflammation: host-directed therapies for tuberculosis. *Front Immunol.* (2016) 7:434. doi: 10.3389/fimmu.2016.00434

Ahmed S, Raqib R, Guð*mundsson GH, Bergman P, Agerberth B, Rekha RS. Host-directed therapy as a novel treatment strategy to overcome tuberculosis: targeting immune modulation. *Antibiotics.* (2020) 9:1–19. doi: 10.3390/antibiotics9010021

Young C, Walzl G, Du Plessis N. Therapeutic host-directed strategies to improve outcome in tuberculosis. *Mucosal Immunol.* (2019) 13:190– 204. doi:10.1038/s41385-019-0226-5

Dallenga T, Linnemann L, Paudyal B, Repnik U, Griffiths G, Schaible UE. Targeting neutrophils for host-directed therapy to treat tuberculosis. *Int J Med Microbiol.* (2017) 308:142–7. doi: 10.1016/j.ijmm.2017.10.001

Mayer-Barber KD, Andrade BB, Oland SD, Amaral EP, Barber DL, Gonzales J, et al. Host-directed therapy of tuberculosis based on interleukin-1 and type I interferon crosstalk. *Nature.* (2016) 5117:99–103. doi: 10.1038/nature 13489

Hu Z, Lowrie DB, Fan X-Y. Statins as adjunctive therapy against tuberculosis (TB): the balance between statin-induced anti-TB effect and trained immunity suppression, *J. Infect. Dis.* (2019) jiz675. doi: 10.1093/infdis/ jiz675

Coussens A, Timms PM, Boucher BJ, Venton TR, Ashcroft AT, Skolimowska KH, et al. 1α,25-dihydroxyvitamin D3 inhibits matrix metalloproteinases induced by *Mycobacterium tuberculosis* infection. *Immunology.* (2009) 127:539–48. doi: 10.1111/j.1365-2567.2008.03024.x

Walker NF, Clark SO, Oni T, Andreu N, Tezera L, Singh S, et al. Doxycycline and HIV infection suppress tuberculosis-induced matrix metalloproteinases. *Am J Respir Crit Care Med.* (2012) 185:989–97. doi: 10.1164/rccm.201110-1769OC

Allen M, Bailey C, Cahatol I, Dodge L, Yim J, Kassissa C, et al. Mechanisms of control of *Mycobacterium tuberculosis* by NK cells: role of glutathione. *Front Immunol.* (2015) 6:1–9. doi: 10.3389/fimmu.2015.00508

Xu X, Jackson PL, Tanner S, Hardison MT, Roda MA, Blalock JE, et al. A self-propagating matrix metalloprotease-9 (MMP-9) dependent cycle of chronic neutrophilic inflammation. *PLoS ONE.* (2011) 6:1– 12. doi: 10.1371/journal.pone.0015781

Overbeek SA, Henricks PA, Srienc AI, Koelink PJ, de Kruijf P, Lim HD, et al. N-acetylated Proline-Glycine-Proline induced G-protein dependent chemotaxis of neutrophils is independent of CXCL8 release. *Eur J Pharmacol.* (2011) 668:428–34. doi: 10.1016/j.ejphar.2011.03.022

Hill JW, Nemoto EM. Matrix-derived inflammatory mediator N-acetyl proline-glycine-proline is neurotoxic and upregulated in brain after ischemic stroke. *J Neuroinflammation.* (2015) 12:1–7. doi: 10.1186/s12974-015-0428-z

Gaggar A, Rowe SM, Hardision M, Blalock JE. Proline-glycine-proline (PGP) and high mobility group box protein-1 (HMGB1): potential mediators of cystic fibrosis airway inflammation. *Open Respir Med J.* (2010) 4:32– 8. doi: 10.2174/1874306401004020032

Wang S, Song R, Wang Z, Jing Z, Wang S, Ma J. S100A8/A9 in inflammation. *Front Immunol.* (2018) 9:1298. doi: 10.3389/fimmu.2018.01298

Scott NR, Zuñiga J, Khader S. S100A8/A9 regulates CD11b expression and neutrophil recruitment during chronic tuberculosis. *J Clin Invest.* (2020). doi: 10.1172/JCI130546. [Epub ahead of print].

2

Development and Validation of a Predictive Model for Severe COVID-19

Zirui Meng[1†], Minjin Wang[1†], Zhenzhen Zhao[1], Yongzhao Zhou[2], Ying Wu[2], Shuo Guo[1], Mengjiao Li[1], Yanbing Zhou[1], Shuyu Yang[1], Weimin Li[2] and Binwu Ying[1*]*

[1] Department of Laboratory Medicine, West China Hospital, Sichuan University, Chengdu, China, [2] Department of Respiratory and Critical Care Medicine, West China Hospital, Sichuan University, Chengdu, China

***Correspondence:**
Binwu Ying
binwuyin@126.com
Weimin Li
weimin003@163.com*

† These authors have contributed equally to this work

Background: Predicting the risk of progression to severe coronavirus disease 2019 (COVID-19) could facilitate personalized diagnosis and treatment options, thus optimizing the use of medical resources.

Methods: In this prospective study, 206 patients with COVID-19 were enrolled from regional medical institutions between December 20, 2019, and April 10, 2020. We collated a range of data to derive and validate a predictive model for COVID-19 progression, including demographics, clinical characteristics, laboratory findings, and cytokine levels. Variation analysis, along with the least absolute shrinkage and selection operator (LASSO) and Boruta algorithms, was used for modeling. The performance of the derived models was evaluated by specificity, sensitivity, area under the receiver operating characteristic (ROC) curve (AUC), Akaike information criterion (AIC), calibration plots, decision curve analysis (DCA), and Hosmer–Lemeshow test.

Results: We used the LASSO algorithm and logistic regression to develop a model that can accurately predict the risk of progression to severe COVID-19. The model incorporated alanine aminotransferase (ALT), interleukin (IL)-6, expectoration, fatigue, lymphocyte ratio (LYMR), aspartate transaminase (AST), and creatinine (CREA). The model yielded a satisfactory predictive performance with an AUC of 0.9104 and 0.8792 in the derivation and validation cohorts, respectively. The final model was then used to create a nomogram that was packaged into an open-source and predictive calculator for clinical use. The model is freely available online at https://severeconid-19predction.shinyapps.io/SHINY/.

Conclusion: In this study, we developed an open-source and free predictive calculator for COVID-19 progression based on ALT, IL-6, expectoration, fatigue, LYMR, AST, and CREA. The validated model can effectively predict progression to severe COVID-19, thus providing an efficient option for early and personalized management and the allocation of appropriate medical resources.

Keywords: COVID-19, severe COVID-19, predictive model, laboratory findings, cytokines, online predictive calculator

INTRODUCTION

The current outbreak of coronavirus disease 2019 (COVID-19) has spread rapidly and widely across the world, causing panic and major public health challenges in the international community (1). COVID-19 presents a wide clinical manifestation, including asymptomatic infection, mild upper respiratory tract illness, and severe viral pneumonia, with respiratory failure. Only a small proportion of the total number of cases progress to a severe condition (~15–20%); however, ~40% of patients with severe disease die (2–5). Although some research has shown that initial therapy with remdesivir or non-invasive positive pressure ventilation (NIPPV) is very efficient for severe cases, there is currently a lack of accepted recommendations for severe patients with regard to individualized treatment (6–8). Therefore, the rapid deterioration of patients with severe COVID-19 deserves special attention. There is an urgent need to develop options for the personalized diagnosis and treatment of such patients, particularly with regard to protecting the relative shortage of medical resources.

Fever, cough, and fatigue are commonly present in patients with mild COVID-19 (9, 10). As the disease progresses further, patients may also experience respiratory failure, acute respiratory distress syndrome, heart failure, metabolic acidosis, and septic shock (11). Besides the well-defined clinical characteristics of COVID-19, previous studies have shown that abnormal laboratory findings and cytokine levels are often associated with disease progression, including coagulation-related markers such as D-dimer and fibrinogen (FIB), neutrophil count, lymphocyte count, and high-sensitivity C-reactive protein (HsCRP) (5, 12–15). In addition, research has identified that a cytokine storm could be the primary driver of severe progression in COVID-19 patients (16, 17). However, the application of these independent indicators is limited by many factors, including insufficient information, individual differences, the experience of the attending physician, and the complexity of disease. Thus, there is an urgent need for advanced multivariable prediction models (18, 19). Although several studies have attempted to develop prediction models, most of the existing models were developed in a single center and based on retrospective data; in some cases, only partial datasets were used, and there was a clear lack of validation. These factors may lead to the omission of key variables and the risk of over-fitting, thus limiting the clinical application of such models. Therefore, there is a critical need to develop more effective prediction models (14, 15, 20, 21).

Here, we prospectively and consecutively enrolled a cohort of COVID-19 patients with a complete set of demographic data, clinical characteristics, laboratory findings, and cytokine information, and we then constructed a multiparameter prediction model for the early identification of severe COVID-19. Our model could help to monitor and guide precision medicine.

METHODS

Participants

COVID-19 patients were prospectively and consecutively enrolled from regional medical institutions by the West China Medical Center between December 20, 2019, and April 10, 2020. The patients were divided into severe and non-severe groups according to the China National Health Commission Guidelines for Diagnosis and Treatment of COVID-19 infection (Versions 5 and 7). Serum samples were collected from patients within 3 days of infection confirmation and stored at −80°C for the subsequent detection of cytokine levels. Demographic data, clinical characteristics, and laboratory findings were acquired from electronic medical records (**Figure 1**). Two independent researchers reviewed the data collection forms.

Diagnostic and Severity Classification Criteria

Patients with pneumonia, typical findings on computed tomography (CT) chest scan, and positive severe acute respiratory syndrome coronavirus 2 (SARS-CoV-2) nucleic acid results, as determined by real-time fluorescent reverse transcription-polymerase chain reaction assessment from bronchoalveolar lavage (BAL) or sputum, were considered as COVID-19 "cases" according to the diagnosis and treatment guidelines released by the China Health and Medical Commission (22). Patients with at least one of the following symptoms during hospitalization were allocated into the severe group: (1) respiratory distress, respiratory rate ≥30 times/min; (2) oxygen saturation ≤93% at rest; and (3) oxygen partial pressure (PaO_2)/oxygen concentration (FiO_2) in arterial blood ≤300 mmHg. All patients were discharged or had died by the time the model was developed.

The Detection of Cytokines

Circulating levels of interferon (IFN)-α2, IFN-β, IFN-γ, tumor necrosis factor (TNF)-α, interleukin (IL)-1α, IL-1β, IL-2, IL-4, IL-6, IL-8, IL-10, IL-17A, IL-17E, IL-17F, IL-22, and IL-33 in serum samples were measured by a multiplexed flow cytometric assay using Human Cytokine Kits on a Luminex® system (MAGPIX® with xPONENT) according to the manufacturer's instructions (MILLIPLEX® Analyst 5.1). All samples were measured in duplicate. Based on standard curves, we calculated the coefficient of variation (CV); this did not exceed 20%.

Construction of the Predictive Model and Internal Validation

Patients from the Chengdu region were divided into a derivation cohort, including a training set for modeling and a testing set for internal validation. Stepwise selection was based on p-values; least absolute shrinkage and selection operator (LASSO) and the Boruta algorithm were used to select variables (23, 24). Stepwise selection, as based on p-values, is a classic regression-based method. A variable's value with a $p < 0.05$ was regarded as significant and was retained. This practice generally achieves a better performance in smaller datasets and has been extensively used in previous research. LASSO regression can compress the coefficients of the features *via* penalty function to obtain optimal constraint models; this practice has been used effectively to avoid over-fitting and co-linearity in classical analysis methods based on significance differences and also enhances the ability of a model to be generalized. Boruta algorithm is a wrapper algorithm

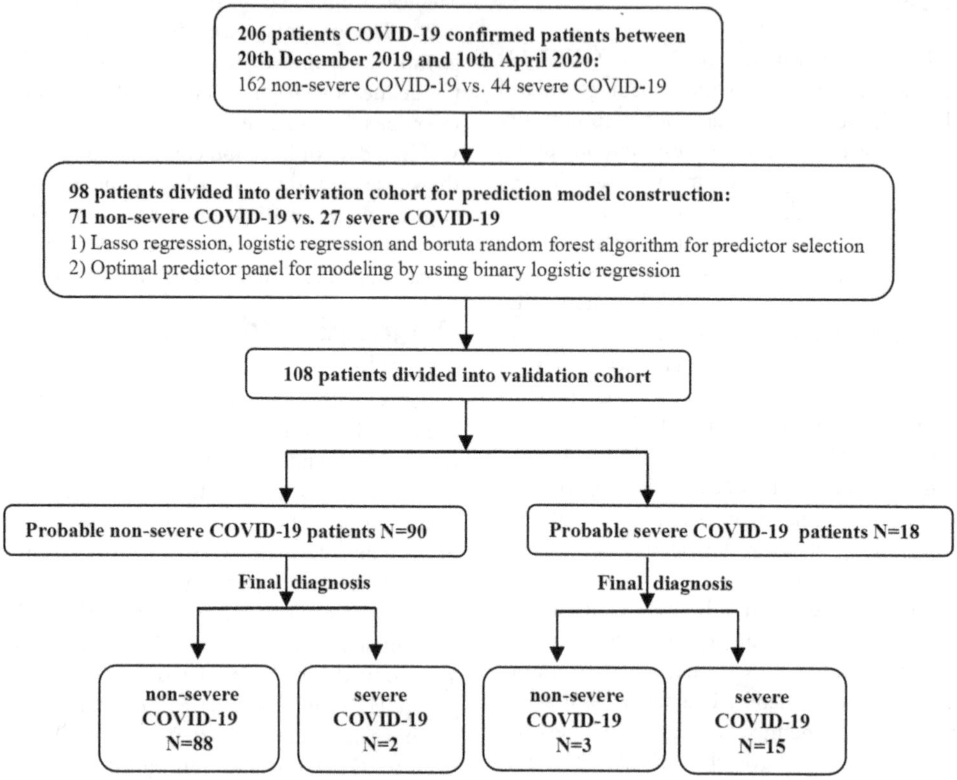

FIGURE 1 | Study flowchart.

that uses random forest classification. This practice can iteratively remove features that prove to be less relevant than random probes and thus aims to retain relevant variables for the function of a response variable. In addition, these two algorithms are particularly suitable for a dataset with a small sample size but with a large number of variables. By using these three different variable selection methods, we were able to select three candidate predictor panels to construct different binary logistic regression models, which were then verified internally by 10-fold cross-validation. The optimal model was then selected by comparing the area under the curve (AUC) and the Akaike information criterion (AIC) in order to generate a nomogram that could be encapsulated as an open-source online predictive calculator.

Independent Validation

The independent validation cohort consisted of patients from outside Chengdu; this was used for external verification to predict the generalization ability of the model by comparing the predicted results with a set of follow-up results to calculate several metrics: sensitivity, specificity, positive predictive value (PPV), and negative predictive value (NPV). AUCs and decision curve analysis (DCA) were used to comprehensively evaluate the model's discrimination and net clinical benefits (25).

Statistical Analysis

Continuous variables and categorical variables are presented as the median (upper and lower quartiles) and as a frequency, respectively. The chi-squared test for categorical variables and the Student *t*-test or Mann–Whitney *U*-test for continuous variables were used to test the data between groups. Pearson correlation was used to determine the linear correlation between two variables. The diagnostic performance of equations was then displayed by AIC and receiver operating characteristic (ROC) curve and quantified by AUCs. An open-source online predictive calculator was then created using the Shiny tool in the R environment (version 1.2.0). All statistical analyses were completed using R 3.5.0 version. All statistical tests were two-tailed, and $p \leq 0.05$ was considered to indicate statistical significance.

Standard Protocol Approvals, Registrations, and Patient Consent

The protocol for this study was approved by the West China Hospital, Sichuan University Medical Ethics Committee (reference no. 193, 2020), and conformed to the principles of the Declaration of Helsinki. Written informed consent was obtained from all participants.

RESULTS

Epidemiological Characteristics

We recruited 206 patients with a confirmed diagnosis of COVID-19; of these, 44 patients progressed to severe COVID-19, and 162 patients were classified as having non-severe COVID-19.

TABLE 1 | Patients' characteristics in training set.

	Non-severe COVID-19 71 patients	Severe COVID-19 27 patients	*P*-value		Non-severe COVID-19 71 patients	Severe COVID-19 27 patients	*P*-value
Demographics				Cytokines			
Age	46 (33, 51)	50 (42, 65)	0.005*	IFN-β	8.87 (8.08, 8.87)	8.87 (8.08, 8.87)	0.403
Sex	53.50%	63.00%	0.4	IFN-γ	10.58 (1.71, 24.88)	17.07 (3.67, 54.26)	0.161
Diabetes	4.20%	29.60%	<0.001*	Laboratory findings			
Hypertension	16.90%	40.70%	0.013*	WBC	5.41 (4.40, 7.15)	6.31 (4.40, 7.67)	0.148
Clinical features				HB	137.00 (126.00, 156.00)	134.00 (125.00, 151.00)	0.239
Temperature	36.7 (36.5, 37.4)	37.2 (36.7, 37.7)	0.115	PLT	180.00 (141.00, 244.00)	146.00 (120.00, 223.00)	0.131
Heart rate	88 (78, 97)	90 (84, 105)	0.196	LYMR	23.80 (18.80, 30.90)	15.20 (5.10, 23.40)	<0.001*
Respiratory rate	20 (20, 21)	20 (20, 22)	0.008*	NEUTR	65.80 (57.60, 71.00)	77.00 (67.20, 87.60)	<0.001*
SBP	130 (120, 140)	139 (123, 150)	0.183	EOSR	0.20 (0.09, 0.90)	0.00 (0.00, 0.20)	0.003*
DBP	82 (77, 89)	84 (76, 94)	0.619	BASOR	0.20 (0.10, 0.30)	0.20 (0.10, 0.30)	0.977
SBP-DBP	48 (42, 58)	50 (44, 63)	0.202	MONOR	8.30 (6.80, 10.80)	7.00 (4.20, 9.10)	0.028*
Fever	60.60%	74.10%	0.212	HCT	39.80 (35.60, 45.40)	36.60 (29.50, 44.10)	0.215
Cough	45.10%	81.50%	0.001*	D-dimer	1.90 (0.32, 62.44)	5.46 (0.83, 31.00)	0.75
Dry cough	25.40%	25.90%	0.954	FIB	3.59 (2.84, 4.32)	4.03 (3.20, 4.86)	0.045*
Expectoration	16.90%	51.90%	<0.001*	APTT	31.82 (27.20, 37.80)	32.70 (31.20, 35.20)	0.578
Dyspnea	2.80%	25.90%	<0.001*	PT	12.40 (11.70, 13.40)	12.70 (11.90, 13.30)	0.559
Asthma	4.20%	18.50%	0.021*	INR	1.02 (0.97, 1.10)	1.05 (1.00, 1.15)	0.379
Chest distress	7.00%	11.10%	0.511	TBIL	10.70 (7.11, 14.90)	6.78 (4.00, 13.35)	0.043*
Nasal obstruction	2.80%	0.00%	$P = 0.378$	DBIL	3.40 (2.20, 4.60)	3.90 (2.64, 6.40)	0.272
Nasal discharge	5.60%	3.70%	$P = 0.698$	IBIL	6.60 (4.50, 11.70)	5.47 (2.70, 9.33)	0.158
Earache	0.00%	3.70%	0.103	ALT	29.50 (18.00, 48.01)	41.17 (21.00, 74.14)	0.147
Sore throat	11.30%	18.50%	0.344	AST	26.00 (19.60, 35.70)	37.00 (23.70, 70.62)	0.022*
Headache	16.90%	7.40%	0.23	TP	75.00 (70.70, 79.00)	68.41 (63.20, 77.30)	0.014*
Myalgia	8.50%	11.10%	0.684	ALB	44.30 (41.00, 46.67)	39.60 (34.90, 44.27)	0.001*
Arthralgia	1.40%	3.70%	0.473	GLB	30.20 (27.06, 33.05)	29.31 (23.80, 32.75)	0.057
Chest wall invagination	0.00%	0.00%	–	TG	1.66 (0.94, 2.28)	1.44 (0.84, 2.37)	0.507
Fatigue	4.20%	25.90%	0.002*	CHOL	4.20 (3.42, 4.80)	3.85 (2.87, 4.58)	0.088
Diarrhea	11.30%	14.80%	0.632	HDL-C	1.20 (1.03, 1.39)	1.04 (0.92, 1.43)	0.231
Cytokines				LDL-C	2.30 (1.84, 2.84)	1.87 (1.33, 2.60)	0.054
IL-1α	2.91 (1.47, 7.80)	7.05 (2.91, 11.53)	0.025*	CK	93.00 (56.80, 216.00)	217.76 (64.00, 314.30)	0.053
IL-1β	1.60 (0.66, 4.86)	3.24 (1.37, 7.80)	0.06	CK-MB	11.83 (5.32, 14.73)	12.34 (3.76, 17.00)	0.688
IL-2	0.21 (0.10, 0.45)	0.36 (0.14, 0.61)	0.343	Glu	5.63 (5.07, 6.97)	6.80 (5.44, 9.15)	0.044*
IL-4	1.94 (0.48, 3.91)	1.73 (0.78, 6.47)	0.181	Na	140.10 (137.10, 143.00)	138.00 (133.14, 141.80)	0.097
IL-6	1.19 (0.66, 3.54)	5.03 (2.12, 18.61)	<0.001*	K	3.97 (3.60, 4.30)	3.94 (3.40, 4.33)	0.519
IL-8	3.72 (2.18, 6.98)	5.56 (3.82, 9.44)	0.074	Ca	2.27 (2.16, 2.39)	2.09 (1.96, 2.19)	<0.001*
IL-10	1.13 (0.34, 2.47)	3.76 (0.92, 14.15)	0.001*	Mg	0.87 (0.82, 0.99)	0.85 (0.79, 1.02)	0.741
IL-17A	0.97 (0.52, 4.12)	1.45 (0.80, 4.37)	0.083	Urea	3.70 (2.90, 5.30)	4.31 (3.30, 7.20)	0.076
IL-17E	28.56 (17.37, 90.70)	24.36 (9.85, 80.88)	0.203	CREA	71.60 (56.00, 83.30)	69.40 (52.00, 192.90)	0.735
IL-17F	7.66 (5.75, 13.53)	7.66 (6.22, 10.75)	0.817	URIC	348.00 (258.00, 427.00)	276.00 (183.00, 379.00)	0.038*
IL-22	36.67 (2.05, 86.54)	11.20 (1.42, 91.01)	0.874	Myo	125.00 (21.89, 583.83)	166.40 (23.72, 1247.00)	0.245
IL-33	8.76 (7.51, 8.76)	8.76 (8.76, 10.11)	0.161	HsCRP	10.00 (2.58, 23.28)	27.60 (6.80, 55.14)	0.004*
TNF-α	41.15 (21.84, 71.55)	45.50 (17.29, 89.73)	0.525	PCT	0.09 (0.04, 4.10)	0.48 (0.04, 7.42)	0.362
IFN-α2	6.46 (4.00, 20.38)	6.46 (4.00, 33.26)	0.92				

*Data are presented as n (%) for categorical variables and as median (upper and lower quartile) for continuous variables. *P < 0.05.*

Patients in the severe group were significantly older (50 *vs.* 46, $p = 0.005$) and had a significantly higher frequency of underlying diseases (diabetes and hypertension) than the non-severe group ($p < 0.001$ and $p = 0.013$, respectively). There were no differences between the two groups in terms of gender (male: 54.940 *vs.* 56.810%, $p = 0.400$). With regard to epidemiological exposure, most of the patients (79.000%) in the severe group had been overseas or had visited Wuhan or surrounding regions within 14 days of disease onset; patients who had been overseas accounted for 50% of the patients with non-severe COVID-19. As of April 28, 2020, the time for the reversal of a negative nucleic acid test result in the non-severe and severe groups was 11 and 18 days (median) except for three patients who died from multiple organ failure (MOF).

Differences in Characteristics and Correlation Analysis

Demographic data, clinical characteristics, laboratory findings, and cytokine levels are shown in **Table 1** and **Supplementary Figures 1, 2**. Several cytokines were significantly elevated in the severe COVID-19 group ($p \leq 0.010$). The predictive value of each single cytokine, and a combined panel of cytokines, were evaluated by ROC curve analysis and quantified by AUC (**Supplementary Figure 3**). Results showed that the AUCs were 0.830, 0.796, 0.729, 0.707, 0.694, 0.667, 0.656, and 0.653 for single IL-10, IL-6, IL-1α, IL-1β, IL-17A, IL-4, TNF-α, and IL-2 and that the binary logistic model had a similar AUC (0.796–0.848). These data indicated that IL-10 and IL-6 may represent potential biomarkers for patients with severe COVID-19. We found significant differences between the severe and non-severe COVID-19 group with regard to a range of clinical characteristics, including respiratory rate, cough, expectoration, dyspnea, asthma, and debilitation. Significant differences were also identified in several laboratory findings; lymphocyte ratio (LYMR), eosinophil ratio (EOSR), monocyte ratio (MONOR), total bilirubin (TBIL), total protein (TP), albumin (ALB), Ca, and URIC were all significantly lower in the severe COVID-19 group, while neutrophil ratio (NEUTR), FIB, aspartate transaminase (AST), glucose (GlU), and HsCRP were all significantly higher. However, the AUCs for these indicators when used to predict severe COVID-19 were all <0.690. Simple logistic analysis was not suited for the severe COVID-19 group, owing to the feature selection of such a large number of indicators.

TABLE 2 | Comprehensive performance of three prediction models.

	Model A	Model B	Model C
Variables	IL-6, LYMR, HsCRP, expectoration, dyspnea	ALT, IL-6, expectoration, fatigue, LYMR, AST, CREA	Dyspnea, diabetes, age, IFN-γ, IL-6, IL-10, LYMR, NEUR, AST, TP, Alb, Ca
AUC	0.8811	0.9104	0.8574
AIC	80.977	76.582	83.909
Cut-off	0.237	0.256	0.468
Specificity	0.831	0.842	0.958
Sensitivity	0.889	0.897	0.667
Hosmer-Lemeshow test (*P*-value)	0.1178	0.4989	0.2986

AIC, Akaike's information criterion; AUC, area under the ROC curve.

We identified significant correlations between each pair for all cytokines except IL-33 and IFN-β. In addition, IL-6, IL-10, and IFN-β were closely associated with certain laboratory indicators of hepatobiliary function. Similarly, hematocrit (HCT), tBIL, direct bilirubin (DBIL), indirect bilirubin (IBIL), TP, creatine kinase (CK), and myoglobin (Myo) were significantly associated with most cytokines except IL-33, which was not correlated with any of the indices.

The Selection of Predictors and Model Construction

Next, we used variation analysis, LASSO regression, and the Boruta algorithm, to select three predictive panels and construct

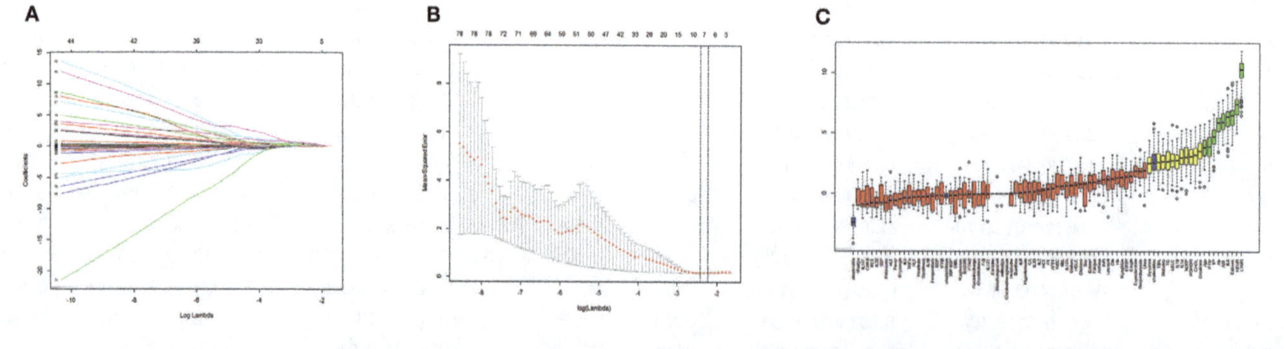

FIGURE 2 | (A) Coefficient diagram of least absolute shrinkage and selection operator (LASSO) variables. Each curve in the figure represents the trajectory of the coefficient of an independent variable. The ordinate represents the value of the coefficient. The lower abscissa, λ, is a parameter that controls the severity of the penalty. The upper abscissa represents the number of non-zero coefficients in the model under the penalty parameter. **(B)** Adjustment parameters in the LASSO model; λ was screened by 10-fold cross-validation. A dashed vertical line was drawn at one standard error (1–SE standard) of the minimum and minimum standards. Λ 0.1 se corresponds to a model with good performance but the fewest number of arguments. **(C)** A variable importance plot according to Boruta feature selection. Blue boxplots correspond to minimal, average, and maximum Z scores of a shadow attribute. The Z-score clearly separates important and non-important attributes. Red, yellow, and green colors represent rejected, suggestive, and confirmed attributes by Boruta selection, respectively.

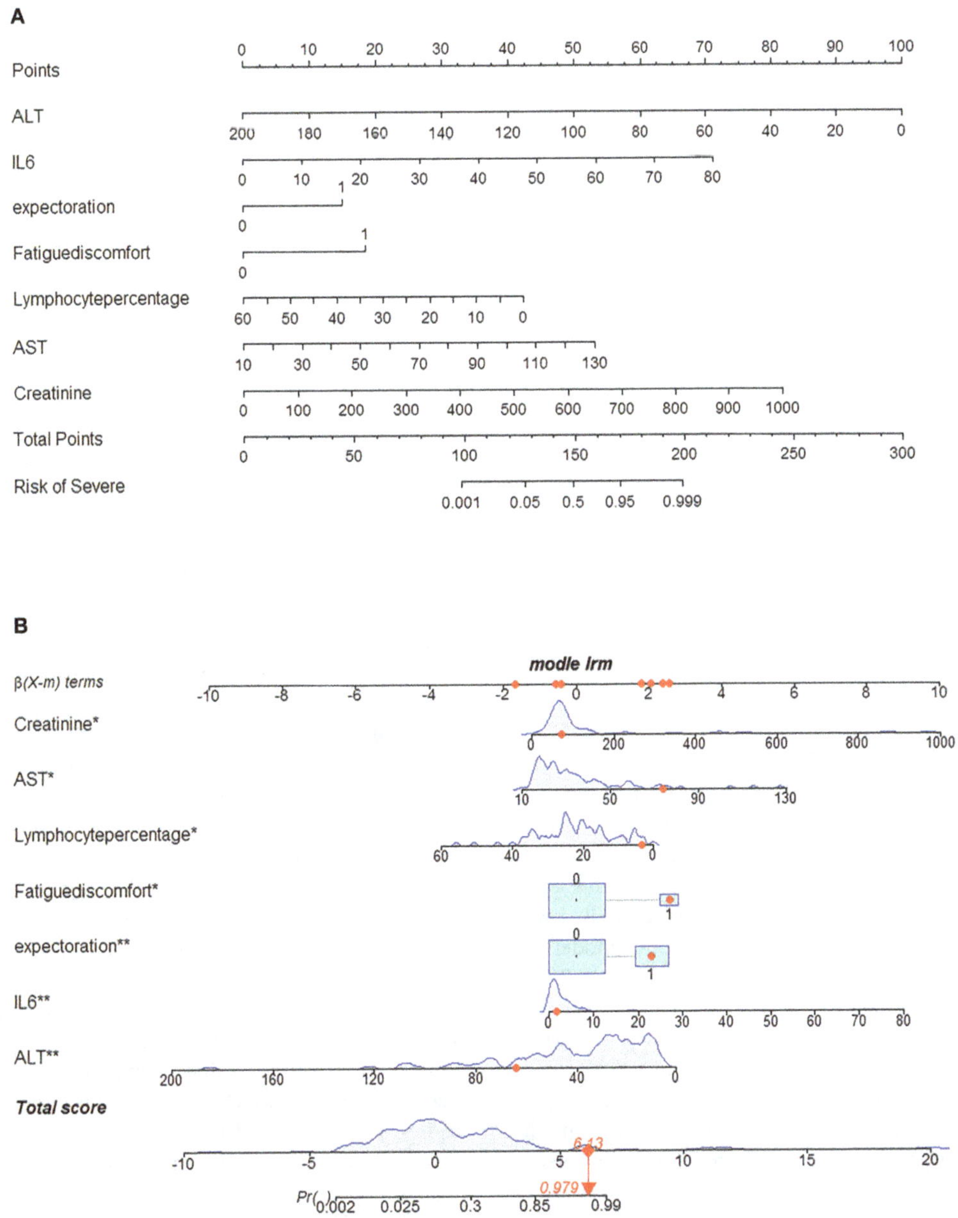

FIGURE 3 | Nomogram for predicting severe coronavirus disease 2019 (COVID-19). **(A)** To use the nomogram for an individual patient, the points (top gridline) for each predictor variable are first assigned and the total points calculated. A vertical line from this value on the Total Points gridline then provides a probability for predicting severe COVID-19. The results of the binary variable are encoded as 0 and 1, representing the absence and presence of this symptom, respectively. The calculation is further illustrated in **(B)**, which shows the results of a patient with certain laboratory findings; the probability of this patient progressing to severe COVID-19 is 97.9%.

corresponding predictive models (predictive models A, B, and C, respectively) (**Table 2**, **Figure 2**). Predictive model B exhibited a better performance than the other two models in terms of sensitivity, specificity, discrimination, calibration, and clinical net benefit. In addition, the predictors included in this model are objective and universal. An optimal model, with seven features, alanine aminotransferase (ALT), IL-6, expectoration, fatigue, LYMR, AST, and serum creatinine (CREA), were used to generate a nomogram (**Figure 3**) and were encapsulated as an open-source online predictive calculator with R/Shiny (https://severeconid-19predction.shinyapps.io/SHINY/).

Validation of the Online Predictive Model

Finally, we predicted the disease progression of the 108 patients in the validation cohort using our model. The model predicted that 18 patients would progress to severe COVID-19 while the remaining 90 would not. Compared with the follow-up results (91 patients with non-severe COVID-19 and 17 patients with

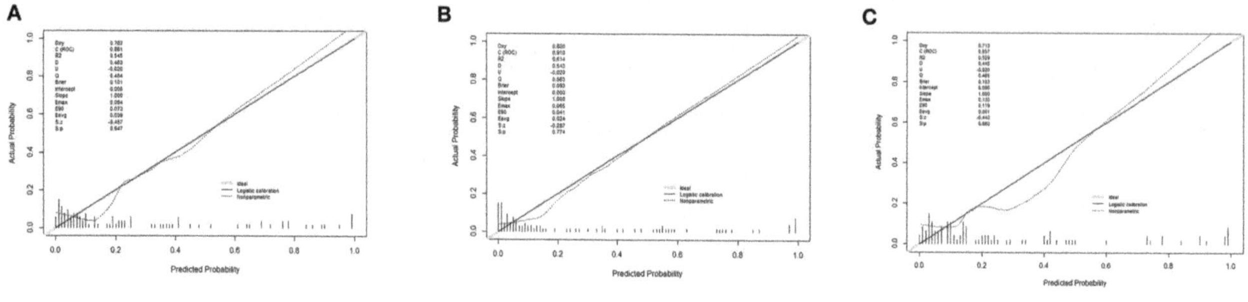

FIGURE 4 | Calibration curves for the three predictive models. **(A)** Predictive model A, **(B)** predictive model B, and **(C)** predictive model C.

severe COVID-19), the sensitivity, specificity, PPV, and NPV of our assay were 0.882 (95% CI; 0.622–0.979), 0.967 (95% CI; 0.890–0.991), 0.833 (95% CI; 0.747–0.896), and 0.978 (95% CI; 0.914–0.996), respectively. The model also achieved excellent discrimination (AUC = 0.879), calibration, and clinical net benefit (**Figures 4, 5**).

DISCUSSION

The accurate and individualized assessment of a patient who may progress to severe COVID-19 will promote the efficiency of clinical intervention and improve the rational use of medical resources. In the present study, we recruited 206 patients (162 patients with non-severe COVID-19 and 44 patients with severe COVID-19). We analyzed a range of indicators associated with severe COVID-19 and developed a novel predictive model that included ALT, IL-6, expectoration, fatigue, LYMR, AST, and CREA. This model proved to have excellent ability to predict the progression of COVID-19 during hospitalization, in both the derivation and validation cohorts.

Our final model was visualized in the form of a nomogram and was then packaged into an open-source and free predictive calculator (https://severeconid-19predction.shinyapps.io/SHINY/). The model represents a powerful tool with which to aid decision-making and guide treatment strategies for target patients who are at high risk of developing severe progression. The model could also be used to facilitate personalized management.

Previous research reported wide differences in the levels of a large number of cytokines from patients with non-severe and severe COVID-19 (26–28). Our present results identified obvious elevations of various cytokines in patients with severe COVID-19, including IL-1α, IL-1β, IFN-γ, TNF-α, IL-2, IL-4, IL-6, IL-10, and IL-17A. Of these cytokines, IL-6 and IL-10 showed the highest fold-change, thus indicating the presence of a strong inflammatory reaction; this could be a sufficient response to trigger a cytokine storm. Univariate logistic analysis showed that a number of cytokines can be used as predictors for patients with severe illness, although their predictive efficacies can vary considerably; these cytokines could not be used individually. We also found that underlying diseases (diabetes and hypertension), initial clinical characteristics (cough, expectoration, dyspnea, asthma, and debilitation), and laboratory findings [LYMR ALT, AST, CK, GlU, and procalcitonin (PCT)] were also significantly associated with disease progression, although these were non-specific. The extensive correlation between cytokines and the clinical response spectrum may be explained by multiple organ damage caused by the over-exuberant inflammatory response in severe COVID-19 (12, 29).

Univariate logistic analysis indicated that using a certain evaluation index could not provide sufficient evidence for the prediction of progression and that modeling by data mining may be a more efficient and viable tool with which to compensate for the lack of a single source of information (30). We used the LASSO algorithm and logistic regression and compared different modeling approaches. Finally, we selected a predictive model that included ALT, IL-6, expectoration, fatigue, LYMR, AST, and CREA. Our model achieved satisfactory predictive performance with AUCs of 0.910 and 0.879 in the derivation and validation cohorts, respectively. We also packaged this model into an open-source online format for clinical use. Although several predictive models have been published previously, these studies were associated with obvious limitations, including the fact that they were retrospective reviews or were associated with suboptimal predictive abilities or were not validated externally (31–33). Taking these limitations into account, our study is superior in several respects. First, we considered potential predictors for severe COVID-19 and included a comprehensive dataset retrospectively. Second, our shrinking model, featuring representative key variables, may exhibit better levels of performance than a complex model. This can be supported by the fact that our predictive model was established by comparing several different methods; the optimal method had a significantly higher AUC than the other models; this finding was reconfirmed in the validation cohort. Third, the predictive model was used to create a nomogram that was then used to generate an open-source online calculator format with visualization and maneuverability function.

There are also some limitations associated with our study that need to be considered. For example, we mainly focused on the changes of symptoms and the levels of key indicators

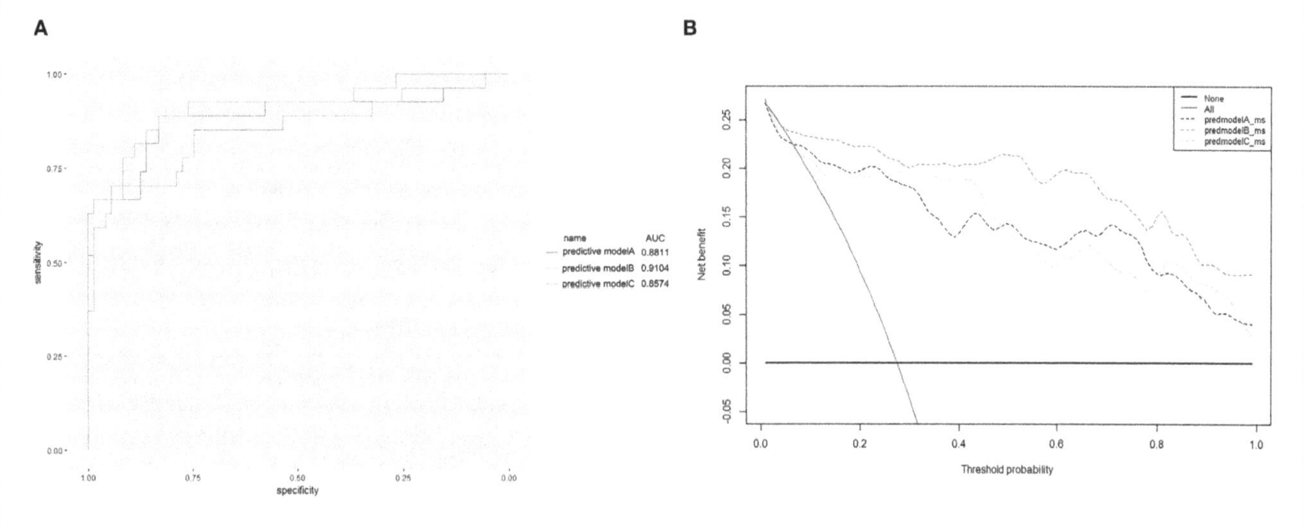

FIGURE 5 | (A) Receiver operating characteristic curves for the three predictive models. The areas under the receiver operating characteristic curves were 0.8811, 0.9104, and 0.8574, for predictive models A, B, and C, respectively. **(B)** The decision curve analysis (DCA) of three predictive models.

in patients after SARS-CoV-2 infection and did not consider the influence of individual differences on the progression of disease. More in-depth investigations and longitudinal dynamic monitoring studies now need to be conducted to explain the specific characteristics of the potential predictors. Furthermore, the predictive model needs to be validated in a larger patient cohort and other populations outside of China.

CONCLUSION

In this study, we developed and validated an online predictive calculator that provides personalized probability for the progression of disease based on seven commonly used variables. The model will be vital for early personalized management, to promote the appropriate allocation of medical resources, and to ensure that patients who may develop severe COVID-19 can receive appropriate treatment as soon as possible.

AUTHOR CONTRIBUTIONS

ZM and MW designed the research and wrote the manuscript. ZZ and YoZ responsible for the recruitment of COVID-19 patients and clinical treatment. YW and SG responsible for the detection of candidate biomarkers. ML, SY, and YaZ responsible for collecting and organizing data. All authors contributed to the article and approved the submitted version.

ACKNOWLEDGMENTS

The authors would like to express their gratitude to EditSprings (https://www.editsprings.com/) for the expert linguistic services provided.

REFERENCES

Yao D, Yan K, Duan J, Zhang X, Zhou L. Coronavirus disease 2019 (COVID- 19): prevention and control in gynecological outpatient clinic. *Front Public Health.* (2020) 8:618494. doi: 10.3389/fpubh.2020.618494

Zhou F, Yu T, Du R, Fan G, Liu Y, Liu Z, et al. Clinical course and risk factors for mortality of adult inpatients with COVID-19 in Wuhan, China: a retrospective cohort study. *Lancet.* (2020) 395:1054–62. doi:10.1016/S0140-6736(20)30566-3

Sun L, Song F, Shi N, Liu F, Li S, Li P, et al. Combination of four clinical indicators predicts the severe/critical symptom of patients infected COVID-19. *J Clin Virol.* (2020) 128:104431. doi: 10.1016/j.jcv.2020.104431

Zheng YL, He YK, Ma XQ, Gao ZC. Feasibility of coronavirus disease 2019 eradication. *Chin Med J.* (2020) 133:1387–9. doi:10.1097/CM9.0000000000000936

Kim SR, Nam SH, Kim YR. Risk factors on the progression to clinical outcomes of COVID-19 patients in South Korea: using national data. *Int J Environ Res Public Health.* (2020) 17:8847. doi: 10.3390/ijerph17238847

Alhazzani W, Moller MH, Arabi YM, Loeb M, Gong MN, Fan E, et al. Surviving sepsis campaign: guidelines on the management of critically ill adults with coronavirus disease 2019 (COVID-19). *Crit Care Med.* (2020). 48:E440–69. doi: 10.1097/CCM.0000000000004363

Hossein-khannazer N, Shokoohian B, Shpichka A, Aghdaei HA, Timashev P, Vosough M. Novel therapeutic approaches for treatment of COVID-19. *J Mol Med.* (2020) 98:789–803. doi: 10.1007/s00109-020-01927-6

Yadav P, Vats R, Bano A, Bhardwaj R. Mesenchymal stem cell immunomodulation and regeneration therapeutics as an ameliorative approach for COVID-19 pandemics. *Life Sci.* (2020) 263:8588. doi: 10.1016/j.lfs.2020.118588

Xu R, Hou KK, Zhang K, Xu HY, Zhang N, Fu H, et al. Performance of two risk-stratification models in hospitalized patients with coronavirus disease. *Front Med-Lausanne.* (2020) 7:518. doi: 10.3389/fmed.2020.00518

Jamwal S, Gautam A, Elsworth J, Kumar M, Chawla R, Kumar P. An updated insight into the molecular pathogenesis, secondary complications and potential therapeutics of COVID-19 pandemic. *Life Sci.* (2020) 257:118105. doi: 10.1016/j.lfs.2020.118105

Wiersinga WJ, Rhodes A, Cheng AC, Peacock SJ, Prescott HC. Pathophysiology, transmission, diagnosis, and treatment of coronavirus disease 2019 (COVID-19) A review. *JAMA-J Am Med Assoc.* (2020) 324:782–93. doi: 10.1001/jama.2020.12839

Tian JB, Yuan XL, Xiao J, Zhong Q, Yang CG, Liu B, et al. Clinical characteristics and risk factors associated with COVID-19 disease severity in patients with cancer in Wuhan, China: a multicentre, retrospective, cohort study. *Lancet Oncol.* (2020) 21:893–903. doi: 10.1016/S1470-2045(20)30309-0

Luo Y, Mao LY, Yuan X, Xue Y, Lin Q, Tang GX, et al. Prediction model based on the combination of cytokines and lymphocyte subsets for prognosis of SARS-CoV-2 infection. *J Clin Immunol.* (2020) 40:960–9. doi: 10.1007/s10875-020-00821-7

Gong J, Ou JY, Qiu XP, Jie YS, Chen YQ, Yuan LX, et al. A tool for early prediction of severe coronavirus disease 2019 (COVID-19): a multicenter study using the risk Nomogram in Wuhan and Guangdong, China. *Clin Infect Dis.* (2020). 71:833–40. doi: 10.1093/cid/ciaa443

Hu CY, Liu ZQ, Jiang YF, Shi OM, Zhang X, Xu KL, et al. Early prediction of mortality risk among patients with severe COVID-19, using machine learning. *Int J Epidemiol.* (2020) 49:1918–29. doi: 10.1101/2020.04.13.20064329

Edalatifard M, Akhtari M, Salehi M, Naderi Z, Jamshidi A, Mostafaei S, et al. Intravenous methylprednisolone pulse as a treatment for hospitalised severe COVID-19 patients: results from a randomised controlled clinical trial. *Eur Respir J.* (2020) 56:2002808. doi: 10.1183/13993003. 02808-2020

Marfia G, Navone S, Guarnaccia L, Campanella R, Mondoni M, Locatelli M, et al. Decreased serum level of sphingosine-1-phosphate: a novel predictor of clinical severity in COVID-19. *Embo Mol Med.* (2021) 13:e13424. doi: 10.15252/emmm.202013424

Michel-Kabamba N, Ngatu NR, Leon-Kabamba N, Katumbo-Mukemo A, Mukuku O, Ngoyi-Mukonkole J, et al. Occupational COVID-19 prevention among congolese healthcare workers: knowledge, practices, PPE compliance, and safety imperatives. *Trop Med Infect Dis.* (2021) 6:6. doi: 10.3390/tropicalmed6010006

Wynants L, Van Calster B, Bonten MMJ, Collins GS, Debray TPA, De Vos M, et al. Prediction models for diagnosis and prognosis of covid-19 infection: systematic review and critical appraisal. *Bmj-Brit Med J.* (2020) 369:m1328. doi:10.1101/2020.03.24.20041020

Li Q, Zhang JL, Ling Y, Li WX, Zhang XY, Lu HZ, et al. A simple algorithm helps early identification of SARS-CoV-2 infection patients with severe progression tendency. *Infection.* (2020) 48:577–84. doi:10.1007/s15010-020-01446-z

Dong YL, Zhou HF, Li MY, Zhang ZL, Guo WN, Yu T, et al. A novel simple scoring model for predicting severity of patients with SARS-CoV-2 infection. *Transbound Emerg Dis.* (2020) 67:2823–9. doi: 10.1111/tbed.13651

Shen B, Yi X, Sun YT, Bi XJ, Du JP, Zhang C, et al. Proteomic and metabolomic characterization of COVID-19 patient sera. *Cell.* (2020) 182:59. doi: 10.1016/j.cell.2020.05.032

MacWilliam D, Kowalewski J, Kumar A, Pontrello C, Ray A. Signaling mode of the broad-spectrum conserved CO_2 receptor is one of the important determinants of odor valence in drosophila. *Neuron.* (2018) 97:1153. doi: 10.1016/j.neuron.2018.01.028

Rubbens P, Schmidt ML, Props R, Biddanda BA, Boon N, Waegeman W, et al. Randomized lasso links microbial taxa with aquatic functional groups inferred from flow cytometry. *Msystems.* (2019) 4:e00093-19. doi: 10.1128/mSystems.00093-19

Muntner P, Colantonio LD, Cushman M, Goff DC, Howard G, Howard VJ, et al. Validation of the atherosclerotic cardiovascular disease pooled cohort risk equations. *JAMA-J Am Med Assoc.* (2014) 311:1406–15. doi: 10.1001/jama.2014.2630

Udomsinprasert W, Jittikoon J, Sangroongruangsri S, Chaikledkaew U. Circulating levels of interleukin-6 and interleukin-10, but not tumor necrosis factor-alpha, as potential biomarkers of severity and mortality for COVID- 19: systematic review with meta-analysis. *J Clin Immunol.* (2021) 41:11–22. doi: 10.1007/s10875-020-00899-z

Ahmad T, Chaudhuri R, Joshi MC, Almatroudi A, Rahmani AH, Ali SM. COVID-19: the emerging immunopathological determinants for recovery or death. *Front Microbiol.* (2020) 11:588409. doi: 10.3389/fmicb.2020.588409

Mannino F, Bitto A, Irrera N. Severe acute respiratory syndrome coronavirus- 2 induces cytokine storm and inflammation during coronavirus disease 19: perspectives and possible therapeutic approaches. *Front Pharmacol.* (2020) 11:592169. doi: 10.3389/fphar.2020.592169

Reznik SE, Tiwari AK, Ashby CR. Edaravone: a potential treatment for the COVID-19-induced inflammatory syndrome? *Pharmacol Res.* (2020) 160:105055. doi: 10.1016/j.phrs.2020.105055

Wang W, Zhang YF, Liu MX, Wang Y, Yang T, Li DS, et al. TIMP2 is a poor prognostic factor and predicts metastatic biological behavior in gastric cancer. *Sci Rep-Uk.* (2018) 8:9629. doi: 10.1038/s41598-018-27897-x

Bello-Chavolla OY, Antonio-Villa NE, Ortiz-Brizuela E, Vargas-Vazquez A, Gonzalez-Lara MF, de Leon AP, et al. Validation and repurposing of the MSL-COVID-19 score for prediction of severe COVID-19 using simple clinical predictors in a triage setting: The Nutri-CoV score. *PLoS ONE.* (2020) 15:244051. doi: 10.1371/journal.pone.0244051

Xiao LS, Li P, Sun FL, Zhang YP, Xu CH, Zhu HB, et al. Development and validation of a deep learning-based model using computed tomography imaging for predicting disease severity of coronavirus disease 2019. *Front Bioeng Biotech.* (2020) 8:898. doi: 10.3389/fbioe.2020.00898

Xiao LS, Zhang WF, Gong MC, Zhang YP, Chen LY, Zhu HB, et al. Development and validation of the HNC-LL score for predicting the severity of coronavirus disease 2019. *Ebiomedicine.* (2020) 57:102880. doi:10.1016/j.ebiom.2020.102880

3

Serum Cytokine Profiling Identifies Axl as a New Biomarker Candidate for Active Eosinophilic Granulomatosis with Polyangiitis

Jianjuan Ma[1,2,3†], Cong Dong[2†], Shushan Wei[2], Minzhi Qiu[2], Penghui Wu[2], Changxing Ou[2], Bomeng Zhang[2], Xueyan Zhang[4], Jie Yan[5], Qingling Zhang[2] and Nanshan Zhong[1,2*]*

[1] *Department of Pathophysiology, School of Basic Medical Sciences, Guizhou Medical University, Guiyang, China,* [2] *Pulmonary and Critical Care Medicine, Guangzhou Institute of Respiratory Health, National Clinical Research Center for Respiratory Disease, National Center for Respiratory Medicine, State Key Laboratory of Respiratory Diseases, The First Affiliated Hospital of Guangzhou Medical University, Guangzhou, China,* [3] *Department of Pediatric Hematology, Affiliated Hospital of Guizhou Medical University, Guiyang, China,* [4] *School of Basic Medical Sciences, The Second Affiliated Hospital, State Key Laboratory of Respiratory Disease, Guangdong Provincial Key Laboratory of Allergy & Clinical Immunology, Guangzhou Medical University, Guangzhou, China,* [5] *The Second Affiliated Hospital, State Key Laboratory of Respiratory Disease, Guangdong Provincial Key Laboratory of Allergy & Clinical Immunology, Guangzhou Medical University, Guangzhou, China*

***Correspondence:**
Nanshan Zhong
nanshan@vip.163.com
Qingling Zhang
zqling68@hotmail.com

† These authors have contributed equally to this work and share first authorship

Background: Eosinophilic granulomatosis with polyangiitis (EGPA) prognosis is generally favorable and is treated with combined corticosteroids/immunosuppressor(s) therapy. However, disease flares increase the number of clinical visits. Therefore, discovering new serum biomarkers for early identification of active EGPA is crucial.

Objective: To identify reliable serum biomarkers to measure EGPA activity.

Methods: The expression of 160 proteins was compared in sera from 15 inactive and 13 active EGPA patients by antibody-based microarray. Network-based analysis identified patterns in the different groups. Differentially expressed proteins (DEPs) in active disease were identified, and the correlation between their serum levels and clinical parameters was assessed. DEPs were further analyzed for GO enrichment and KEGG pathways. Finally, DEP marker candidates were validated by ELISA and Bio-plex as well as against a second cohort of 22 inactive and 18 active EGPA patients.

Results: The active group presented higher peripheral and sputum eosinophil counts, FeNO, and FEV1 (% predicted) ($P < 0.05$). Network-based analysis showed scattered expression patterns in active subjects, but no significant bias in inactive subjects. Significant differences were observed in serum levels of 19 candidate markers, all of which were higher in active EGPA ($P < 0.05$). KEGG analysis indicated that DEPs were mainly involved in the MAPK, PI3K-Akt, RAS and Rap1 related pathways. Nine out of 19 candidate markers were positively correlated with peripheral eosinophil counts including FGF-7, SCF, GDNF, β-NGF, IGFBP-4, Axl, PIGF, Insulin, NT-4, ErbB3, OPN and BMP-4 ($r = 0.693$, $r = 0.692$, $r = 0.687$, $r = 0.683$, $r = 0.671$, $r = 0.606$, $r = 0.571$, $r = 0.570$, $r = 0.516$, respectively; $P < 0.05$), while two, CD14 and MCP-3, were negatively correlated ($r = -0.644$ and $r = -0.515$; $P < 0.05$). The higher expression of Axl, OPN, HCC-4, GDNF, and MCP-3 in active EGPA subjects was confirmed by ELISA and Custom Multiplex Bio-plex analyses.

Conclusion: The serum protein profiles were significantly different between active and inactive EGPA. The expression of the candidate proteins correlated with peripheral blood eosinophil count. Serum Axl, OPN, HCC-4, GDNF, and MCP-3 levels were consistently higher in active EGPA, independent of the assessment methods. Finally, Axl had the largest AUC, indicating that this cytokine may serve as novel biomarker for the diagnosis of active EGPA.

Keywords: eosinophilic granulomatosis with polyangiitis, antibody array, biomarkers, active, serum

INTRODUCTION

Eosinophilic granulomatosis with polyangiitis (EGPA), formerly called Churg-Strauss syndrome, is a systemic necrotizing vasculitis affecting small- and medium-size vessels; it is characterized by asthma, peripheral eosinophilia, eosinophil-rich inflammation, and vascular and/or extravascular granulomas. Since 1951, when EGPA was first reported by Churg and Strauss, there have been several definitions and classification criteria for EGPA (Churg and Strauss, 1951). In 1990, the American College of Rheumatology (ACR) proposed the first EGPA classification criteria including the following six items (Lightfoot et al., 1990; Masi et al., 1990): (1) asthma; (2) paranasal sinus abnormality; (3) peripheral blood eosinophilia (>10%); (4) unfixed pulmonary infiltration; (5) mononeuropathy or polyneuropathy; and (6) extravascular eosinophils on histology. When four or more items are satisfied, a patient can be classified as EGPA. The sensitivity and specificity of the 1990 ACR criteria for EGPA have been reported were 85% and 99.75% respectively (Masi et al., 1990).

However, there are no definitive diagnosis criteria for EGPA. EGPA diagnosis remains clinical and is based on the existence of vasculitis. Moreover, discriminating disease activity from worsening underlying asthma is challenging. Thus, biomarkers to diagnose EGPA disease flares would be extremely valuable. Further, to improve EGPA management, researchers have attempted to identify biomarkers that discriminate active and inactive EGPA. Some studies have established associations between common laboratory readouts, e.g., serum IgE, erythrocyte sedimentation rate and C-reactive protein (CRP) (Peter C. Grayson et al., 2015), and disease activity, but these have limitations as longitudinal biomarkers to monitor disease activity. In addition, the eosinophil cationic protein was correlated with disease activity in small series. Other studies examined several novel biomarkers, e.g., CCL17/TARC (Dallos et al., 2010; Dejaco et al., 2015), IgG4 (Augusto Vaglio et al., 2012; Dejaco et al., 2015) and CCL26/eotaxin-3 (Polzer et al., 2008; Dejaco et al., 2015; Zagvozdkina et al., 2016), but their use for routine diagnosis has not yet been implemented. These findings suggest that novel biomarkers to monitor disease activity in EGPA are still needed.

High throughput protein expression studies, such as microarray analyses, are increasingly used to identify changes in protein profiles during the onset and progression of complex diseases. In this study, we integrated microarray data from EGPA and sought to identify protein expression profiles and signaling pathways that can mark pathogenetic changes in active EGPA. This study led to the identification of new diagnostic markers and therapeutic targets.

METHODS

Study Design and Subjects

In the current study, we conducted a prospective observational study in which 2 groups of patients were recruited, including 31 patients with active EGPA, and 37 patients with inactive EGPA, all treated at the Department of Allergy and Clinical Immunology at The First Affiliated Hospital of Guangzhou Medical University, China. Among them, an exploration subgroup included 15 inactive patients and 13 active patients. Other 22 inactive patients and 18 active patients were recruited in the validation study.

All EGPA subjects met four or more ACR items (Masi et al., 1990), including (1) asthma; defined as a history of wheezing or diffuse high- pitched rales on expiration; (2) peripheral blood eosinophilia (>10%); (3) mononeuropathy or polyneuropathy; defined as the development of mononeuropathy, multiple mononeuropathies, or polyneuropathy (i.e., glovel stocking distribution) attributable to a systemic vasculitis; (4) unfixed pulmonary infiltration; defined as migratory or transitory pulmonary infiltrates on radiographs (not including fixed infiltrates), attributable to a systemic vasculitis; (5) paranasal sinus abnormality; defined as a history of acute or chronic paranasal sinus pain or tenderness or radiographic opacification of the paranasal sinuses and (6) extravascular eosinophils on histology; defined as biopsy including artery, arteriole, or venule, showing accumulations of eosinophils in extravascular areas. All EGPA subjects had vasculitis manifestations and met ACR criteria. Disease activity was assessed at diagnosis using the original 1994 Birmingham Vasculitis Activity Score (BVAS) (Luqmani et al., 1994) and was recorded in the database. Patients with a score under 15 were recruited to the inactive group, whereas they joined the active group above a score of 15. All subjects underwent a standardized clinical assessment, including pulmonary function test, sputum induction, inflammatory cell differentiation test, allergy status or serum(Se)-specific-IgE measurement, fractional exhaled nitric oxide (FeNO), anti-neutrophil cytoplasmic antibodies (ANCA) test and complete blood count (CBC).

The study was approved by the Ethics Review Board of the First Affiliated Hospital of Guangzhou Medical University

[Medical research ethics review 2018,No.35]. All participants provided written informed consent.

Lung Function

Lung function was measured by spirometer (MasterScreen PFT; Jaeper™, CareFusion, Hoechberg, Germany), in accordance with the American Thoracic Society/European Respiratory Society guidelines (Miller et al., 2005). Parameters, including percent of predicted forced vital capacity (FVC%) and forced expiratory volume in 1 second of predicted (FEV_1%), percent of predicted peak expiratory flow (PEF%) and maximum mid expiratory flow (MMEF75/25), were recorded.

Blood Sample

Five milliliters of venous blood sample were collected into vacutainer tubes containing no additive. Sera were prepared by centrifugation and stored at −80°C for protein microarray analysis, ELISA and Bio-Plex assay.

Protein Microarray Analysis

RayBiotech Human Cytokine Antibody Array 3000 (RayBiotech, Inc., Cat# QAH-CAA-3000) was used to analyze serum protein profiles. This antibody array simultaneously detects 160 human cytokines shared between 4 non-overlapping arrays (**Supplementary Table 1**). The samples were read by the Guangzhou Biotech Company. The experimental procedure was carried out in accordance with the manufacturer's instructions. Briefly, antibody pre-coated array membranes were incubated with coating buffer for 30 min. The blocking buffer was then decanted and replaced with dilutions of the samples, for overnight incubation at 4°C under shaking. The next day, the membranes were washed and incubated with a mix of biotin-conjugated antibodies for 2 h. The biotin-conjugated antibodies were removed, and Streptavidin-Fluor was added to each subarray. The incubation chambers were covered with adhesive film and incubated for 2 h. After washing, signals were read with a GenePix 4000B system (Axon Instruments, Foster City, CA, United States). GenePix Pro 6.0 software (Axon Instruments) was used for densitometric analysis of the spots. The values were normalized to the signals obtained for the positive controls of each sample. The total normalized fluorescence values of the replicates were averaged and are expressed as the fold increase compared to the control samples.

Gene Ontology and KEGG Pathway Analysis

The Database for Annotation, Visualization and Integrated Discovery (DAVID[1]) is an online biological information database for gene functional analysis (Huang et al., 2007). To predict the possible functions of the overlapping differentially expressed proteins (DEPs) and their neighboring genes, and the potential pathways in which they intervene, we performed Gene Ontology (GO) enrichment and KEGG pathway analyses in DAVID. $P < 0.05$ was considered statistically significant.

[1]https://david.ncifcrf.gov/

ELISA

ELISA kits (Thermo/Invitrogen Carlsbad, CA, United States) were used to validate the results obtained from the antibody arrays, following the manufacturer's instructions. Briefly, serum samples were diluted at different dilution factors based on individual serum biomarker characteristics. Samples were coated on the plates for 1 to 2.5 h at room temperature. The plates were washed, and a biotin-conjugated antibody specific for each kit was added and incubated for 1 h under gentle shaking. Horse Radish Peroxidase (HRP)-conjugated streptavidin was added to catalyze the 3,3′,5,5′-Tetramethylbenzidine (TMB) chromogenic reagent. Finally, the catalytic reaction was stopped by addition of sulfuric acid. At each step, the reactional volume in each well was of 100 μl. Finally, the OD450 was read using a microplate reader (Multiskan GO, Thermo Scientific, Carlsbad, CA, United States).

TABLE 1 | Clinical manifestations in patients with EGPA.

Subjects' characteristics	Inactive (*n* = 31)	Active (*n* = 37)	*P*-value
Age, mean ± SD years*	42.1 ± 12.7	42.8 ± 18.1	0.903
Gender (female, %)#	58	53	0.063
Body Mass Index*	21.9 ± 2.9	19.8 ± 1.6	0.055
Smoking history (>10 packs/year, *n*)*	11	13	0.603
Atopic status (*n*)*	15	21	0.804
Asthma diagnosis (*n*)*	31	37	–
Duration of asthma (years)*	5.2 ± 4.8	4.1 ± 2.7	0.466
Presence of rhinosinusitis (%)#	91	93	0.828
Peripheral eosinophil count*	5.8 ± 5.2	20.3 ± 9.8	**0.000**
Sputum eosinophil percent (%)#	5.4 ± 8.0	40.7 ± 30.1	**0.000**
Parameters of lung function			
·FEV1% Pred*	76.3 ± 22.6	57.7 ± 18.5	**0.030**
·FVC % Pred*	87.3 ± 21.2	82.1 ± 15.9	0.497
·FEV1/FVC*	77.8 ± 18.9	55.8 ± 15.9	0.066
·PEF% Pred*	77.5 ± 35.7	61.0 ± 11.7	0.158
·MMEF75/25*	22.6 ± 22.7	27.6 ± 22.7	0.526
FeNO (ppb)*	39.3 ± 26.3	87.6 ± 53.2	**0.015**
Organ involvement			
·Arthralgia/Arthritis, n (%)#	0	0	1.000
·Myalgia/Myostits, n (%)#	3 (9.6)	3 (8.8)	0.959
·Skin, *n* (%)#	12 (38.7)	19 (53.4)	0.087
·Ear/nose/throat, *n* (%)#	128 (80.6)	31 (83.8)	0.828
·Cardiovascular Events, *n* (%)#	0 (0)	3 (8.1)	0.060
·Gastrointestinal, *n* (%)#	5 (16.1)	10 (27.2)	0.128
·Pulmonary, *n* (%)#	31 (100)	37 (100)	–
·Kidney, *n* (%)#	3 (9.6)	5 (13.5)	0.603
·Peripheral neuropathy, *n* (%)#	5 (16.1)	5 (13.5)	0.939
BVAS score*	6 ± 2.95	20.0 ± 3.7	**0.000**

*Data expressed as mean ± standard deviation, median (interquartile range) or number (%). The P-value was calculated from the χ2 test and ANOVA, between the 2 groups. FVC, forced vital capacity; FEV1, forced expiratory volume in 1 s; PEF% Pred, percent of predicted peak expiratory flow; MMEF75/25, maximum mid expiratory flow; FeNO, fractional exhaled nitric oxide; BVAS, Birmingham Vasculitis Activity Score. *Values are expressed as means ± SEM, #Values are expressed as percentage. Bold values means P-value < 0.05.*

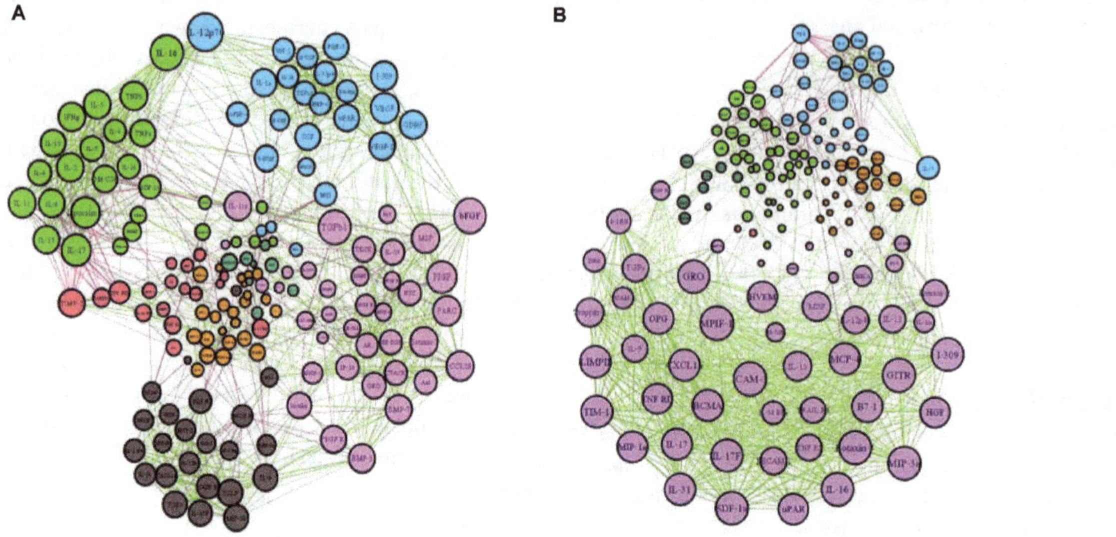

FIGURE 1 | Network-based analysis of protein expression in active and inactive EGPA. The network graphs were constructed with the expression data of 160 proteins. Each protein is represented by a specific node whose color represents a specific cluster. Different colors represent the different weighting degrees of nodes and edges. The size of the node is proportional to the to the number of connections (i.e., degree). Edges between nodes represent a statistically significant association ($P < 0.05$). Edge thickness represents the strengths of association between two nodes (correlation coefficient, Spearman's correlation). The correlation coefficient is represented by a color code, green and purple indicating positive and negative relationships, respectively. **(A)** Inactive EGPA; **(B)** Active EGPA

Bio-Plex Assay

The levels of 13 cytokines were assessed in the sera by the Custom Multiplex Kit featuring Axl, GDNF, HB-EGF, MCP-3, NGF beta, PDGF-BB, PlGF-1 and SCF (Thermo/invitrogen Carlsbad, CA, United States; Cat#PPX-08), and the Custom Multiplex Kit featuring BMP-4, ErbB3, IGFBP-4, Insulin and NT-4 (Thermo/invitrogen Carlsbad, CA, United States; Cat# LSAHM-05). The experimental procedure was carried out according to the manufacturer's instructions. Briefly, beads coated with capture antibodies were incubated with premixed standards or sample supernatants for 120 min at room temperature under 500-rpm agitation. Following incubation, premixed detection antibodies were added and incubated for 30 min at room temperature under 500-rpm agitation. After washing, Phycoerythrin (PE)-conjugated streptavidin was added and incubated as before. After washing, the beads were resuspended in Bio-Plex cytokine assay buffer and read on the Bio-Plex 200 system using Low PMT setting. Data were analyzed with Bio-Plex Manager^{TM} software version 2.0.

Statistical Analysis and Visualization

Statistical analysis was performed using the SPSS software package (version 22.0; IBM Corp., Armonk, NY, United States). Continuous variables are expressed as number (%) or means $\pm$ standard deviation (SD). Comparisons between groups were made using the *t*-test or Mann-Whitney *U*-test for continuous endpoints, and the χ^2 test for categorical endpoints. *P*-values were corrected using the Benjamini-Hochberg false discovery rate (FDR). Correlations were assessed using Pearson's or Spearman's correlation test. A *P*-value of < 0.05 was considered significant.

Network analysis based on the Spearman analysis was performed using Gephi V0.9.2 open source software[2] output showing the 160 serum soluble proteins from the different subjects. Each serum soluble protein is represented by a specific node whose color represents a specific cluster. The size of the node is proportional to the sum of the edges that connects to them. Edges connecting nodes represent statistically significant correlations ($P < 0.05$). The edge's thickness represents the strengths of their association (Spearman's correlation). We used the existence of modules represented by highly interlinked to pological clusters in the network using the computational algorithm proposed by Blonde et al. (Lancichinetti and Fortunato, 2009) and included in the Gephi statistical module. Modularity is the fraction of the edges that fall within the given groups of nodes minus the expected fraction if the edges were distributed at random. The value of the modularity lies in the range of -1 to 1. If positive then the number of edges within groups exceeds the number expected on the basis of chance.

RESULTS

Patient Characteristics

After screening, we recruited 37 patients with inactive EGPA and 31 patients with active EGPA. All subjects had a definitive EGPA diagnosis, presented more than two organs involvement, and tested negative for ANCAs. There were no significant clinical differences among all EGPA subjects regarding lung function indices (FVC (% predicted), FEV1/FVC, PEF (% predicted), MMEF75/25) and organ involvement ($P > 0.05$). However, the

[2]https://gephi.org/

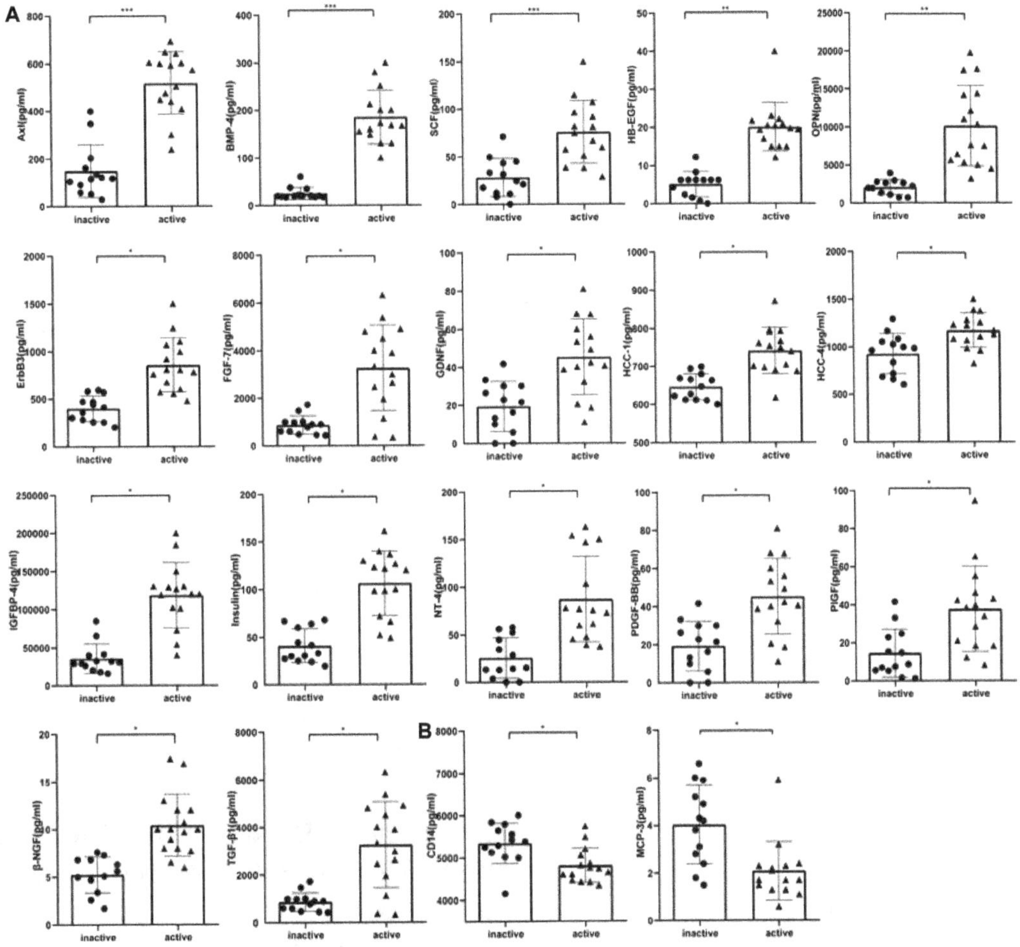

FIGURE 2 | Serum levels of proteins differentially expressed in inactive and active EGPA assessed by antibody-based protein microarray. **(A)** Serum concentration of seventeen proteins were higher in active EGPA than that in inactive EGPA. **(B)** Two proteins were higher in inactive EGPA than that in active EGPA. Statistical significance was calculated by unpaired nonparametric Mann-Whitney test. * p.adj < 0.05, ** p.adj < 0.01, and *** p.adj < 0.001 indicates statistical significance between two groups (FDR correction). Data were present as Median with interquartile range. Dot symbols: inactive disease; triangle symbols: active disease.

EGPA active group presented higher peripheral and sputum eosinophil counts, FeNO and FEV1 (% predicted) ($P = 0.000$, $P = 0.000$, $P = 0.015$, $P = 0.030$, respectively). The demographics and characteristics of the subjects are shown in **Table 1**.

Network-Based Analysis

The patterns of serum proteins in active and inactive EGPA patients were characterized by network-based analysis (**Figure 1**). The active network graphs comprise 152 nodes, each representing a serum protein concentration, and a total of 1174 links representing correlations between nodes scoring a P-value < 0.05. The active EGPA network contains 4 clusters of highly interlinked nodes: cluster 1 gathers 51 nodes (purple) corresponding to 51 serum proteins (**Supplementary Table 2**); cluster 2, 21 nodes (or serum proteins; orange), cluster 3, 28 nodes (or serum proteins; blue); and cluster 4, 42 nodes (or serum proteins; green). The inactive network graphs comprise 160 nodes, each representing a serum protein concentration, and a total of 1209 links representing correlations between nodes scoring a P-value < 0.05. The inactive EGPA network contains 4 clusters of highly interlinked nodes: cluster 1 gathers 37 nodes (purple) corresponding to 37 serum proteins (**Supplementary Table 3**); cluster 2, 23 nodes (or serum proteins; brown), cluster 3, 24 nodes (or serum proteins; blue); and cluster 4, 27 nodes (or serum proteins; green). In active EGPA, cluster 1 has the largest number of nodes, suggesting that the proteins in cluster 1 are most closely related to other clusters, which may be related to disease activity. Specifically, featured cytokines associate with endothelial (PECAM-1, HVEM, VCAM-1, ICAM-3), immune cells including macrophage (CXCL16, MIP-3a, MPIF1,MIP-3b,MCP-4), eosinophil (Eotaxin-2,Eotaxin-3,CCL28), lymphocyte (TARC, GITR,IL-31, IL-17F, IL-9,IL-17,IL-16,IL-15, IL-13,IL-10 Rb, IL-18 BPa,IL21R) in cluster1 might robustly suggest that EGPA active stage involves the activation of multiple immune cells and vascular endothelium. But in inactive EGPA, the size of the nodes in the four clusters is similar, which indicates that during the inactive stage the proteins in the clusters are in balance with each other and might maintain the body's homeostasis.

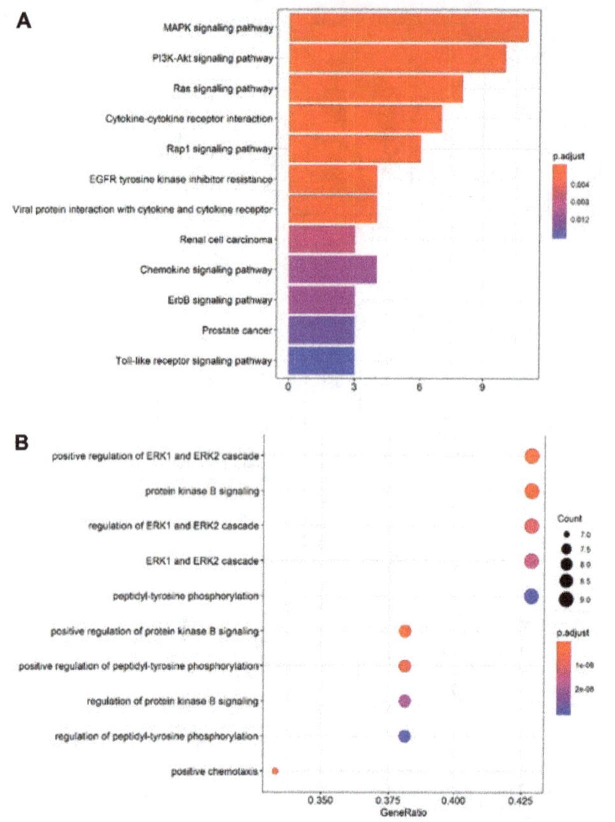

FIGURE 3 | Gene Ontology (GO) and Kyoto Encyclopedia of Genes and Genomes (KEGG) pathway enrichment analyses of the proteins differentially expressed in active and inactive EGPA. **(A)**Top 10 KEGG pathways represented by the DEPs. **(B)** Top 10 GO Term biological processes represented by the DEPs.

Comparison of the Serum Levels of 160 Proteins in Inactive and Active EGPA

To identify accurate and predictive biomarkers of disease activity, we first compared the serum levels of 160 serum proteins in active and inactive EGPA. Twenty-one serum proteins displayed differential levels between active and inactive disease ($P < 0.05$) (**Supplementary Table 4**, unpaired nonparametric Mann-Whitney test). To further strengthen our selection criteria, *P*-values were corrected using the Benjamini-Hochberg false discovery rate (FDR). Finally, 19 DEPs were identified (**Figure 2**). These DEPs can mainly be divided into three categories: growth factors and related receptors (BMP4, SCF, HB-EGF, OPN, FGF-7, TGF-β, IGFBP4, insulin, PDGF-BB, PIGF, ErbB3), many of which have firmly correlation with vascular remodeling; neurotrophic factor (GDNF, NT-4, β-NGF) and chemokines (HCC-1; HCC-4, CD14, MCP-3). The results probably demonstrated that multifaceted biological events engaged including neurotrophic, immune cells, and vascular activation during active disease phage. Following via using short-listed proteins, i.e., scoring FDR < 0.5, we performed KEGG pathway and GO enrichment analyses to gain insights into the potential functions involved in the clinical evolution of EGPA. Five major signaling pathways were represented by the DEPs during active EGPA, i.e., MAPK signaling pathway, PI3K-Akt signaling pathway, RAS signaling pathway, cytokine-cytokine receptor interaction and Rap1 signaling pathway. Four major biological processes were found, i.e., positive regulation of ERK1 and ERK2 cascade, protein kinase B signal, regulation of ERK1 and ERK2 cascade, ERK1 and ERK2 cascade and positive regulation of peptide-tyrosine phosphorylation (**Figure 3**).

Correlations Between the Serum Level of the DEPs and Peripheral Eosinophil Cell Count in Patients With Inactive and Active EGPA

To evaluate the clinical relevance of the variation in serum level of the candidate proteins, we performed a correlation analysis between protein levels and peripheral eosinophil counts in all patients. Importantly, 15 serum proteins were significantly correlated with peripheral eosinophil count ($P < 0.05$) (**Figure 4**).Precisely, 13 of the proteins positively correlated with eosinophil count, while another two proteins (CD14 and MCP3) negatively correlated with eosinophil count. Results were objectively credible because CD14 and MCP3 are two chemokines with monocyte/macrophage. And The results might suggest that eosinophils participated in the process of vascular remodeling during EGPA active phage.

Correlations Between the Serum Level of the DEPs and BVAS With Inactive and Active EGPA

To evaluate the relationship between DEPs and disease activity, we performed a correlation analysis between protein levels and BVAS in all patients. Nine the DEPs were significantly correlated with BVAS($P < 0.05$) (**Figure 5**). Serum level of Axl, IGFBP4, PIGF, OPN, SCF, β-NGF, and NT-4 (**Figure 5A**)positively correlated with BVAS, while MCP-3 and CD14 (**Figure 5B**) negatively.

Evaluation of the Sensitivity and Specificity of the Candidate Protein Biomarkers

Receiver operating characteristic (ROC) analysis is the standard approach to evaluate the sensitivity and specificity of diagnostic procedures (Song, 1997). We evaluated the sensitivity and specificity of the 15 differentially expressed serum proteins by ROC curve analysis ($P < 0.001$) (**Figure 6; Supplementary Table 5**). Axl has the largest AUC (0.94), specificity was 100% and sensitivity was 86.7%.

Validation of the Differential Expression of the Biomarker Candidates by ELISA and Custom Multiplex Bio-plex Assay

To further consolidate the data on the variation of candidate biomarkers levels between inactive and active EGPA, we measured serum levels of the 19 DEPs by ELISA and Custom

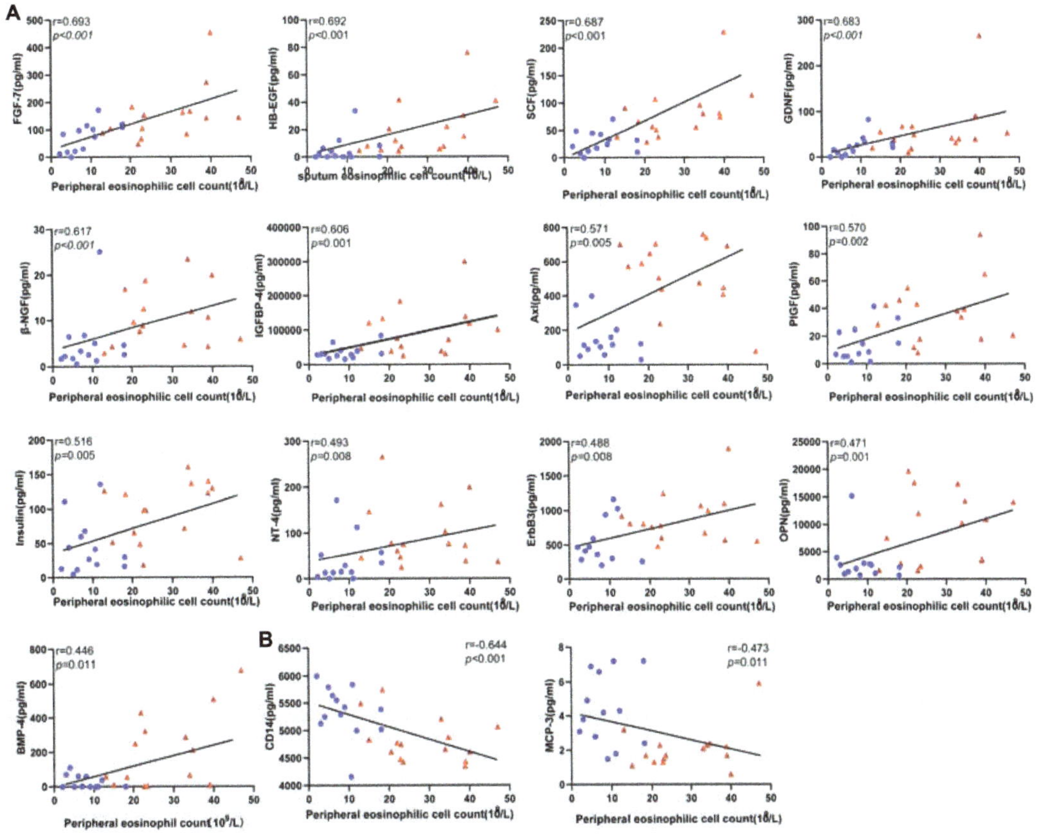

FIGURE 4 | Correlations between the level of the differentially expressed protein candidates and peripheral eosinophil count in EGPA patients (Spearman correlation). Only the significant correlations are shown in dot plots. Fifteen protein markers had serum levels correlated with eosinophil cell counts. **(A)** Thirteen protein markers had a level of expression positively correlated with blood eosinophil count. **(B)** Two protein markers had level of expression negatively correlated with blood eosinophil count. Blue dots represent data from patients with inactive disease. Red triangles represent data from patients with active disease. *P*-values and Spearman correlation coefficients are displayed.

Multiplex assay (**Figure 7A**). The variation of serum levels of Axl, GDNF, HCC-4, MCP-3 and OPN were consistent with the array results, confirming their differential expression in inactive and active EGPA (**Figures 7B–F**).

Follow-up of Serum Level of Axl

Furthermore, to confirm the faithfully clinical diagnosis significance of Axl, we followed up the longitudinal Axl expressions for paired 12 enrolled patients in active and remission disease stage. Specifically, the serum Axl levels decreased significantly in the inactive disease compared with the baseline. Moreover, 10/12 patients showed descending tendency, suggesting that the high expression of Axl is related to the disease activity.(**Figure 8**).

DISCUSSION

In EGPA, identifying active disease is often challenging, especially when non-specific symptoms occur, such as worsening asthma or rhinosinusitis. The development of predictive biomarkers would greatly improve the ability to identify patients likely to enter an active phase of the disease. To this aim, we screened 160 soluble proteins to identify those presenting differential serum levels in inactive and active EGPA, and tested their associations with clinical characteristics. Network-based analysis defined 4 clusters of serum proteins characteristic of patients with active disease, and containing 51, 21, 28, and 42 serum proteins, respectively. Among the 160 screened proteins, 19 were significantly upregulated in the sera of patients with active disease compared with sera from patients in the inactive phase ($P < 0.05$). Spearman's correlation analysis indicated that 16 of these DEFs were significantly correlated with peripheral eosinophil count in active and inactive EGPA patients ($P < 0.05$). Finally, we verified the differential levels of the candidate markers by ELISA and bio-plex assay. With these methods, Axl, OPN, HCC-4, GDNF and MCP-3 were further validated, and among them, Axl scored the largest AUC, indicating its superior diagnostic value above the other candidates. Thus, our study uncovered Axl as a candidate biomarker to discriminate active from inactive disease in EGPA.

Eosinophilic granulomatosis with polyangiitis is considered a Th2-mediated disease. Previous studies on the differential expression of serum ECP, CCL17/ TARC, eotaxin-3, periostin and IgG4, representing Th2 features, were reported to correlate

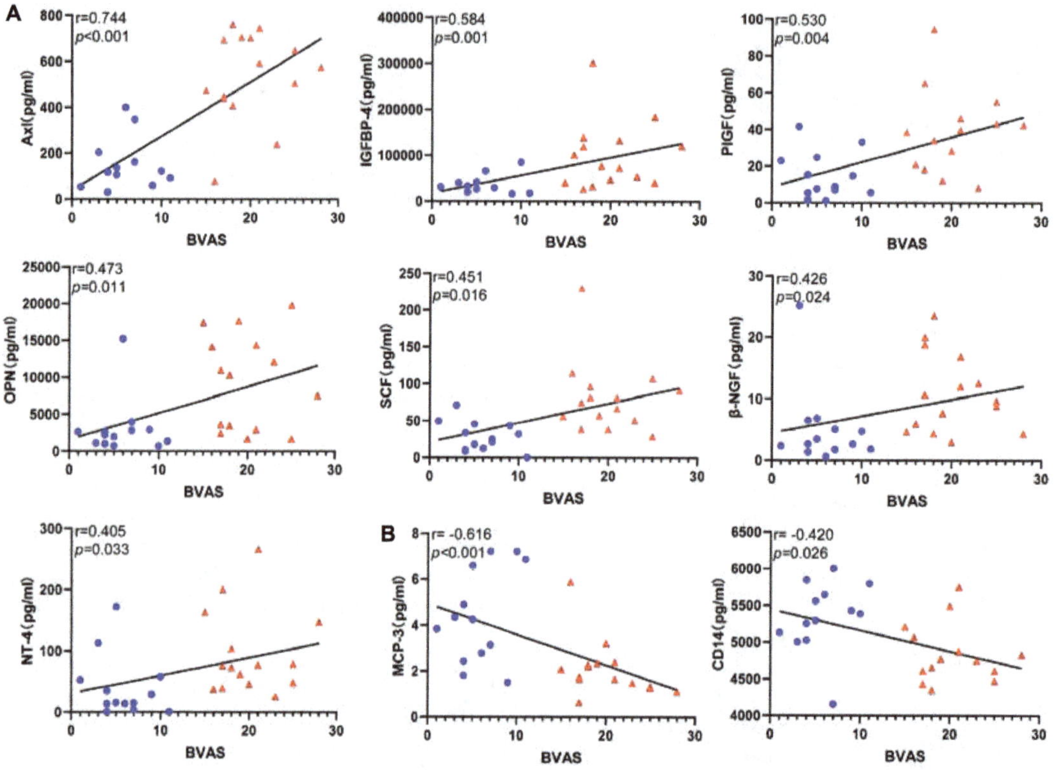

FIGURE 5 | Correlations between the level of the differentially expressed protein candidates and BVAS(Spearman correlation). Only the significant correlations are shown in dot plots. Fifteen protein markers had serum levels correlated with BVAS **(A)** Thirteen protein markers had a level of expression positively correlated with BVAS. **(B)** Two protein markers had level of expression negatively correlated with BVAS. Blue dots represent data from patients with inactive disease. Red triangles represent data from patients with active disease. *P*-values and Spearman correlation coefficients are displayed.

with disease activity, but could not distinguish between different phases of the disease (Guilpain et al., 2007; Dallos et al., 2010; Vaglio et al., 2012; Rhee et al., 2018). The clinical value of absolute eosinophil count, serum IgE, ESR and CRP also showed their limitations as longitudinal biomarkers of disease activity or predictors of flare in EGPA (Grayson et al., 2015). Therefore, it is urgent to uncover new serum biomarkers of active and inactive EGPA. The clinical phenotype of EGPA cannot be explained by exaggerated Th2 response alone. Pagnoux et al. (2019) explored a panel of 54 serum cytokines and chemokines involved in Th1/Th2, Th9/Th17/Th22/Treg, and inflammatory responses, but did not detect clear differences in the serum levels of these proteins, indistinguishable between active or inactive EGPA. Some of the non-differential proteins found in this previous study were also non-differential in our study. However, contrary to what Pagnoux and colleagues reported, we found the MCP-3 level was significantly different between active and inactive EGPA. The reason for this discrepancy remains unclear. In our study, all patients were treated with glucocorticoid, and 75% (51 / 68) of them were treated with glucocorticoid combined with immunosuppressors. In the cohort studied by Pagnoux et al. (2019), only 45% (18/40) of the patients were treated with glucocorticoids. These different treatments likely affected the expression of serum cytokines. In addition, ethnic differences cannot be excluded to explain the different results. Our findings also suggest that, whereas most emphasis has been given to eosinophils and some cytokines in the pathophysiology of EGPA, more attention should be paid to a possible role of monocytes/macrophages. Decision making for treatments should not rely solely on cytokine level.

Network analysis was used to compare the expression profiles of 160 soluble serum proteins in patients with active and inactive EGPA. Result showed that serum samples with different disease activity have a distinguishable expression pattern, suggesting that distinct disease activity have different target proteins.

Pathogenesis of EGPA remains largely unknown. However, like many other autoimmune diseases, genetic predisposition and environmental factors appear to contribute to the development of EGPA (Nguyen and Guillevin, 2018). Eosinophilic inflammation and ANCA-mediated vasculitis are both cardinal features of EGPA (Furuta et al., 2019). Our study found that peripheral blood eosinophils, induced sputum eosinophils and FeNO were significantly higher in patients with active EGPA than in those with inactive disease. The reasons for these differences were mainly related to the pathogenesis of the disease itself. IL-5, a main eosinophil activator, seems involved in EGPA pathogenesis. IL-5 is produced by Th2 cells and induces the differentiation and maturation of human eosinophils (Sanderson, 1988). Following activation, eosinophils release granules containing stored cytotoxic proteins and toxins such as eosinophil-derived

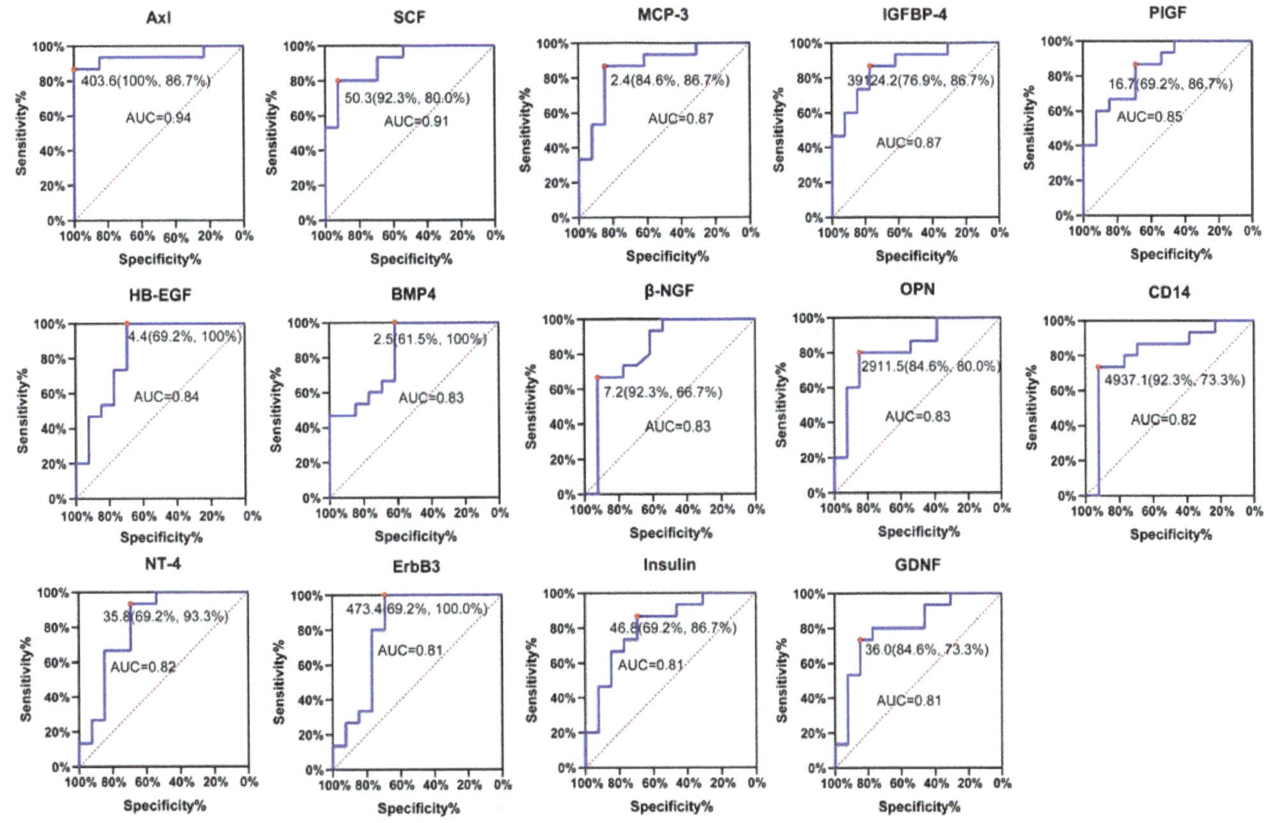

FIGURE 6 | Receiver operating characteristic (ROC) analysis of candidate proteins. ROC curve showing the sensitivity and specificity for various cutoff values of the protein. Red dot indicates sensitivity at the specificity. ROC, receiver operating characteristic; AUC, area under the ROC curve.

neurotoxin, major basic protein (MBP), eosinophil peroxidase, and eosinophil cationic protein (ECP), all causing tissue damage (Guilpain et al., 2006). These pathophysiological differences explain the differential network between active and inactive EGPA. There were 19 DEPs between active and inactive EGPA, and some of these DEPs were related to eosinophil count in peripheral blood. This suggests that the differences between the two groups may be related to eosinophilic inflammation. To better understand the potential biological functions of these DEPS in active EGPA, GO and KEGG pathways analyses were performed. This analysis revealed the prominence of biological pathways involving ERK1 and ERK2. These proteins are related protein-serine/threonine kinases that participate in the Ras-Raf-MEK-ERK signal transduction cascade, regulating a broad variety of processes including cell adhesion, cell cycle progression, cell migration, cell survival, differentiation, metabolism, proliferation, and transcription (Roskoski, 2012). Robins et al. (2011) proposed ERK1/ERK2 MAPK cascade as a novel and attractive target in severe asthma, because this pathway is resistant to glucocorticoids, while it contributes the inflammation by neutrophil recruitment. This observation supports that the ERK1/ERK2 MAPK cascade may be also functionally involved in the active phase of EGPA, but this hypothesis needs further confirmation. Previous studies comparing biomarkers in serum of patients with active and inactive EGPA did not address the signaling pathways and biological functions related to the different biomarkers. In this study, GO and KEGG analyses were used for the first time to further explore the biological functions and signaling pathways of DEPs, and discover the possible mechanisms and biological roles involving the cytokines in active EGPA. It is expected that follow-up on these candidate pathways in *in vitro* and *in vivo* experiments will help better explain disease etiology and variations underlying different phases of EGPA.

The concentration of Axl and IGFBP-4 were significantly correlated with eosinophil counts in peripheral blood and sputum (**Supplementary Figure 1**). The reasons for this difference may be explained by the fact that the samples used for differential screening were from the peripheral blood, and not from the respiratory tract. Thus, differences may exist between the pathogenesis of the acute phase in peripheral blood and in the respiratory tract. ROC analysis showed that Axl had the highest diagnostic efficiency and significantly correlation with eosinophil counts in both peripheral blood and induced sputum, and meanwhile it has a significantly correlation with BVAS. Axl serum levels were significantly diminished in follow-up inactive patients. Therefore, Axl may be a better biomarker to distinguish active and inactive EGPA. Furthermore, Axl combined with BMP-4 and SCF could improve the diagnostic sensitivity (93.3%) (**Supplementary Figure 2**).

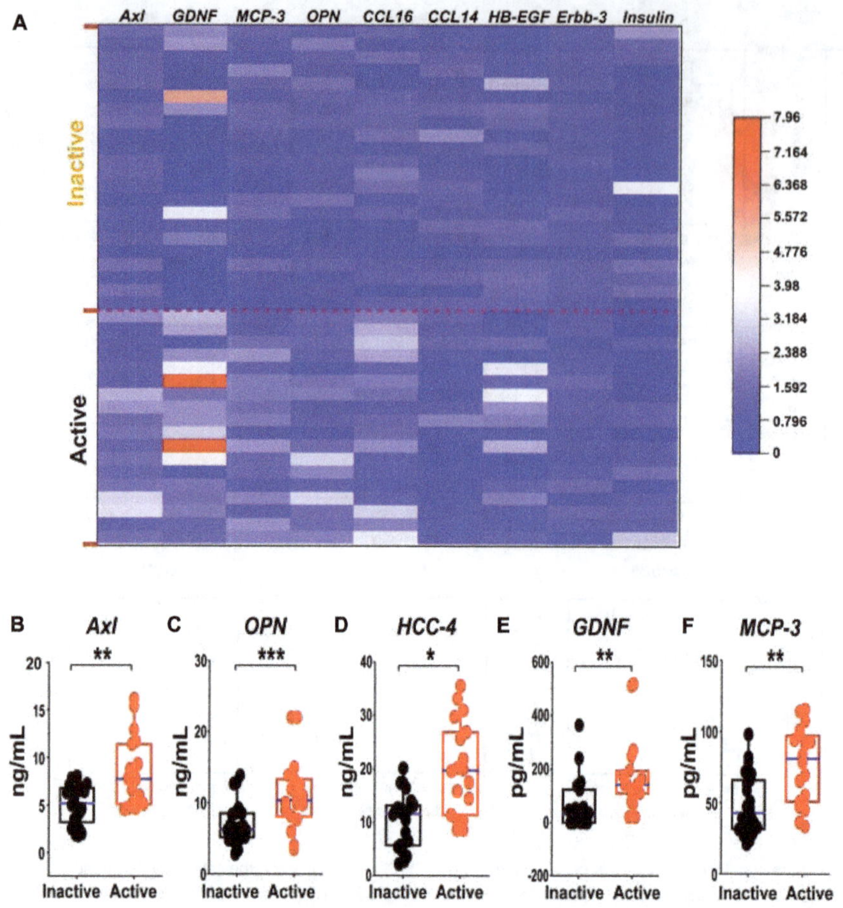

FIGURE 7 | Validation of the differential expression of the serum protein marker candidates for active GEPA by ELISA and Custom Multiplex. **(A)** Heatmap comparison of the expression level of the serum protein marker candidates in inactive and active EGPA by ELISA and Bio-plex. Nine of 13 were highly expressed. **(B-F)** Scatter plots representing the median values of the expression level of the serum protein marker candidates in inactive and active EGPA assessed ELISA and Bio-plex. Five of 9 were significant difference in the group. The P values were calculated by nonparametric t-test and are noted $^{*}P < 0.05$, $^{**}P < 0.01$, $^{***}P < 0.001$, versus inactive group. Black dots represent data from patients with inactive disease. Red dots represent data from patients with active disease.

Axl is a receptor tyrosine kinase that transduces signals from the extracellular matrix to the cytoplasm by binding the growth factor GAS6. Thus, Axl regulates many physiological processes including cell survival, cell proliferation, migration and differentiation (Korshunov, 2012; Brown et al., 2016). GAS6/Axl signaling plays a role in processes such as endothelial cell survival during acidification by preventing apoptosis, optimal cytokine signaling during human natural killer cell development, hepatic regeneration, gonadotropin-releasing hormone neuron survival and migration, platelet activation, or regulation of thrombotic responses (Sasaki et al., 2006). The mechanism underlying Axl upregulation is not clear but continuous stimulation of macrophages by apoptotic debris may increase its expression and release (Lee and Chun, 2019). Axl is critical for phagocytosis of apoptotic cells and regulation of the immune system (Di Stasi et al., 2020).

Shuai Wang et al. (2021) found that, consistent with ACE2, SARS-CoV-2 can cause infection through the Axl receptor of the lung epithelium, while knocking out Axl significantly reduces the effect of SARS-CoV-2 on H1299 lung cells and human primary lung epithelial cells. Besides, Milena S. Espindola et al. (2018) found that Axl activation is obviously related to the process of pulmonary fibrosis, and pulmonary fibrosis is significantly reduced after Axl inhibition. These studies showed that Axl plays very important roles in inflammatory diseases. Therefore, further investigations on the role of the Gas6/Axl pathway in EGPA and the development of specific antagonists targeting this pathway are necessary.

The present study has limitations. First, we limited our investigation to the study of the level of expression of 160 soluble proteins in peripheral blood of patients with active and inactive subjects. Although this approach validated our strategy of identification of a new marker for active EGPA, it could be extended to whole proteomes, using broader proteomics screening. Thus, while we identified candidate cytokine markers, our study did not provide a comprehensive view on the proteomic differences distinguishing active and inactive EGPA. Second, although we uncovered correlations between some of the differentially expressed proteins and clinical features, we did not further explore the molecular mechanisms linking the

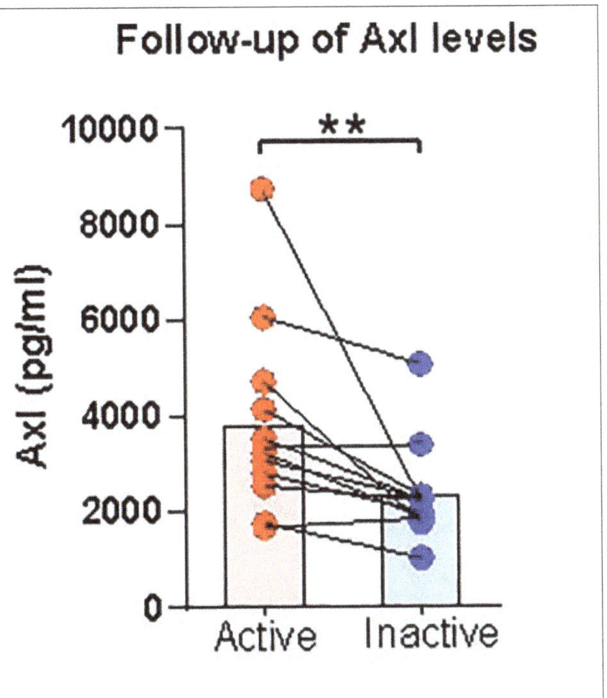

FIGURE 8 | Follow-up serum level of Axl in patients after treatment. Serum levels of Axl in paired active and inactive patients. Axl serum levels were significantly diminished in inactive patients. The *P*-values were calculated by nonparametric t-test and are noted $^{**}P < 0.01$, versus inactive group. Red dots represent data from patients with active disease. Blue dots represent data from patients with inactive disease.

protein markers to the pathology. Functional approaches will be endeavored in the future, using a broader range of clinical samples (e.g., sputum, bronchoalveolar lavage, *etc.*), to further verify the consistency of the results, and validate the use of the biomarker candidates in diagnostic and prognosis. The development of *in vitro* models and/or *in vivo* animal models of the disease will help verify the reliability of the functional results.

In conclusion, we identified a new cytokine, Axl, related to active EGPA, and demonstrated a high degree of correlation between its serum level and peripheral blood and induced sputum eosinophil counts. This is the first report of this biomarker in EGPA. Further studies involving higher numbers of clinical samples will help strengthen its clinical value for the diagnosis and prognosis of active EGPA and other vasculitis.

AUTHOR CONTRIBUTIONS

JM and CD performed the experiments and drafted the manuscript. SW, MQ, PW, CO, and BZ interpreted the patient data and collected the samples. XZ and JY co-designed the experiment strategy. NZ and QZ critically revised the manuscript. All authors read and approved the final manuscript.

ACKNOWLEDGMENTS

We thank LetPub (www.letpub.com) for its linguistic assistance and scientific consultation during the preparation of this manuscript.

SUPPLEMENTARY MATERIAL

Supplementary Figure 1 | Correlations between Axl or IGFBP-4 protein levels and sputum eosinophilic cell count in EGPA patients (Spearman correlation). Only the significant correlations are shown in dot plots. Two protein markers had serum levels correlated with eosinophil cell counts. Blue dots represent data from patients with inactive disease. Red triangles represent data from patients with active disease. P values and Spearman correlation coefficients are displayed.

Supplementary Figure 2 | ROC combination analysis of Axl, BMP-4 and SCF. Combination ROC curve showing the sensitivity and specificity for cutoff values of Axl with BMP-4 and SCF. Red dot indicates sensitivity at the specificity. ROC, receiver operating characteristic; AUC, area under the ROC curve.

Supplementary Table 1 | Information of 160 soluble proteins.

Supplementary Table 2 | The nodes or serum proteins of each cluster of network in active EGPA.

Supplementary Table 3 | The nodes or serum proteins of each cluster of network in inactive EGPA.

Supplementary Table 4 | Differentially expressed proteins from unpaired nonparametric Mann-Whitney test.

Supplementary Table 5 | Summary of the ROC curve analysis.

REFERENCES

Brown, M., Black, J. R., Sharma, R., Stebbing, J., and Pinato, D. J. (2016). Gene of the month: Axl. *J. Clin. Pathol.* 69, 391–397. doi: 10.1136/jclinpath-2016-203629

Churg, J., and Strauss, L. (1951). Allergic granulomatosis, allergic angiitis, and periarteritis nodosa. *Am. J. Pathol.* 27, 277–301.

Dallos, T., Heiland, G. R., Strehl, J., Karonitsch, T., Gross, W. L., Moosig, F., et al. (2010). CCL17/thymus and activation-related chemokine in Churg-Strauss syndrome. *Arthritis Rheum.* 62, 3496–3503. doi: 10.1002/art.27678

Dejaco, C., Oppl, B., Monach, P., Cuthbertson, D., Carette, S., Hoffman, G., et al. (2015). Serum biomarkers in patients with relapsing eosinophilic granulomatosis with polyangiitis (Churg-Strauss). *PLoS One* 10:e121737. doi: 10.1371/journal.pone.0121737

Di Stasi, R., De Rosa, L., and D'Andrea, L. D. (2020). Therapeutic aspects of the Axl/Gas6 molecular system. *Drug Discov. Today* 25, 2130–2148. doi: 10.1016/j.drudis.2020.09.022

Espindola, M. S., Habiel, D. M., Narayanan, R., Jones, I., Coelho, A. L., Murray, L. A., et al. (2018). Targeting of TAM receptors ameliorates fibrotic mechanisms in idiopathic pulmonary fibrosis. *Am. J. Respir. Crit. Care Med.* 197, 1443–1456. doi: 10.1164/rccm.201707-1519OC

Furuta, S., Iwamoto, T., and Nakajima, H. (2019). Update on eosinophilic granulomatosis with polyangiitis. *Allergol. Int.* 68, 430–436. doi: 10.1016/j.alit.2019.06.004

Grayson, P. C., Monach, P. A., Pagnoux, C., Cuthbertson, D., Carette, S., Hoffman, G. S., et al. (2015). Value of commonly measured laboratory tests as biomarkers of disease activity and predictors of relapse in eosinophilic granulomatosis with polyangiitis. *Rheumatology* 54, 1351–1359. doi: 10.1093/rheumatology/keu427

Guilpain, P., Auclair, J. F., Tamby, M. C., Servettaz, A., Mahr, A., Weill, B., et al. (2007). Serum eosinophil cationic protein: a marker of disease activity in Churg-Strauss syndrome. *Ann. N. Y. Acad. Sci.* 1107, 392–399. doi: 10.1196/annals.1381.041

Guilpain, P., Guillevin, L., and Mouthon, L. (2006). [Eosinophil granule cationic proteins: eosinophil activation markers]. *Rev. Med. Internet* 27, 406–408. doi: 10.1016/j.revmed.2006.01.008

Huang, D. W., Sherman, B. T., Tan, Q., Kir, J., Liu, D., Bryant, D., et al. (2007). DAVID bioinformatics resources: expanded annotation database and novel algorithms to better extract biology from large gene lists. *Nucleic Acids Res.* 35, W169–W175. doi: 10.1093/nar/gkm415

Korshunov, V. A. (2012). Axl-dependent signalling: a clinical update. *Clin. Sci.* 122, 361–368. doi: 10.1042/CS20110411

Lancichinetti, A., and Fortunato, S. (2009). Community detection algorithms: a comparative analysis. *Phys. Rev. E Stat. Nonlin. Soft Matter Phys.* 80(5 Pt 2), 56117. doi: 10.1103/PhysRevE.80.056117

Lee, C. H., and Chun, T. (2019). Anti-inflammatory role of TAM family of receptor tyrosine kinases via modulating macrophage function. *Mol. Cells* 42, 1–7. doi: 10.14348/molcells.2018.0419

Lightfoot, R. J., Michel, B. A., Bloch, D. A., Hunder, G. G., Zvaifler, N. J., McShane, D. J., et al. (1990). The american college of rheumatology 1990 criteria for the classification of polyarteritis nodosa. *Arthritis Rheum.* 33, 1088–1093. doi: 10.1002/art.1780330805

Luqmani, R. A., Bacon, P. A., Moots, R. J., Janssen, B. A., Pall, A., Emery, P., et al. (1994). Birmingham Vasculitis Activity Score (BVAS) in systemic necrotizing vasculitis. *QJM* 87, 671–678.

Masi, A. T., Hunder, G. G., Lie, J. T., Michel, B. A., Bloch, D. A., Arend, W. P., et al. (1990). The American College of Rheumatology 1990 criteria for the classification of Churg-Strauss syndrome (allergic granulomatosis and angiitis). *Arthrit. Rheum.* 33, 1094–1100. doi: 10.1002/art.1780330806

Miller, M. R., Hankinson, J., Brusasco, V., Burgos, F., Casaburi, R., Coates, A., et al. (2005). Standardisation of spirometry. *Eur. Respir. J.* 26, 319–338. doi: 10.1183/09031936.05.00034805

Nguyen, Y., and Guillevin, L. (2018). Eosinophilic granulomatosis with polyangiitis (Churg-Strauss). *Semin. Respir. Crit. Care Med.* 39, 471–481. doi: 10.1055/s-0038-1669454

Pagnoux, C., Nair, P., Xi, Y., Khalidi, N. A., Carette, S., Cuthbertson, D., et al. (2019). Serum cytokine and chemokine levels in patients with eosinophilic granulomatosis with polyangiitis, hypereosinophilic syndrome, or eosinophilic asthma. *Clin. Exp. Rheumatol.* 37(Suppl. 117), 40–44.

Polzer, K., Karonitsch, T., Neumann, T., Eger, G., Haberler, C., Soleiman, A., et al. (2008). Eotaxin-3 is involved in Churg-Strauss syndrome–a serum marker closely correlating with disease activity. *Rheumatology* 47, 804–808. doi: 10.1093/rheumatology/ken033

Rhee, R. L., Holweg, C., Wong, K., Cuthbertson, D., Carette, S., Khalidi, N. A., et al. (2018). Serum periostin as a biomarker in eosinophilic granulomatosis with polyangiitis. *PLoS One* 13:e205768. doi: 10.1371/journal.pone.0205768

Robins, S., Roussel, L., Schachter, A., Risse, P. A., Mogas, A. K., Olivenstein, R., et al. (2011). Steroid-insensitive ERK1/2 activity drives CXCL8 synthesis and neutrophilia by airway smooth muscle. *Am. J. Respir. Cell Mol. Biol.* 45, 984–990. doi: 10.1165/rcmb.2010-0450OC

Roskoski, R. J. (2012). ERK1/2 MAP kinases: structure, function, and regulation. *Pharmacol. Res.* 66, 105–143. doi: 10.1016/j.phrs.2012.04.005

Sanderson, C. J. (1988). Interleukin-5: an eosinophil growth and activation factor. *Dev. Biol. Stand.* 69, 23–29.

Sasaki, T., Knyazev, P. G., Clout, N. J., Cheburkin, Y., Gohring, W., Ullrich, A., et al. (2006). Structural basis for Gas6-Axl signalling. *EMBO J.* 25, 80–87. doi: 10.1038/sj.emboj.7600912

Song, H. H. (1997). Analysis of correlated ROC areas in diagnostic testing. *Biometrics* 53, 370–382.

Vaglio, A., Strehl, J. D., Manger, B., Maritati, F., Alberici, F., Beyer, C., et al. (2012). IgG4 immune response in Churg-Strauss syndrome. *Ann. Rheum. Dis.* 71, 390–393. doi: 10.1136/ard.2011.155382

Wang, S., Qiu, Z., Hou, Y., Deng, X., Xu, W., Zheng, T., et al. (2021). AXL is a candidate receptor for SARS-CoV-2 that promotes infection of pulmonary and bronchial epithelial cells. *Cell Res.* 31, 126–140. doi: 10.1038/s41422-020-00460-y

Zagvozdkina, E. S., Moiseev, S. V., and Novikov, P. I. (2016). Eotaxin-3 as a biomarker of activity in established eosinophilic granulomatosis with polyangiitis. *J. Rheumatol.* 43, 2082–2083. doi: 10.3899/jrheum.160576

4

Matrix Metalloproteinase-12 is Required for Granuloma Progression

Arjun Mohan[1], Nicole Neequaye[1], Anagha Malur[1], Eman Soliman[1,2], Matthew McPeek[1], Nancy Leffler[1], David Ogburn[1], Debra A. Tokarz[3], Warren Knudson[4], Sina A. Gharib[5], Lynn M. Schnapp[6], Barbara P. Barna[1] and Mary Jane Thomassen[1*]

[1] Division of Pulmonary, Critical Care and Sleep Medicine, Department of Medicine, Brody School of Medicine- East Carolina University, Greenville, NC, United States, [2] Department of Pharmacology and Toxicology, Faculty of Pharmacy, Zagazig University, Zagazig, Egypt, [3] Department of Population Health and Pathobiology, College of Veterinary Medicine, North Carolina State University, Raleigh, NC, United States, [4] Department of Anatomy and Cell Biology, Brody School of Medicine- East Carolina University, Greenville, NC, United States, [5] Division of Pulmonary, Critical Care and Sleep Medicine, Computational Medicine Core, Center for Lung Biology, Department of Medicine, University of Washington, Seattle, WA, United States, [6] Allergy, Pulmonary and Critical Care Medicine, Department of Medicine, University of Wisconsin-Madison School of Medicine and Public Health, Madison, WI, United States

***Correspondence:**
Mary Jane Thomassen
thomassenm@ecu.edu

Background: Sarcoidosis is a chronic inflammatory disease of unknown cause characterized by granuloma formation. Mechanisms for chronic persistence of granulomas are unknown. Matrix Metalloproteinase-12 (MMP12) degrades extracellular matrix elastin and enables infiltration of immune cells responsible for inflammation and granuloma formation. Previous studies report increased MMP12 in sarcoidosis patients and association between MMP12 expression and disease severity. We also observed elevated MMP12 in our multiwall carbon nanotube (MWCNT) murine model of granulomatous inflammation. Here we hypothesized that MMP12 is important to acute and late phases of granuloma pathogenesis. To test this hypothesis, we analyzed granulomatous and inflammatory responses of *Mmp12 knock-out* (KO) mice at 10 (acute) and 60 days (late) after MWCNT instillation.

Methods: C57BL/6 (wildtype) and *Mmp12* KO mice underwent oropharyngeal instillation of MWCNT. Lungs were harvested at 3, 10, 20, and 60 days post instillation for evaluation of MMP12 expression and granulomatous changes. Bronchoalveolar lavage (BAL) cells were analyzed 60 days after MWCNT instillation for expression of mediators thought to play a role in sarcoid granulomatosis: peroxisome proliferator-activated receptor-gamma (PPARγ), interferon-gamma (IFN-γ), and CCL2 (MCP-1).

Results: Pulmonary granuloma appearance at 10 days after MWCNT instillation showed no differences between wildtype and *Mmp12* KO mice. In contrast, by 60 days after MWCNT instillation, *Mmp12* KO mice revealed markedly attenuated granuloma formation together with elevated PPARγ and reduced IFNγ expression in BAL cells compared to wildtype. Unexpectedly, *Mmp12* KO mice further demonstrated increased alveolar macrophages with increased CCL2 at 60 days.

Conclusions: The striking reduction of granuloma formation at day 60 in *Mmp12* KO mice suggests that MMP12 is required to maintain chronic granuloma pathophysiology. The increased PPARγ and decreased IFNγ findings suggest that these mediators also may be involved since previous studies have shown that PPARγ suppresses IFNγ and PPARγ deficiency amplifies granuloma formation. Interestingly, a role of MMP12 in granuloma resolution is also suggested by increases in both macrophage influx and CCL2. Overall, our results strongly implicate MMP12 as a key factor in granuloma persistence and as a possible therapeutic target in chronic pulmonary sarcoidosis.

Keywords: sarcoidosis, MMP12, PPARγ, MWCNT, granuloma, inflammation

INTRODUCTION

Sarcoidosis is a prototypic granulomatous inflammatory disorder which predominantly affects the lungs and thoracic lymph nodes (1). Recent studies show that average sarcoidosis-associated mortality has increased by approximately 3% per year in the United States (2, 3). Unfortunately, large gaps in our understanding of sarcoidosis pathogenesis have hindered research and development of novel therapies. Animal models may be helpful for exploring select pathways and directing research toward higher yield mechanisms. Our multiwall carbon nanotube (MWCNT) based murine model of granulomatous inflammation was first described in 2011 (4). The model replicates human disease at multiple biological levels including key mediators such as IFN-γ and PPARγ. The transcription factor, PPARγ is a regulator of glucose and lipid metabolism but is also recognized as a negative regulator of macrophage activation (5). Alveolar macrophages from healthy individuals express constitutively high PPARγ levels but PPARγ is deficient in alveolar macrophages from sarcoid patients (6). Our previous studies with the MWCNT model indicated decreased PPARγ (7). Further studies with macrophage-specific *Pparγ* knock out (KO) mice revealed enhanced granulomatous disease as evidenced by increased granuloma size and incidence (7). Interestingly, previous studies indicated that IFNγ represses PPARγ in human alveolar macrophages (8), suggesting a reciprocal relationship.

MMP12, also known as macrophage metalloelastase is a member of a family of extracellular endopeptidases (9, 10). MMPs were originally thought to be mainly responsible for turnover and degradation of extracellular matrix components. However, in recent years it has become clear that MMPs mediate many crucial functions in immunity and repair including cell migration, leukocyte activation and anti-microbial defense (9, 10). Furthermore, many of the earlier *in vitro* studies may not accurately reflect the *in vivo* situation (11). As Giannandrea and Parks note in their review, degradation studies with individual substrates show that isolated MMPs have redundancy *in vitro*, but *in vivo* functions of specific MMPs are limited and unique (11). MMP12 was first implicated as a mediator in sarcoidosis pathogenesis in 2009 (12). In those studies, lung tissues from sarcoidosis patients showed increased (>25-fold) *Mmp12* gene expression. Interestingly, MMP12 expression was highest near areas of active granulomatous inflammation, and MMP12 levels in bronchoalveolar fluid (BALF) correlated with disease severity. These findings make MMP12 biology an area of acute interest in sarcoidosis pathogenesis.

Using gene network analysis we previously demonstrated that MMP12 was one of the most highly expressed genes in MWCNT-exposed mice as well as in sarcoidosis patients, suggesting that MMP12 is a putative driver of granulomatous disease (detailed microarray information and raw data have been deposited in Gene Expression Omnibus[1] [GSE 100500 and GSE75023 (13, 14)]. We therefore hypothesized that MMP12 is critical to granuloma formation. Because conclusions made from *in vitro* studies have proven to be poor predicators of *in vivo* pathogenesis, an animal model which replicates many of the features of sarcoidosis is essential. To test this hypothesis, we compared *in vivo* granuloma genesis in *Mmp12* gene KO versus wild type mice after exposure to MWCNT.

MATERIALS AND METHODS

Multiwall Carbon Nanotube Model

All studies were conducted in conformity with Public Health Service (PHS) Policy on humane care and use of laboratory animals and were approved by the institutional animal care and use committee. C57BL/6J wild-type, *Mmp12* KO mice (Jackson Laboratories, Bar Harbor, ME, United States) and macrophage-specific *Pparγ* KO (15) received a single oropharyngeal instillation of MWCNT (100 μg) in PBS/35%surfactant (Ony Inc, Amherst, NY, United States) (4). Briefly, mice were sedated with isofluorane and by gently pulling forward the mouse tongue the epiglottis was exposed and a 50 μl volume was instilled using a pipette. MWCNTs (900–1201, lot-GS1802, SES Research, Houston, TX, United States) were freshly prepared and have been described previously (16). Sham controls received vehicle alone. Animals were sacrificed at 3, 10, 20, and 60 days post instillation and evaluated as previously described (4).

Histological Analysis

Lungs were dissected and fixed in PBS-buffered 10% formalin. Paraffin embedded slides were sectioned at 7 μm, and stained with hematoxylin and eosin (H&E) or Gomori's trichrome stain as previously described (4, 16). A previously described semiquantitative scoring system (7, 16, 17) was used to calculate a relative comparison of the numbers and quality of granulomas formed in MWCNT-instilled mice. Trichrome stain was evaluated using modified Ashcroft method (16, 18).

Lymph Nodes

Tracheobronchial lymph node volume, identified based on Van den Broeck et al., was determined using the formula

[1]https://www.ncbi.nlm.nih.gov/geo

(Length × Width^2)π/6, as previously described (16). Lymph nodes were fixed overnight in PBS-buffered 10% formalin and paraffin embedded. Representative Hemotoxylin/Eosin histological images were taken for each condition, time point and mouse strain using a Zeiss Axio Imager A1.

Characterization of Bronchoalveolar Lavage Cells

BAL cells were obtained as previously described (15, 16). Total cell counts and differential counts were evaluated (**Table 1**). Cells were stored at −80°C for gene expression, and BAL fluid was aliquoted and frozen for protein analysis.

RNA Purification and Gene Expression From BAL Cells

Total RNA was extracted from frozen BAL cells using miRNeasy Micro kit, (217084) (Qiagen, Germantown, MD, United States), according to manufacturer's protocol. Mouse specific primers and probes were obtained from Qiagen, for *Mmp12* (PPM03619F), *Ccl2* (PPM03151G), *Pparγ* (PPM05108B), and

TABLE 1 | BAL cell characteristics of C57Bl/6 and *Mmp12* KO mice 60 day.

	Treatment	*N*	Total cell count (×10^5)	AM (X10^5)	LYM (×10^5)	PMN (×10^5)
C57Bl/6	PBS/Surf	10	8.0 ± 2.9	7.7 ± 2.8 [97]	0.3 ± 0.3 [3]	0.06 ± 0.09 [1]
C57Bl/6	MWCNT	10	9.8 ± 2.5	8.9 ± 2.0 [92]	0.7 ± 0.5 [6]	0.2 ± 0.2 [2]
Mmp12 KO	PBS/Surf	10	7.7 ± 2.5	7.5 ± 2.5 [97]	0.1 ± 0.1 [2]	0.05 ± 0.1 [1]
Mmp12 KO	MWCNT	10	12.0 ± 4.1*	11.1 ± 4.0 [92]*	0.4 ± 0.2 [4]	0.5 ± 0.4 [4]*

*AM, alveolar macrophages; LYM, lymphocytes; PMN, neutrophils. *Means ± SD, $p \leq 0.05$ compared to PBS/Surf vs MWCNT in MMP12 KO. [ ] Percentage.*

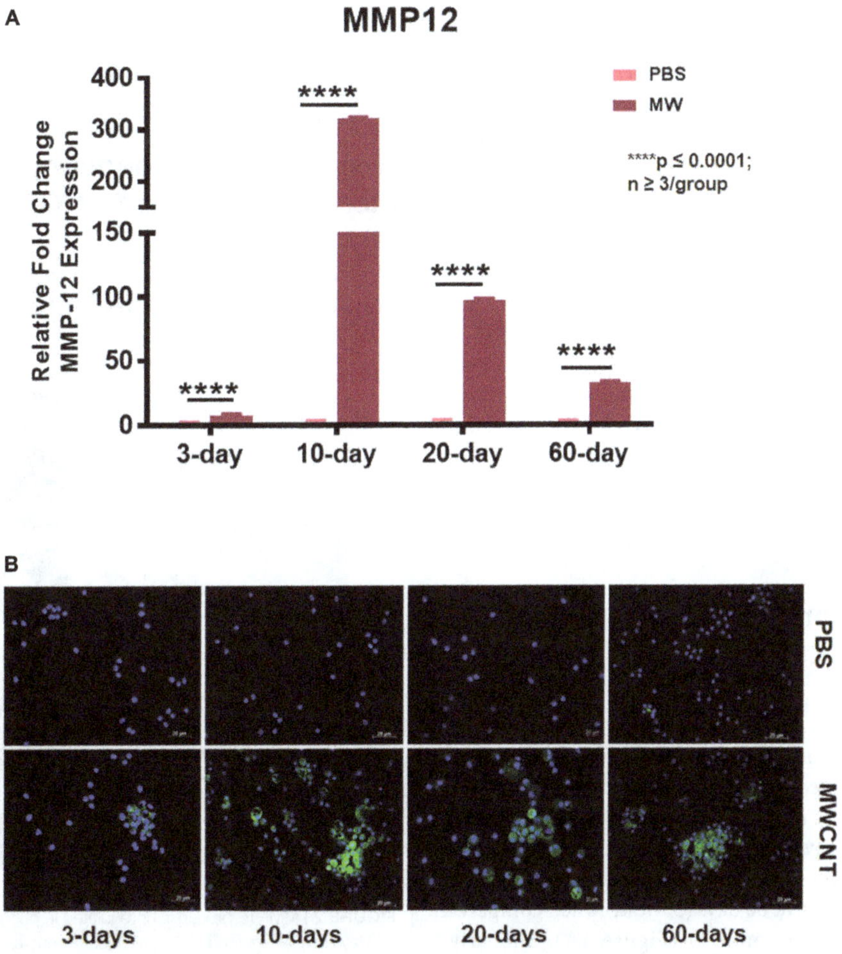

FIGURE 1 | *Mmp12* gene expression and protein are upregulated in BAL cells of MWCNT-instilled C57BL/6. **(A)** *Mmp12* gene expression is increased at 3 days, with a peak at 10 days, and remains significantly upregulated at 60 days post MWCNT-instillation ($p \leq 0.05$; $n \geq 3$ per group). **(B)** Immunofluorescent anti-MMP12 staining was minimal at 3 days, with a peak at 10 days and persistence through 60 days (representative of $n = 3$).

IFNγ (PPM03121A). GAPDH (PPM02946E) was used as a housekeeping gene. Quantitative-PCR was performed on complementary DNA synthesized with the RT2 First Strand Kit and evaluated on the StepOnePlus PCR system (Thermo Fisher Scientific, Waltham, MA, United States) in comparison to GAPDH using the $2^{-\Delta\Delta CT}$ method (19).

Protein Analyses of BAL Fluid

CCL2 was assayed in BALF by ELISA ([MJE00B] R&D systems Minneapolis, MN, United States), as per manufacturer's protocol.

Immunostaining of BAL Cells and Frozen Tissue

Cytospin slides of BAL cells were fixed with 4% paraformaldehyde-PBS, permeabilized with Triton X-100, blocked and stained with anti-PPARγ at 1:250 dilution (Sc-7196) (Santa Cruz Biotechnology, Dallas, TX, United States), and Alexa 488 (1:1000) (Invitrogen, Carlsbad, CA, United States) or anti-IFNγ 1:200 (sc-57207) (Santa Cruz Biotechnology, Dallas, TX, United States) with secondary antibody Alexa Texas Red 569 (15).

Frozen lung tissue sections (7 μm) were fixed with 4% paraformaldehyde–PBS, permeabilized with Triton X-100, blocked with normal goat serum in PBS/Triton X-100 for nonspecific binding and stained with anti-MMP12 antibody (Sc-390863) (Santa Cruz Biotechnology, Dallas, TX, United States), 1:250 dilution, followed by Alexa conjugated goat anti-rabbit IgG 488 (Invitrogen, Carlsbad, CA, United States). Slides were counter-stained with DAPI (Vector Laboratories, Burlingame, CA, United States) to facilitate nuclear localization. Slides were imaged on Zeiss confocal LSM700.

Statistical Analyses

Data were analyzed by Student's *t*-test or one-way analysis of variance (ANOVA) using Prism 7 software (GraphPad, Inc., San Diego, CA, United States).

RESULTS

MWCNT Instillation Increases MMP12 Expression in BAL Cells of Wild-Type Mice

To explore MMP12 involvement in granuloma development, we examined the time course of *Mmp12* expression. C57BL/6J wildtype mice were instilled with MWCNT and BAL cells were collected after 3, 10, 20, and 60 days. Quantitative RT-PCR (qRT-PCR) of BAL cells revealed significant increases in *Mmp12* mRNA expression at 3 days (7.6-fold) with a peak at 10 days (322-fold) and sustained elevation at 60 days (33-fold) when compared to PBS-instilled mice (sham controls) (**Figure 1A**). Similarly, immunofluorescence showed MMP12 protein expression to be upregulated in wildtype BAL cells (**Figure 1B**). MMP12 appeared most prominent at 10 days post instillation and persisted to 60 days. In lung tissues from wildtype animals, expression of MMP12 protein was also upregulated around granulomas at 60-days after MWCNT instillation (**Figure 2**).

Progression of Granuloma Formation Is Attenuated in MWCNT-Instilled *Mmp12* KO Mice

The effects of MMP12 on granuloma formation were examined in *Mmp12* KO and wildtype mice instilled with MWCNT. Pulmonary histological changes were observed in both *Mmp12* KO and wildtype mice at 3, 10, 20, and 60 days post MWCNT instillation compared to PBS controls (**Figure 3A**). Granulomas formed in wildtype mice were detected as early as 10 days post instillation. These early granulomas were poorly formed, but by 60 days post instillation, granulomas appeared to be well defined. Surprisingly, no histological differences in granuloma formation were noted acutely in *Mmp12* KO mice compared to wildtype at days 3 and 10. In contrast, by 20 days after MWCNT instillation, granulomas in *Mmp12* KO mice appeared to be resolving and by 60 days were smaller and less well-formed. None of the time points showed evidence of necrosis or caseation. Histological analyses at 60-days post instillation (**Figure 3B**) were scored based upon size and frequency of granulomas. Scores were significantly ($p = 0.01$) less in *Mmp12* KO mice. Trichrome staining revealed no fibrosis in MWCNT-instilled *Mmp12* KO mice (data not shown).

Mediastinal Lymphadenopathy Is Attenuated in *Mmp12* KO Mice at 60 Days

MWCNT promoted an exacerbated lymphadenopathy in wildtype mice (**Figure 4A**). We hypothesized that as granulomas

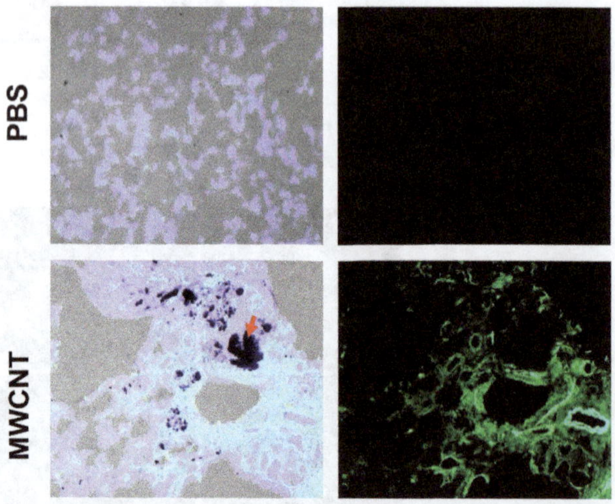

FIGURE 2 | MMP12 protein is upregulated in pulmonary granulomas of 60-day MWCNT-instilled C57BL/6 mice. Representative bright-field and immunofluorescence images for MMP12 protein indicate very minimal to no staining in PBS instilled mice, but increased protein around granulomas in MWCNT-instilled C57BL/6 at 60-days. Black aggregates in (lower left, red arrows) bright-field images are MWCNT accumulations in the tissue.

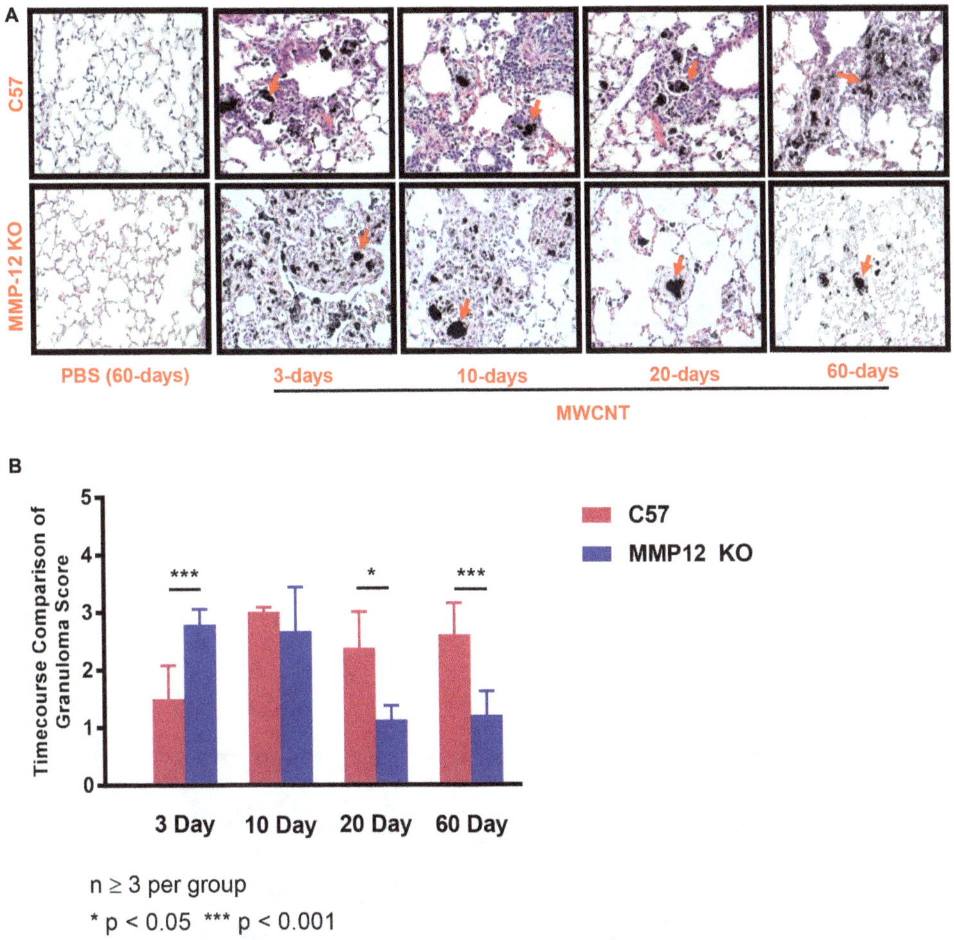

FIGURE 3 | Granulomas from *Mmp12* KO mice are resolving at 60 days. **(A)** Histological examination of H&E-stained lung tissue sections from MMCNT-instilled C57BL/6 and *Mmp12* KO mice indicate loosely formed granulomas as early as 3 days in *Mmp12* KO mice with resolution beginning at 20 days in contrast to C57BL/6. Representative bright field images illustrating granuloma formation in MWCNT-instilled mice at 60 days show decreased size and number of granulomas in *Mmp12* KO compared to C57BL/6 mice. Red arrows indicate deposition of MWCNT in the lung. **(B)** Granuloma scoring (mean ± SEM) of *Mmp12* KO as compared to C57BL/6. *Mmp12* KO lung scores were significantly less than those of C57BL/6 at 60 days (***$p < 0.001$). Sections were evaluated by two independent observers from $n = 6$ lungs for each group.

in *Mmp12* KO mice were diminished at 60 days, mediastinal lymphadenopathy would also be attenuated in these mice. As predicted, MWCNT-instilled *Mmp12* KO mice exhibited reduced mediastinal lymph node sizes compared to wildtype at 60 days after instillation (**Figure 4**). It should be noted that at 10 days, there were no differences in mediastinal lymph node volume between wildtype and *Mmp12* KO mice. Granulomas were not present in the lymph nodes of either wildtype or *Mmp12* KO mice (**Figure 4B**). However, MWCNT are present in wildtype and *Mmp12* KO mice at 10 days and MWCNT deposition is increased in both at 60 days.

MWCNT-Instilled *Mmp12* KO Mice at 60 Days Have Increased Macrophage Influx in BAL

Surprisingly, despite the resolution of granulomatous inflammation at 60 days, MWCNT-instilled *Mmp12* KO mice had significantly ($p \leq 0.05$) increased numbers of macrophages in BAL fluid compared to *Mmp12* PBS controls or MWCNT-instilled wildtypes (**Table 1**). These results suggest that macrophage influx may be involved in the resolution of granulomatous inflammation.

MMP12 Deficiency Does Not Affect CCL2 Expression in BAL Cells and Fluids

Because of the increased number of macrophages in BAL fluid of MWCNT-instilled *Mmp12* KO mice at 60 days despite the granuloma resolution, we investigated the monocyte/macrophage chemokine CCL2. Unexpectedly, *Ccl2* gene expression in BAL cells was not different in MWCNT-instilled *Mmp12* KO mice compared to wildtype despite the histological resolution (**Figure 5A**). In order to determine whether CCL2 was elevated in alveolar spaces, BAL fluid was analyzed. CCL2 protein was elevated in BAL fluids from

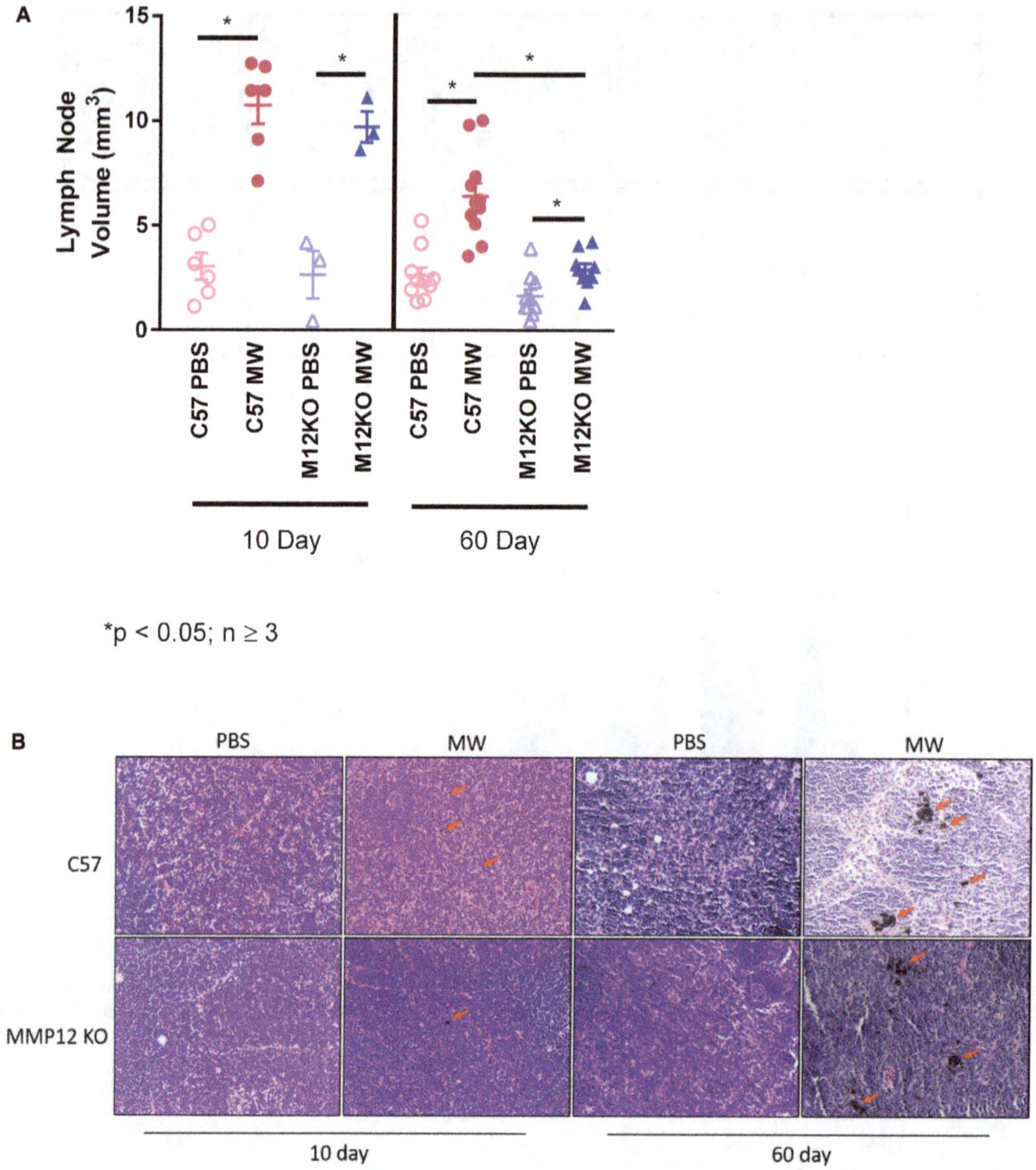

FIGURE 4 | Mediastinal Lymph node volume is decreased at 60-days in MWCNT-instilled *Mmp12* KO mice. **(A)** At 10 days lymph node volumes were not significantly different between MWCNT-instilled C57BL/6 and *Mmp12* KO mice. However, at 60 days, lymph node volumes from MWCNT-instilled *Mmp12* KO mice were significantly decreased compared to C57BL/6 (*$p \leq 0.05$, $n \geq 3$/group). **(B)** Carbon particle deposition can be seen in both C57BL/6 and *Mmp12* KO mice at 10 days (red arrows) and is more prominent at 60-day (red arrows) as compared to respective lymph nodes from PBS-instilled mice.

MWCNT-instilled *Mmp12* KO and wildtype mice compared to PBS-instilled controls and increased levels did not differ between the two mouse strains (**Figure 5B**).

PPARγ Expression Is Increased in *Mmp12* KO Mice Compared to Wild Type

We postulated that MMP12 levels might be higher in PPARγ KO mice. As shown in **Figure 6**, MMP12 expression was significantly elevated in BAL cells of PBS-instilled *Pparγ* KO mice and further increased after MWCNT instillation compared to wildtype. These findings suggested a PPARγ regulatory role in MMP12 expression. Based on these data, we hypothesized that PPARγ might be elevated in BAL cells from *Mmp12* KO mice since granuloma formation was decreased. At 60 days, *Mmp12* KO BAL cells from MWCNT-instilled mice exhibited elevated PPARγ expression in contrast to wild-type where PPARγ was decreased (**Figure 7A**). In order to confirm whether PPARγ was active in *Mmp12* KO mice, BAL cells were stained with anti-PPARγ antibody. Wildtype mice instilled with MWCNT exhibited decreased PPARγ protein. PBS-instilled *Mmp12* KO mice showed increased PPARγ protein, which further increased after MWCNT instillation (**Figure 7B**).

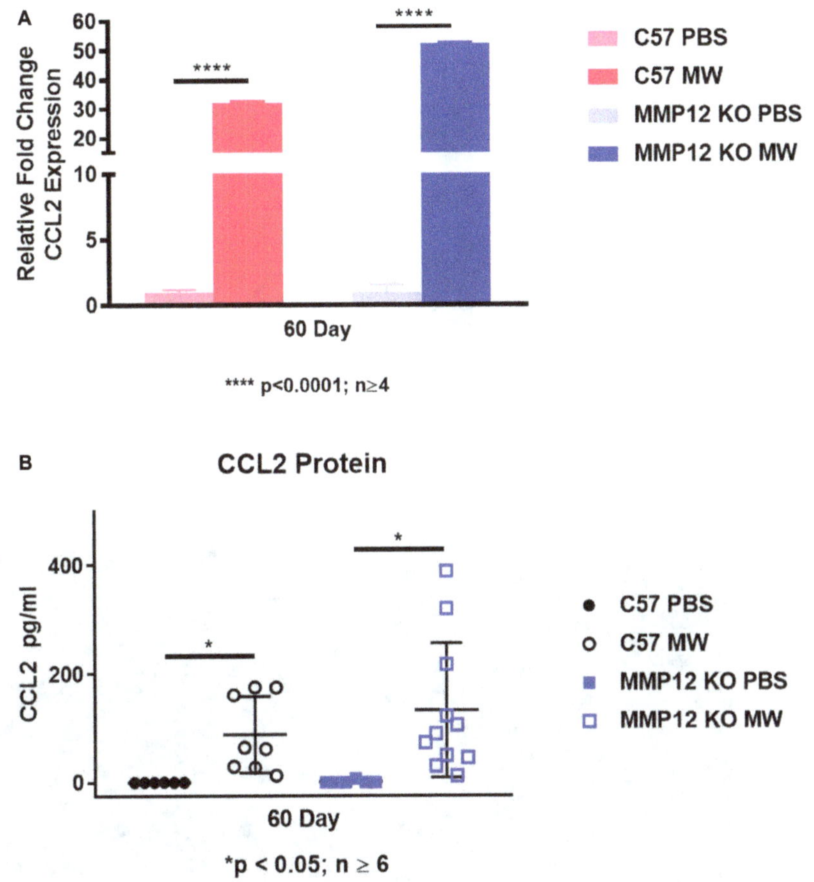

FIGURE 5 | *Ccl2* gene expression and protein are elevated in both C57BL/6 and *Mmp12* KO mice at 60 days after MWCNT instillation. **(A)** *Ccl2* gene expression is increased in BAL cells of both C57BL/6 and *Mmp12* KO MWCNT-instilled mice compared to PBS controls (****$p < 0.0001$; $n \geq 4$). **(B)** CCL2 protein from the BAL fluid is increased in both C57BL/6 and *Mmp12* KO MWCNT-instilled mice compared to PBS (*$p \leq 0.05$; $n \geq 6$).

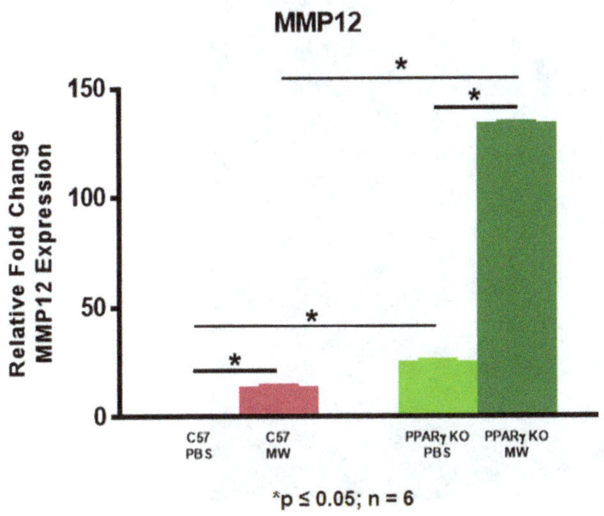

FIGURE 6 | MMP12 is elevated in MWCNT-instilled *Pparγ* KO BAL cells. *Mmp12* gene expression in *Pparγ* KO mice is significantly increased intrinsically, and further increased after MWCNT instillation compared to C57BL/6 (*$p \leq 0.05$; n = 6/group).

IFN-γ Gene and Protein Expression Are Not Increased in MWCNT-Instilled *Mmp12* KO Compared to Wild Type

We investigated IFN-γ expression in the MWCNT murine model and found that IFN-γ gene expression was decreased in MWCNT-instilled *Mmp12* KO mice compared to wild type (**Figure 8A**). IFN-γ protein was evaluated by immunostaining of BAL cytospins to confirm the differences. MWCNT-instilled wildtype mice demonstrated prominent IFN-γ protein expression. In contrast MWCNT-instilled *Mmp12* KO mice exhibited almost no detectable IFN-γ (**Figure 8B**).

DISCUSSION

The current findings in the murine MWCNT granuloma model highlight the importance of MMP12 in granuloma pathophysiology and complement findings in sarcoidosis. Our previous and current reports demonstrate that inflammation and granuloma formation in the MWCNT model are associated with a marked increase in MMP12 expression as early as 10 days post instillation with a significant increase persisting

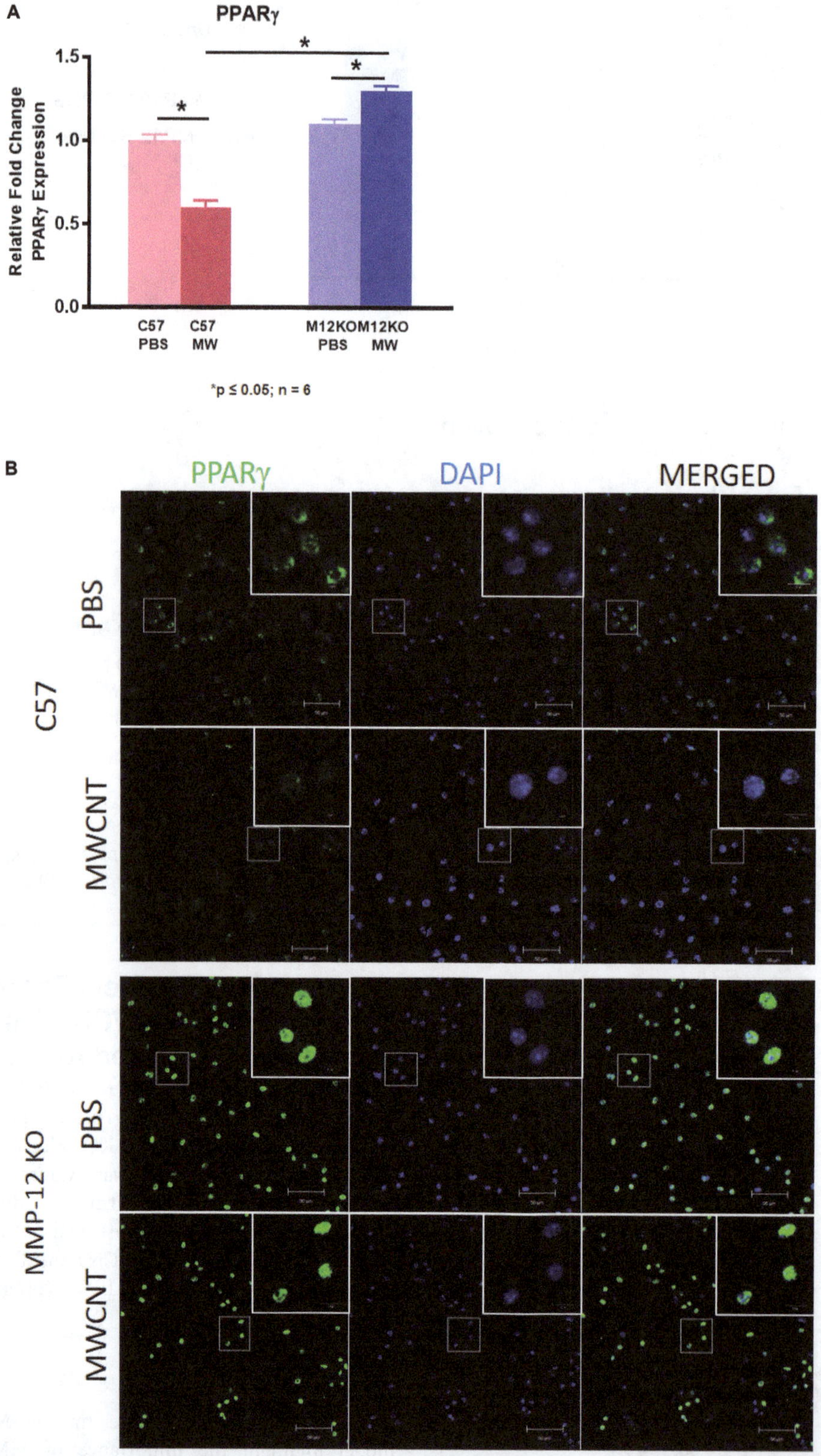

FIGURE 7 | *Pparγ* gene expression and protein are increased in 60-day MWCNT-instilled *Mmp12* KO mice compared to C57BL/6. **(A)** *Pparγ* gene expression is decreased in MWCNT-instilled C57BL/6 mice compared to PBS controls. In contrast, *Pparγ* is significantly increased in MWCNT-instilled *Mmp12* KO mice compared to PBS controls (*$p \leq 0.05$; $n \geq 6$ /group). **(B)** Immunofluorescent anti-PPARγ staining of BAL cells from PBS-instilled mice show constitutive PPARγ protein as indicated by green fluorescence, while MWCNT-instilled C57BL/6 show decreased expression. PBS instilled *Mmp12* KO mice show intrinsically high levels of PPARγ protein, and with MWCNT, PPARγ protein remains highly expressed (representative figure of $n = 3$).

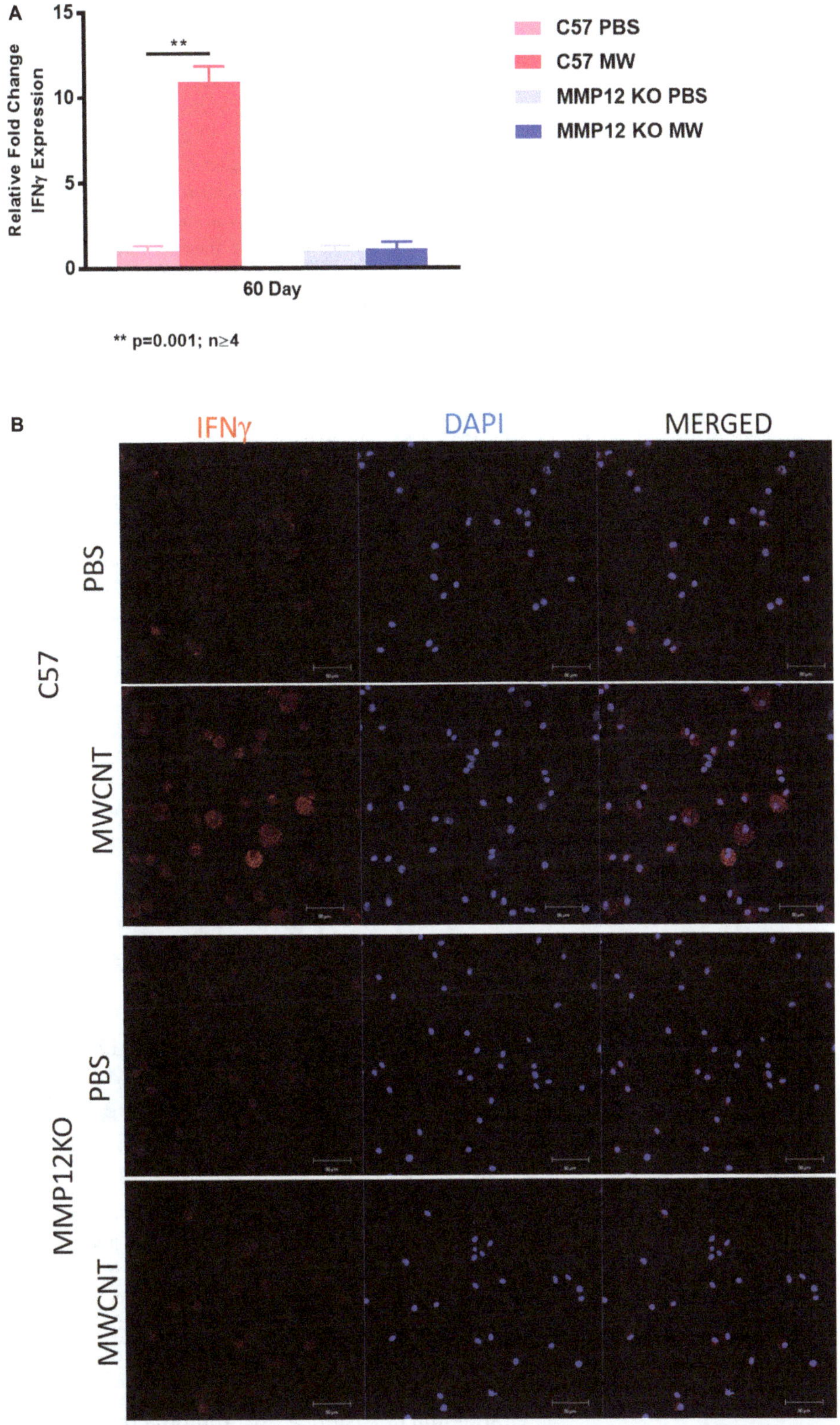

FIGURE 8 | IFNγ gene expression and protein are not increased in MWCNT-instilled *Mmp12* KO compared to C57BL/6. **(A)** *Ifnγ* gene expression is significantly (**$p = 0.001$; $n \geq 4$) increased in C57BL/6 mice instilled with MWCNT compared to PBS controls. In *Mmp12* KO mice, *Ifnγ* gene expression is not increased by MWCNT instillation compared to PBS controls. **(B)** Immunofluorescent anti-IFNγ staining of BAL cells from PBS-instilled mice show minimal IFNγ protein, while MWCNT-instilled C57BL/6 show marked IFNγ protein as indicated by red fluorescence. Both PBS and MWCNT-instilled *Mmp12* KO mice showed minimal staining for IFNγ protein (representative figure of $n = 3$).

to 60 days (4). These data suggest that MMP12 is required for the chronic stages of inflammation associated with granuloma formation. In sarcoidosis, MMP12 constitutes one of the most highly expressed genes in granulomatous lung tissues (12). Our previous comparative transcriptional survey of alveolar macrophages from sarcoidosis patients and MWCNT-instilled mice also revealed marked MMP12 elevation in both species (13). Numerous previous studies have also shown that MMP12, an elastase enzyme predominantly produced by macrophages, is an important mediator of both acute and chronic lung injury and directly involved in development of inflammatory responses (9, 10). MMP12 mechanisms involve degradation of the extracellular matrix protein, elastin, into fragments which can act as a chemoattractant for macrophage recruitment (20).

The monocyte/macrophage chemokine CCL2 has been linked to granuloma formation in other animal model systems (21) and transcriptional studies also indicated elevated expression in both MWCNT instilled mice and sarcoidosis patients (13, 14). Elevation of CCL2 in BAL cells was unexpected in *Mmp12* KO mice at 60 days after MWCNT instillation when granulomas had resolved. In our previous studies, CCL2, which is produced by macrophages, was consistently elevated in parallel with MWCNT-induced granuloma formation (4, 7). Upregulation of CCL2 in BAL fluid is also characteristic of patients with pulmonary sarcoidosis (22, 23). We noted that an influx of BAL macrophages accompanied the granuloma resolution in *Mmp12* KO mice at 60 days. Whether this is driven by CCL2 is unclear. Recent studies have suggested that CCL2 functions may extend beyond its original characterization as a chemoattractant [reviewed in Gschwandtner et al. (24)]. Additional functions attributed to CCL2 have included adhesion, polarization, and effector molecule secretion, and many are context-dependent and may be synergistic with other inflammatory stimuli (24). Gene expression analyses in both MWCNT-instilled mice and sarcoidosis indicated a multitude of elevated inflammatory mediators that may modify CCL2 effects (12, 13). Additional studies will be required to define the complex role of CCL2 in MMP12 regulation.

The current findings also noted a lack of IFN-γ upregulation in 60-day MWCNT-instilled *Mmp12* KO mice in contrast with wildtypes in which IFN-γ was significantly increased as noted in previous MWCNT studies (7, 25). Elevated IFN-γ in sarcoidosis patients with pulmonary disease has been well-reported in the

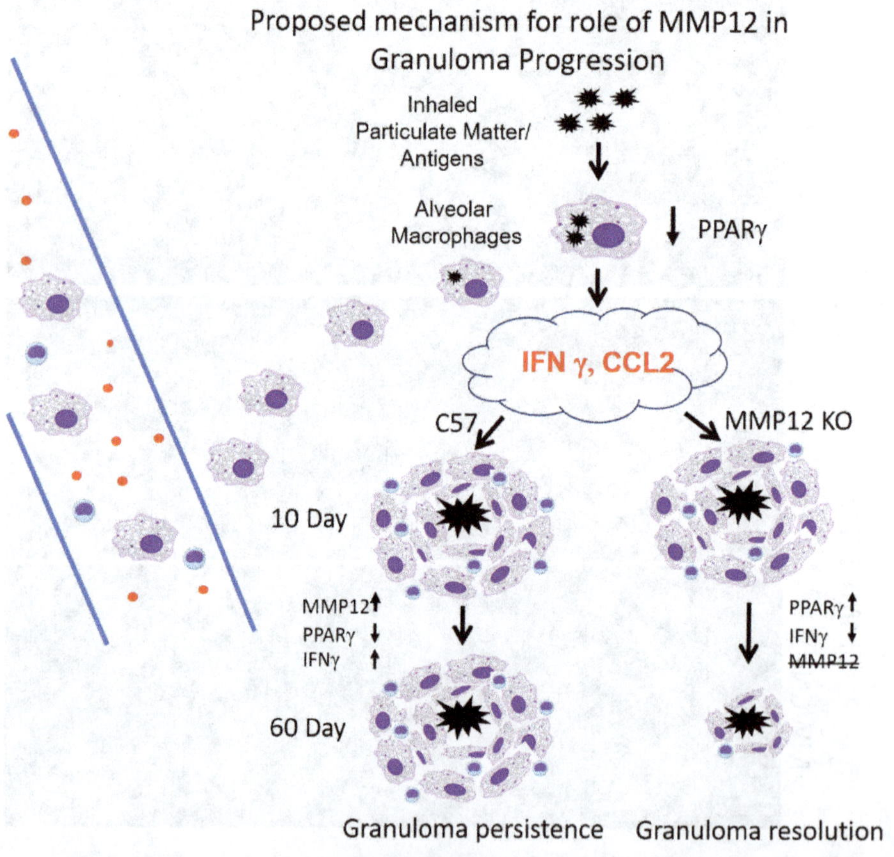

FIGURE 9 | Proposed mechanism for role of MMP12 in granuloma progression. Initial exposure to inhaled particulate matter/and or antigens triggers secretion of several cytokines (CCL2, IFNγ), with further recruitment of alveolar macrophages/monocytes and T cells. Once on site, macrophages produce additional cytokines which promote the formation of multinucleated giant cells and retention of T cells. With MMP12 upregulation (C57/Bl6) persistent PPARγ decrease and IFNγ increase results in granuloma persistence. Whereas as in the absence of MMP12 (*Mmp12 KO*) PPARγ increases and IFNγ decreases resulting in granulomas resolution.

literature (26, 27, 28). Upregulated expression of IFN-γ signaling pathways was also found in both MWCNT-instilled wildtype mice and sarcoidosis patients in our recent transcriptional survey of alveolar macrophages from both groups (13, 14). Thus, the current studies emphasize an association between IFN-γ and granulomatous changes in the lung. In contrast to absence of IFN-γ, expression of PPARγ was elevated in *Mmp12* KO mice at 60 days post MWCNT instillation. PPARγ is a nuclear receptor that regulates expression of genes involved in lipid homeostasis and inflammation in immune cells especially macrophages (29, 30). Interestingly, PPARγ and IFN-γ exhibit mutually antagonistic properties (8, 31) which may explain, in part, our observations. However, further studies are needed to better elucidate the interconnected role of IFN-γ – PPARγ pathways in *Mmp12* KO mice.

Our previous studies demonstrated that PPARγ deficiency exacerbates granuloma formation in the MWCNT murine granuloma model (7). The relationship between PPARγ and MMP12 in granuloma formation has not been previously described, and the current data show for the first time an inverse relationship between PPARγ and MMP12 in mediating pulmonary granulomatous inflammation. MMP12 expression is increased by PPARγ deficiency as shown by the MWCNT experiments in PPARγ KO mice. In *Mmp12* KO mice, both PPARγ expression and activity increased with MWCNT instillation, suggesting that MMP12 deficiency enhances PPARγ. Overall, our data suggest that PPARγ pathways may contribute to the reduction of granuloma formation in *Mmp12* KO mice.

Evidence from the present study and previous studies (4, 7, 16, 25) is summarized in **Figure 9**. We propose that an initial exposure to inhaled particulate matter and/or various antigens (which may include bacterial components such as mycobacterial peptides) triggers the alveolar macrophage secretion of several cytokines (CCL2, IFNγ) with further recruitment of alveolar macrophages/monocytes and T cells. Once on site, macrophages produce additional cytokines which promote the formation of multinucleated giant cells and retention of T cells. With MMP12 upregulation (C57/Bl6), persistent PPARγ decrease and IFNγ increase results in granuloma persistence. Whereas in the absence of MMP12 (*Mmp12 KO*), PPARγ increases and IFNγ decreases, resulting in granuloma resolution.

Decades of research suggest that the etiology of sarcoidosis may be multifactorial and complex, as illustrated by the multiple environmental factors which have been associated with sarcoidosis disease development [reviewed by Judson (32)]. Studies of lung tissues from sarcoid patients have found silica, aluminum, and titanium as well as carbon nanotubes (33). Fibrotic granulomatous lung disease together with elevated CCL2 and MMP12 gene expression as we have described in the wildtype murine MWCNT model have been reported in a rat model of chronic silicosis (34). This model, however, lacks some key sarcoidosis features such as elevated IFN-γ and also does not exhibit any MMP12 protein, unlike the MWCNT model in which high levels of MMP12 protein were detected in both alveolar macrophages and lung tissues from MWCNT-instilled mice. A recent review of available animal models of sarcoidosis concluded that no single model faithfully reproduces all aspects of sarcoidosis pathology (35), but the models may help in evaluating selective sarcoidosis pathways that can be reproduced in the models.

CONCLUSION

This study demonstrates that MMP12 deficiency reduces pulmonary granuloma progression and highlights a critical role for MMP12 in the chronicity of granulomatous inflammation. Potential mechanisms involved in granuloma resolution require further exploration, including identifying how the down-regulation of IFN-γ results in elevated PPARγ, and a better understanding of how CCL2 promotes macrophage recruitment. Deciphering MMP12–orchestrated mechanisms in granuloma formation can lead to novel approaches for treating sarcoidosis.

AUTHOR CONTRIBUTIONS

NN, ES, MM, NL, DO, and DT: acquisition of data. AMo, AMa, WK, BB, SG, LS, and MJT: concept and design. BB, AMa, and MJT: analysis, interpretation, and drafting of manuscript for important intellectual content. All authors contributed to the article and approved the submitted version.

REFERENCES

Baughman RP, Teirstein AS, Judson MA, Rossman MD, Yeager H, Bresnitz EA, et al. Clinical characteristics of patients in a case control study of sarcoidosis. *Am J Respir Crit Care Med.* (2001) 164:1885–9.

Swigris JJ, Olson AL, Huie TJ, Fernandez-Perez ER, Solomon J, Sprunger D, et al. Sarcoidosis-related mortality in the United States from 1988 to 2007. *Am J Respir Crit Care Med.* (2011) 183:1524–30. doi: 10.1164/rccm.201010-1679oc

Kearney GD, Obi ON, Maddipati V, Mohan A, Malur A, Carter JC, et al. Sarcoidosis deaths in the United States: 1999-2016. *Respir Med.* (2019) 149:30–5. doi: 10.1016/j.rmed.2018. 11.010

Huizar I, Malur A, Midgette YA, Kukoly C, Chen P, Ke PC, et al. Novel murine model of chronic granulomatous lung inflammation elicited by carbon nanotubes. *Am J Respir Cell Mol Biol.* (2011) 45:858–66. doi: 10.1165/rcmb. 2010-0401oc

Ricote M, Li AC, Willson TM, Kelly CJ, Glass CK. The peroxisome proliferator-activated receptor-γ is a negative regulator of macrophage activation. *Nature.* (1998) 391:79–82. doi: 10.1038/34178

Culver DA, Barna BP, Raychaudhuri B, Bonfield TL, Abraham S, Malur A, et al. Peroxisome proliferator-activated receptor gamma activity is deficient in alveolar macrophages in pulmonary sarcoidosis. *Am J Respir Cell Mol Biol.* (2004) 30:1–5. doi: 10.1165/rcmb.2003-0304rc

Huizar I, Malur A, Patel J, McPeek M, Dobbs L, Wingard C, et al. The role of PPARgamma in carbon nanotube-elicited granulomatous lung inflammation. *Respir Res.* (2013) 14:7. doi: 10.1186/1465-9921-14-7

Barna BP, Culver DA, Abraham S, Malur A, Bonfield TL, John N, et al. Depressed peroxisome proliferator-activated receptor gamma (PPARgamma) is indicative of severe pulmonary sarcoidosis: possible involvement of interferon gamma (IFN-gamma). *Sarcoidosis Vasc Diffuse Lung Dis.* (2006) 23:93–100.

Parasa VR, Muvva JR, Rose JF, Braian C, Brighenti S, Lerm M. Inhibition of tissue matrix metalloproteinases interferes with mycobacterium tuberculosis- induced granuloma formation and reduces bacterial load in a human lung tissue model. *Front Microbiol.* (2017) 8:2370. doi: 10.3389/fmicb.2017.02370

Fingleton B. Matrix metalloproteinases as regulators of inflammatory processes. *Biochim Biophys Acta Mol Cell Res.* (2017) 1864:2036–42. doi: 10.1016/j. bbamcr.2017.05.010

Giannandrea M, Parks WC. Diverse functions of matrix metalloproteinases during fibrosis. *Dis Model Mech.* (2014) 7:193–203. doi: 10.1242/dmm.012062

Crouser ED, Culver DA, Knox KS, Julian MW, Shao G, Abraham S, et al. Gene expression profiling identifies MMP-12 and ADAMDEC1 as potential pathogenic mediators of pulmonary sarcoidosis. *Am J Respir Crit Care Med.* (2009) 179:929–38. doi: 10.1164/rccm.200803-490oc

Mohan A, Malur A, McPeek M, Barna BP, Schnapp LM, Thomassen MJ, et al. Transcriptional survey of alveolar macrophages in a murine model of chronic granulomatous inflammation reveals common themes with human sarcoidosis. *Am J Physiol Lung Cell Mol Physiol.* (2018) 314:L617–25.

Gharib SA, Malur A, Huizar I, Barna BP, Kavuru MS, Schnapp LM, et al. Sarcoidosis activates diverse transcriptional programs in bronchoalveolar lavage cells. *Respir Res.* (2016) 17:93.

Malur A, Mccoy AJ, Arce S, Barna BP, Kavuru MS, Malur AG, et al. Deletion of PPARγ in alveolar macrophages is associated with a Th-1 pulmonary inflammatory response. *J Immunol.* (2009) 182:5816–22. doi: 10.4049/jimmunol.0803504

Malur A, Mohan A, Barrington RA, Leffler N, Malur A, Muller-Borer B, et al. PPARgamma deficiency exacerbates fibrotic response to mycobacteria peptide in murine sarcoidosis model. *Am J Respir Cell Mol Biol.* (2019) 61:198–208. doi: 10.1165/rcmb.2018-0346oc

McPeek M, Malur A, Tokarz DA, Lertpiriyapong K, Gowdy KM, Murray G, et al. Alveolar macrophage ABCG1 deficiency promotes pulmonary granulomatous inflammation. *Am J Respir Cell Mol Biol.* (2019) 61:332–40. doi: 10.1165/rcmb.2018-0365oc

Hubner RH, Gitter W, El Mokhtari NE, Mathiak M, Both M, Bolte H, et al. Standardized quantification of pulmonary fibrosis in histological samples. *Biotechniques.* (2008) 44:507–11. doi: 10.2144/000112729

Livak KJ, Schmittgen TD. Analysis of relative gene expression data using real-time quantitative PCR and the 2(-Delta Delta C(T)) method. *Methods.* (2001) 25:402–8. doi: 10.1006/meth.2001.1262

Houghton AM. Matrix metalloproteinases in destructive lung disease. *Matrix Biol.* (2015) 44-46:167–74. doi: 10.1016/j.matbio.2015.02.002

Lu B, Rutledge BJ, Gu L, Fiorillo J, Lukacs NW, Kunkel SL, et al. Abnormalities in monocyte recruitment and cytokine expression in monocyte chemoattractant protein 1-deficient mice. *J Exp Med.* (1998) 187:601–8. doi: 10.1084/jem.187.4.601

Palchevskiy V, Hashemi N, Weigt SS, Xue YY, Derhovanessian A, Keane MP, et al. Immune response CC chemokines CCL2 and CCL5 are associated with pulmonary sarcoidosis. *Fibrogenesis Tissue Repair.* (2011) 4:10.

Barna BP, Huizar I, Malur A, McPeek M, Marshall I, Jacob M, et al. Carbon nanotube-induced pulmonary granulomatous disease: twist1 and alveolar macrophage m1 activation. *Int J Mol Sci.* (2013) 14:23858–71. doi: 10.3390/ijms141223858

Gschwandtner M, Derler R, Midwood KS. More than just attractive: how CCL2 influences myeloid cell behavior beyond chemotaxis. *Front Immunol.* (2019) 10:2759. doi: 10.3389/fimmu.2019.02759

Malur A, Barna BP, Patel J, McPeek M, Wingard CJ, Dobbs L, et al. Exposure to a mycobacterial antigen, ESAT-6, exacerbates granulomatous and fibrotic changes in a multiwall carbon nanotube model of chronic pulmonary disease. *J Nanomed Nanotechnol.* (2015) 6:340. doi: 10.4172/2157-7439.1000340

Robinson BW, McLemore TL, Crystal RG. Gamma interferon is spontaneously released by alveolar macrophages and lung T lymphocytes in patients with pulmonary sarcoidosis. *J Clin Invest.* (1985) 75:1488–95. doi: 10.1172/jci111852

Asano M, Minagawa T, Ohmichi M, Hiraga Y. Detection of endogenous cytokines in sera or in lymph nodes obtained from patients with sarcoidosis. *Clin Exp Immunol.* (1991) 84:92–6. doi: 10.1111/j.1365-2249.1991.tb08129.x

Ramstein J, Broos CE, Simpson LJ, Ansel KM, Sun SA, Ho ME, et al. Interferon-γ-producing Th17.1 cells are increased in sarcoidosis and more prevalent than Th1 cells. *Am J Respir Crit Care Med.* (2015) 193:1281–91. doi: 10.1164/rccm.201507-1499OC

Ohshima K, Mogi M, Horiuchi M. Role of peroxisome proliferator- activated receptor-gamma in vascular inflammation. *Int J Vasc Med.* (2012) 2012:508416.

Tyagi S, Gupta P, Saini AS, Kaushal C, Sharma S. The peroxisome proliferator-activated receptor: a family of nuclear receptors role in various diseases. *J Adv Pharm Technol Res.* (2011) 2:236–40. doi: 10.4103/2231-4040.90879

Cunard R, Eto Y, Muljadi JT, Glass CK, Kelly CJ, Ricote M. Repression of IFN-gamma expression by peroxisome proliferator-activated receptor gamma. *J Immunol.* (2004) 172:7530–6.

Judson MA. Environmental risk factors for sarcoidosis. *Front Immunol.* (2020) 11:1340. doi: 10.3389/fimmu.2020.01340

Wu M, Gordon RE, Herbert R, Padilla M, Moline J, Mendelson D, et al. Case report: lung disease in World Trade Center responders exposed to dust and smoke: carbon nanotubes found in the lungs of World Trade Center patients and dust samples. *Environ Health Perspect.* (2010) 118:499–504. doi: 10.1289/ehp.0901159

Langley RJ, Mishra NC, Pena-Philippides JC, Rice BJ, Seagrave JC, Singh SP, et al. Fibrogenic and redox-related but not proinflammatory genes are upregulated in Lewis rat model of chronic silicosis. *J Toxicol Environ Health A.* (2011) 74:1261–79. doi: 10.1080/15287394.2011.595669

Sellares J, Strambu I, Crouser ED, Freudenberg MA, Gulati M, Hart S, et al. New advances in the development of sarcoidosis models: a synopsis of a symposium sponsored by the foundation for sarcoidosis research. *Sarcoidosis Vasc Diffuse Lung Dis.* (2018) 35:2–4.

5

Identification of the Core MicroRNAs and Potential Molecular Mechanisms in Sarcoidosis using Bioinformatics Analysis

Yuan Cao[1†], *Hua Zhang*[2†], *Lulu Zheng* [1] *and Qiao Li*[3*]

[1] Department of Pulmonary and Critical Care Medicine, The Second Affiliated Hospital of Xi'an Jiaotong University (Xibei Hospital), Xi'an, China, [2] Department of Respiratory Medicine, Zhangjiakou First Hospital, Zhangjiakou, China, [3] Clinical Laboratory, The Affiliated Children Hospital of Xi'an Jiaotong University, Xi'an, China

Correspondence:
Qiao Li
liqiao@csu.edu.cn

† These authors have contributed equally to this work and share first authorship

Sarcoidosis is a systemic heterogeneous inflammatory disease; however, the etiology and pathogenesis of sarcoidosis are still unknown. Herein, we investigated the core microRNAs and potential molecular mechanisms in sarcoidosis. The DE-miRNAs were diagnosed using the LIMMA software package. DIANA-mirPath was employed to perform pathway and GO enrichment analysis of the DE-miRNAs. PPI networks and miRNA-target gene regulatory networks were used to obtain insight into the actions of DE-miRNAs. Expression of the hub genes along with miRNAs was validated in clinical specimens. Overall, 266 DE-miRNAs were screened. Among these DE-miRNAs, hsa-miR-144, hsa-miR-126, as well as hsa-miR-106a were the upmost upregulated miRNAs; hsa-miR-151-3p, hsa-miR-320d, and hsa-miR-324-3p were the top downregulated miRNAs. *NR3C1*, *ZBTB7A*, *NUFIP2*, *BZW1*, *ERGIC2*, and *VEGFA* were mapped as the most targeted hub genes in the upregulation of miRNAs, and *MCL1* and *SAE1* were the most targeted hub genes in the downregulation of miRNA. *VEGFA* and *NR3C1* were selected and potentially modulated by hsa-miR-20b, hsa-miR-126, and hsa-miR-106a. In sarcoidosis pathological tissue, hsa-miR-126 was highly expressed, and VEGFA and NR3C1 were overexpressed. In conclusion, our results revealed the dysregulation of hsa-miR-126 and a potential regulatory mechanism for pathogenesis in sarcoidosis.

Keywords: sarcoidosis, bioinformatics analysis, microRNA-126, VEGFA, NR3C1

INTRODUCTION

Sarcoidosis is a systemic heterogeneous inflammatory disease that usually leads to a multisystemic granulomatous disorder (Iannuzzi et al., 2007; Jain et al., 2020). It can affect any organ; however, at least 90% of cases occur in intrathoracic lymph nodes, as well as the lungs (Ungprasert et al., 2019). The annual incidence of sarcoidosis changes with race and ethnicity and is highest in African Americans (17 to 35/100,000) and lowest in Asians (1/100,000). However, the incidence may be underestimated, as almost 50% of the sarcoidosis patients are asymptomatic, especially those in the early stage of the disease. Epidemiologic studies have reported that the maximum incidence of sarcoidosis occurs in female non-smokers with an average age of 30 (Jain et al., 2020).

The characteristic pathologic lesion of pulmonary sarcoidosis is a non-necrotizing granuloma (Iannuzzi et al., 2007). The etiology and pathogenesis of sarcoidosis are still unknown, and genetic susceptibility, autoimmunity, and environmental factors are all considered to be involved in the development of sarcoidosis.

MicroRNAs (miRNAs) are small, single-stranded, non-coding RNAs approximately 22 nucleotides long, some of which have been discovered to perform significant modulatory functions in animals through targeting the messages of protein-coding genes for translational inhibition. Research has documented that changes in the expression levels of miRNAs participate in multiple pathologies, as well as diseases. A previous study evaluated the expression trend of multiple miRNAs in sarcoidosis, and selected miRNAs were identified. However, regulatory miRNAs, their target genes, and the correlated protein expression have seldom been explored (Pattnaik et al., 2020). In this regard, we examined the microarray data of the gene expression profile of GSE26409 by a series of biological informatics approaches. The potential target genes of the upmost up-regulated, as well as down-regulated miRNAs were prognosticated by miRTarBase, and their potential functions were evaluated by DIANA-mirPath. Then, a protein–protein interaction (PPI) and miRNA-gene modulatory network were established by Cytoscape. Moreover, we validated the expression status of these hub genes and their modulated microRNAs in sarcoidosis samples by immunohistochemistry (IHC) along with fluorescence *in situ* hybridization (FISH). Based on a gene chip array, we used biological information technology to reveal the potential pathway in the etiology of sarcoidosis and yield additional information for its diagnosis, prognosis and treatment.

MATERIALS AND METHODS

Microarray Data

The microarray GSE26409 cohort was selected for further study and abstracted from the National Center for Biotechnology Information GEO (Gene Expression Omnibus) website[1], which is available online. This data set was based on the GPL9040 platform (febit Homo Sapiens miRBase 13.0) and included 45 samples from sarcoidosis patients and 55 from normal controls.

Screening for DE-miRNAs

First, normalization of the downloaded data was performed using the Normalize Between Array function in the Bioconductor R package "LIMMA" (available online: http://www.bioconductor.org/). Then, the unpaired Student's t-test was employed in comparing the sarcoidosis group with the control group. The cut-off criterion for screening differentially expressed miRNAs (DE-miRNAs) were $p < 0.05$ along with $|$ fold change (FC)$| > 1$. Additionally, the GEO2R online analytic tool based on GEO data platform was employed further to validate the DE-miRNAs.

[1]http://www.ncbi.nlm.nih.gov/geo

Prediction of Target Genes of DE-miRNAs

MiRTarBase (available online: http://mirtarbase.mbc.nctu.edu.tw/php/index.php) is extensively employed to search for miRNA target genes. The microRNA-target interactions in this database were experimentally validated. Herein, miRTarBase was employed to identify the target genes of DE-miRNAs.

GO Annotation and KEGG Pathway Enrichment Analyses of DE-miRNAs

DIANA-mirPath (available online: https://microrna.gr/miRPathv3/) constitutes a miRNA pathway analysis web-platform that provides accurate statistics and at the same time accommodates advanced pipelines (Vlachos et al., 2015). The functional, as well as pathway enrichment of the candidate miRNAs were explored and annotated by mirPath v2.0 based on the database Tarbase v7. The GO (Gene Ontology) was annotated through the DIANA-mirPath online tool on the selected DE-miRNAs. The KEGG (Kyoto Encyclopedia of Genes and Genomes) pathway analysis of DE-miRNAs was also performed by using DIANA-mirPath. $p < 0.05$ signified statistical significance.

PPI Network Integration

To analyze the connection among proteins, the identify target genes of the upmost 5 most up and downregulated DE-miRNAs were uploaded to the STRING data resource[2], and the results were visualized in Cytoscape 3.7.1 (Damian et al., 2015). Furthermore, we screened the significant nodes or hub genes based on degree, and then the miRNA-hub gene networks were mapped with Cytoscape 3.7.1.

Immunohistochemistry (IHC)

Immunohistochemistry was used to further validate the paraffin sections of mediastinal lymph node tissues from pulmonary sarcoidosis patients and tuberculosis patients (control group), which came from the Second Affiliated Hospital of Xi'an Jiaotong University, with ethical approval. All specimens were obtained by endobronchial ultrasound-guided transbronchial needle aspiration (EBUS-TBNA), and all the patients in the study group and the control group have been screened, and those with cardiovascular and cerebrovascular diseases, endocrine, infectious diseases, tumor diseases, etc., have been excluded. The diagnosis was made based on guidelines (Costabel and Hunninghake, 1999). The tissue paraffin sections were first deparaffinized with dimethylbenzene and ethyl alcohol for 15 min, repaired by boiling for 8 min in the repairing solution with EDTA (pH 9.0), digested for 10 min by 3% H_2O_2 at 37°C, washed with PBS solution and blocked for 30 min with 3% BSA at room temperature (RT). Afterward, the sections were overnight-incubated with the primary antibody (NR3C1, VEGFA) at 4°C (Abcam, Cambridge, United States). The next day, the tissues were inoculated with the horseradish-peroxidase (HRP) and incubated at RT for 60 min and incubated with diaminobenzidine

[2]http://string-db.org/

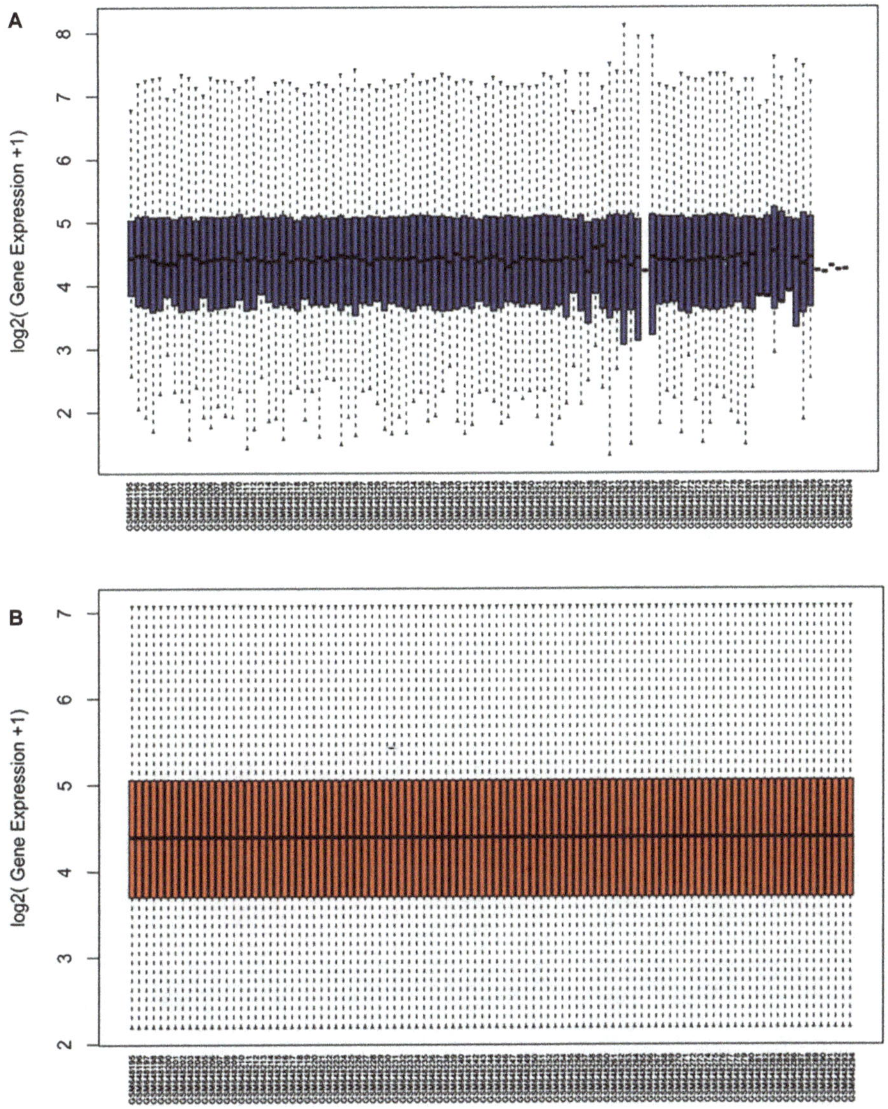

FIGURE 1 | Normalization of dataset GSE26409 **(A)** raw data of GSE26409; **(B)** standardization of GSE26409.

(DAB) color liquid after washing. Afterward, the tissues were counterstained using Harris hematoxylin, 1% hydrochloric acid alcohol, and lithium carbonate blue sequentially, and then visualized using an optical microscope (10×, 40×, Nikon, Japan) after routine cleaning and drying.

Fluorescence *in situ* Hybridization (FISH)

In situ hybridization was carried out on the clinical samples using a FISH kit (Servicebio, Wuhan, China). First, tissue paraffin sections were deparaffinated with dimethylbenzene and 100% ethyl alcohol for 15 min, repaired by boiling for 8 min, digested by protein kinase K at 37°C for 10 min, washed 2× with a saline-sodium citrate (2× SSC) solution and dried before hybridization. Then, the prepared tissues were prehybridized at 37°C for 60 min, and hybridized with a hsa-miR-126, hsa-miR-20b, or hsa-miR-106a oligodeoxynucleotide probe (Shenggong, Shanghai, China) in the hybridization solution at 37°C overnight in the dark. Hsa-miR-126 probe: 5′-FAM-UCGUACCGUGAGUAAUAAUGCG-FAM-3′ (Entrez Gene 574032, Xq26.2); hsa-miR-20b probe: 5′-FAM- CTACCTG CACTATGAGCACTTTG-FAM-3′ (Entrez Gene 406913, 9q3 4.3); hsa-miR-106a: 5′-FAM-ATCTGCACTGTCAGCACTTTA-FAM-3′ (Entrez Gene 406899, Xq26.2). The next day, the tissues were washed by 2× SSC solution and 3% BSA employed to block the tissues for 30 min at RT, then counterstained with anti-digoxigenin antibody and DAPI (4′,6-diamidino-2-phenylindole, dihydrochloride), all from Servicebio, and imaged using a fluorescence microscope (400×, Nikon, Japan) and measured using Image-J software at two to three fields after routine cleaning and drying. Mean fluorescence intensity (MFI) was calculated. All measured intensities were normalized to the respective channel in control tissues.

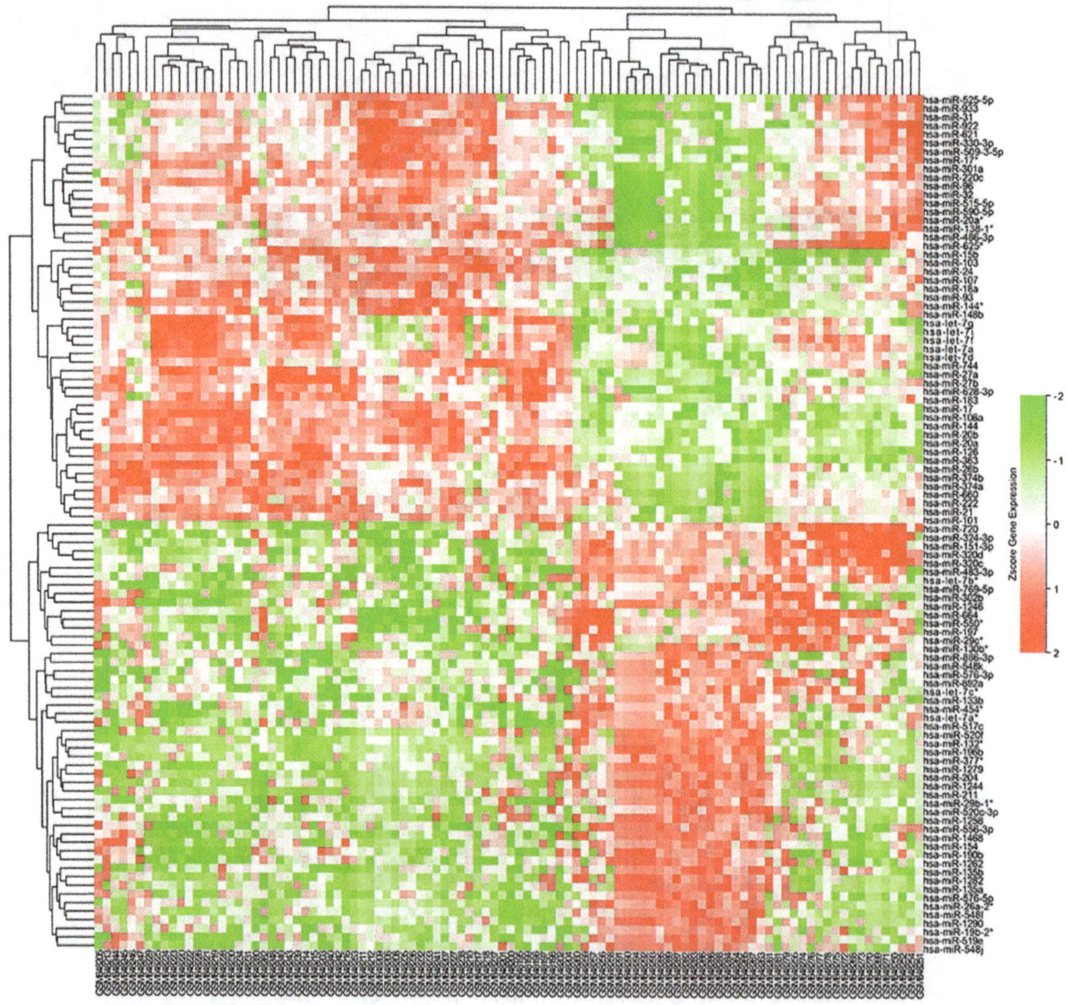

FIGURE 2 | Heatmap of DE-miRNAs: DE miRNAs (differentially expressed miRNAs) in 45 cases of sarcoidosis and 55 cases of normal controls.

RESULTS

Identification of DE-miRNAs and Prediction of Target Genes

The microarray GSE26409 cohort was acquired from the GEO website, and this cohort consisted of 45 cases of sarcoidosis (GSM648250-GSM648294) and 55 normal controls (GSM648195-GSM648249). After normalization (**Figure 1**), processing of the data was conducted via unpaired *t*-test, with the cutoff criterion of $P < 0.05$ along with $|\log2FC| > 1$). Overall, 266 DE-miRNAs were finally screened (**Figures 2, 3**), which constituted 132 and 134 upregulated and downregulated miRNAs, respectively. The top ten most upregulated, as well as downregulated miRNAs are indicated in **Table 1**. On the basis of the fold change (FC), hsa-miR-144, hsa-miR-126, and hsa-miR-106a were the upmost 3 upregulated miRNAs and hsa-miR-151-3p, hsa-miR-320d, and hsa-miR-324-3p were the upmost 3 downregulated miRNAs. For the three upregulated miRNAs, 580 potential target genes were investigated, and 543 genes were predicted for the 3 downregulated miRNAs via the miRTarBase platform.

Functional Enrichment Analysis

To determine the enriched pathways and process enrichment of these target genes, we afterward carried out a KEGG pathway enrichment and GO functional annotation. The KEGG pathway analysis included non-small cell lung cancer, proteoglycans in cancer, viral carcinogenesis, *etc.* (**Figure 4A**, **Table 2**). We selected 3 GO categories consisting of biological pathway (BP), cellular component (CC), along with molecular function (MF) for functional annotation. The top ten GO terms of the target genes of the 10 upmost up-regulated DE-miRNAs are indicated in **Figures 4B–D** and **Table 3**, including the responses to stress, catabolic process, gene expression, *etc.* in the BP category; cellular component, nucleoplasm, cytosol, *etc.* in the CC category; and enzyme binding, nucleic acid binding transcription factor activity, RNA binding, *etc.* in the MF category. Subsequently, the target genes of the ten

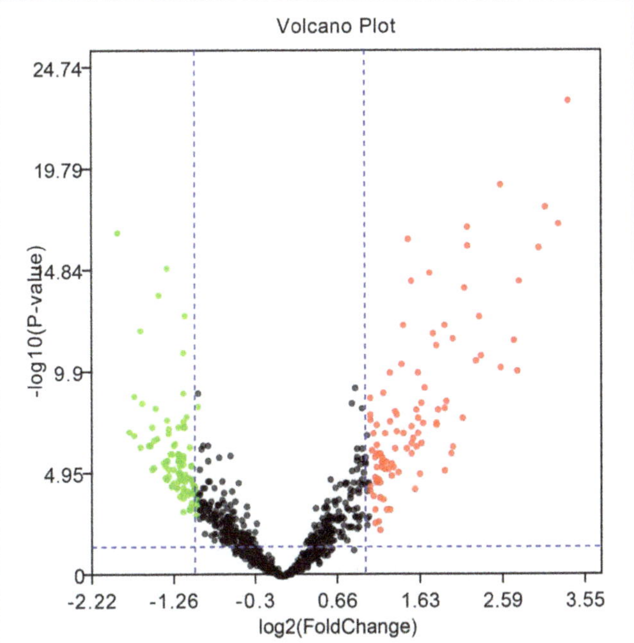

FIGURE 3 | Volcano diagram of the DE-miRNAs. The black dots designate the genes with no remarkable difference. The red dots and green dots designate up-regulated and down-regulated genes selected according to | fold change| > 1.0 along with a corrected $p < 0.05$.

upmost downregulated DE-miRNAs were analyzed in the same way, and the results are shown in **Figures 5A–D** and **Tables 4, 5.**

Development and Analysis of the PPI Network and miRNA-Target Network

The STRING online data resource was used to develop the PPI network complex of the filtered target genes of the 5 upmost upregulated and downregulated miRNAs. By using Cystoscope software, the hub nodes were screened out and further developed the miRNA-hub gene network (**Supplementary Figures 1, 2**). After simplification, a concise relationship between miRNAs and hub genes was achieved. As shown in **Figure 6A**, *NR3C1*, *ZBTB7A*, *NUFIP2*, *BZW1*, *ERGIC2*, *VEGFA*, *BTG2*, and *BCL2L11* were the eight most targeted hub genes in the upregulation of miRNAs. Among these, four hub genes could potentially be modulated by the upregulation of hsa-miR-144. Six hub genes and eight hub genes could potentially be modulated by hsa-miR-126 and hsa-miR-106a, respectively. Eight and five hub genes could potentially be modulated by hsa-miR-20b and hsa-miR-363, respectively. Moreover, *MCL1* and *SAE1* were the two most targeted hub genes in the downregulation of miRNA. *MCL1* could potentially be targeted by hsa-miR-30d, hsa-miR-320d, and hsa-miR-151-3p; *SAE1* could potentially be regulated by hsa-miR-324-3p, hsa-miR-30d, as well as hsa-miR-151-3p (**Figure 6B**).

To further identify reliable hub genes, the targeted hub genes of miRNAs were screened in the gene nodes of the PPI network, and only two overlapping genes (*NR3C1*, *VEGFA*) were found with a relatively high degree (19 and 18, respectively) in the up and downregulated hub genes. After combining the above results, *NR3C1* and *VEGFA* were selected and potentially modulated by hsa-miR-126, hsa-miR-20b, and hsa-miR-106a. Of note, these three miRNAs might be potential regulators in manipulating the pathogenesis and development of sarcoidosis.

TABLE 1 | Top ten up-regulated and down-regulated differentially expressed miRNAs between sarcoidosis and normal control.

Row names(tT)	logFC	AveExpr	*t*	*P* Value	Adj. *P* Val	B	Regulated
hsa-miR-144	3.550863	9.313051	13.49568	9.40E-25	4.05E-22	45.78095	Up-Regulated
hsa-miR-126	3.320719	9.096936	13.12656	5.97E-24	1.72E-21	43.9572	Up-Regulated
hsa-miR-106a	2.530724	11.62744	11.24603	8.78E-20	1.90E-17	34.4828	Up-Regulated
hsa-miR-20b	3.063342	10.19364	10.80117	8.78E-19	1.52E-16	32.20948	Up-Regulated
hsa-miR-363	3.221189	10.27816	10.42804	6.08E-18	8.75E-16	30.29805	Up-Regulated
hsa-miR-15b	1.469123	13.24834	10.08452	3.62E-17	3.47E-15	28.53664	Up-Regulated
hsa-miR-103	2.156385	11.94484	9.951238	7.24E-17	6.25E-15	27.85326	Up-Regulated
hsa-miR-20a	2.986091	10.55733	9.923751	8.35E-17	6.55E-15	27.71235	Up-Regulated
hsa-miR-27a	1.718716	7.379181	9.366076	1.51E-15	1.00E-13	24.85707	Up-Regulated
hsa-miR-17	2.75136	11.48185	9.189665	3.75E-15	2.31E-13	23.95629	Up-Regulated
hsa-miR-151-3p	−2.12643	9.873969	−13.827	1.81E-25	1.56E-22	47.40578	Down-Regulated
hsa-miR-320d	−1.93278	10.06991	−10.2473	1.56E-17	1.68E-15	29.37113	Down-Regulated
hsa-miR-324-3p	−1.36532	9.917577	−9.47768	8.45E-16	6.08E-14	25.42768	Down-Regulated
hsa-miR-720	−1.46921	12.4055	−8.86408	2.02E-14	1.02E-12	22.29872	Down-Regulated
hsa-miR-30d	−1.15751	13.04519	−8.42283	1.94E-13	9.15E-12	20.06631	Down-Regulated
hsa-miR-550	−1.67819	9.709234	−8.11338	9.40E-13	3.69E-11	18.51341	Down-Regulated
hsa-miR-132	−2.22146	4.350623	−7.72266	6.76E-12	2.16E-10	16.57212	Down-Regulated
hsa-miR-320b	−1.17778	11.65868	−7.62165	1.12E-11	3.46E-10	16.07431	Down-Regulated
hsa-miR-30c	−1.16476	11.15127	−6.68633	1.11E-09	2.51E-08	11.56764	Down-Regulated
hsa-miR-483-3p	−1.75494	5.540333	−6.5849	1.80E-09	3.78E-08	11.09214	Down-Regulated

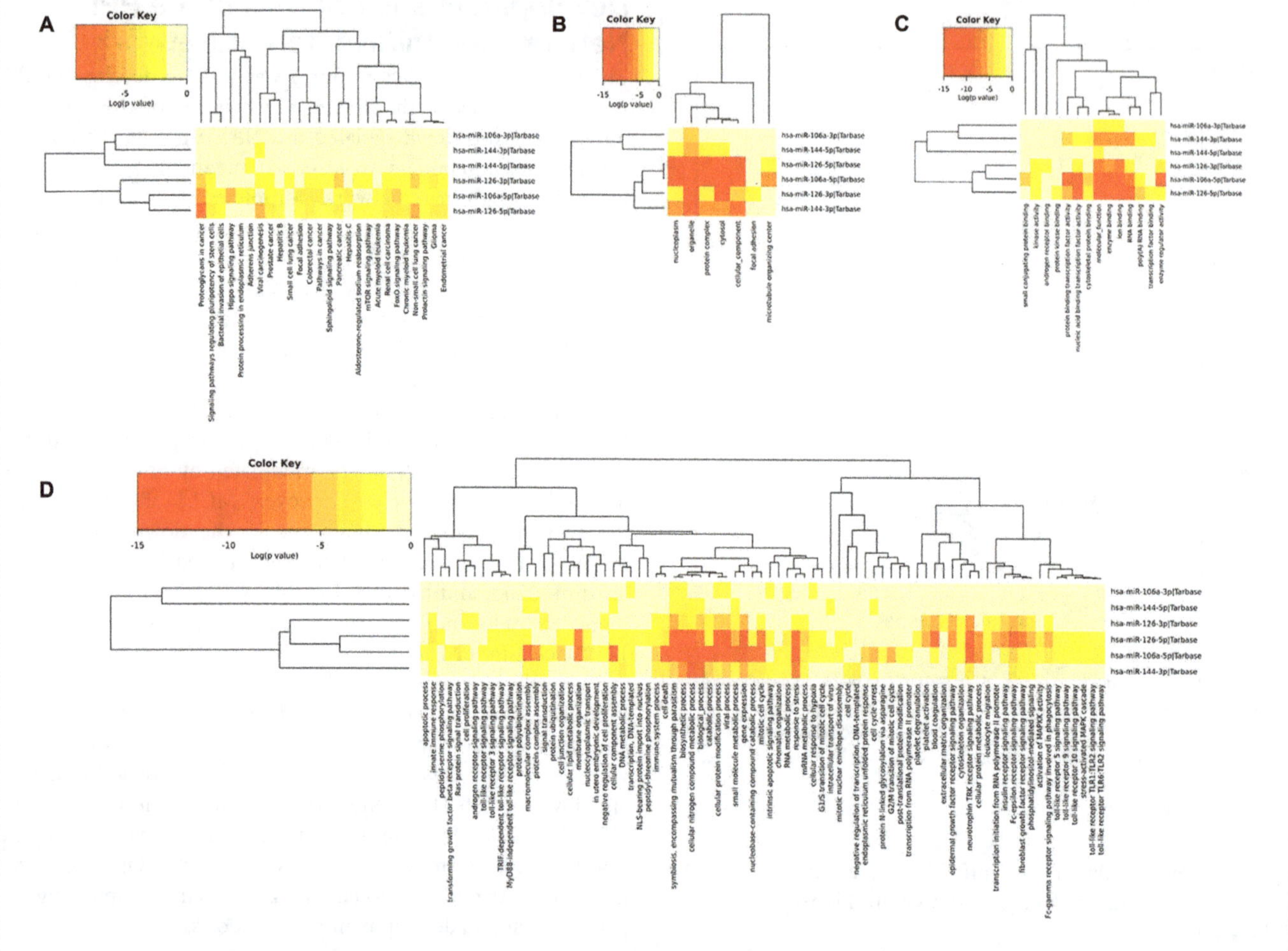

FIGURE 4 | Functional enrichment of the target genes of the upmost 10 most up-regulated miRNAs. **(A)** enriched Kyoto encyclopedia of genes and genomes (KEGG) pathways of these target genes; **(B)** enriched cellular component (CC) of these target genes; **(C)** enriched molecular function (MF) of these target genes, **(D)** enriched biological process (BP) of these target genes.

Verification of the Expression of Hub Genes and miRNAs in Clinical Specimens

To validate the expression of *VEGFA* and *NR3C1*, we performed IHC to examine 12 mediastinal lymph node tissues from pulmonary sarcoidosis patients and 13 mediastinal lymph node tissues from tuberculosis patients. Ten of the twelve sections showed moderate to strong dark brown staining of VEGFA in both the epithelioid cells and lymphocytes (**Figures 7C,D**), and negative to very weak staining for control group (**Figures 7A,B**). Nine of the twelve sections presented weak to moderate staining expression of NR3C1 (**Figures 7G,H**) comparing the control sections which present negative to very weak staining (**Figures 7E,F**).

The expression contents of hsa-miR-126, hsa-miR-20b, and hsa-miR-106a were further analyzed via FISH on the 12 mediastinal lymph node tissues of pulmonary sarcoidosis patients versus the 13 control tissues. Typical results were shown in **Figure 8**. The staining revealed strong enrichment of hsa-miR-126 along the edge of the non-caseating granulomas (**Figure 8B**), presenting higher expression than the controls (**Figure 8A**), while hsa-miR-20b (**Figures 8D,E**) and hsa-miR-106a had low expression (**Figures 8G,H**) in both groups. Quantification of fluorescence for hsa-miR-126, hsa-miR-20b, and hsa-miR-106a were measured, and it demonstrated that hsa-miR-126 significantly increased in mediastinal lymph node tissues of pulmonary sarcoidosis patients (**Figures 8C,F,I**).

DISCUSSION

Sarcoidosis, a multisystem disease, is typified by non-caseating granulomas. Up to 50% of sarcoidosis cases are diagnosed by chest radiographs during a routine examination. Clinically, approximately 1/4 of pulmonary sarcoidosis cases are atypical with non-specific clinical symptoms, atypical radiological manifestations, and non-unique pathology, which easily lead to misdiagnosis (Aryal and Nathan, 2019). The etiology and pathogenesis are still uncertain. Although intensive studies have revealed genetic factors, inflammation, and immune responses in the risk and clinical development of sarcoidosis, the regulation

TABLE 2 | KEGG pathway analysis of unregulated DE-miRNAs in sarcoidosis.

KEGG pathway	*p*-value	Genes	miRNAs
Proteoglycans in cancer (hsa05205)	7.77E-16	PIK3R2, PIK3CD, CTNNB1, AKT1, PIK3CA, SDC2, VEGFA, MAPK1, ITGB1, PTCH1, WNT5A, PIK3R2, FRS2, RDX, KRAS, FZD4, PIK3CD, CCND1, CTNNB1, AKT1, FLNB, GAB1, PIK3CA, SDC2, PDPK1, VEGFA, MAPK1, GRB2, MDM2, RPS6KB1, PDCD4, ITGB1, EZR, CBL, NRAS, CAV1, ROCK2, FRS2, IGF1R, RHOA, PPP1R12B, CAV2, FZD3, PPP1R12A, CCND1, CTNNB1, FLNB, TIMP3, PIK3R1, SOS1, DDX5, GAB1, AKT3, CDKN1A, VEGFA, MAPK1	hsa-miR-126-3p, hsa-miR-126-5p, hsa-miR-106a-5p
Viral carcinogenesis (hsa05203)	8.91E-08	CCND2, YWHAB, DDX3X, CASP3, JUN, EP300, USP7, HIST2H2BE, GTF2A1, PIK3R2, HIST1H2BD, PIK3CD, GTF2H3, CCNE1, PIK3CA, IL6ST, HDAC8, MAPK1, ATF2, RASA2, DLG1, PIK3R2, CDK1, KRAS, CDK6, PMAIP1, PIK3CD, CCND1, YWHAZ, HDAC2, RBPJ, ACTN4, CCNE1, PIK3CA, USP7, MAPK1, CREBBP, GRB2, JAK1, MDM2, CCND3	hsa-miR-144-3p, hsa-miR-126-3p, hsa-miR-126-5p
Non-small cell lung cancer (hsa05223)	4.87E-07	E2F1, PIK3R2, PIK3CD, E2F3, AKT1, PIK3CA, MAPK1, RXRA, PIK3R2, KRAS, CDK6, PIK3CD, CCND1, E2F3, AKT1, PIK3CA, PDPK1, MAPK1, GRB2, E2F1, NRAS, STK4, CCND1, PIK3R1, RB1, SOS1, AKT3, MAPK1, RASSF5	hsa-miR-126-3p, hsa-miR-126-5p, hsa-miR-106a-5p
Pancreatic cancer (hsa05212)	5.51E-06	E2F1, PIK3R2, PIK3CD, E2F3, AKT1, PIK3CA, VEGFA, MAPK1, PIK3R2, KRAS, CDK6, PIK3CD, CCND1, E2F3, AKT1, PIK3CA, VEGFA, MAPK1, TGFBR2, JAK1, STAT3, E2F1, SMAD3, CCND1, SMAD4, MAPK8, PIK3R1, RB1, AKT3, VEGFA, MAPK1, TGFBR2, JAK1	hsa-miR-126-3p, hsa-miR-126-5p, hsa-miR-106a-5p
Colorectal cancer (hsa05210)	9.75E-06	PIK3R2, PIK3CD, CTNNB1, AKT1, PIK3CA, MAPK1, GSK3B, PIK3R2, BCL2, KRAS, PIK3CD, CCND1, CTNNB1, AKT1, PIK3CA, MAPK1, TGFBR2, TCF7L1, SMAD3, RHOA, APPL1, CCND1, SMAD4, CTNNB1, MAPK8, PIK3R1, AKT3, LEF1, MAPK1, TGFBR2	hsa-miR-126-3p, hsa-miR-126-5p, hsa-miR-106a-5p
Glioma (hsa05214)	1.33E-05	PIK3R2, KRAS, CDK6, PIK3CD, CCND1, E2F3, AKT1, PIK3CA, MAPK1, GRB2, MDM2, PDGFRA, E2F1, NRAS, IGF1R, CCND1, PIK3R1, RB1, SOS1, AKT3, CDKN1A, MAPK1	hsa-miR-126-3p, hsa-miR-126-5p, hsa-miR-106a-5p
FoxO signaling pathway (hsa04068)	1.34E-05	IRS2, PIK3R2, STK11, PIK3CD, AKT1, PLK2, IRS1, PIK3CA, MAPK1, SGK1, IRS2, CCNB1, SIRT1, PIK3R2, KRAS, PIK3CD, CCND1, AKT1, IRS1, PRKAA1, BCL6, PRKAB2, SOD2, PIK3CA, USP7, PDPK1, MAPK1, CREBBP, GRB2, CCNG2, TGFBR2, MDM2, RBL2, STAT3, CCNB1, NRAS, STK4, SIRT1, SETD7, CCND2, STK11, SMAD3, IGF1R, NLK, CCND1, SMAD4, MAPK8, PLK2, PIK3R1, SOS1, IRS1, PRKAB2, CSNK1E, AKT3, SOD2, CDKN1A, MAPK1, CCNG2, TGFBR2	hsa-miR-126-3p, hsa-miR-126-5p,hsa-miR-106a-5p
Renal cell carcinoma (hsa05211)	1.64E-05	CRK, CUL2, PIK3R2, RAP1A, ETS1, KRAS, PIK3CD, AKT1, GAB1, PIK3CA, VEGFA, MAPK1, CREBBP, GRB2, NRAS, CRK, PAK2, ARNT, ETS1, EPAS1, EGLN3, PIK3R1, SOS1, GAB1, AKT3, VEGFA, MAPK1, EGLN1	hsa-miR-126-3p,hsa-miR-126-5p,hsa-miR-106a-5p
Chronic myeloid leukemia (hsa05220)	4.95E-05	E2F1, CRK, PIK3R2, CTBP2, PIK3CD, E2F3, AKT1, PIK3CA, MAPK1, KRAS, CDK6, CCND1, HDAC2, GRB2, TGFBR2, MDM2, CBL, NRAS, RUNX1, SMAD3, SMAD4, PIK3R1, RB1, SOS1, AKT3, CDKN1A	hsa-miR-126-3p, hsa-miR-126-5p, hsa-miR-106a-5p
Pathways in cancer (hsa05200)	5.12E-05	E2F1, CRK, PIK3R2, GNA13, ETS1, CTBP2, PIK3CD, CTNNB1, E2F3, AKT1, CCNE1, PIK3CA, ITGA6, VEGFA, MAPK1, ADCY9, RXRA, GSK3B, ITGB1, CRK, PTCH1, CUL2, WNT5A, PIK3R2, GNA13, ETS1, BCL2, KRAS, CDK6, FZD4, PIK3CD, CCND1, CTNNB1, E2F3, AKT1, HDAC2, CCNE1, PIK3CA, VEGFA, MAPK1, CREBBP, GRB2, TGFBR2, JAK1, MDM, STAT3, PDGFRA, E2F1, ITGB1, CXCL8, CBL, CXCR4, NRAS, STK4, CRK, RUNX1, ROCK2, TCF7L1, ARNT, ETS1, SMAD3, IGF1R, RHOA, APPL1, FZD3, TPM3, EPAS1, CCND1, SMAD4, CTNNB1, COL4A2, MAPK8, EGLN3, PIK3R1, RB1, SOS1, HSP90B1, AKT3, LEF1, CDKN1A, ITGA6, VEGFA, MAPK1, TGFBR2, JAK1, EGLN1, COL4A1, RASSF5	hsa-miR-126-3p, hsa-miR-126-5p, hsa-miR-106a-5p

of miRNAs is rarely involved. Our study indicated that multiple complex signal transduction pathways and factors participate in the pathogenic mechanisms of sarcoidosis. The microarray and bioinformatics analysis provides us with a comprehensive map of the biological functions and interactions of sarcoidosis-related genes, this will not only provide us with pivotal information to reveal the pathogenesis of the disease, but also help us to find novel preventive and therapeutic interventions.

Herein, we explored the gene expression profile of GSE26409 consisting of 45 sarcoidosis blood samples and 55 normal blood samples, to identify the molecular mechanism of sarcoidosis. Totally,266 DE-miRNAs were filtered, consisting of 132 upregulated and 134 downregulated miRNAs. Among these, hsa-miR-144, hsa-miR-126 along with hsa-miR-106a were the most upregulated miRNAs; hsa-miR-151-3p, hsa-miR-320d, and hsa-miR-324-3p were the most downregulated miRNAs. At the molecular level, prediction of the miRNA target genes was performed, then GO annotation and associated cascades were analyzed. Furthermore, by constructing the protein–protein interaction (PPI) networks, *NR3C1*, *ZBTB7A*, *NUFIP2*, *BZW1*, *ERGIC2*, *VEGFA*, *BTG2*, and *BCL2L11* were mapped as the most targeted hub genes in the upregulation of miRNAs, and *MCL1* and *SAE1* were the most targeted hub genes in the downregulation of miRNA. *NR3C1* and *VEGFA* were selected and are potentially modulated by hsa-miR-126, hsa-miR-20b, and hsa-miR-106a. To validate the bioinformatics analysis data, immunohistochemistry along with fluorescence *in situ* hybridization were employed to assess gene expression in clinical specimens. Among the identified miRNAs involved in sarcoidosis, hsa-miR-126 was highly expressed, and the two target genes VEGFA and NR3C1 were also highly expressed in lymph node samples of sarcoidosis.

TABLE 3 | GO analysis of unregulated DE-miRNAs associated with sarcoidosis.

GO Category	Gene function (Term)	Gene count	miRNAs	*p*-value
BP	Response to stress (GO:0006950)	313	hsa-miR-144-3p, hsa-miR-126-3p, hsa-miR-126-5p, hsa-miR-106a-5p	<1e-325
BP	Catabolic process (GO:0009056)	249	hsa-miR-144-3p, hsa-miR-126-3p, hsa-miR-126-5p, hsa-miR-106a-5p	<1e-325
BP	Gene expression (GO:0010467)	119	hsa-miR-144-3p, hsa-miR-126-3p, hsa-miR-126-5p, hsa-miR-106a-5p	<1e-325
BP	Fc-epsilon receptor signaling pathway (GO:0038095)	38	hsa-miR-144-3p, hsa-miR-126-3p, hsa-miR-126-5p, hsa-miR-106a-5p	<1e-325
BP	Neurotrophin TRK receptor signaling pathway (GO:0048011)	58	hsa-miR-144-3p, hsa-miR-126-3p, hsa-miR-126-5p, hsa-miR-106a-5p	<1e-325
BP	Cellular protein modification process (GO:0006464)	376	hsa-miR-144-3p, hsa-miR-126-3p, hsa-miR-126-5p, hsa-miR-106a-3p, hsa-miR-106a-5p	<1e-325
BP	Biological_process (GO:0008150)	1711	hsa-miR-144-3p, hsa-miR-144-5p, hsa-miR-126-3p, hsa-miR-126-5p, hsa-miR-106a-5p	<1e-325
BP	Viral process (GO:0016032)	101	hsa-miR-144-3p, hsa-miR-126-3p, hsa-miR-126-5p, hsa-miR-106a-3p, hsa-miR-106a-5p	<1e-325
BP	Cellular nitrogen compound metabolic process (GO:0034641)	647	hsa-miR-144-3p, hsa-miR-144-5p, hsa-miR-126-3p, hsa-miR-126-5p, hsa-miR-106a-5p	<1e-325
BP	biosynthetic process (GO:0009058)	536	hsa-miR-144-3p,hsa-miR-144-5p, hsa-miR-126-3p, hsa-miR-126-5p, hsa-miR-106a-3p, hsa-miR-106a-5p	< 1e-325
CC	cellular component (GO:0005575)	1729	hsa-miR-144-3p, hsa-miR-126-3p, hsa-miR-126-5p, hsa-miR-106a-5p	< 1e-325
CC	nucleoplasm (GO:0005654)	196	hsa-miR-144-3p, hsa-miR-144-5p, hsa-miR-126-3p, hsa-miR-126-5p, hsa-miR-106a-5p	< 1e-325
CC	cytosol (GO:0005829)	419	hsa-miR-144-3p, hsa-miR-144-5p, hsa-miR-126-3p, hsa-miR-126-5p, hsa-miR-106a-5p	< 1e-325
CC	protein complex (GO:0043234)	483	hsa-miR-144-3p, hsa-miR-144-5p, hsa-miR-126-3p, hsa-miR-126-5p, hsa-miR-106a-5p	< 1e-325
CC	organelle (GO:0043226)	1324	hsa-miR-144-3p, hsa-miR-144-5p, hsa-miR-126-3p, hsa-miR-126-5p, hsa-miR-106a-3p, hsa-miR-106a-5p	< 1e-325
CC	microtubule organizing center (GO:0005815)	64	hsa-miR-126-5p, hsa-miR-106a-5p	3.37E-06
CC	focal adhesion (GO:0005925)	13	hsa-miR-126-3p	0.013148
MF	nucleic acid binding transcription factor activity (GO:0001071)	161	hsa-miR-144-3p, hsa-miR-126-3p, hsa-miR-126-5p, hsa-miR-106a-5p	< 1e-325
MF	RNA binding (GO:0003723)	266	hsa-miR-144-3p, hsa-miR-126-3p, hsa-miR-126-5p, hsa-miR-106a-5p	< 1e-325
MF	enzyme binding (GO:0019899)	233	hsa-miR-144-3p, hsa-miR-126-3p, hsa-miR-126-5p, hsa-miR-106a-3p, hsa-miR-106a-5p	< 1e-325
MF	ion binding (GO:0043167)	756	hsa-miR-144-3p, hsa-miR-126-3p, hsa-miR-126-5p, hsa-miR-106a-3p, hsa-miR-106a-5p	< 1e-325
MF	molecular_function (GO:0003674)	1767	hsa-miR-144-3p, hsa-miR-144-5p, hsa-miR-126-3p, hsa-miR-126-5p, hsa-miR-106a-3p, hsa-miR-106a-5p	< 1e-325
MF	protein binding transcription factor activity (GO:0000988)	90	hsa-miR-144-3p, hsa-miR-126-5p, hsa-miR-106a-5p	2.22E-16
MF	enzyme regulator activity (GO:0030234)	109	hsa-miR-126-3p, hsa-miR-126-5p, hsa-miR-106a-5p	3.56E-12
MF	poly(A) RNA binding (GO:0044822)	205	hsa-miR-144-3p, hsa-miR-126-5p, hsa-miR-106a-5p	6.95E-08
MF	cytoskeletal protein binding (GO:0008092)	102	hsa-miR-144-3p, hsa-miR-126-5p, hsa-miR-106a-5p	1.82E-07
MF	transcription factor binding (GO:0008134)	46	hsa-miR-144-3p, hsa-miR-126-5p	0.000592

The GO annotation and KEGG pathway analysis have identified more cancer related pathways that were closely related to upregulated DE-miRNAs in sarcoidosis, which including proteoglycans in cancer, viral carcinogenesis, non-small cell lung cancer, pancreatic cancer, colorectal cancer, glioma, etc. The relationship between sarcoidosis

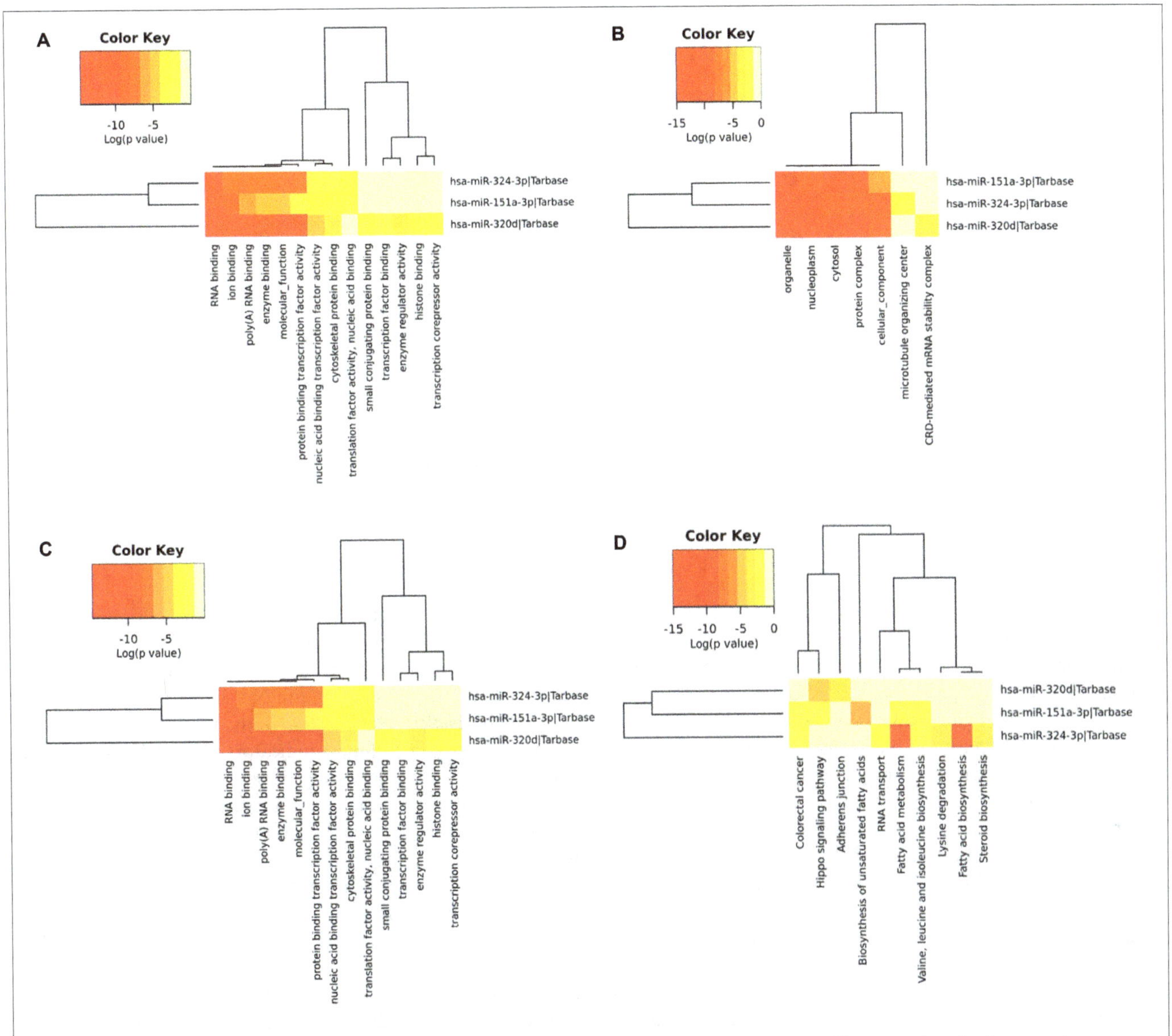

FIGURE 5 | Functional enrichment of the target genes of the upmost ten most down-regulated miRNAs. **(A)** enriched Kyoto encyclopedia of genes and genomes (KEGG) pathways of these target genes; **(B)** enriched cellular component (CC) of these target genes; **(C)** enriched molecular function (MF) of these target genes; **(D)** enriched biological process (BP) of these target genes.

and cancer is complex, and meta-analyses have concluded that an increased risk of neoplasia in sarcoidosis (El Jammal et al., 2020). Fatty acid biosynthesis and metabolism also participated in the biological functions of miRNA in sarcoidosis. The mismatch of myocardial fatty acid metabolism and myocardial perfusion under positron emission tomography computed tomography (PET-CT) could diagnosis and detection of myocardial injury in cardiac sarcoidosis (Momose et al., 2015).

VEGFA (Vascular endothelial growth factor-A) is a PDGF/VEGF growth factor family member, and by triggering the proliferation, as well as the migration of vascular endothelial cells, it is vital for physiological and pathological of angiogenesis (Tamura et al., 2019). A previous clinical study confirmed that the serum levels of VEGF were higher in sarcoidosis subjects than in normal controls (Mirsaeidi et al., 2018). Further research evaluated the VEGFA level in serum, as well as bronchoalveolar lavage (BAL) and found similar results: VEGFA was remarkably higher in individuals with sarcoidosis relative to the healthy controls ($p = 0.0002$). The results also showed that the immunoexpression of VEGFA was higher in serum in contrast to the BAL fluid. However, the levels of VEGFA had no correlation with the clinical phenotype (acute onset or insidious onset), stage, or lung function (Piotrowski et al., 2015). Immunohistochemistry analyses on VATS (video-assisted thoracoscopic surgery) lung biopsy samples of sarcoidosis lesions were very consistent with our findings that VEGF was upregulated compared to the control group (Tzouvelekis et al., 2012).

TABLE 4 | KEGG pathway analysis of downregulated DE-miRNAs in sarcoidosis.

KEGG pathway	*p*-value	Genes	miRNAs
Fatty acid biosynthesis (hsa00061)	<1e-325	FASN	hsa-miR-324-3p
Fatty acid metabolism (hsa01212)	1.12E-09	PTPLB, ELOVL5, SCD, ACACA, FASN, CPT2	hsa-miR-151a-3p, hsa-miR-324-3p
Hippo signaling pathway (hsa04390)	6.90E-05	APC, PPP2CA, PPP1CC, SNAI2, YWHAB, CCND1, SMAD4, PPP2CB, LATS1, PARD6B, PPP2CA, YWHAG, CCND2, GLI2, SMAD3, WWTR1, CDH1, CTNNB1, CSNK1E, WNT2, SMAD7, LATS1	hsa-miR-151a-3p, hsa-miR-320d
Biosynthesis of unsaturated fatty acids (hsa01040)	0.000417325	PTPLB, ELOVL5, SCD	hsa-miR-151a-3p
Colorectal cancer (hsa05210)	0.001949491	BRAF, APC, RHOA, PIK3R3, CCND1, SMAD4, MSH6, GSK3B, PIK3CB, BIRC5, CCND1, SMAD4, CTNNB1	hsa-miR-151a-3p, hsa-miR-324-3p
Adherens junction (hsa04520)	0.00509092	SMAD3, TJP1, CDH1, CTNNB1, RAC1, INSR, SSX2IP, MAPK1	hsa-miR-320d
RNA transport (hsa03013)	0.01706858	PAIP1, NUP160, EIF3B, NUP214, RNPS1, EIF2B3, EIF4B, EIF4G1, EEF1A1, NDC1, EIF4, BP2, NUP155, RAN, EIF4G2	hsa-miR-324-3p
Lysine degradation (hsa00310)	0.02839269	WHSC1L1, ALDH3A2, SETD2, ASH1L, KMT2C	hsa-miR-324-3p
Steroid biosynthesis (hsa00100)	0.02915267	DHCR24	hsa-miR-324-3p
Valine, leucine and isoleucine biosynthesis (hsa00290)	0.04059014	BCAT2	hsa-miR-151a-3p, hsa-miR-324-3p

NR3C1 (Nuclear receptor subfamily 3 group C member-1) codes for the glucocorticoid receptor and extensively participates in cellular proliferation, differentiation of target tissues, as well as inflammatory responses. Mutations that occurred in NR3C1 are related to generalized glucocorticoid resistance. Glucocorticoids (GCs) are the most common therapeutic agents in clinical use, and due to the fundamental regulatory roles in suppression of inflammation, GCs were widely used for autoimmune and inflammatory diseases (Gharesouran et al., 2018). GWAS (Genome-wide association studies) have found that SNPs (single nucleotide polymorphisms) located in *NR3C1* were positively replicated in the corticosteroid drug pathway of asthma (Keskin et al., 2019). After evaluating the SNPs of *NR3C1* in *in vivo* and *in vitro* models, the results showed that it was closely associated with hypersensitivity to glucocorticoids in asthma (Cuzzoni et al., 2012). In this study, *NR3C1* was upregulated in sarcoidosis and expressed in pathological specimens, which may be related to the sensitivity of sarcoidosis to glucocorticoid therapy. Simultaneously, we found that NR3C1 is not always highly expressed, which may be related to the insensitivity of some sarcoidosis patients to glucocorticoid treatment in clinical practice. It can finally be seen that the DNA polymorphism reflects the heterogeneity of the disease.

At present, the role of miRNA in sarcoidosis remains unclear. Kiszałkiewicz et al. investigated the expression of ten screened miRNAs in 94 pulmonary sarcoidosis patients and 50 controls, and remarkable differences were discovered between the sarcoidosis patients and healthy controls in the expression of diverse detected miRNAs in peripheral blood lymphocytes (miR-27b, miR-let-7f, miR-15b, miR-192, miR-130a miR-221, miR-222). Three miRNAs were merely reported to differ in BALF cells (miR-15b, miR-192, as well as miR-221) (Kiszałkiewicz et al., 2016). A subgroup analysis further observed several correlations among the levels of expression of miRNA, lung function parameters (FVC, FEV_1/FVC), and selected laboratory molecular markers (CD4+/CD8+, serum Ca^{2+} concentration). The results showed only gender was not related to the expression of miRNA in BALF (Kiszałkiewicz et al., 2016). Nevertheless, in our study, we did not evaluate the relationship of some clinical indicators to miRNAs expression. We summarized the following reasons. Firstly, the expression of miRNA in peripheral blood is affected by various factors throughout the body, so is the alveolar lavage fluid. For patients with lung infection, COPD, asthma, and tumors, the detected miRNA itself is not accurate enough, subsequently, error in correlation analysis is even greater. Secondly, for early stage sarcoidosis, the lung function is hardly affected, especially FVC, FEV1/FVC, and diffusion function parameters. And, changes in lung function cannot reflect the true situation of patients with sarcoidosis. Thirdly, our study is a retrospective study, not all included patients had lung function tests and samples of alveolar lavage fluid, thus, some of these parameters could not be tested.

To elucidate the function of miRNAs in sarcoidosis, Jazwa et al. (2015) compared the expression levels of selected inflammatory miRNAs in patients with sarcoidosis and healthy individuals. After screening the miRNA transcriptome, miR-34a was isolated from sarcoidosis patients in peripheral blood mononuclear cells, which suggested that it may be involved in the pathology of sarcoidosis. Additionally, miR-155 was shown to be one of the miRNAs that are differentially expressed in macrophages, which are considered to have a role in formation of granuloma in sarcoidosis (Zhang et al., 2013). A study on the mechanism of miRNA in pulmonary sarcoidosis proved that miR-34a along with miR-155 enhance the secretion of interferon-gamma and negatively modulate SIRT-1, therefore inhibiting NF-κB transcription, as well as deacetylate the p53 protein, ultimately inactivating

TABLE 5 | GO analysis of downregulated DE-miRNAs associated with sarcoidosis.

GO Category	Gene function (Term)	Gene count	miRNAs	*p*-value
BP	Cellular protein modification process (GO:0006464)	231	hsa-miR-151a-3p, hsa-miR-320d, hsa-miR-324-3p	<1e-325
BP	Biosynthetic process (GO:0009058)	363	hsa-miR-151a-3p, hsa-miR-320d, hsa-miR-324-3p	<1e-325
BP	Gene expression (GO:0010467)	110	hsa-miR-151a-3p, hsa-miR-320d, hsa-miR-324-3p	<1e-325
BP	Cellular nitrogen compound metabolic process (GO:0034641)	461	hsa-miR-151a-3p, hsa-miR-320d, hsa-miR-324-3p	<1e-325
BP	Symbiosis, encompassing mutualism through parasitism (GO:0044403)	72	hsa-miR-151a-3p, hsa-miR-320d, hsa-miR-324-3p	7.99E-14
BP	Viral process (GO:0016032)	65	hsa-miR-151a-3p, hsa-miR-320d, hsa-miR-324-3p	1.59E-13
BP	Mitotic cell cycle (GO:0000278)	57	hsa-miR-151a-3p, hsa-miR-320d, hsa-miR-324-3p	3.04E-12
BP	Cell death (GO:0008219)	104	hsa-miR-151a-3p, hsa-miR-320d, hsa-miR-324-3p	9.11E-12
BP	Neurotrophin TRK receptor signaling pathway (GO:0048011)	40	hsa-miR-151a-3p, hsa-miR-320d, hsa-miR-324-3p	4.37E-11
BP	Biological_process (GO:0008150)	1138	hsa-miR-151a-3p, hsa-miR-320d, hsa-miR-324-3p,	1.42E-10
CC	Cellular_component (GO:0005575)	1189	hsa-miR-151a-3p, hsa-miR-320d, hsa-miR-324-3p	<1e-325
CC	Nucleoplasm (GO:0005654)	157	hsa-miR-151a-3p, hsa-miR-320d, hsa-miR-324-3p	<1e-325
CC	Cytosol (GO:0005829)	279	hsa-miR-151a-3p, hsa-miR-320d, hsa-miR-324-3p	<1e-325
CC	Organelle (GO:0043226)	889	hsa-miR-151a-3p, hsa-miR-320d, hsa-miR-324-3p	<1e-325
CC	Protein complex (GO:0043234)	349	hsa-miR-151a-3p, hsa-miR-320d, hsa-miR-324-3p	<1e-325
CC	CRD-mediated mRNA stability complex (GO:0070937)	5	hsa-miR-320d	0.006458676
CC	Microtubule organizing center (GO:0005815)	20	hsa-miR-324-3p	0.00699504
MF	Protein binding transcription factor activity (GO:0000988)	73	hsa-miR-151a-3p, hsa-miR-320d, hsa-miR-324-3p	<1e-325
MF	Molecular_function (GO:0003674)	1174	hsa-miR-151a-3p, hsa-miR-320d, hsa-miR-324-3p	<1e-325
MF	RNA binding (GO:0003723)	223	hsa-miR-151a-3p, hsa-miR-320d, hsa-miR-324-3p	<1e-325
MF	Enzyme binding (GO:0019899)	144	hsa-miR-151a-3p, hsa-miR-320d, hsa-miR-324-3p	<1e-325
MF	Ion binding (GO:0043167)	478	hsa-miR-151a-3p, hsa-miR-320d, hsa-miR-324-3p	<1e-325
MF	Poly(A) RNA binding (GO:0044822)	195	hsa-miR-151a-3p, hsa-miR-320d, hsa-miR-324-3p	<1e-325
MF	Nucleic acid binding transcription factor activity (GO:0001071)	93	hsa-miR-151a-3p, hsa-miR-320d, hsa-miR-324-3p	7.76E-07
MF	Cytoskeletal protein binding (GO:0008092)	76	hsa-miR-151a-3p, hsa-miR-320d, hsa-miR-324-3p	1.46E-05
MF	Translation factor activity, nucleic acid binding (GO:0008135)	15	hsa-miR-151a-3p, hsa-miR-324-3p	0.000339
MF	Enzyme regulator activity (GO:0030234)	38	hsa-miR-320d	0.002755

p53-regulated transcription and apoptosis (Kachamakova-Trojanowska et al., 2018). On the other hand, by establishing a murine model, Barna et al. (2016) found that elevated miRNA-33 promoted the formation of granuloma through the inhibition of the alveolar macrophage lipid transporters ABCA1 and ABCG1.

In our study, the lymphatic tissue of tuberculosis patients was used as a control group. This is why we raise the

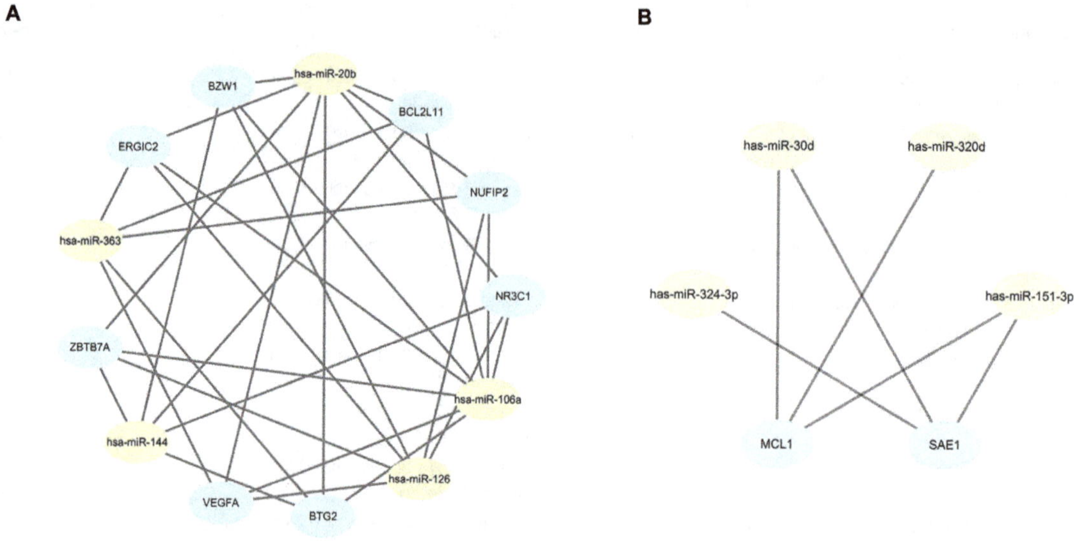

FIGURE 6 | Simplified miRNA-gene network. **(A)** miRNA-gene network of upregulated miRNAs after simplified by interaction at degree ≥ 4; **(B)** miRNA-gene network of downregulated miRNAs after simplified by interaction at degree ≥ 3.

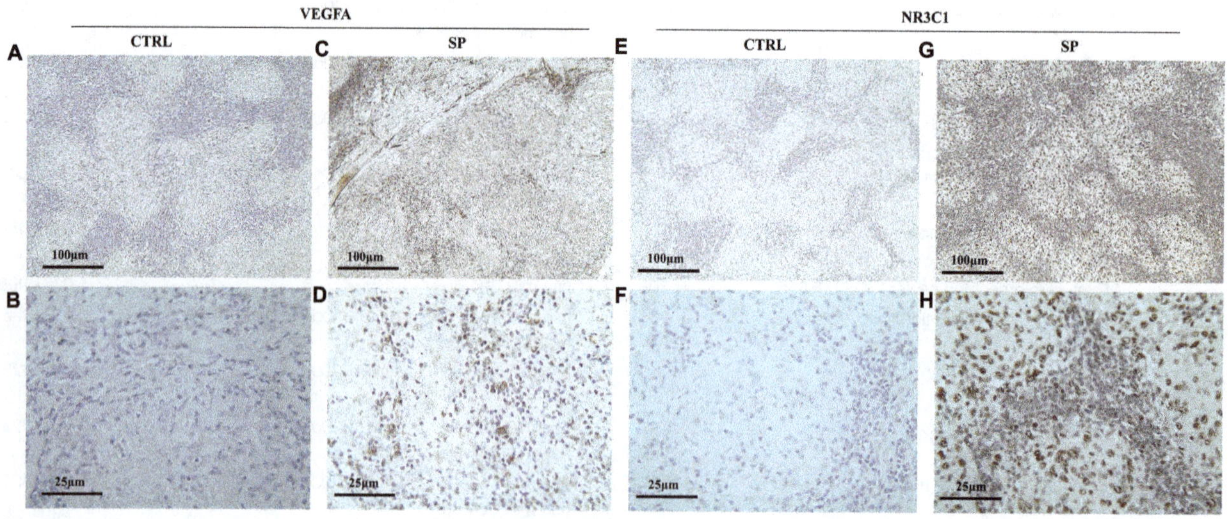

FIGURE 7 | Immunohistochemical methods were employed to assess the cellular localization and expression levels of NR3C1 and VEGFA in mediastinal lymph node tissues of pulmonary sarcoidosis (SP group, n = 12) and tuberculosis (CRTL group, n = 13). **(A–D)** VEGFA (+); **(E–H)** NR3C1 (+). (10×: ACEG; 40×: BDFH).

question from clinic and return to clinic through this research. Pulmonary sarcoidosis and tuberculosis are the most difficult to distinguish in clinical practice. Even if they have the gold standard of pathological diagnosis, it still needs experienced pathologists to give a definite diagnosis. Sometimes, for the small tissue, it can interfere with the definitive diagnosis of sarcoidosis. At the same time, the treatments for these two diseases are completely opposite. For treatment of sarcoidosis requires glucocorticoids, but the use of glucocorticoids for tuberculosis often causes the spread of disease. More significantly, the mediastinal lymph node of healthy people is not enlarged, and it is not available or difficult to obtain, which also violates ethical principles. Therefore, we used lymphatic tissue of tuberculosis as control group in this study.

There are still several limitations in this study. First of all, in the section of clinical specimen verification, the sample size we included is still small. Although immunohistochemistry and FISH have obtained positive results, a large sample study is still needed to further corroborate our results. Secondly, the specific regulatory mechanism of miR-126 in the pathogenesis and development of sarcoidosis still needs to be explored *in vitro* and *in vivo*. Finally, the incidence of sarcoidosis in different races is slightly different. In this study,

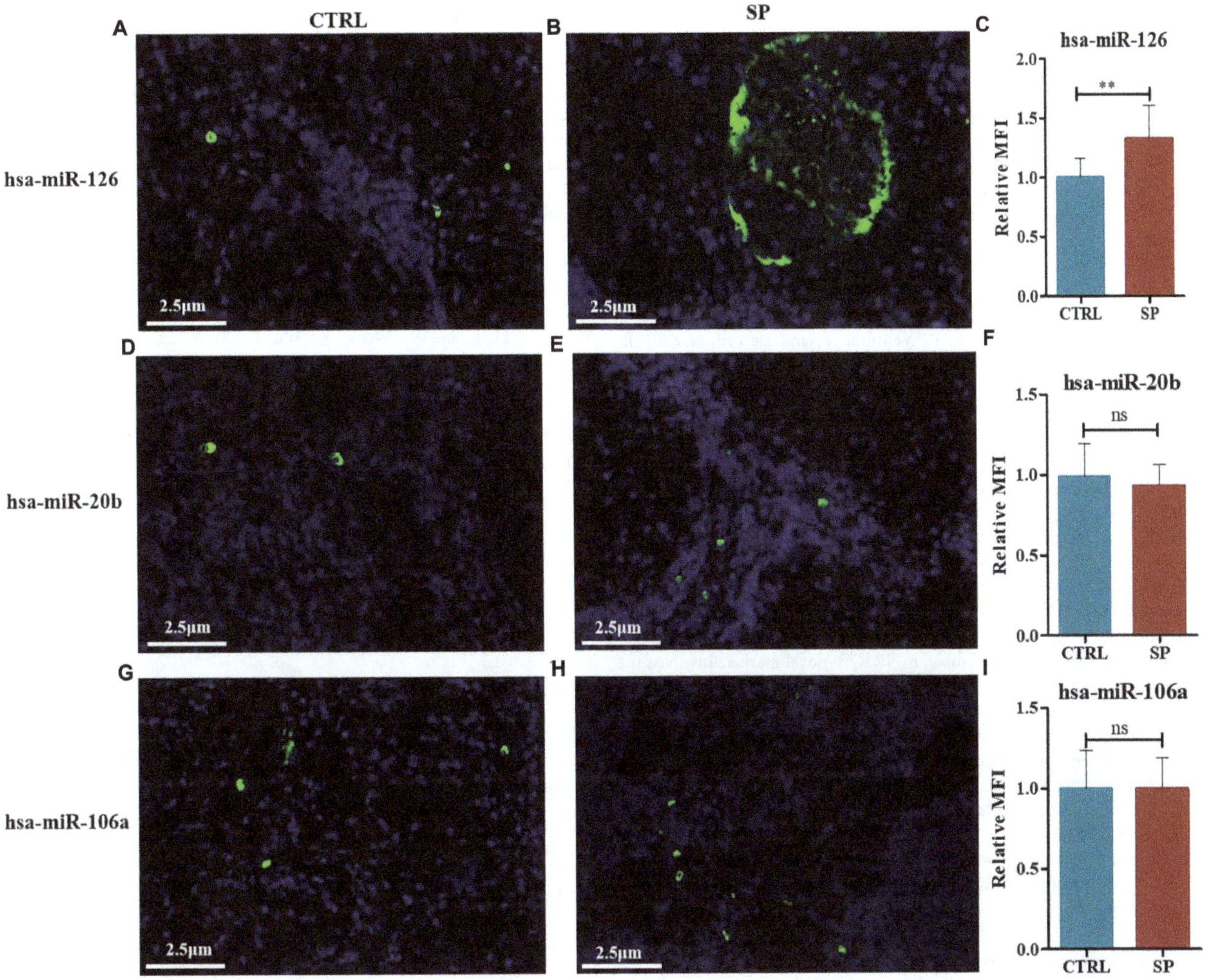

FIGURE 8 | FISH methods were conducted to detect the expression levels of hsa-miR-126, hsa-miR-20b, as well as hsa-miR-106a in mediastinal lymph node tissues of pulmonary sarcoidosis (SP group, $n = 12$, 400×) and tuberculosis (CRTL group, $n = 13$, 400×). **(A–C)** hsa-miR-126 (+); **(D–F)** hsa-miR-20b (+); **(G–I)**: hsa-miR-106a (+). Data have been represented as mean ± SD, $^{**}p < 0.01$. MFI: mean fluorescence; ns: no significant.

we only included Asian individuals. This may bring certain limitations to our results.

From our results, we found that VEGFA and NR3C1 were overexpressed in the pathological tissue of sarcoidosis, which was mainly regulated by hsa-miR-126. To our knowledge, miRNAs are small non-coding RNAs that function as negative gene expression regulators. However, emerging evidences have shown that its function was switching from repression to activation, and its gene-activation function can up-regulate translation in nuclear (Vasudevan et al., 2007; Xiao et al., 2017). The GO annotation of our study comprised the molecular function on current biological knowledge of miRNA in sarcoidosis, which showed nucleic acid binding transcription factor activity has a pronounced gene count. This novel finding was also worth exploring for the study of the role of miRNAs in the regulation of sarcoidosis.

In summary, this work sheds further light on understanding the pathogenesis of sarcoidosis and might indicate novel diagnostic markers and treatment targets in the clinical practice of sarcoidosis. Nevertheless, further studies should be conducted to clarify the role of miRNAs and their related pathways in the pathogenesis of sarcoidosis.

AUTHOR CONTRIBUTIONS

YC, HZ, and QL performed the experiments, contributed to data analyses, as well as wrote the manuscript. YC, HZ, and LZ conceptualized the study design, contributed equally to data analyses and experimental materials. All authors contributed to the article and approved the submitted version.

REFERENCES

Aryal, S., and Nathan, S. D. (2019). Contemporary optimized practice in the management of pulmonary sarcoidosis. *Ther. Adv. Respir. Dis.* 13:1753466619868935. doi: 10.1177/1753466619868935

Barna, B. P., Mcpeek, M., Malur, A., Fessler, M. B., Wingard, C. J., Dobbs, L., et al. (2016). Elevated MicroRNA-33 in sarcoidosis and a carbon nanotube model of chronic granulomatous disease. *Am. J. Respir. Cell Mol. Biol.* 54, 865–871. doi: 10.1165/rcmb.2015-0332OC

Costabel, U., and Hunninghake, G. W. (1999). ATS/ERS/WASOG statement on sarcoidosis. sarcoidosis statement committee. american thoracic society. European respiratory society. world association for sarcoidosis and other granulomatous disorders. *Eur. Respir. J.* 14, 735–737. doi: 10.1034/j.1399-3003.1999.14d02.x

Cuzzoni, E., De Iudicibus, S., Bartoli, F., Ventura, A., and Decorti, G. (2012). Association between BclI polymorphism in the NR3C1 gene and in vitro individual variations in lymphocyte responses to methylprednisolone. *Br. J. Clin. Pharmacol.* 73, 651–655. PMID:NOPMIDdoi: 10.1111/j.1365-2125.2011.04130.x

Damian, S., Andrea, F., Stefan, W., Kristoffer, F., Davide, H., Jaime, H. C., et al. (2015). STRING v10: protein-protein interaction networks, integrated over the tree of life. *J. Nucleic Acids Res.* 43:D447.

El Jammal, T., Pavic, M., Gerfaud-Valentin, M., Jamilloux, Y., and Sève, P. (2020). Sarcoidosis and cancer: a complex relationship. *Front. Med.* 7:594118. doi: 10.3389/fmed.2020.594118

Gharesouran, J., Taheri, M., Sayad, A., Ghafouri-Fard, S., Mazdeh, M., and Omrani, M. D. (2018). The growth arrest-specific transcript 5 (GAS5) and nuclear receptor subfamily 3 group C member 1 (NR3C1): novel markers involved in multiple sclerosis. *Int. J. Mol. Cell Med.* 7, 102–110. doi: 10.22088/ijmcm.Bums.7.2.102

Iannuzzi, M. C., Rybicki, B. A., and Teirstein, A. S. (2007). Sarcoidosis. *N. Engl. J. Med.* 357, 2153–2165. doi: 10.1056/NEJMra071714

Jain, R., Yadav, D., Puranik, N., Guleria, R., and Jin, J.-O. (2020). Sarcoidosis: causes, diagnosis, clinical features, and treatments. *J. Clin. Med.* 9:1081. doi: 10.3390/jcm9041081

Jazwa, A., Kasper, L., Bak, M., Sobczak, M., Szade, K., Jozkowicz, A., et al. (2015). Differential inflammatory microRNA and cytokine expression in pulmonary sarcoidosis. *Arch. Immunol. Ther. Exp.* 63, 139–146. doi: 10.1007/s00005-014-0315-9

Kachamakova-Trojanowska, N., Jazwa-Kusior, A., Szade, K., Kasper, L., Soja, J., Andrychiewicz, A., et al. (2018). Molecular profiling of regulatory T cells in pulmonary sarcoidosis. *J. Autoimmun.* 94, 56–69. doi: 10.1016/j.jaut.2018.07.012

Keskin, O., Farzan, N., Birben, E., Akel, H., Karaaslan, C., Maitland-Van Der Zee, A. H., et al. (2019). Genetic associations of the response to inhaled corticosteroids in asthma: a systematic review. *Clin. Transl. Allergy* 9:2. doi: 10.1186/s13601-018-0239-2

Kiszałkiewicz, J., Piotrowski, W. J., Pastuszak-Lewandoska, D., Górski, P., Antczak, A., Górski, W., et al. (2016). Altered miRNA expression in pulmonary sarcoidosis. *BMC Med. Genet.* 17:2. doi: 10.1186/s12881-016-0266-6

Mirsaeidi, M., Omar, H. R., Calzadilla, A., Khatib, A. E., Whitney, P., Sweiss, N., et al. (2018). Circulatory TGF-beta1 is significantly higher in early stage of pulmonary sarcoidosis. *Sarcoidosis Vasculitis Diffuse Lung Dis.* 35, 213–217. doi: 10.36141/svdld.v35i3.6112

Momose, M., Fukushima, K., Kondo, C., Serizawa, N., Suzuki, A., Abe, K., et al. (2015). Diagnosis and detection of myocardial injury in active cardiac sarcoidosis–significance of myocardial fatty acid metabolism and myocardial perfusion mismatch. *Circ. J.* 79, 2669–2676. doi: 10.1253/circj.CJ-15-0681

Pattnaik, B., Sryma, P. B., Mittal, S., Agrawal, A., Guleria, R., and Madan, K. (2020). MicroRNAs in pulmonary sarcoidosis: a systematic review. *Respir Investig.* 58, 232–238. doi: 10.1016/j.resinv.2020.02.008

Piotrowski, W. J., Kiszałkiewicz, J., Górski, P., Antczak, A., Górski, W., Pastuszak-Lewandoska, D., et al. (2015). Immunoexpression of TGF-β/Smad and VEGF-A proteins in serum and BAL fluid of sarcoidosis patients. *BMC Immunol.* 16:58. doi: 10.1186/s12865-015-0123-y

Tamura, R., Tanaka, T., Akasaki, Y., Murayama, Y., Yoshida, K., and Sasaki, H. (2019). The role of vascular endothelial growth factor in the hypoxic and immunosuppressive tumor microenvironment: perspectives for therapeutic implications. *Med. Oncol.* 37:2. doi: 10.1007/s12032-019-1329-2

Tzouvelekis, A., Ntolios, P., Karameris, A., Koutsopoulos, A., Boglou, P., Koulelidis, A., et al. (2012). Expression of hypoxia-inducible factor (HIF)-1a-vascular endothelial growth factor (VEGF)-inhibitory growth factor (ING)-4- axis in sarcoidosis patients. *BMC Res. Notes* 5:654. doi: 10.1186/1756-0500-5-654

Ungprasert, P., Ryu, J. H., and Matteson, E. L. (2019). Clinical manifestations, diagnosis, and treatment of sarcoidosis. *Mayo Clin. Proc. Innov. Qual. Outcomes* 3, 358–375. doi: 10.1016/j.mayocpiqo.2019.04.006

Vasudevan, S., Tong, Y., and Steitz, J. A. (2007). Switching from repression to activation: microRNAs can up-regulate translation. *Science* 318, 1931–1934. doi: 10.1126/science.1149460

Vlachos, I. S., Zagganas, K., Paraskevopoulou, M. D., Georgakilas, G., Karagkouni, D., Vergoulis, T., et al. (2015). DIANA-miRPath v3.0: deciphering microRNA function with experimental support. *Nucleic Acids Res.* 43, W460–W466. doi: 10.1093/nar/gkv403

Xiao, M., Li, J., Li, W., Wang, Y., Wu, F., Xi, Y., et al. (2017). MicroRNAs activate gene transcription epigenetically as an enhancer trigger. *RNA Biol.* 14, 1326–1334. doi: 10.1080/15476286.2015.1112487

Zhang, Y., Zhang, M., Zhong, M., Suo, Q., and Lv, K. (2013). Expression profiles of miRNAs in polarized macrophages. *Int. J. Mol. Med.* 31, 797–802. doi: 10.3892/ijmm.2013.1260

6

Management of Coronavirus Disease 2019 Patients with Lung Cancer: Experience from a Thoracic Oncology Center

David Barros Coelho[1,2], Vanessa Santos[1], David Araújo[1], Hélder Novais Bastos[1,2,3], Adriana Magalhães[1], Venceslau Hespanhol[1,2,3], Henrique Queiroga[1,2], Natália Cruz-Martins[2,3,4] and Maria Gabriela O. Fernandes[1,2,3]*

[1] Pulmonology Department, Centro Hospitalar Universitário São João, Porto, Portugal, [2] Faculdade de Medicina, University of Porto, Porto, Portugal, [3] Institute for Research and Innovation in Health (i3S), University of Porto, Porto, Portugal, [4] Laboratory of Neuropsychophysiology, Faculty of Psychology and Education Sciences, University of Porto, Porto, Portugal

***Correspondence:**
David Barros Coelho
david.b.c@hotmail.com

Background: Cancer patients appear to be at a higher risk of complications from coronavirus disease 2019 (COVID-19). Specific data related to lung cancer (LC) patient management, active treatment, and/or recent diagnosis are still very limited. Here, we aimed to investigate the clinical presentation, baseline features, and clinical outcomes of LC patients with COVID-19.

Methods: A retrospective case study was performed at Centro Hospitalar Universitário de São Joao, a tertiary hospital in the North of Portugal. Data from LC patients diagnosed with COVID-19 were collected during the first 10 months of the COVID-19 pandemic (March 2020–January 2021).

Results: Twenty-eight patients with active LC were diagnosed with COVID-19, being adenocarcinoma the most common histological type present (n = 13, 46.4%). Sixteen patients had metastatic stage IV LC (61.5%). Twenty-five patients (89.3%) had relevant comorbidities including hypertension (39.3%) and chronic obstructive pulmonary disease (32.1%). For patients undergoing antineoplastic treatment, the median time from the last chemotherapy administration to COVID-19 diagnosis was of 16 days (interquartile range = 13–41 days). Half of patients were previously on corticosteroid therapy. Twenty patients (71.4%) needed hospitalization, 18 received oxygen therapy (64.3%), 3 (10.7%) of them received high-flow nasal cannula with good tolerability, and 1 (3.6%) needed non-invasive ventilation. Hydroxychloroquine and antibiotics were given to 4 (14.3%) and 12 (42.9%) patients, respectively. Seven patients (25%) died at a median time of 5 days following COVID-19 diagnosis.

Conclusion: This is one of the first studies reporting the adverse outcomes associated with COVID-19 in LC patients at same time that adds evidence regarding the need to create protocols and guidelines to reduce the infection risk in such patients.

Keywords: COVID-19, lung cancer, infection, thoracic oncology, clinical management

INTRODUCTION

Coronavirus disease 2019 (COVID-19) is a viral infection triggered by severe acute respiratory syndrome coronavirus 2 (SARS-CoV-2), with high pulmonary impairment. Although the first cases were reported in Hubei, China, in December 2019, the disease spread rapidly around the world and was recognized as a global pandemic by the World Health Organization (WHO) (Guan et al., 2020; Johns Hopkins University, 2020). Among the main patients with features that confer a higher risk of a serious disease state and a higher mortality rate resulting from infection are the elderly and those with underlying comorbidities (Guan et al., 2020; Johns Hopkins University, 2020).

Regarding oncology, data on clinical outcomes in cancer patients are still scarce, although published case reports indicate that cancer leads to worse outcomes. For example, a study conducted in China found that cancer patients were at higher risk of COVID-19 with a worse prognosis than those without cancer (de Marinis et al., 2020; Liang et al., 2020; Passaro et al., 2020; Yu et al., 2020). In addition, the first report from a global database (TERAVOLT) revealed a 33% mortality rate and a low proportion of patients in intensive care or mechanical ventilation (Garassino et al., 2020), an aspect that has already been highlighted by smaller studies (de Marinis et al., 2020; Liang et al., 2020; Passaro et al., 2020; Yu et al., 2020). In this sense, it is important to understand the clinical context and epidemiological features of cancer patients in order to create or even improve the existing protocols in cancer centers to deal with lung cancer (LC) patients in the COVID-19 era. In addition, and given the scarcity of specific data on LC patient management in active treatment and/or with recent diagnosis, it is also of utmost importance to better understand the global scope to develop clinical guidelines in this regard. Anyway, considering the disease burden, age, comorbidities, smoking, and even the immunosuppression state to which such patients are exposed, we hypothesize that they face a higher risk of COVID-19–related complications and even death. Thus, the present study aims to analyze the incidence of cases and the impact of infection control measures in LC patients at a thoracic oncology center.

MATERIALS AND METHODS

A retrospective case study was carried out at the Centro Hospitalar Universitário de São João (CHUSJ), a tertiary hospital in the Oporto region, located at the Northern Portugal. In fact, the Oporto region was the epicenter at the time of the first COVID-19 outbreak in Portugal, as it was in the second wave. The first national cases were reported in this region and, according to data from Portuguese public health authorities, six of the 10 most affected municipalities were in the Porto region during the first 2 months of the pandemic.

The Department of Thoracic Oncology is part of the CHUSJ Oncology Unit. Briefly, it is located in an adjacent building to CHUSJ, where consultations, examinations, and radiotherapy and chemotherapy are performed. In this study, data were collected from LC patients with COVID-19 diagnosis in Portugal from March 2020 to January 2021. Active cancer was defined as LC diagnosed or treated in the previous 6 months or recurrent/metastatic cancer.

During this period, a contingency plan was developed by the CHUSJ and the Department of Thoracic Oncology, aiming to (1) reduce the in-person consultation, establishing telemedicine for non-essential care; (2) COVID-19 screening in patients starting treatment (chemotherapy or radiotherapy); (3) regular and adequate cleaning of surfaces and objects in the Oncology Daycare Unit; and (4) patient engagement in social distancing and proper hand cleaning techniques.

Demographic and clinical features, laboratory findings, and chest computed tomography (CT) or chest X-ray images were collected and analyzed.

Coronavirus disease 2019 diagnosis was based on the criteria published by the WHO and confirmed by reverse transcriptase–polymerase chain reaction assay of nasal and/or pharyngeal specimens. Patients with confirmed COVID-19 diagnosis were treated according to the emergency room policy, and ward treatment and follow-up were done by a dedicated team led by the Infectious Diseases Unit.

The study protocol was approved by the ethics committee of CHUSJ.

RESULTS

A total of 28 patients with active LC were retrospectively identified and analyzed. Baseline demographic and clinical characteristics of patients are summarized in **Table 1**. Most patients were male (n = 20, 71.4%), with median age of 68 years [interquartile range (IQR) = 57–76 years]. All cases presented between March 21, 2020, and January 4, 2021.

Regarding LC histological type, adenocarcinoma was the most common (n = 13, 46.4%), followed by squamous cell carcinoma (n = 7, 25.0%). Most had stage IV metastatic LC (n = 16, 61.5%), whereas four had stage IIIb (15.4%). The remaining histological types and staging are represented in **Table 1**.

Two patients (7.1%) had a prior history of another cancer, including lymphoma (recently treated with rituximab) and colon cancer. Eleven patients (39.3%) had hypertension, and nine (32.1%) had chronic obstructive pulmonary disease (COPD) (two of them requiring long-term oxygen therapy). Other relevant comorbidities included hypercholesterolemia (n = 7), diabetes (n = 3), and heart failure (n = 3). One patient had organizing pneumonia (OP) undergoing steroid treatment (**Table 1**).

Most patients were on active treatment (n = 20, 71.4%). The anticancer therapy is detailed in **Table 1**. The median time from the last administration of chemotherapy to COVID-19 diagnosis was of 16 days (IQR = 13–41 days). The patients from the first COVID-19 wave (n = 5) had a median time of last treatment to diagnosis of 4 days, whereas the remaining had 18 days (IQR = 13–41 days).

TABLE 1 | Characterization of lung cancer (LC) patients with coronavirus disease 2019 (COVID-19) diagnosis.

Disease features	
Median age (IQR), years	73 (64–76)
Male sex, no. (%)	20 (71.4%)
Smoking status, no. (%)	
Non-smoker	6 (23.1%)
Former smoker	9 (34.6%)
Smoker	11 (42.3%)
Comorbidities, no. (%)	
HBP	11 (39.3%)
COPD	9 (32.1%)
Dyslipidemia	7 (25.0%)
Atrial fibrillation	4 (16.0%)
Cardiac failure	4 (16.0%)
Diabetes	3 (10.7%)
Psoriasis	2 (7.1%)
OSA	2 (7.1%)
Alcoholism	2 (7.1%)
Asthma	1 (3.6%)
Stroke	1 (3.6%)
Laryngeal carcinoma	1 (3.6%)
Hypothyroidism	1 (3.6%)
GERD	1 (3.6%)
Ankylosing spondylitis	1 (3.6%)
Colon cancer	1 (3.6%)
Organizing pneumonia	1 (3.6%)
Peripheral arterial disease	1 (3.6%)
Scleroderma	1 (3.6%)
Lymphoma	1 (3.6%)
Non-significant	3 (10.7%)
Histology, no. (%)	
Adenocarcinoma	13 (46.4%)
Squamous cell carcinoma	7 (25.0%)
Small cell lung cancer	3 (10.7%)
Non–small cell lung carcinoma	1 (3.6%)
Neuroendocrine	1 (3.6%)
Poorly differentiated carcinoma	2 (7.1%)
Glomic tumor	1 (3.6%)
Staging, no. (%)	
IV 16/26 (61.5%)	16 (61.5%)
IIIb 4/26 (15.4%)	4 (15.4%)
Ia 1/26 (3.8%)	1 (3.8%)
IIa 1/26 (3.8%)	1 (3.8%)
IIIa 1/26 (3.8%)	1 (3.8%)
IIIb 1/26 (3.6%)	1 (3.6%)
Median time since LC diagnosis (IQR), months	6 (1–13)
Last LC treatment, no. (%)	
No treatment/recent diagnosis	8 (28.6%)
Carboplatin-vinorelbine	4 (14.3%)
Carboplatin-pemetrexed	3 (10.7%)
Atezolizumab	2 (7.1%)
Docetaxel	2 (7.1%)
Durvalumab	2 (7.1%)
Etoposide	2 (7.1%)
Gencitabine	1 (3.6%)
Carboplatin-Paclitxel	1 (3.6%)
Caboplatin-gemcitabine	1 (3.6%)
Nivolumab	1 (3.6%)
Carboplatin + etoposide	1 (3.6%)
Time since last treatment (days)	16 (13–41)

IQR, interquartile range; HBP, high blood pressure; COPD, chronic obstructive pulmonary disease; OSA, obstructive sleep apnea; GERD, gastroesophageal reflux; LC, lung cancer.

Most patients (11/22) were under corticosteroid therapy, namely, for symptom relief and OP treatment. Three patients (60%) were receiving doses ≥20 mg/day because of OP (n = 1), vena cava syndrome (n = 1), and for preparing chemotherapy (n = 1).

Regarding COVID-19, patients mostly presented with dyspnea (n = 12, 42.9%) and cough (n = 6, 21.4%). Seven patients (25.0%) were diagnosed as a screening for treatment, whereas two patients were screened because of hospital admissions for other reasons (e.g., uncontrolled pain and hemoptysis). The median time since symptom onset until COVID-19 diagnosis was of 2 days (IQR = 0–4 days). More information regarding symptoms at presentation is detailed in **Table 2**.

Laboratory findings on admission are shown in **Table 2**. Regarding data from blood cells count, neutrophilia was present in 17 (70.8%) of patients, whereas 16 (66.7%) had lymphopenia (80%). All patients had increased levels of C-reactive protein.

A total of 16 patients (57.1%) had a thorax image at presentation or shortly after diagnosis of COVID-19. The CT scan of patients revealed the presence of bilateral ground-glass opacities, and three patients evidenced consolidations suggestive of coinfection, in addition to baseline radiological manifestations of LC, such as pleural effusion and lung masses. **Figure 1** represents examples of chest CT scan of patients.

Regarding therapeutic intervention, 18 patients (64.3%) received supplemental oxygen, including three (10.7%) who received high-flow nasal cannula at time of intensive care unit admission due to type 1 respiratory failure. One patient (3.6%) needed non-invasive ventilation, and one (3.6%) had continuous positive airway pressure with supplemental oxygen. No patient received mechanical ventilation or extracorporeal membrane oxygenation.

Empirical SARS-CoV-2 treatment with hydroxychloroquine was administered in four cases (14.3%), one of them with concomitant azithromycin. These patients were all treated in the first 3 months. Twelve patients (42.9%) needed empirical antibiotics (two of them in the context of febrile neutropenia). Nine patients (32.1%) were treated with corticosteroids, all in-hospital. One patient remained on corticotherapy at the same dose because of previous OP diagnosis, with CT scan still showing consolidations consistent with the previous diagnosis. This patient developed pulmonary thromboembolism, with no

TABLE 2 | Characterization of symptoms, management, and outcomes of COVID-19 in LC patients.

Characterization of COVID-19	
Median symptoms duration (IQR), days	2 (0–4)
Symptoms	
Dyspnea	13 (46.3%)
Cough	9 (32.1%)
Sputum	4 (14.3%)
Anorexia	2 (7.1%)
Odynophagia	1 (3.6%)
Hemoptysis	1 (3.6%)
Prostration	1 (3.6%)
Screening before LC treatment	7 (25.0%)
Biochemical results, median (IQR)	
White blood cells, $\times 10^3/\mu L$	6.31 (4.2–10.9)
Neutrophils/lymphocytes/eosinophils, $\times 10^3/\mu L$	3.9; 0.8; 0.01
Hemoglobin, g/dL	11.4 (1.9)
Platelets, $\times 10^3/\mu L$	173 (140–356)
C-reactive protein, mg/L	61 (33–164)
Treatment, no. (%)	
Supplementary oxygen	18 (64.3%)
Antibiotics	12 (42.9%)
Steroids	9 (32.1%)
HDQ	4 (14.3%)
HFNC	3 (10.7%)
NIV	1 (3.6%)
CPAP	1 (3.6%)
No treatment	10 (35.7%)
Outcome, no. (%)	
Death	7 (25.0%)

IQR, interquartile range; NIV, non-invasive ventilation; HFNC, high-flow nasal cannula; HDQ, hydroxychloroquine; LC, lung cancer; CPAP, continuous positive airway pressure.

signs of right-sided heart failure and with good recovery after hypocoagulation with low-molecular-weight heparin.

Regarding clinical outcomes, seven patients died (25.0%) after a median time of 5 days since the COVID-19 diagnosis (min–max = 0–116 days). The patients who died had metastatic and progressive LC (stage IV); four of them (80.0%) were previously on steroids.

DISCUSSION

The COVID-19 pandemic has dramatically changed the population's daily life and health support, with an increased risk reported for cancer patients. This current scenario has put in a higher emphasis the need for continuous changes and adaptations of previous routines in oncology care units.

In our sample, a high lethality rate was observed. When considering the cases of the first wave (between March and May), in fact, at the end of April, the rate of COVID-19–positive cases for the general population was 0.24%, linked to a lethality rate of 4.0%. However, in our case, the rate per LC patient was 1.12%, where 60% of patients died. Such differences can be attributed, in particular, to the oncological process features, age, treatment regimen, and patients' comorbidities. For example, in the TERAVOLT study, it was found that, in LC patients, poor prognosis was associated with advanced age (>65 years), comorbidities, Eastern Cooperative Oncology Group performance status grade 2 (ECOG2), steroids (>10 mg of prednisolone), anticoagulants, chemotherapy, and chemotherapy plus immunotherapy (Garassino et al., 2020). In this sample, half of patients were on steroid therapy for different reasons. We could speculate that the worse outcome could also be attributed to the immunosuppression state induced by steroids. Indeed, this aspect further raises the need for a careful intervention in these patients, where the use of lower doses of steroids may be an alternative in cancer patients at high risk of COVID-19.

Additionally, one patient was diagnosed with pulmonary thromboembolism. Cancer is a prothrombotic state that *per se* can explain this finding. However, in COVID-19–derived pneumonia, coagulopathy and disseminated intravascular coagulation are common complications and the most common causes of death (Helms et al., 2020; Wu et al., 2020), with the possible benefit of using heparin in selected acute respiratory distress syndrome patients with coagulopathy (Tang et al., 2020). It is therefore essential to monitor LC patients for the development of pulmonary thrombosis, as they are at an even greater risk of thrombotic events.

In this series, all casualties happened in patients with stage IV LC. This suggests that an advanced and progressive lung disease may be responsible for the worst outcomes. Several reasons may explain the worse prognosis observed to these LC patients, such as the immunosuppression status, male gender, smoking, and the presence of cardiovascular and chronic lung diseases, including the COPD (Cai, 2020; Passaro et al., 2020). LC patients often have recurrent respiratory symptoms, which can eventually delay the recognition of a viral infection for both the patient and the clinician. In our sample, the most common symptoms were dyspnea and cough, which can be wrongly attributed to the disease progression, especially at advanced cancer stages. Thus, regular testing, particularly before treatments and when patients regularly visit the hospital for consultation, should be performed, as they are crucial for early detection, at the same time, which also helps to avoid interventions that can aggravate the disease.

Another key issue is to assess the indication for antineoplastic treatment. In this way, a proper discussion in a multidisciplinary team, which can be done by videoconference and other emerging platforms, can help the clinician to adopt the most appropriate therapeutic option, with a consequent reduction in the risk of infection. In fact, this should be a priority in the decision-making process, if case-by-case risk–benefit assessment is high. In reality, what is intended here is to emphasize that the interruption of the necessary and effective anticancer therapy should not be an option, except for low-priority cases, on a case-by-case analysis. The European Society for Medical Oncology (ESMO) has published specific online guidelines for the different therapeutic regimens that should be considered for LC treatment, dividing them into high (should not be delayed), medium (should not be delayed for more than 6 weeks), and low (the patient's condition is stable enough that services can be suspended during

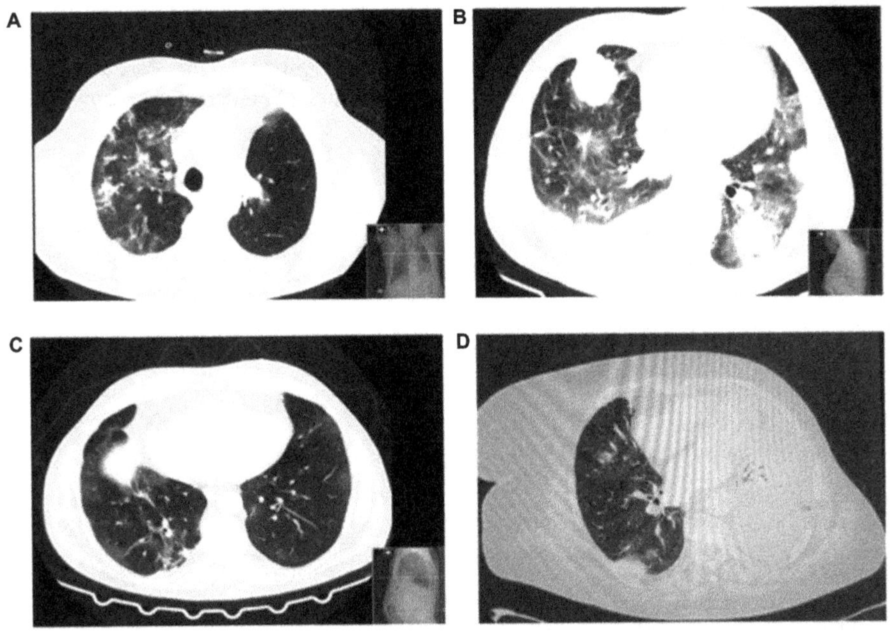

FIGURE 1 | Patients' chest CT scans. **(A)** Bilateral predominantly peripheral ground-glass opacities. Asymmetrical consolidations in the right lobes suggestive of concomitant bacterial infection. Left upper lobe lobectomy signs (consistent with recent surgery). **(B)** Patient with multiple findings related to coronavirus disease 2019 (COVID-19) and the underlying lung cancer: bilateral ground-glass opacities, pulmonary mass and pleural implant, right pleural effusion. **(C)** Chest CT: bilateral ground-glass opacities, both central and peripheral, some with nodular shape. Some "band" consolidative opacities in the right upper lobe, middle lobe, and lower inferior lobe opacities suggestive of residual processes. **(D)** Left large-volume pleural effusion with left lung atelectasis. Diffuse ground-glass opacities. Small right pleural effusion. No signs of pulmonary thromboembolism.

the pandemic, or the intervention is unlikely to have a marked benefit) priority.

On the other side, and also worth of note is that hospital transmission was considered a possibility in two of the cases, as they underwent treatment at the daycare oncology unit 4 days before the symptoms developed. However, an epidemiologic link has not been found. Other retrospective studies have indicated the occurrence of hospital transmission in COVID-19 patients. For example, in a retrospective case study in China with 138 patients, 41.3% of patients were reported to have acquired SARS-CoV-2 during hospitalization, five in the oncology department (Wang et al., 2020).

In our particular case, since the beginning of the COVID-19 outbreak, and in line with recommendations from international and national societies, such as ESMO and Direção Geral da Saúde, a specific protocol has been designed to be applied to reduce the patients' access to the oncology unit, promoting telephone screening and consultation. All patients have been screened for COVID-19 symptoms and temperature upon arrival at the entrance to the oncology unit, since the beginning of April. In addition, all patients and staff use a surgical mask inside the hospital. As a result, from May to June 2020, there was no new diagnosis of COVID-19 among LC patients at our institution. This reduction can be in part due to policies adopted to reduce the spread of nosocomial infections. At national level, the peak in the number of active cases was at mid-May (May 15); so, the lack of new cases during the month of May seems to be related to the successful preventive measures implemented. On the other hand, seven patients had a diagnosis as part of screening for oncologic treatment (chemotherapy or radiotherapy), which could have prevented more serious complications had the patients done treatment. This probably explains the findings regarding time, from the last cancer treatment to the COVID-19 diagnosis, having increased from 4 days in the first wave to 16 days in the following months.

As main study limitations, the reduced sample size is the most prominent one, which limits the conclusions regarding clinical presentation and outcomes to the general population of patients with LC. However, this single-center experience majorly intends to highlight the measures related to infection control and its effects on reducing the likelihood of getting infected by SARS-CoV-2 in our patients. Therefore, this analysis adds to the evidence that strict rules to prevent SARS-CoV-2 infection among LC patients are particularly relevant.

CONCLUSION

In view of the high vulnerability of LC patients, the death risk associated with COVID-19 is imminent. Thus, and given the data presented in this report, there is urgency in implementing and maintaining protocols at the oncology unit to minimize the viral infection spread and to reduce the consequences in SARS-CoV-2–infected patients.

AUTHOR CONTRIBUTIONS

All authors listed have made a substantial, direct and intellectual contribution to the work, and approved it for publication.

ACKNOWLEDGMENTS

NC-M acknowledges the Portuguese Foundation for Science and Technology under the Horizon 2020 Program (PTDC/PSI-GER/28076/2017).

REFERENCES

Cai, H. (2020). Sex difference and smoking predisposition in patients with COVID-19. *Lancet Respir. Med.* 8:e20. doi: 10.1016/S2213-2600(20)30117-X

de Marinis, F., Attili, I., Morganti, S., Stati, V., Spitaleri, G., Gianoncelli, L., et al. (2020). Results of multilevel containment measures to better protect lung cancer patients from COVID-19: the IEO model. *Front. Oncol.* 10:665. doi: 10.3389/fonc.2020.00665

Garassino, M. C., Whisenant, J. G., Huang, L.-C., Trama, A., Torri, V., Agustoni, F., et al. (2020). COVID-19 in patients with thoracic malignancies (TERAVOLT): first results of an international, registry-based, cohort study. *Lancet Oncol.* 21, 914–922. doi: 10.1016/S1470-2045(20)30314-4

Guan, W., Ni, Z., Hu, Y., Liang, W., Ou, C., He, J., et al. (2020). Clinical characteristics of coronavirus disease 2019 in China. *N. Engl. J. Med.* 382, 1708–1720. doi: 10.1056/NEJMoa2002032

Helms, J., Tacquard, C., Severac, F., Leonard-Lorant, I., Ohana, M., Delabranche, X., et al. (2020). High risk of thrombosis in patients with severe SARS-CoV-2 infection: a multicenter prospective cohort study. *Intensive Care Med.* 46, 1089–1098. doi: 10.1007/s00134-020-06062-x

Johns Hopkins University (2020). *Coronavirus COVID-19 Global Cases by the Center for Systems Science and Engineering (CSSE) at Johns Hopkins University (JHU).* Baltimore, MD: Johns Hopkins Univ.

Liang, W., Guan, W., Chen, R., Wang, W., Li, J., Xu, K., et al. (2020). Cancer patients in SARS-CoV-2 infection: a nationwide analysis in China. *Lancet Oncol.* 21, 335–337. doi: 10.1016/S1470-2045(20)30096-6

Passaro, A., Peters, S., Mok, T. S. K., Attili, I., Mitsudomi, T., and de Marinis, F. (2020). Testing for COVID-19 in lung cancer patients. *Ann. Oncol.* 31, 832–834. doi: 10.1016/j.annonc.2020.04.002

Tang, N., Bai, H., Chen, X., Gong, J., Li, D., and Sun, Z. (2020). Anticoagulant treatment is associated with decreased mortality in severe coronavirus disease 2019 patients with coagulopathy. *J. Thromb. Haemost.* 18, 1094–1099. doi: 10.1111/jth.14817

Wang, D., Hu, B., Hu, C., Zhu, F., Liu, X., Zhang, J., et al. (2020). Clinical characteristics of 138 hospitalized patients with 2019 novel coronavirus-infected pneumonia in Wuhan, China. *JAMA* 323, 1061–1069. doi: 10.1001/jama.2020.1585

Wu, C., Chen, X., Cai, Y., Xia, J., Zhou, X., Xu, S., et al. (2020). Risk factors associated with acute respiratory distress syndrome and death in patients with coronavirus disease 2019 pneumonia in Wuhan, China. *JAMA Intern. Med.* 180, 934–943. doi: 10.1001/jamainternmed.2020.0994

Yu, J., Ouyang, W., Chua, M. L. K., and Xie, C. (2020). SARS-CoV-2 transmission in patients with cancer at a tertiary care hospital in Wuhan, China. *JAMA Oncol.* 6, 1108–1110. doi: 10.1001/jamaoncol.2020.0980

7

Adaptive Immunity in Pulmonary Sarcoidosis and Chronic Beryllium Disease

Sarah A. Greaves[1], *Shaikh M. Atif*[1] *and Andrew P. Fontenot*[1,2*]

[1] *Department of Medicine, University of Colorado Anschutz Medical Campus, Aurora, CO, United States,* [2] *Department of Immunology and Microbiology, University of Colorado Anschutz Medical Campus, Aurora, CO, United States*

***Correspondence:**
Andrew P. Fontenot
andrew.fontenot@cuanschutz.edu

Pulmonary sarcoidosis and chronic beryllium disease (CBD) are inflammatory granulomatous lung diseases defined by the presence of non-caseating granulomas in the lung. CBD results from beryllium exposure in the workplace, while the cause of sarcoidosis remains unknown. CBD and sarcoidosis are both immune-mediated diseases that involve Th1-polarized inflammation in the lung. Beryllium exposure induces trafficking of dendritic cells to the lung in a mechanism dependent on MyD88 and IL-1α. B cells are also recruited to the lung in a MyD88 dependent manner after beryllium exposure in order to protect the lung from beryllium-induced injury. Similar to most immune-mediated diseases, disease susceptibility in CBD and sarcoidosis is driven by the expression of certain MHCII molecules, primarily *HLA-DPB1* in CBD and several *HLA-DRB1* alleles in sarcoidosis. One of the defining features of both CBD and sarcoidosis is an infiltration of activated CD4+ T cells in the lung. CD4+ T cells in the bronchoalveolar lavage (BAL) of CBD and sarcoidosis patients are highly Th1 polarized, and there is a significant increase in inflammatory Th1 cytokines present in the BAL fluid. In sarcoidosis, there is also a significant population of Th17 cells in the lungs that is not present in CBD. Due to persistent antigen exposure and chronic inflammation in the lung, these activated CD4+ T cells often display either an exhausted or anergic phenotype. Evidence suggests that these T cells are responding to common antigens in the lung. In CBD there is an expansion of beryllium-responsive TRBV5.1+ TCRs expressed on pathogenic CD4+ T cells derived from the BAL of CBD patients that react with endogenous human peptides derived from the plexin A protein. In an acute form of sarcoidosis, there are expansions of specific TRAV12-1/TRBV2 T cell receptors expressed on BAL CD4+ T cells, indicating that these T cells are trafficking to and expanding in the lung in response to common antigens. The specificity of these pathogenic CD4+T cells in sarcoidosis are currently unknown.

Keywords: human, T cells, MHC, lung, T cell receptors, sarcoidosis

INTRODUCTION

Granulomatous lung diseases represent a diverse set of disorders that are caused by both infectious and non-infectious agents that induce granuloma formation in the lung. Infectious organisms that induce granulomas include *Mycobacteria* sp. and various fungal organisms, while non-infectious etiologies include hypersensitivities, particulate exposures, and autoimmune reactions, among others [reviewed in (1)]. Because the clinical manifestations of many of these diseases are similar, the differential diagnosis is broad, and it is sometimes difficult to obtain diagnostic certainty. Sarcoidosis and chronic beryllium disease (CBD) are both non-infectious granulomatous lung diseases defined by the presence of non-caseating granulomas, comprised primarily of lymphocytes, epithelioid cells, giant cells, and macrophages (2–4). Although sarcoidosis can affect many organ systems, it involves the lungs in ~95% of cases (3), while CBD is typically limited to the pulmonary system.

Sarcoidosis is a disease of unknown etiology that occurs in individuals of all age, sex, and ethnic backgrounds. The highest prevalence of sarcoidosis is found in Sweden and the United States (5). CBD results from exposure to beryllium, which is a rare alkaline earth metal with exposures occurring through inhalation in the workplace, particularly in the United States (6). The adverse health effects of beryllium have long been described (7), and despite the implementation of beryllium exposure standards (8) cases of beryllium-induced disease continue to occur. The clinical manifestations of both CBD and sarcoidosis can be highly variable. In sarcoidosis, symptoms range from coughing to loss of lung function [reviewed in (9)]. Some patients develop an acute form of the disease that is self-resolving, while others develop a chronic condition that can substantially affect their quality of life. The average mortality rate for sarcoidosis patients is 3.6 per million, although this is highly variable depending on age, sex, and ethnicity (5). The first stage of beryllium-induced disease is beryllium sensitization (BeS), which involves beryllium-specific immune responses in the blood with no clinical manifestations (10). A subset of BeS patients eventually develop CBD, depending on quantity of beryllium exposure and genetic susceptibility of the individual (11, 12). If left untreated, CBD can progress to lung fibrosis, with one-third of patients historically progressing to respiratory failure (13).

Both diseases are characterized by an infiltration of activated CD4+ T cells in the lung. In CBD patients, these T cells recognize beryllium, while in sarcoidosis their specificity is unknown. Certain MHCII molecules, primarily *HLA-DPB1* in CBD and several *HLA-DRB1* alleles in sarcoidosis, increase disease susceptibility (14–17). Recently, there has also been evidence to suggest that B cells and antibody responses are involved in the pathogenesis of CBD and sarcoidosis (18–20). This review focuses on how different aspects of the immune system influence the progression of these diseases.

INNATE IMMUNE RESPONSES IN CBD AND SARCOIDOSIS

Innate immune cell populations are involved in propagating inflammation in both CBD and sarcoidosis (**Table 1**). Alveolar macrophages (AMs) comprise a major cell population in a healthy lung and are crucial for maintaining lung immunity (21). AMs are altered in sarcoidosis, with protein profiling revealing 80 differentially-expressed proteins in AMs of sarcoidosis patients compared to control subjects, including increased expression of two major phagocytic pathways (22). Activation of the mTORC1 pathway by deletion of the TSC2 gene in macrophages promoted excessive granuloma formation in mice (23). In sarcoidosis patients, mTORC1 activation and macrophage proliferation are associated with disease progression (23). Additionally, the number of monocytes undergoing phagocytosis in the blood of sarcoidosis patients is heightened compared to control subjects (24), and circulating monocytes also display higher TLR2 and TLR4 expression (25). Bronchoalveolar lavage (BAL) cells from sarcoidosis patients produce more TNF-α and IL-6 in response to TLR2 agonists than healthy controls, while PBMCs from sarcoidosis patients had impaired TLR2 responses (26, 27). Serum amyloid A (SAA) proteins are a group of acute phase inflammatory response proteins that are significantly elevated in the granulomas of sarcoidosis patients and localize to macrophages and giant cells within the granulomas (28). In a murine model of granulomatous lung inflammation SAA amplified inflammatory responses via TLR2 signaling (28). It has also recently been shown that SAAs promote Th17 induced inflammation (29), which will be discussed in the T cell section below. Certain MyD88 polymorphisms are also associated with the development of sarcoidosis (30). While these studies have led some to speculate that the abnormal inflammation in sarcoidosis is caused by aberrant monocyte and macrophage activity and TLR responses, the evidence for specific antigenic stimuli, as discussed below, indicates that there is an interplay between the innate and adaptive immune responses that drives the inflammation and granuloma formation.

Similar to sarcoidosis, beryllium exposure and the development of granulomatous inflammation in CBD patients results from activation of both innate and adaptive immunity. Although beryllium is a part of an antigenic complex that generates an adaptive immune response in genetically-susceptible, beryllium-exposed workers, it also serves as an adjuvant to prime innate immunity (31–33). As compared to mice immunized with parasitic antigens alone, mice immunized with a combination of beryllium and parasitic antigens had enhanced control of the infection through increased production of IFN-γ in lymph nodes and spleen (34). PMBCs and dendritic cells (DCs) exhibit increased production of inflammatory chemokines after exposure to beryllium, and TNF-α was produced by beryllium-stimulated PBMCs independent of disease-associated HLA molecules (35, 36). In murine models of CBD, beryllium exposure promoted trafficking of DCs to lung-draining lymph nodes and enhanced expression of costimulatory molecules, CD80 and CD86, on DCs that was dependent on MyD88 signaling (37). Furthermore, it was recently demonstrated that exposure to beryllium hydroxide ($Be(OH)_2$) resulted in the release of IL-1α and DNA into the airways, which subsequently acted as damage-associated molecular patterns (DAMPS) by engaging IL-1R1 and TLR9 to induce migration of DCs into lung-draining lymph nodes and the subsequent generation of memory CD4+ T cells (38). Thus,

Abbreviations: CBD, chronic beryllium disease; AM, alveolar macrophage; DC, dendritic cell; DAMP, damage associated molecular pattern; BeO, beryllium oxide; BAL, bronchoalveolar lavage; ELA, ectopic lymphoid aggregate; TRAV, TCR alpha variable region; TRBV, TCR beta variable region; SAA, serum amyloid A.

TABLE 1 | Immune characteristics of chronic beryllium disease and sarcoidosis.

	Sarcoidosis	Chronic beryllium disease
Innate Immunity	Increased TLR2 and TLR4 expression on monocytes Alveolar macrophages display increased phagocytosis Increased mTORC1 activation and macrophage proliferation PMBCs show impaired TLR2 responses MyD88 polymorphisms are associated with disease	Beryllium has adjuvant properties that prime innate immunity PMBCs and DCs have increased production of inflammatory cytokines Increased CD80 and CD86 on DCs Beryllium generates DAMPs to induce migration of DCs to lung
B cells/antibody responses	Increased IgA Anti-vimentin antibodies in BAL fluid	B cells recruited to lung dependent on MyD88 and organized into ELAs B cell depletion enhances lung injury
HLA susceptibility	*HLA-DRB1*11:01* (US) *HLA-DRB1*15:01* (US) *HLA-DRB1*03:01* (Sweden)	*HLA-DPB1*02:01* *HLA-DPB1*17:01*
Cytokine profiles	Increased Th1 polarized cytokines including TNF-α, IL-6, IFN-γ, IL-1, IL-2, IL-12	Increased Th1 polarized cytokines including IFN-γ, TNF-α, IL-2, IL-1
CD4+ T cells	CD4+ T cell alveolitis Majority Th1 polarized Th17 and Th17.1 CD4+ T cells also present Elevated PD-1 expression, dysfunctional TCR responses	CD4+ T cell alveolitis Majority Th1 polarized No evidence of Th2 or Th17 CD4+ T cells present Increased PD-1 and CTLA-4 expression Predominantly effector memory phenotype
Public TCRs	TCRs with TRAV12-1/TRBV2 are most frequent in HLA-DR3 Löfgren's syndrome patients	TRBV5.1 beryllium specific TCRs are expressed in majority of HLA-DP2 patients Public TCRs recognize HLA-DP2/beryllium/plexin A peptide complex

beryllium exposure has a crucial effect on innate cell function that contributes to disease development and progression.

B CELL INVOLVEMENT IN CBD AND SARCOIDOSIS

CBD and sarcoidosis have historically been thought of as T cell-driven inflammatory diseases. Until recently, the role of B cells in CBD was completely unknown. Our group recently demonstrated the importance of B cells in protecting the lung from beryllium oxide (BeO)-induced injury (**Table 1**). Using a murine model of CBD that mimics the human disease, we established that activated follicular B cells are recruited to the lung after beryllium exposure and are organized into ectopic lymphoid aggregates (ELAs) (20). B cell depletion eradicated these ELAs and enhanced lung injury, indicating that B cells play an important protective role in BeO-induced lung injury (20). In addition, BeO-induced B cell recruitment to the lung is dependent on MyD88 signaling (20). B cells also accumulate in the lungs of CBD patients, indicating that this protective role may translate to human disease (20). Further studies are needed to determine the exact mechanism of B cell-mediated protection in the lung after BeO exposure.

Although there is no evidence of B cells playing a direct role in disease pathogenesis in sarcoidosis, several studies have reported altered antibody responses in these patients. Particularly in patients with pulmonary sarcoidosis, there is a direct correlation between the number of T cells in the BAL and the proportion of BAL cells that secrete IgG, which is not apparent in control subjects (39). Additionally, increased numbers of memory B cells producing IgA are found in patients with sarcoidosis, raising the possibility that IgA could be involved in granuloma formation (40). Antibodies toward autoantigens have been found in only a small proportion of sarcoidosis patients, making it unclear whether autoimmune responses play a role in disease pathogenesis (18). Recent data show that in patients with an acute, self-resolving form of sarcoidosis, Löfgren's syndrome, there are increased quantities of anti-vimentin antibodies in the BAL fluid (19). Vimentin is a self-antigen that has been found in the lungs of sarcoidosis patients (41), although more validation is required to determine whether immune responses to vimentin are involved in disease initiation and progression. Overall, the role of B cells in sarcoidosis needs to be more thoroughly investigated to establish their role in this disease.

T CELLS IN CBD AND SARCOIDOSIS

A defining feature of both CBD and pulmonary sarcoidosis is an infiltration of pathogenic CD4+ T cells in the lung (42–47) (**Table 1**, **Figure 1**). CD4+ T cells in the BAL fluid of CBD patients are predominantly antigen-experienced T cells expressing CD45RO and lacking CD62L and CCR7 (48). Large numbers of these cells (in some cases, >30%) are responsive to beryllium sulfate ($BeSO_4$) in culture, secreting Thl cytokines, including IFN-γ and TNF-α and lesser quantities of IL-2 (48). CD4+ T cell responses to beryllium are dependent upon major histocompatibility complex class II (MHCII) molecules, but independent of CD28 costimulation, indicative of an effector memory T cell phenotype (48, 49). There is no evidence that beryllium-responsive Th2 or Th17 CD4+ T cells or CD8+ T cells are present in the lungs of CBD patients or that these cells play a role in beryllium-induced disease (48, 50).

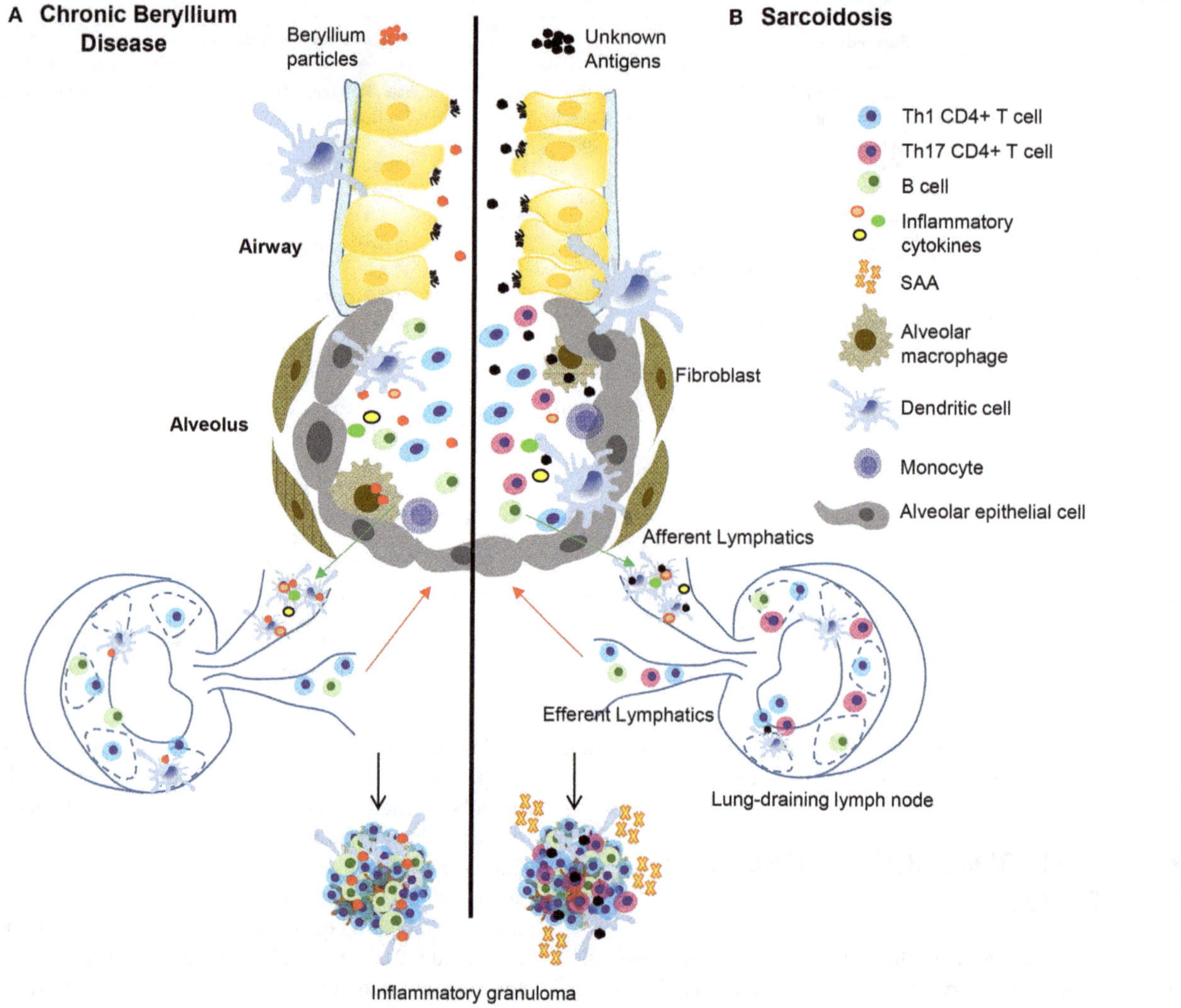

FIGURE 1 | Immunopathogenesis of chronic beryllium disease and sarcoidosis. In CBD **(A)**, beryllium particles enter the lung and generate an immune response. In sarcoidosis **(B)** unknown antigens induce an immune response after entering the lung. In CBD, beryllium particles cause the release of DAMPs in the airways, which promote activation and migration of DCs. Either beryllium **(A)** or unknown antigens **(B)** are taken up by alveolar macrophages and dendritic cells in the lung and are transported to lung-draining lymph nodes. In the lymph nodes, antigen specific CD4+ T cells are stimulated by activated antigen-presenting cells expressing certain HLA molecules dependent on disease (see **Table 1**). T-B cell interactions also occur in the lymph nodes and commitment of B cells to antibody production takes place in the germinal centers. Antibodies and activated B and T cells circulate back to the lung to generate an adaptive immune response against the target antigen. In CBD, Th1 CD4+ T cells that display an effector memory phenotype are the primary cell type, but there is also an infiltration of activated B cells in the lungs that help form granulomatous structures **(A)**. In sarcoidosis and CBD, Th1 CD4+ T cells make up the majority of the cell population in the lungs. In sarcoidosis, but not CBD, there are also Th17 and Th17.1 cells present. SAAs are also present in pulmonary granulomas of sarcoidosis patients, but not CBD, where they contribute to the inflammatory milieu and induce proliferation of pathogenic, inflammatory Th17 cells. In both diseases, there is an abundance of Th1 inflammatory cytokines secreted by T cells and innate cells that propagate the inflammatory environment, including TNF-α, IFN-γ, IL-1, and IL-2.

CD4+ T cells from the BAL of sarcoidosis patients are also highly Th1 polarized. This enhanced Th1 polarization is driven by increased expression of inflammatory cytokines, such as IFN-γ, IL-1, IL-2, IL-6, IL-12, and TNF-α in addition to others, while Th2 cytokines have not been detected (51–53). Unlike CBD, there is no known inciting particle(s) or antigen(s) in sarcoidosis. However, in light of the infiltration of Th1-polarized CD4+ T cells in the lung, it is widely accepted that these T cells are trafficking to and proliferating in the lung in response to an unknown antigen. In contrast to findings in the BAL of sarcoidosis patients where a CD4+ T cell alveolitis (20–60% total cell count) exists (42), T cell lymphopenia in the peripheral blood is characteristic of the disease (54). CD4+ T cells with a Th17 phenotype and T cells expressing both IL-17 and IFN-γ (i.e., Th17.1 cells) have been found in lung tissue and BAL from patients with sarcoidosis (55, 56). A study recently demonstrated that there is a significant increase in CCR6+ Th17.1 cells in both the BAL fluid and mediastinal lymph nodes of sarcoidosis patients compared to controls and that these cells contribute to IFN-γ production (57). Additionally, Th17.1 cells in the BAL fluid are found in higher proportions in sarcoidosis patients with active disease vs. patients undergoing disease resolution, suggesting that these cells could be playing a role in disease progression (57). Interestingly, a recent study highlighted the importance of SAA in the differentiation of pathogenic Th17 cells in certain inflammatory conditions (29). SAA expression is increased in the lungs of sarcoidosis patients (28), so it is possible that SAAs contribute to the expansion of Th17 cells observed in these patients. Furthermore, SAAs in the lungs of sarcoidosis patients are significantly higher than that of CBD patients (28), which could explain the lack of Th17 cells in CBD.

As a consequence of constant antigen exposure in both sarcoidosis and CBD, pathogenic CD4+ T cells develop an anergic and/or exhausted phenotype as a mechanism to decrease chronic T cell activation and subsequent inflammation. Pulmonary CD4+ T cells from sarcoidosis spontaneously secrete IL-2 *ex vivo*, but when given TCR stimulation, these cells express less IL-2 and IFN-γ relative to CD4+ T cells from various other lung diseases and healthy control subjects, consistent with an anergic/exhausted phenotype (58). Additionally, sarcoidosis CD4+ T cells have a reduced proliferative capacity and higher levels of apoptosis, along with increased PD-1 expression, which is often associated with persistent antigen exposure to limit chronic T cell activation (59, 60). A recent study demonstrated that PD-1 expression was highest on sarcoidosis CD4+ T cells with a Th17 phenotype (61). Furthermore, PD-1+ Th17 CD4+ cells produce high levels of TGFB-1, a key factor in the development in fibrosis (61). PD-1 blockade significantly reduced TGFB-1 produced by Th17 CD4+ T cells from sarcoidosis patients and reduced their ability to induce collagen-1 production in a fibroblast cell line (61). These data demonstrate that T cell dysfunction in sarcoidosis is seemingly due to persistent antigen exposure, thus discovering the etiologic antigens driving this disease will be important for therapies directed at reducing antigen exposure.

BAL CD4+ T cells in CBD also have elevated PD-1 expression and blockade of the PD-1 pathway increases proliferation of beryllium-responsive CD4+ T cells (62). Interestingly, a subsequent study showed that CTLA-4, another T cell co-inhibitory receptor, was upregulated on BAL CD4+ T cells in CBD, but its expression was not capable of reducing beryllium-stimulated T cell proliferation (63). Taken together, these findings show that persistent antigen exposure drives an exhausted T cell phenotype in both CBD and sarcoidosis. Despite the immune systems attempt to dampen T cell-mediated immune activation, the cells are still able to promote chronic inflammation and disease progression in non-infectious granulomatous lung disease.

GENETIC SUSCEPTIBILITY TO CBD AND SARCOIDOSIS

Similar to most immune-mediated diseases, MHCII molecules are strongly associated with both sarcoidosis and CBD (**Table 1**). Saltini et al. (44) demonstrated that BAL CD4+ T cells from CBD patients recognize beryllium in an MHCII-restricted manner. Genetic susceptibility was strongly linked to HLA-DPB1 alleles with a glutamic acid (E) at position 69 of the β-chain (βGlu69), with the most prevalent βGlu69-containing allele being *HLA-DPB1*02:01* (14). Multiple studies have corroborated these findings, documenting the presence of βGlu69-containing *DPB1* alleles in 73–95% of BeS and CBD patients compared to 30–48% of exposed controls [reviewed in (64)]. A differential risk of disease development is also associated with certain rare βGlu69-containing *DPB1* alleles, such as *HLA-DPB1*17:01* (15, 65–67). Thus, CBD is a classic example of a disorder resulting from gene-by-environment interactions, where both components are required for the development of granulomatous inflammation. In this regard, the probability of CBD increases with HLA-DP βGlu69 copy number and increasing workplace exposure to beryllium (12), suggesting that genetic and exposure factors may have an additive effect on the risk of disease development (11).

Similar to CBD, genetics and environmental exposures are involved in the initiation of sarcoidosis. Because sarcoidosis is a more heterogeneous disease that occurs worldwide and the etiologic antigen(s) are currently unknown, genetic studies are important to determine common disease characteristics. However, many genetic studies involving sarcoidosis patients demonstrate that even commonalities among subsets of patients differ between ethnic and regional groups, suggesting that there are multiple factors involved in the progression of sarcoidosis. A large-scale ACCESS study that collected patient data in the United States from 1996 to 1999 demonstrated that siblings of sarcoidosis patients are about 5-fold more likely to develop the disease than unrelated control subjects (68), suggesting that genetic factors influence disease susceptibility. As suspected by the accumulation of CD4+ T cells in the BAL of sarcoidosis subjects, the dominant genetic associations in sarcoidosis are linked to HLA. While both HLA class I and class II genes are associated with the development of sarcoidosis, the strongest correlations are shown with class II genes, although these differ between ethnic and regional groups [reviewed in (69)]. In the United States, *HLA-DRB1*11:01* and *HLA-DRB1*15:01* are both associated with sarcoidosis (16). The most striking genetic association in sarcoidosis is present in Löfgren's syndrome in Scandinavian patients. Löfgren's syndrome is an acute form of sarcoidosis associated with a favorable prognosis that presents with a specific set of inflammatory symptoms including bilateral hilar lymphadenopathy, fever, erythema nodosum, and ankle arthritis (70). The majority of Löfgren's syndrome patients express *HLA-DRB1*03:01*, with most of these patients resolving their disease within 2 years (70). Specific αβTCR variable region genes are also highly associated with Löfgren's syndrome, as discussed below. These studies clearly demonstrate that genetic susceptibility due to expression of certain MHCII molecules in both CBD and sarcoidosis is a crucial aspect of disease pathogenesis.

PUBLIC T CELLS IN BAL OF CBD AND SARCOIDOSIS DRIVING DISEASE PATHOGENESIS

As discussed in the previous section, specific MHCII expression is crucial for disease development in both CBD and sarcoidosis.

CD4+ T cells recognize peptide epitopes in an MHCII-restricted manner (71). In CBD, MHCII molecules require beryllium for antigen presentation to pathogenic T cells (48). The positively-charged beryllium particle is coordinated in the MHCII groove along with specific naturally-occurring peptides to complete the beryllium-dependent T cell ligand (72, 73). BAL CD4+ T cells from CBD patients have unique oligoclonal populations that are enriched for certain TCR β-chain motifs (46, 74). Furthermore, there are public (i.e., expressed in the majority of HLA-DP2-expressing CBD patients) beryllium-responsive TCRβ variable region (TRBV) 5.1+ TCRs expressed on CD4+ T cells derived from the BAL of CBD patients, and the frequency of these public beryllium-responsive TCRs inversely correlate with loss of lung function, suggesting that these public T cells are pathogenic in nature (75). Falta et al. (76) discovered beryllium-dependent mimotopes (i.e., peptides that mimic the naturally-occurring epitope) that bound to HLA-DP2 in the presence of beryllium and are recognized by pathogenic TRBV5.1+ CD4+ T cells expanded in the lungs of HLA-DP2+ CBD patients. Our group further discovered that an endogenous human peptide derived from plexin A proteins binds to the HLA-DP2/Be complex and stimulates these same pathogenic CD4+ T cells from CBD patients (76). CD4+ T cells specific for the HLA-DP2-plexin A4/beryllium complex comprise ~5% of beryllium-responsive CD4+ T cells in the lung (76).

Although the inciting antigen(s) in sarcoidosis is unknown, there is strong evidence suggesting that the disease is driven by antigen-specific CD4+ T cells in the lungs of patients. The most conclusive evidence comes from Löfgren's syndrome. The majority of Löfgren's syndrome patients in Sweden express *HLA-DRB1*03:01* (HLA-DR3) (17), and expression of HLA-DR3 was strongly associated with disease resolution and an excellent prognosis (70). Additionally, HLA-DR3-expressing Löfgren's syndrome patients exhibit oligoclonal expansions of CD4+ T cells in the BAL that express TCRα variable region (TRAV) 12-1, and the quantity of these cells in the BAL correlates with disease remission (77–79). Importantly, this expansion of TRAV12-1+ CD4+ T cells is only seen in patients with active disease, and upon disease resolution, these cells are greatly reduced, highlighting their importance in disease pathogenesis (80). Using deep sequencing approaches, our group recently demonstrated that TRAV12-1 preferentially pairs with TCRβ variable region (TRBV) 2 in BAL CD4+ T cells from Löfgren's syndrome patients and that TRAV12-1 and TRBV2 are the most expanded variable regions relative to control subjects (81). Additionally, there are specific TRAV12-1/TRBV2 CDR3 motifs expressed on BAL CD4+ T cells of multiple Löfgren's syndrome patients, indicating that these T cells are trafficking to and expanding in the lung in response to the same antigen.

ANTIGENIC DRIVERS OF SARCOIDOSIS

One of the most active areas of sarcoidosis research is focused on determining the etiologic antigens that drive the recruitment of CD4+ T cells to the lungs of sarcoidosis patients. One problem hindering this endeavor is the lack of understanding of the origin of the inciting antigens, whether it is a foreign or self-antigen, or even a product of environmental exposure. Although there is some evidence for each of these categories, nothing has been conclusive enough to determine a cause of disease. The most detailed studies involving an autoantigen focus on vimentin, a filamentous protein of which the cytoskeleton is composed (82). Vimentin has been eluted from HLA-DR molecules expressed on BAL cells from some patients with sarcoidosis, and vimentin-specific autoantibodies are found in BAL fluid of sarcoidosis patients (19, 41, 83). More validation is required to determine whether immune responses to vimentin are involved in disease initiation and progression.

Due to the similarities between the clinical features of sarcoidosis and certain pulmonary infections, it has long been thought that there may be an infectious agent driving sarcoidosis etiology. The most substantial evidence linking a microorganism to sarcoidosis pathogenesis involves *Mycobacteria sp.* Several meta-analyses demonstrate that the odds of finding mycobacterial DNA by PCR in the lungs of sarcoidosis patients is ~5–20% greater than in control subjects (84, 85). However, the data collected in these studies is very heterogeneous, and *Mycobacteria sp.* are not detected in the majority of sarcoidosis patients.

To investigate whether there were any functional implications that mycobacterial infections induce sarcoidosis, several groups have measured T cell responsiveness to mycobacterial candidate antigens in sarcoidosis patients. A higher number of T cells in the blood of sarcoidosis patients produce IFN-γ after stimulation with a *M. tuberculosis* antigen catalase peroxidase (mKatG) (86). Additionally, T cells derived from the BAL fluid of sarcoidosis patients respond to mKatG along with an additional mycobacterial antigen, early secreted antigen protein (ESAT-6) (87). Furthermore, one study detected protein derived from mKatG in ~50% of tissue samples from sarcoidosis patients (88), and IgG antibodies were detected in ~50% of sarcoidosis serum samples (88). Despite this evidence, sarcoidosis patients show no signs active mycobacterial infections even during immunosuppressive treatments. There are also no mycobacterial-specific CD4+ T cell clones identified from sarcoidosis patients to date.

Cutibacterium acnes (previously *Propionibacterium acnes*) infections are also associated with sarcoidosis. *C. acnes* is a commensal bacteria that is commonly found on the skin of healthy individuals. By quantitative PCR, DNA from *C. acnes* is found in the majority of lymph nodes obtained from sarcoidosis patients (89). However, *C. acnes* is also found in a large percentage of lymph nodes isolated from healthy control subjects (90), making it difficult to ascertain whether the presence of *C. acnes* in sarcoidosis patients is a consequence of the disease or normal colonization of commensal bacteria.

In addition to infectious agents, it has also been postulated that there are environmental factors involved in the progression of sarcoidosis. Stage I sarcoidosis occurs more frequently in the Spring, and the lowest incidence of disease diagnosis occurs in the Winter, suggesting that airborne allergens or other seasonal particulates may be involved in disease progression (91). There are positive associations between the development of sarcoidosis and certain environmental and occupational exposures, such as insecticides and mold/mildew (92). "Sarcoid-like" granulomatous pulmonary disease occurred in rescue workers that were exposed to airborne particulates during the World Trade Center collapse (93). Recently, it was reported that patients exposed to occupational silica during work in the iron production industry in Sweden have a significantly higher incidence of sarcoidosis than unexposed individuals (94). Whether these exposures are driving sarcoidosis by activating specific CD4+ T cells in the lung or are merely inducing an inflammatory environment that makes individuals more susceptible to disease is currently unknown.

CONCLUSIONS

The immunology of sarcoidosis and CBD are quite similar, based on a predominance of CD4+ T cells in the lung, a Th1 polarized immune response, and a pathologic hallmark of granulomatous inflammation. As such, the presence of a known antigen in CBD can further our understanding of the driving factors involved in sarcoidosis pathogenesis. In CBD, our group has performed unbiased antigen discovery approaches that focused on the related and expanded CD4+ T cell subsets in the BAL of patients with active disease and have delineated several beryllium-dependent T cell ligands. It is possible that a similar unbiased antigen discovery approach utilizing expanded CD4+ T cell clones in the lungs of sarcoidosis patients may lead to the discovery of the inciting antigens that drive CD4+ T cell alveolitis and granulomatous inflammation in sarcoidosis.

AUTHOR CONTRIBUTIONS

SG, SA, and AF wrote the article. SA contributed to designing the figure and table for the article. All authors contributed to article revisions.

REFERENCES

Ohshimo S, Guzman J, Costabel U, Bonella F. Differential diagnosis of granulomatous lung disease: clues and pitfalls: number 4 in the Series "Pathology for the clinician" Edited by Peter Dorfmuller and Alberto Cavazza. *Eur Respir Rev.* (2017) 26:170012. doi: 10.1183/16000617.0012-2017

Newman LS, Kreiss K, King TE Jr, Seay S, Campbell PA. Pathologic and immunologic alterations in early stages of beryllium disease. Re-examination of disease definition and natural history. *Am Rev Respir Dis.* (1989) 139:1479–86. doi: 10.1164/ajrccm/139.6.1479

Baughman RP, Teirstein AS, Judson MA, Rossman MD, Yeager H Jr, Bresnitz EA, et al. Clinical characteristics of patients in a case control study of sarcoidosis. *Am J Respir Crit Care Med.* (2001) 164:1885–9. doi:10.1164/ajrccm.164.10.2104046

Kosjerina Z, Zaric B, Vuckovic D, Lalosevic D, Djenadic G, Murer B. The sarcoid granuloma: 'epithelioid' or 'lymphocytic-epithelioid' granuloma? *Multidiscip Respir Med.* (2012) 7:11. doi: 10.4081/mrm.2012.598

Arkema EV, Cozier YC. Epidemiology of sarcoidosis: current findings and future directions. *Ther Adv Chronic Dis.* (2018) 9:227–40. doi: 10.1177/2040622318790197

Henneberger PK, Goe SK, Miller WE, Doney B, Groce DW. Industries in the United States with airborne beryllium exposure and estimates of the number of current workers potentially exposed. *J Occup Environ Hyg.* (2004) 1:648–59. doi: 10.1080/15459620490502233

Hardy HL, Tabershaw IR. Delayed chemical pneumonitis occurring in workers exposed to beryllium compounds. *J Ind Hyg Toxicol.* (1946) 28:197–211.

Eisenbud M. Origins of the standards for control of beryllium disease (1947-1949). *Environ Res.* (1982) 27:79–88. doi: 10.1016/0013-9351(82)9 0059-7

Chen ES, Moller DR. Sarcoidosis–scientific progress and clinical challenges. *Nat Rev Rheumatol.* (2011) 7:457–67. doi: 10.1038/nrrheum.2011.93 Newman LS, Mroz MM, Balkissoon R, Maier LA. Beryllium sensitization progresses to chronic beryllium disease: a longitudinal study of disease risk. *Am J Respir Crit Care Med.* (2005) 171:54–60. doi:10.1164/rccm.200402-190OC

Richeldi L, Kreiss K, Mroz MM, Zhen B, Tartoni P, Saltini C. Interaction of genetic and exposure factors in the prevalence of berylliosis. *Am J Ind Med.* (1997) 32:337–40.

Van Dyke MV, Martyny JW, Mroz MM, Silveira LJ, Strand M, Fingerlin TE, et al. Risk of chronic beryllium disease by HLA-DPB1 E69 genotype and beryllium exposure in nuclear workers. *Am J Respir Crit Care Med.* (2011) 183:1680–8. doi: 10.1164/rccm.201002-0254OC

Newman LS, Lloyd J, Daniloff E. The natural history of beryllium sensitization and chronic beryllium disease. *Environ Health Perspect.* (1996) 104(Suppl. 5):937–43. doi: 10.1289/ehp.96104s5937

Richeldi L, Sorrentino R, Saltini C. HLA-DPB1 glutamate 69: a genetic marker of beryllium disease. *Science.* (1993) 262:242–4. doi: 10.1126/science.8105536

Wang Z, White PS, Petrovic M, Tatum OL, Newman LS, Maier LA, et al. Differential susceptibilities to chronic beryllium disease contributed by different Glu69 HLA-DPB1 and -DPA1 alleles. *J Immunol.* (1999) 163:1647–53.

Rossman MD, Thompson B, Frederick M, Maliarik M, Iannuzzi MC, Rybicki BA, et al. HLA-DRB11101: a significant risk factor for sarcoidosis in blacks and whites. *Am J Hum Genet.* (2003) 73:720–35. doi: 10.1086/378097

Grunewald J. HLA associations and Löfgren's syndrome. *Expert Rev Clin Immunol.* (2012) 8:55–62. doi: 10.1586/eci.11.76

Kobak S, Yilmaz H, Sever F, Duran A, Sen N, Karaarslan A. The prevalence of antinuclear antibodies in patients with sarcoidosis. *Autoimmune Dis.* (2014) 2014:351852. doi: 10.1155/2014/351852

Kinloch AJ, Kaiser Y, Wolfgeher D, Ai J, Eklund A, Clark MR, et al. *In situ* humoral immunity to vimentin in HLA-DRB103^{+} patients with pulmonary sarcoidosis. *Front Immunol.* (2018) 9:1516. doi: 10.3389/fimmu.2018.01516

Atif SM, Mack DG, McKee AS, Rangel-Moreno J, Martin AK, Getahun A, et al. Protective role of B cells in sterile particulate-induced lung injury. *JCI Insight.* (2019) 5:125494. doi: 10.1172/jci.insight.125494

Rubins JB. Alveolar macrophages: wielding the double-edged sword of inflammation. *Am J Respir Crit Care Med.* (2003) 167:103–4. doi: 10.1164/rccm.2210007

Kjellin H, Silva E, Branca RM, Eklund A, Jakobsson PJ, Grunewald J, et al. Alterations in the membrane-associated proteome fraction of alveolar macrophages in sarcoidosis. *Sarcoidosis Vasc Diffuse Lung Dis.* (2016) 33:17–28. Available online at: https://mattioli1885journals.com/index. php/sarcoidosis/article/view/4180

Linke M, Pham HT, Katholnig K, Schnoller T, Miller A, Demel F, et al. Chronic signaling via the metabolic checkpoint kinase mTORC1 induces macrophage granuloma formation and marks sarcoidosis progression. *Nat Immunol.* (2017) 18:293–302. doi: 10.1038/ni.3655

Dubaniewicz A, Typiak M, Wybieralska M, Szadurska M, Nowakowski S, Staniewicz-Panasik A, et al. Changed phagocytic activity and pattern of Fcgamma and complement receptors on blood monocytes in sarcoidosis. *Hum Immunol.* (2012) 73:788–94. doi: 10.1016/j.humimm.2012.05.005

Wiken M, Grunewald J, Eklund A, Wahlstrom J. Higher monocyte expression of TLR2 and TLR4, and enhanced pro-inflammatory synergy of TLR2 with NOD2 stimulation in sarcoidosis. *J Clin Immunol.* (2009) 29:78–89. doi: 10.1007/s10875-008-9225-0

Gabrilovich MI, Walrath J, van Lunteren J, Nethery D, Seifu M, Kern JA, et al. Disordered Toll-like receptor 2 responses in the pathogenesis of pulmonary sarcoidosis. *Clin Exp Immunol.* (2013) 173:512–22. doi: 10.1111/cei. 12138

Julian MW, Shao G, Schlesinger LS, Huang Q, Cosmar DG, Bhatt NY, et al. Nicotine treatment improves Toll-like receptor 2 and Toll-like receptor 9 responsiveness in active pulmonary sarcoidosis. *Chest.* (2013) 143:461–70. doi: 10.1378/chest.12-0383

Chen ES, Song Z, Willett MH, Heine S, Yung RC, Liu MC, et al. Serum amyloid A regulates granulomatous inflammation in sarcoidosis through Toll-like receptor-2. *Am J Respir Crit Care Med.* (2010) 181:360–73. doi: 10.1164/rccm.200905-0696OC

Lee JY, Hall JA, Kroehling L, Wu L, Najar T, Nguyen HH, et al. Serum amyloid A proteins induce pathogenic Th17 cells and promote inflammatory disease. *Cell.* (2020) 180:79–91 e16. doi: 10.1016/j.cell.2019.11.026

Daniil Z, Mollaki V, Malli F, Koutsokera A, Antoniou KM, Rodopoulou P, et al. Polymorphisms and haplotypes in MyD88 are associated with the development of sarcoidosis: a candidate-gene association study. *Mol Biol Rep.* (2013) 40:4281–6. doi: 10.1007/s11033-013-2513-7

Behbehani K, Beller DI, Unanue ER. The effects of beryllium and other adjuvants on Ia expression by macrophages. *J Immunol.* (1985) 134:2047–9.

Hall JG. Studies on the adjuvant action of beryllium. IV The preparation of beryllium containing macromolecules that induce immunoblast responses *in vivo*. *Immunology.* (1988) 64:345–51.

Denham S, Hall JG. Studies on the adjuvant action of beryllium. III The activity in the plasma of lymph efferent from nodes stimulated with beryllium. *Immunology.* (1988) 64:341–4.

Lee JY, Atochina O, King B, Taylor L, Elloso M, Scott P, et al. Beryllium, an adjuvant that promotes gamma interferon production. *Infect Immun.* (2000) 68:4032–9. doi: 10.1128/IAI.68.7.4032-4039.2000

Amicosante M, Berretta F, Franchi A, Rogliani P, Dotti C, Losi M, et al. HLA-DP-unrestricted TNF-alpha release in beryllium-stimulated peripheral blood mononuclear cells. *Eur Respir J.* (2002) 20:1174–8. doi: 10.1183/09031936.02.02232001

Hong-Geller E, Pardington PE, Cary RB, Sauer NN, Gupta G. Chemokine regulation in response to beryllium exposure in human peripheral blood mononuclear and dendritic cells. *Toxicology.* (2006) 218:216–28. doi:10.1016/j.tox.2005.10.016

McKee AS, Mack DG, Crawford F, Fontenot AP. MyD88 dependence of beryllium-induced dendritic cell trafficking and CD4$^+$ T-cell priming. *Mucosal Immunol.* (2015) 8:1237–47. doi: 10.1038/mi.2015.14

Wade MF, Collins MK, Richards D, Mack DG, Martin AK, Dinarello CA, et al. TLR9 and IL-1R1 promote mobilization of pulmonary dendritic cells during beryllium sensitization. *J Immunol.* (2018) 201:2232–43. doi: 10.4049/jimmunol.1800303

Hunninghake GW, Crystal RG. Mechanisms of hypergammaglobulinemia in pulmonary sarcoidosis. Site of increased antibody production and role of T lymphocytes. *J Clin Invest.* (1981) 67:86–92. doi: 10.1172/JCI1 10036

Kamphuis LS, van Zelm MC, Lam KH, Rimmelzwaan GF, Baarsma GS, Dik WA, et al. Perigranuloma localization and abnormal maturation of B cells: emerging key players in sarcoidosis? *Am J Respir Crit Care Med.* (2013) 187:406–16. doi: 10.1164/rccm.201206-1024OC

Wahlstrom J, Dengjel J, Persson B, Duyar H, Rammensee HG, Stevanovic S, et al. Identification of HLA-DR-bound peptides presented by human bronchoalveolar lavage cells in sarcoidosis. *J Clin Invest.* (2007) 117:3576–82. doi: 10.1172/JCI32401

Hunninghake GW, Crystal RG. Pulmonary sarcoidosis: a disorder mediated by excess helper T-lymphocyte activity at sites of disease activity. *N Engl J Med.* (1981) 305:429–34. doi: 10.1056/NEJM198108203050804

Rossman MD, Kern JA, Elias JA, Cullen MR, Epstein PE, Preuss OP, et al. Proliferative response of bronchoalveolar lymphocytes to beryllium. A test for chronic beryllium disease. *Ann Intern Med.* (1988) 108:687–93. doi: 10.7326/0003-4819-108-5-687

Saltini C, Winestock K, Kirby M, Pinkston P, Crystal RG. Maintenance of alveolitis in patients with chronic beryllium disease by beryllium-specific helper T cells. *N Engl J Med.* (1989) 320:1103–9. doi:10.1056/NEJM198904273201702

Saltini C, Kirby M, Trapnell BC, Tamura N, Crystal RG. Biased accumulation of T lymphocytes with "memory"-type CD45 leukocyte common antigen gene expression on the epithelial surface of the human lung. *J Exp Med.* (1990) 171:1123–40. doi: 10.1084/jem.171.4.1123

Fontenot AP, Falta MT, Freed BM, Newman LS, Kotzin BL. Identification of pathogenic T cells in patients with beryllium-induced lung disease. *J Immunol.* (1999) 163:1019–26.

Grunewald J, Eklund A. Role of CD4+ T cells in sarcoidosis. *Proc Am Thorac Soc.* (2007) 4:461–4. doi: 10.1513/pats.200606-130MS

Fontenot AP, Canavera SJ, Gharavi L, Newman LS, Kotzin BL. Target organ localization of memory CD4$^+$ T cells in patients with chronic beryllium disease. *J Clin Invest.* (2002) 110:1473–82. doi: 10.1172/JCI0215846

Fontenot AP, Gharavi L, Bennett SR, Canavera SJ, Newman LS, Kotzin BL. CD28 costimulation independence of target organ versus circulating memory antigen-specific CD4+ T cells. *J Clin Invest.* (2003) 112:776–84. doi:10.1172/JCI200318317

Tinkle SS, Kittle LA, Schumacher BA, Newman LS. Beryllium induces IL-2 and IFN-gamma in berylliosis. *J Immunol.* (1997) 158:518–26.

Homolka J, Muller-Quernheim J. Increased interleukin 6 production by bronchoalveolar lavage cells in patients with active sarcoidosis. *Lung.* (1993) 171:173–83. doi: 10.1007/BF00183946

Terao I, Hashimoto S, Horie T. Effect of GM-CSF on TNF-alpha and IL-1- beta production by alveolar macrophages and peripheral blood monocytes from patients with sarcoidosis. *Int Arch Allergy Immunol.* (1993) 102:242–8. doi: 10.1159/000236532

Moller DR, Forman JD, Liu MC, Noble PW, Greenlee BM, Vyas P, et al. Enhanced expression of IL-12 associated with Th1 cytokine profiles in active pulmonary sarcoidosis. *J Immunol.* (1996) 156:4952–60.

Sweiss NJ, Salloum R, Gandhi S, Alegre ML, Sawaqed R, Badaracco M, et al. Significant CD4, CD8, and CD19 lymphopenia in peripheral blood of sarcoidosis patients correlates with severe disease manifestations. *PLoS ONE.* (2010) 5:e9088. doi: 10.1371/annotation/a75007e1-492a-4bcb-80a8-28b4d432c099

Facco M, Cabrelle A, Teramo A, Olivieri V, Gnoato M, Teolato S, et al. Sarcoidosis is a Th1/Th17 multisystem disorder. *Thorax.* (2011) 66:144–50. doi: 10.1136/thx.2010.140319

Ramstein J, Broos CE, Simpson LJ, Ansel KM, Sun SA, Ho ME, et al. IFN-gamma-producing T-helper 17.1 cells are increased in sarcoidosis and are more prevalent than T-helper type 1 cells. *Am J Respir Crit Care Med.* (2016) 193:1281–91. doi: 10.1164/rccm.201507-1499OC

Broos CE, Koth LL, van Nimwegen M, In 't Veen J, Paulissen SMJ, van Hamburg JP, et al. Increased T-helper 17.1 cells in sarcoidosis mediastinal lymph nodes. *Eur Respir J.* (2018) 51:170112. doi:10.1183/13993003.01124-2017

Oswald-Richter KA, Richmond BW, Braun NA, Isom J, Abraham S, Taylor TR, et al. Reversal of global CD4+ subset dysfunction is associated with spontaneous clinical resolution of pulmonary sarcoidosis. *J Immunol.* (2013) 190:5446–53. doi: 10.4049/jimmunol.1202891

Hawkins C, Shaginurova G, Shelton DA, Herazo-Maya JD, Oswald-Richter KA, Rotsinger JE, et al. Local and systemic CD4$^+$ T cell exhaustion reverses with clinical resolution of pulmonary sarcoidosis. *J Immunol Res.* (2017) 2017:3642832. doi: 10.1155/2017/3642832

Sharpe AH, Pauken KE. The diverse functions of the PD1 inhibitory pathway. *Nat Rev Immunol.* (2018) 18:153–67. doi: 10.1038/nri.2017.108

Celada LJ, Kropski JA, Herazo-Maya JD, Luo W, Creecy A, Abad AT, et al. PD-1 up-regulation on CD4$^+$ T cells promotes pulmonary fibrosis through STAT3-mediated IL-17A and TGF-beta1 production. *Sci Transl Med.* (2018) 10:eaar8356. doi: 10.1126/scitranslmed.aar8356

Palmer BE, Mack DG, Martin AK, Gillespie M, Mroz MM, Maier LA, et al. Up-regulation of programmed death-1 expression on beryllium-specific CD4+ T cells in chronic beryllium disease. *J Immunol.* (2008) 180:2704–12. doi:10.4049/jimmunol.180.4.2704

Chain JL, Martin AK, Mack DG, Maier LA, Palmer BE, Fontenot AP. Impaired function of CTLA-4 in the lungs of patients with chronic beryllium disease contributes to persistent inflammation. *J Immunol.* (2013) 191:1648–56. doi: 10.4049/jimmunol.1300282

Balmes JR, Abraham JL, Dweik RA, Fireman E, Fontenot AP, Maier LA, et al. An official American Thoracic Society statement: diagnosis and management of beryllium sensitivity and chronic beryllium disease. *Am J Respir Crit Care Med.* (2014) 190:e34–59. doi: 10.1164/rccm.201409-1722ST

Rossman MD, Stubbs J, Lee CW, Argyris E, Magira E, Monos D. Human leukocyte antigen Class II amino acid epitopes: susceptibility and progression markers for beryllium hypersensitivity. *Am J Respir Crit Care Med.* (2002) 165:788–94. doi: 10.1164/ajrccm.165.6.2104002

Maier LA, McGrath DS, Sato H, Lympany P, Welsh K, Du Bois R, et al. Influence of MHC class II in susceptibility to beryllium sensitization and chronic beryllium disease. *J Immunol.* (2003) 171:6910–8. doi:10.4049/jimmunol.171.12.6910

Silveira LJ, McCanlies EC, Fingerlin TE, Van Dyke MV, Mroz MM, Strand M, et al. Chronic beryllium disease, HLA-DPB1, and the DP peptide binding groove. *J Immunol.* (2012) 189:4014–23. doi: 10.4049/jimmunol.12 00798

Rybicki BA, Iannuzzi MC, Frederick MM, Thompson BW, Rossman MD, Bresnitz EA, et al. Familial aggregation of sarcoidosis. A case-control etiologic study of sarcoidosis (ACCESS). *Am J Respir Crit Care Med.* (2001) 164:2085– 91. doi: 10.1164/ajrccm.164.11.2106001

Iannuzzi MC, Rybicki BA. Genetics of sarcoidosis: candidate genes and genome scans. *Proc Am Thorac Soc.* (2007) 4:108–16. doi:10.1513/pats.200607-141JG

Grunewald J, Eklund A. Löfgren's syndrome: human leukocyte antigen strongly influences the disease course. *Am J Respir Crit Care Med.* (2009) 179:307–12. doi: 10.1164/rccm.200807-1082OC

Marrack P, Kappler J. The T cell receptor. *Science.* (1987) 238:1073–9. doi:10.1126/science.3317824

Dai S, Murphy GA, Crawford F, Mack DG, Falta MT, Marrack P, et al. Crystal structure of HLA-DP2 and implications for chronic beryllium disease. *Proc Natl Acad Sci USA.* (2010) 107:7425–30. doi: 10.1073/pnas.1001772107

Clayton GM, Wang Y, Crawford F, Novikov A, Wimberly BT, Kieft JS, et al. Structural basis of chronic beryllium disease: linking allergic hypersensitivity and autoimmunity. *Cell.* (2014) 158:132–42. doi: 10.1016/j.cell.2014. 04.048

Fontenot AP, Kotzin BL, Comment CE, Newman LS. Expansions of T-cell subsets expressing particular T-cell receptor variable regions in chronic beryllium disease. *Am J Respir Cell Mol Biol.* (1998) 18:581–9. doi: 10.1165/ajrcmb.18.4.2981

Bowerman NA, Falta MT, Mack DG, Wehrmann F, Crawford F, Mroz MM, et al. Identification of multiple public TCR repertoires in chronic beryllium disease. *J Immunol.* (2014) 192:4571–80. doi: 10.4049/jimmunol. 1400007

Falta MT, Pinilla C, Mack DG, Tinega AN, Crawford F, Giulianotti M, et al. Identification of beryllium-dependent peptides recognized by CD4+ T cells in chronic beryllium disease. *J Exp Med.* (2013) 210:1403–18. doi: 10.1084/jem.20122426

Grunewald J, Janson CH, Eklund A, Ohrn M, Olerup O, Persson U, et al. Restricted V alpha 2.3 gene usage by CD4+ T lymphocytes in bronchoalveolar lavage fluid from sarcoidosis patients correlates with HLA-DR3. *Eur J Immunol.* (1992) 22:129–35. doi: 10.1002/eji.1830220120

Grunewald J, Olerup O, Persson U, Ohrn MB, Wigzell H, Eklund A. T-cell receptor variable region gene usage by CD4+ and CD8+ T cells in bronchoalveolar lavage fluid and peripheral blood of sarcoidosis patients. *Proc Natl Acad Sci USA.* (1994) 91:4965–9. doi: 10.1073/pnas.91. 11.4965

Grunewald J, Berlin M, Olerup O, Eklund A. Lung T-helper cells expressing T-cell receptor AV2S3 associate with clinical features of pulmonary sarcoidosis. *Am J Respir Crit Care Med.* (2000) 161:814–18. doi:10.1164/ajrccm.161.3.9906001

Planck A, Eklund A, Grunewald J. Markers of activity in clinically recovered human leukocyte antigen-DR17-positive sarcoidosis patients. *Eur Respir J.* (2003) 21:52–7. doi: 10.1183/09031936.03.00059103

Mitchell AM, Kaiser Y, Falta MT, Munson DJ, Landry LG, Eklund A, et al. Shared alphabeta TCR Usage in Lungs of Sarcoidosis Patients with Löfgren's Syndrome. *J Immunol.* (2017) 199:2279–90. doi: 10.4049/jimmunol. 1700570

Coulombe PA, Wong P. Cytoplasmic intermediate filaments revealed as dynamic and multipurpose scaffolds. *Nat Cell Biol.* (2004) 6:699–706. doi: 10.1038/ncb0804-699

Heyder T, Kohler M, Tarasova NK, Haag S, Rutishauser D, Rivera NV, et al. Approach for identifying human leukocyte antigen (HLA)-DR bound peptides from scarce clinical samples. *Mol Cell Proteomics.* (2016) 15:3017–29. doi: 10.1074/mcp.M116.060764

Gupta D, Agarwal R, Aggarwal AN, Jindal SK. Molecular evidence for the role of mycobacteria in sarcoidosis: a meta-analysis. *Eur Respir J.* (2007) 30:508–16. doi: 10.1183/09031936.00002607

Esteves T, Aparicio G, Garcia-Patos V. Is there any association between Sarcoidosis and infectious agents?: a systematic review and meta- analysis. *BMC Pulm Med.* (2016) 16:165. doi: 10.1186/s12890-016- 0332-z

Chen ES, Wahlstrom J, Song Z, Willett MH, Wiken M, Yung RC, et al. T cell responses to mycobacterial catalase-peroxidase profile a pathogenic antigen in systemic sarcoidosis. *J Immunol.* (2008) 181:8784–96. doi: 10.4049/jimmunol.181.12.8784

Oswald-Richter KA, Culver DA, Hawkins C, Hajizadeh R, Abraham S, Shepherd BE, et al. Cellular responses to mycobacterial antigens are present in bronchoalveolar lavage fluid used in the diagnosis of sarcoidosis. *Infect Immun.* (2009) 77:3740–8. doi: 10.1128/IAI.00142-09

Song Z, Marzilli L, Greenlee BM, Chen ES, Silver RF, Askin FB, et al. Mycobacterial catalase-peroxidase is a tissue antigen and target of the adaptive immune response in systemic sarcoidosis. *J Exp Med.* (2005) 201:755–67. doi:10.1084/jem.20040429

Eishi Y, Suga M, Ishige I, Kobayashi D, Yamada T, Takemura T, et al. Quantitative analysis of mycobacterial and propionibacterial DNA in lymph nodes of Japanese and European patients with sarcoidosis. *J Clin Microbiol.* (2002) 40:198–204. doi: 10.1128/JCM.40.1.198-204.2002

Ishige I, Eishi Y, Takemura T, Kobayashi I, Nakata K, Tanaka I, et al. Propionibacterium acnes is the most common bacterium commensal in peripheral lung tissue and mediastinal lymph nodes from subjects without sarcoidosis. *Sarcoidosis Vasc Diffuse Lung Dis.* (2005) 22:33–42.

Demirkok SS, Basaranoglu M, Akbilgic O. Seasonal variation of the onset of presentations in stage 1 sarcoidosis. *Int J Clin Pract.* (2006) 60:1443–50. doi: 10.1111/j.1742-1241.2006.00773.x

Newman LS, Rose CS, Bresnitz EA, Rossman MD, Barnard J, Frederick M, et al. A case control etiologic study of sarcoidosis: environmental and occupational risk factors. *Am J Respir Crit Care Med.* (2004) 170:1324–30. doi: 10.1164/rccm.200402-249OC

Izbicki G, Chavko R, Banauch GI, Weiden MD, Berger KI, Aldrich TK, et al. World Trade Center "sarcoid-like" granulomatous pulmonary disease in New York City Fire Department rescue workers. *Chest.* (2007) 131:1414–23. doi: 10.1378/chest.06-2114

Vihlborg P, Bryngelsson IL, Andersson L, Graff P. Risk of sarcoidosis and seropositive rheumatoid arthritis from occupational silica exposure in Swedish iron foundries: a retrospective cohort study. *BMJ Open.* (2017) 7:e016839. doi: 10.1136/bmjopen-2017-016839

8

Management and Prognosis of Interstitial Lung Disease with Lung Cancer (ILD-LC): A Real-World Cohort from Three Medical Centers in China

Xie Xiaohong[1†], Wang Liqiang[1†], Li Na[2†], Lin Xinqing[1], Qin Yinyin[1], Liu Ming[1], Ouyang Ming[1], Han Qian[1], Luo Qun[1], Li Shiyue[1], Li Chunyan[3], Wang Xiaoqian[3], Yang Shuanying[2], Huang Wei[2], Liu Mei[2], Wang Ping[4] and Zhou Chengzhi[1]**

[1] State Key Laboratory of Respiratory Disease, National Clinical Research Center of Respiratory Disease, The First Affiliated Hospital of Guangzhou Medical University, Guangzhou Institute of the Respiratory Health, Guangzhou Medical University, Guangzhou, China, [2] Department of Respiratory and Critical Care Medicine, The Second Affiliated Hospital of Xi'an Jiaotong University, Xi'an, China, [3] Department of Respiratory and Critical Care Medicine, The First Medical Center of PLA General Hospital, Beijing, China, [4] Department of Respiratory and Critical Care Medicine, The Eighth Medical Center of PLA General Hospital, Beijing, China

***Correspondence:**
Wang Ping
taoybs_wp@163.com
Zhou Chengzhi
zhouchengzhi@gird.cn;
doctorzcz@163.com

† These authors have contributed equally to this work and share first authorship

Background and Objective: Interstitial lung disease with lung cancer (ILD-LC) is rare and its management has not been fully described. This study aimed to investigate the management and prognosis of ILD-LC patients in China.

Methods: The present analysis is a retrospective real-world cohort study. Clinical data of ILD-LC patients were obtained from 3 hospitals in China. The overall survival (OS) of patients was analyzed. Univariate and multivariate regression analyses were performed.

Results: One hundred eighty-four ILD-LC patients included were biased toward male (85.3%), smokers (75.5%), idiopathic pulmonary fibrosis (IPF) (58.2%) patients with comorbidities (67.9%) and ECOG-PS score of 1 (65.2%). Most patients were advanced peripheral non-small cell lung cancer. The initial anti-cancer regimen for ILD-LC is mainly chemotherapy, and patients with early-stage LC prefer surgery. In the anti-cancer cohort, the number of ILD-LC patients who underwent the 2nd and 3rd or more anti-cancer regimens were 78 (55.7%) and 32 (22.8%), respectively. In the non-anticancer cohort, the median OS was 3.5 months. In the early-stage cohort, the median OS was 14.2 months in the systematic therapy group; however, the median OS was not reached in the surgery group. In the advanced-stage cohort with systematic therapy, the median OS was 7.2 months. Interstitial pneumonia (IIP) and anti-angiogenesis were associated with OS in the univariate analysis, whereas anti-angiogenesis was an independent protective factor for advanced LC with ILD.

Conclusion: Patients with ILD-LC have very poor prognosis. Appropriate anti-tumor treatment can prolong the survival time of patients who can tolerate it. Targeted therapy and immunotherapy are alternative treatments for LC patients with mild ILD. For ILD patients with advanced LC, antiangiogenic regimens significantly improve the prognosis of the disease.

Keywords: interstitial lung disease, lung cancer, ILD-LC, prognosis, anti-angiogenesis treatment

INTRODUCTION

Interstitial lung disease (ILD), especially idiopathic pulmonary fibrosis (IPF) and connective tissue disease (CTD)-ILD, is a risk factor for lung cancer. The incidence of lung cancer is 4.4–48% in IPF patients, while 5.5–9.0% in CTD-ILD patients (Raghu et al., 2004; Tomassetti et al., 2015; Enomoto et al., 2016; Jung et al., 2018; Watanabe et al., 2018). Risk factors for developing ILD with lung cancer (ILD-LC) include male sex, older age, smoking, combined pulmonary fibrosis and emphysema (CPFE) (Usui et al., 2011; Watanabe et al., 2018). In addition, CTD-ILD without immunosuppressive therapy may be a risk factor for cancer (Watanabe et al., 2018).

Recently, the clinical profile of patients with ILD-LC was described. The ILD-LC population comprises individuals who are male, elderly, smokers, have IPF and are at advanced stage of LC (Minegishi et al., 2009). High-resolution computed tomography (HRCT) shows that the tumors are mainly in peripheral areas around ILD (Minegishi et al., 2009; Yoo et al., 2019). Squamous cell carcinoma was considered to be the most common pathological type of ILD-LC (Tomassetti et al., 2015; Watanabe et al., 2018), but there was an increasing trend for adenocarcinoma and small cell carcinoma nowadays (Saijo et al., 2017).

The IPF guidelines recommend that IPF be considered in treatment decisions for LC in IPF-LC patients (Cottin et al., 2017; Homma et al., 2018). However, the LC guidelines have not yet been established for the treatment of these patients. Surgery is recommended for early-stage lung cancer patients with ILD (Homma et al., 2018); however, there is still controversy over whether active anti-tumor strategies are suitable for inoperable ILD-LC patients with pulmonary dysfunction and poor PS score. The acute exacerbation (AE) of ILD (AE-ILD) is the main reason for the difficulty in treating patients with anti-cancer therapy (Minegishi et al., 2011a,b; Sekine et al., 2016; Hanibuchi et al., 2018; Asahina et al., 2019; Fujimoto et al., 2019; Kenmotsu et al., 2019). Although there are a few prospective studies involving chemotherapy and immunotherapy (Minegishi et al., 2009; Naccache et al., 2018), the current researches on inoperable ILD-LC focus on describing the treatments and AE-ILD retrospectively in a small population. Reducing AE-ILD is urgent, and several studies have shown that anti-angiogenic drugs such as nintedanib and bevacizumab can reduce the risk of chemotherapy-related AE-ILD (Richeldi et al., 2014; Hamada et al., 2019). However, there are more anti-angiogenic drugs, such as apatinib, anlotinib and recombinant human endostatin, etc., which have an unknown effect in reducing AE-ILD.

To date, there is no large-scale research on the treatment and prognosis of ILD-LC in China. Besides, the treatment of lung cancer has undergone tremendous changes, so the management of ILD-LC needs to be further described. To better understand the current management and prognosis of ILD-LC in China, we conducted a retrospective study to provide a feasible reference for the follow-up treatment for ILD-LC in real clinical practice.

PATIENTS AND METHODS

Patients and Diagnostic Criteria

A systematic search was conducted in the databases of three medical centers, The First Affiliated Hospital of Guangzhou Medical University, Chinese People's Liberation Army General Hospital, and The Second Affiliated Hospital of Xi'an Jiaotong University, located in Southeast, North, and Northwest China. All included cases presented with ILD on chest HRCT scan and were histologically diagnosed with LC from January 1, 2009 to October 1, 2019. Those with missing clinical data, other malignant tumors, drug-related ILD, and cancerous lymphangitis were excluded.

Patients eligible were grouped into idiopathic interstitial pneumonia (IIP) and CTD-ILD groups based on HRCT findings and clinical courses. We classify IIP into two groups: the IPF pattern and non-IPF groups. The IPF pattern group consisted of patients diagnosed as IPF histologically or clinically according to the American Thoracic Society/European Respiratory Society (ATS/ERS) criteria. IPF diagnosed without pathology is mainly based on clinical manifestations and typical chest CT findings: basal and peripheral predominant reticular abnormalities with traction bronchiectasis and honeycombing (ATS and ERS, 2002).

Data Collection

Data such as demographic characteristics, as well as information on smoking history, comorbidities, the subtype of ILD, pulmonary function test, time to diagnose LC, histology according to World Health Organization (WHO) tumor classification, stage group using the 8th edition of the TNM classification, and regimens for anti-cancer, was obtained retrospectively from the medical record. Two independent pulmonologists evaluated the chest HRCT images taken during the diagnosis of ILD-LC that met the criteria. The imaging evaluation mainly distinguishes the IPF pattern which is mentioned above. The location of the mass is recorded as either peripheral or central. The peripheral location is defined as <3 cm from the pleura. The disagreement between the 2 reviewers has been resolved by consensus.

Statistical Analysis

SPSS software version 24 (IBM) was used for statistical analysis and Graphpad Prism version 8 for graphing. Patient demographics were compared using the unpaired t-test for continuous variables and Pearson's χ^2 test for categorical variables. Overall survival (OS) was defined as the time from the date of diagnosis of primary lung cancer to the date of death from any cause. Patients who were alive or had been lost to follow-up at the time of analysis were considered censored. Kaplan-Meier was used for survival analysis and the log-rank test was used to assess differences between groups. Cox's proportional hazards regression analysis was used to identify significant variables that affect the survival of advanced ILD-LC patients and to estimate hazard ratios

(HR) and 95% confidence intervals (CI) for predictors of survival. All tests were two-tailed, and $p < 0.05$ was considered statistically significant.

RESULTS

Patient Characteristics

A total of 236 patients with ILD-LC were identified, and 184 were eventually enrolled in the study (**Figure 1**). The baseline characteristics of all patients, the anti-cancer group and the non-anticancer group are shown in **Table 1**. Overall, at the time of LC diagnosis, the majority of the patients were male (85.3%) and smokers (75.5%) with a median age of 68 years (range, 44–90 years). The main subtype of ILD was IPF (58.2%). Most patients were stage III/IV peripheral NSCLC with comorbidities (67.9%) and ECOG-PS scores of 1 (65.2%). There were differences in age, ECOG-PS, and smoking status between the anti-cancer and non-anticancer groups. Patients in the non-anticancer group had older age and worse ECOG-PS scores.

The Distribution of Various Anti-cancer Regimens at Different Treatment Stages in ILD-LC

Most patients with ILD-LC could not undergo multiple courses of anti-cancer regimens (**Table 2**). Compared with the initial treatment, the number of patients underwent the 2nd and 3rd or more anti-cancer regimens were 78 (55.7%) and 32 (22.8%), respectively. Chemotherapy accounted for the largest proportion of all treatment stages. In addition to chemotherapy, surgery (17.9%) and radiotherapy (28.2%) were the most common in the first-stage treatment and the second- stage treatment, respectively. Besides, anti-angiogenic therapy (25.0%) is preferred in the third and above stage therapies.

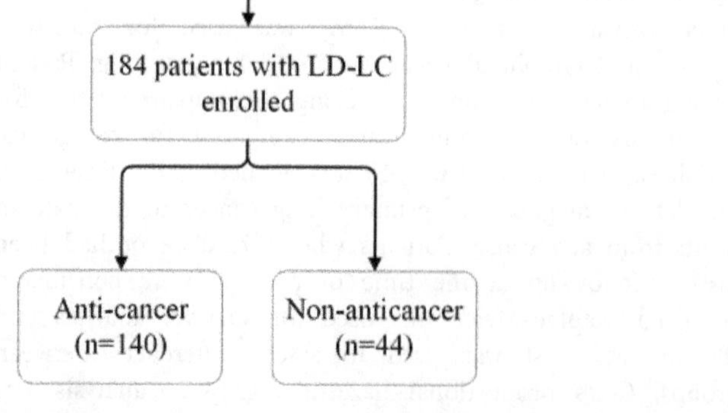

FIGURE 1 | Flowchart of the ILD-LC patients selecting process.

The Choice of Anti-cancer Regimens Based on Histological Type, Clinical-Stage, the Subtype of ILD, and ECOG-PS Score

The anti-cancer regimen for ILD-LC is similar to that for lung cancer alone (**Table 3**). Patients who underwent surgery were early-stage non-small cell lung cancer patients with good ECOG-PS scores and non-IPF can be found for a higher proportion of these patients. Patients with good ECOG-PS score, small cell lung cancer, advanced stage lung cancer, and non-IPF are more inclined to choose chemotherapy. Radiotherapy is mainly used for stage III/IV squamous cell carcinoma and small cell carcinoma with an ECOG-PS score of 1, and IPF accounts for more. Targeted therapy is mainly used for IIP patients with an ECOG-PS score of 2–3 and stage III/IV adenocarcinoma. Immune checkpoint inhibitors have also been used in our ILD-LC patients, who are characterized by advanced IIP-LC with better ECOG-PS scores.

Survival Data and Prognostic Factors

Patients were followed-up until May 2020. Thirty-four of the one hundred eighty-four patients were lost to follow-up and 23 were still alive. The median follow-up time was 27 months. In the overall population, the median OS for anti-cancer cohort and non-anticancer cohort were 11.1 vs. 3.5 (HR 0.3014, 95%CI: 0.1771 to 0.5130). In the non-anticancer cohort, the 6-month and 1-year OS rates were 25 and 6.8%, respectively. Furthermore, we divided the patients in the anti-cancer cohort into two groups: the early-stage (stage I-IIIA) group ($n = 48$) and the advanced stage (stage IIIB-IV) cohort ($n = 92$). In the early-stage group, 25 patients received surgery and 23 received systematic therapy. The advanced stage group all received systematic therapy. Among the surgical patients, 7 cases died, 13 cases survived, and 5 cases were lost to follow-up. The median OS was not reached for patients who underwent surgery, and the 1, 2, and 3-year OS rates were 80.0, 68.0, and 36.0%, respectively. The median OS for the early-stage group that underwent systematic therapy was 14.2 m, the 1 and 2-year OS rate was 47.8%, and 17.4%, respectively. The median OS of the advanced-stage cohort that underwent systematic therapy was 7.2 m, and the 1-year OS rate was 20.7% (**Figure 2**). Sixteen advanced-stage LC patients were receiving targeted therapy with a median OS of 6.5 months, while 9 of them with EGFR mutations receiving targeted therapy in the first stage have a median OS of 16.2 months. The median OS of 6 patients with advanced-stage LC receiving immunotherapy was 8.8 months.

Analysis of prognostic factors was conducted to identify significant variables that affect the OS of the advanced stage group (**Table 4**). Gender, age, smoking status, anatomical type, histological type, stage, the subtype of ILD, the sequence of tumor occurrence, and anti-cancer regimens were included in the study. Univariate analysis revealed that patients with CTD-ILD and antiangiogenic therapy had a significantly better prognosis.

TABLE 1 | Characteristics of anti-cancer and non-anticancer patients with interstitial lung disease and lung cancer (ILD-LC).

Characteristics	All patients ($N = 184$)	Anti-cancer ($N = 140$)	Non-anticancer ($N = 44$)	*p*-value
Gender, male, *n* (%)	157 (85.3)	121 (86.4)	36 (81.8)	0.451
Age, median (range), year	68.0 (44–90)	66.0 (44–90)	70.5 (46–89)	0.005
ECOG-PS				0.001
1	120 (65.2)	99 (70.7)	21 (47.7)	
2	57 (31.0)	39 (27.9)	18 (40.9)	
3	7 (3.8)	2 (1.4)	5 (11.4)	
Smoking status, current or former, *n* (%)	139 (75.5)	111 (79.2)	28 (63.6)	0.035
Smoking index	885 ± 514	881 ± 500	901 ± 577	0.850
Comorbidities, yes, *n* (%)	125(67.9)	93 (66.4)	32 (72.7)	0.435
Histology				0.36
Squamous cell carcinoma	58 (31.5)	42 (30.0)	16 (36.4)	
Adenocarcinoma	69 (37.5)	50 (35.7)	19 (43.2)	
Other NSCLC	17 (9.2)	15 (10.7)	2 (4.5)	
Small cell carcinoma	40 (21.7)	33 (23.6)	7 (15.9)	
Clinical stage				0.536
I	19 (10.3)	17 (12.1)	2 (4.5)	
II	12 (6.5)	9 (6.4)	3 (6.8)	
III	52 (28.3)	38 (27.1)	14 (31.8)	
IV	101 (54.9)	76 (54.3)	25 (56.8)	
Anatomical type				0.776
Peripheral	145 (78.8)	111 (79.3)	34 (77.3)	
Central	39 (21.2)	29 (20.7)	10 (22.7)	
Subtype of ILD				0.107
IPF	107 (58.2)	78 (55.7)	29 (65.9)	
non-IPF	56 (30.4)	48 (34.3)	8 (18.2)	
CTD-ILD	21 (11.4)	14 (10.0)	7 (15.9)	
Time to diagnose LC				0.781
After ILD	87 (47.3)	67 (47.9)	20 (45.5)	
Simultaneous	97(52.7)	73 (52.1)	24 (54.5)	
Disorder of ventilation function (*n*)	68	47	21	0.071
Normal	15 (22.1)	14 (29.8)	1 (4.8)	
Restrictive	32 (47.1)	20 (42.6)	12 (57.1)	
Mixed	21 (30.9)	13 (27.6)	8 (38.1)	
Degree of ventilation function (*n*)	68	47	21	0.521
Normal or Mild	42 (61.8)	31 (66.0)	11 (52.4)	
Moderate	17 (25.0)	10 (21.3)	7 (33.3)	
Severe	9 (13.2)	6 (12.8)	3 (14.3)	
Degree of diffusion capacity (*n*)	61	43	18	0.077
Normal or mild	24 (39.3)	20 (46.5)	4 (22.2)	
Moderate and severe	37 (60.7)	23 (53.5)	14 (77.8)	

ECOG-PS, Eastern Cooperative Oncology Group-Performance Status; ILD, interstitial lung disease; IPF, idiopathic pulmonary fibrosis; CTD, connective tissue disease; NSCLC, non-small cell lung cancer; LC, lung cancer. The p-values refer to comparisons between the anti-cancer and non-anti-cancer groups.

Anti-angiogenic therapy was the independent factor in the Cox regression model. Patients with anti-angiogenic therapy have significantly longer OS compared to those without anti-angiogenesis, with a median OS of 9.3 vs. 6.1 m (HR: 0.5002, 95% CI: 0.2866 to 0.8731, $p = 0.0148$).

DISCUSSION

The current descriptions of the treatment and prognosis of ILD-LC are mainly derived from retrospective studies involving a small population, which are insufficient and limited. Here, we conducted a multicenter retrospective study involving 184 ILD-LC patients, with the aim of understanding the clinical profile, management, and prognosis of ILD-LC patients in China. Consistent with previous studies (Minegishi et al., 2009; Tomassetti et al., 2015), patients with ILD-LC in our cohort are mainly elderly, smokers, male. They also had IIP, peripheral NSCLC, poor ECOG-PS, and comorbidities. Half of the patients were diagnosed with lung cancer and ILD at the same time, and most of them had mild to moderate restrictive ventilatory dysfunction and moderate to severe diffuse dysfunction.

TABLE 2 | Initial and follow-up anti-cancer regimens for patients with ILD-LC.

Stage of treatment[#]	Totol	1st- (n,%[&])	2nd- (n,%)	≥3rd-or more (n,%)
N	140	140 (100.0)	78 (55.7)	32 (22.8)
Surgery	25	25 (17.9)	0 (0)	0 (0)
Chemotherapy	109	89 (63.6)	45 (57.7)	23 (71.9)
Interventional therapy	6	2 (1.4)	3 (3.8)	1 (3.1)
Radiotherapy	35	10 (7.1)	22 (28.2)	3 (9.4)
Anti-angiogenic therapy[※]	29	13 (9.3)	10 (12.8)	8 (25.0)
Targeted therapy[£]	20	12 (8.6)	8 (10.3)	3 (9.4)
Immunotherapy	8	5 (3.6)	3 (3.8)	1 (3.1)
Others[€]	7	7 (5.0)	0 (0)	0 (0)

[#] *Patients can receive more than one anti-cancer regimens at every stage of treatment.*
[&] *The proportion of a regimen in the treatment stage to total events of the regimen.*
[※] *Anti-angiogenic agents include 11 cases of bevacizumab, 3 cases of apatinib, 5 cases of anlotinib, 9 cases of nintedanib, 1 case of recombinant human endostatin.*
[£] *There were 11 patients with EGFR mutations, 10 in the first stage and 1 in the second stage. Two patients in the first stage received EGFR-TKIs without confirming the EGFR status. The remaining patients in the second- and above stage were at an unknown EGFR status for lacking records.*
[€] *Oral anti-cancer drugs.*

The management of ILD-LC is important and necessary but has not been fully described. The published articles hardly discuss the differences in choosing anti-cancer or not in patients with ILD-LC. In our study, 44 (23.9%) of 184 patients chose the best supportive care (BSC) without anti-cancer regimens. We found that older age, worse ECOG-PS scores, and poor lung function may be reasons for patients choosing the BSC. Furthermore, the anti-cancer regimens in our cohort are similar to that of patients with lung cancer only. However, the challenge in clinical practice is that AE induced by anti-cancer regimens may interrupt the treatment of LC and even cause the death of patients (Minegishi et al., 2009; Amundson et al., 2019). We did not summarize the AE-ILD in most patients for the lack of clinical data. Therefore, the number of patients who underwent anti-cancer treatment at different stages was used to reflect the tolerance of these patients to anti-cancer treatment. There were 55.7% of patients administered second- and above stage treatments in our study, while 36.3% (32 of 88 in anticancer) in Minegishi et al. (2009). However, only 22.8% of ILD-LC patients underwent a third or more anti-cancer treatment in the anti-cancer group. All this means that many patients have lost the opportunity to receive more anti-cancer treatments because of ILD.

Appropriate anti-cancer measures for ILD-LC are reasonable, which makes patients live longer. Surgery is important and recommended for the management of early-stage LC with ILD due to the high survival rate (Omori et al., 2015; Sato et al., 2015; Homma et al., 2018). We also concluded that the 3-year OS rates of surgery cohort were 36.0%. However, postoperative AE-ILD is a serious complication for patients with surgery. There was one patient who experienced postoperative AE-ILD and died within 2 months in our study. Sato et al. (2014) showed that 9.3% of 1,763 patients suffered postoperative AE-ILD with a mortality rate of 43.9%. Minegishi et al. (2009) reported that 8 of 35 patients who underwent surgery experienced postoperative AE-ILD, and 3 died of AE. Surgical procedures, male sex, history of exacerbation, preoperative steroid use, serum sialylated carbohydrate antigen KL-6 levels, preoperative percent vital capacity plus serum LDH

TABLE 3 | Treatment options for the anti-cancer cohort of ILD-LC stratified according to histological type, clinical stage, subtype of ILD, and ECOG-PS score.

	N	Surgery[&]	Chemotherapy	Interventional therapy	Radiotherapy	Anti-angiogenic therapy	Targeted therapy	Immunotherapy	Others
Histology									
Squamous cell carcinoma[#]	42	10 (23.8)	31 (73.8)	3 (7.1)	16 (38.1)	6 (14.3)	2 (4.7)	4 (9.5)	5 (11.9)
Adenocarcinoma	50	8 (16.0)	36 (72.0)	0 (0)	5 (10.0)	14 (28.0)	15 (30.0)	1 (2.0)	1 (2.0)
Other NSCLC	15	4 (26.7)	11 (73.3)	1 (6.7)	2 (13.3)	3 (20.0)	3 (20.0)	1 (6.7)	1 (6.7)
Small cell carcinoma	33	3 (9.1)	31 (93.9)	2 (6.1)	12 (36.4)	6 (18.2)	0 (0)	2 (6.1)	0 (0)
Clinical stage									
I	17	14 (82.4)	10 (58.8)	0 (0)	5 (29.4)	3 (17.6)	1 (5.9)	1 (5.9)	2 (11.8)
II	9	5 (55.6)	8 (88.9)	0 (0)	2 (22.2)	1 (11.1)	0 (0)	0 (0)	0 (0)
III	38	6 (15.8)	30 (78.9)	1 (2.6)	13 (34.2)	8 (21.1)	4 (10.5)	2 (5.3)	3 (7.9)
IV	76	0 (0)	61 (80.3)	5 (6.6)	15 (19.7)	17 (22.4)	15 (19.7)	5 (6.6)	2 (2.6)
ILD classification									
IPF	78	12 (15.4)	60 (76.9)	3 (3.8)	15 (19.2)	17 (21.8)	13 (16.7)	4 (5.1)	6 (7.7)
non-IPF	48	11 (22.9)	40 (83.3)	3 (6.3)	16 (33.3)	6 (12.5)	6 (12.5)	4 (8.3)	1 (2.1)
CTD-ILD	14	2 (14.3)	9 (64.3)	0 (0)	4 (28.6)	6 (42.9)	1 (7.1)	0 (0)	0 (0)
ECOG-PS									
1	99	23 (23.2)	81 (81.8)	2 (2.0)	35 (35.3)	21 (21.2)	8 (8.1)	7 (7.1)	6 (6.1)
2	39	2 (5.1)	27 (69.2)	3 (7.7)	0 (0)	7 (17.9)	12 (30.8)	1 (2.6)	1 (2.6)
3	2	0 (0)	0 (0)	1 (50)	0 (0)	1 (50)	0 (0)	0 (0)	0 (0)

ECOG-PS, Eastern Cooperative Oncology Group-Performance Status; ILD, interstitial lung disease; IPF, idiopathic pulmonary fibrosis; CTD, connective tissue disease; NSCLC, non-small cell lung cancer.
[#] *Patients in each stratification may receive one or more treatments.*
[&] *The proportion of a regimen in each stratification to the total number of the stratification.*

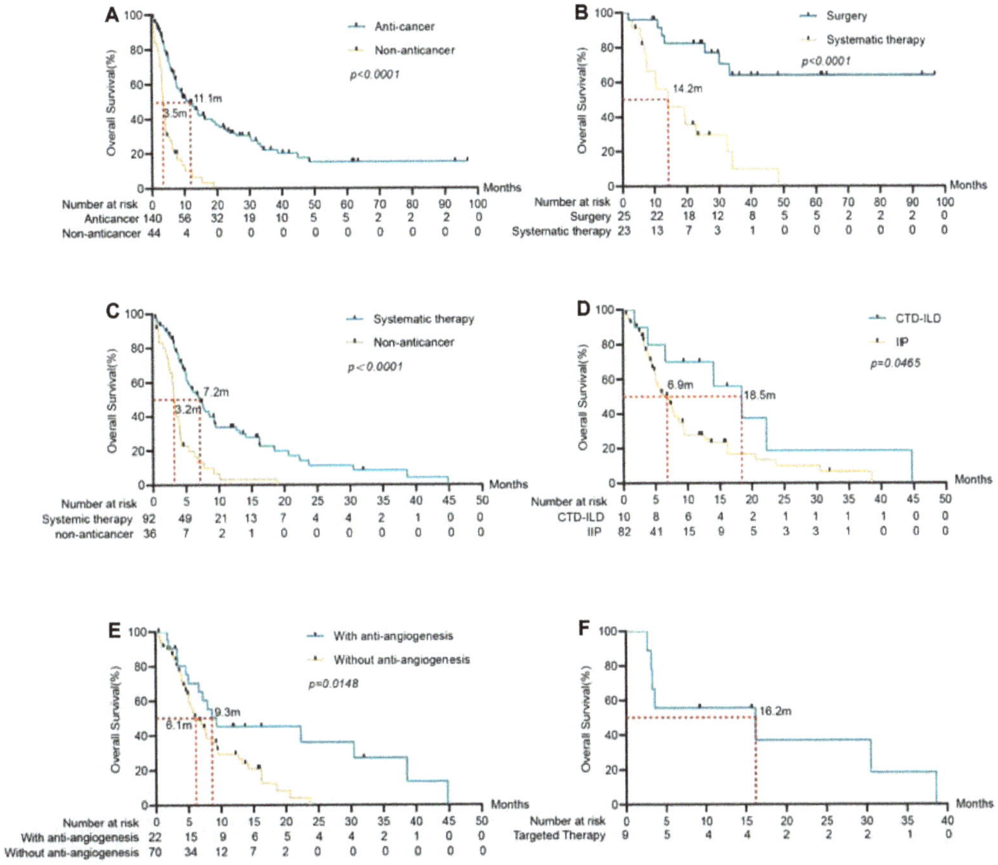

FIGURE 2 | Survival analysis of ILD-LC patients in different groups. **(A)** Anti-cancer group (n = 140) vs. non-anticancer group (n = 44), the mOS of the anti-cancer group was significantly longer than that of the non-anticancer group. **(B)** Surgery group (n = 25) and systematic therapy group (n = 23) in early-stage LC with ILD. **(C)** Systematic therapy group (n = 92) vs. non-anticancer group in advanced stage LC with ILD. **(D)** For patients in advanced stage LC with ILD, OS was associated with the subtype of ILD (p = 0.0465). **(E)** OS was associated with anti-angiogenesis (p = 0.0148). **(F)** Patients received targeted therapy in advanced stage LC with ILD and the mOS was 16.2 months.

values were risk factors for postoperative AE-ILD after in patients with ILD (Shintani et al., 2010; Sato et al., 2014).

Systematic therapy for inoperable or recurrent LC with ILD is still controversial due to the AE-ILD. As mentioned above, most patients fail to receive multi-stage anti-cancer treatments in our study. However, consistent with the published researches (Kawahara et al., 2019), the present study showed that patients with advanced-stage LC benefit from systematic therapy in OS compared to those without anti-cancer treatment. The options of systematic treatment are diverse, and there is no optimal treatment for ILD-LC. Consistent with the previous study, chemotherapy was the most commonly chosen in our patients. However, the chemotherapy regimen for less AE is still inconclusive and chemotherapy-related exacerbation of ILD was between 9 and 42.8% (Watanabe et al., 2013; Kenmotsu et al., 2015). A series of prospective studies conducted in Japan showed that nab-paclitaxel plus carboplatin in NSCLC and etoposide plus carboplatin in SCLC were safe for patients with mild or moderate ILD (Minegishi et al., 2011a,b; Kenmotsu et al., 2019).

Radiotherapy plays a critical role in unresectable SCLC and NSCLC but should be used with caution in ILD-LC due to severe radiation pneumonia or AE-ILD (Yamaguchi et al., 2013; Glick et al., 2018). There were 35 patients with mild ILD administered with radiotherapy in our study, and 2 of them suffered grade 3 radiation pneumonia and AE-ILD respectively. The patient with radiation pneumonia received nintedanib monotherapy for more than a year and is still alive. While the patient with AE-ILD received BSC and died with an OS of 8 months. Radiotherapy-related grade 2–5 pneumonitis of patients with ILD-LC was 15.8% (Yamaguchi et al., 2013). Hagiwara et al. (2020) conducted a nationwide survey of radiotherapy in Japan for ILD-LC and found that 5(7.5%) of 67 patients suffered AE-ILD and 1 died of radiation-induced AE. Kobayashi et al. (2018) revealed that 17 (46%) of 37 patients treated with chemoradiotherapy developed grade 3 and above AE-ILD within 1 year after the last irradiation. Therefore, radiotherapy should be applied cautiously considering the serious side effects.

For patients with driver genes and mutations, tyrosine kinase inhibitors (TKIs) are more effective than traditional chemotherapy. However, the risk of TKI-induced ILD and AE-ILD remind us that TKIs should be applied cautiously in ILD-LC (Shi et al., 2014; Shah, 2016; Gemma et al., 2019). In our cohort,

TABLE 4 | Clinical characteristics, univariate and multivariate analysis of 92 advanced lung cancer with ILD for overall survival.

Group	No. patients (%)	Overall survival: Univariate analysis: P	Overall survival: Multivariate analysis: P
Gender (male, %)	77 (83.7)	0.058	0.065
Age (≥65, %)	58 (63.0)	0.071	0.163
Smoking status (yes, %)	72 (78.3)	0.47	*
Comorbidities (yes, %)	64 (69.6)	0.103	0.113
Histology (NSCLC, %)	68 (73.9)	0.647	*
Clinical stage (IV, %)	72 (78.3)	0.323	*
Anatomical type (peripheral, %)	70 (76.1)	0.659	*
ECOG-PS (1, %)	62 (67.4)	0.551	*
Subtype of ILD (IIP, %)	82 (89.1)	**0.046**	0.138
Time to diagnose LC (simultaneous, %)	52 (56.5)	0.17	0.122
Interventional therapy (yes, %)	3 (3.3)	*	*
Radiotherapy (yes, %)	21 (22.8)	0.16	0.133
Chemotherapy (yes, %)	74 (80.4)	0.659	*
Anti-angiogenic therapy (yes, %)	22 (23.9)	**0.015**	**0.011**
Targeted therapy (yes, %)	16 (17.4)	0.736	*
Immunotherapy (yes, %)	6 (6.5)	*	*
Others (yes, %)	5 (5.4)	*	*

ECOG-PS, Eastern Cooperative Oncology Group-Performance Status; ILD, interstitial lung disease; CTD, connective tissue disease; NSCLC, non-small cell lung cancer; IIP, idiopathic interstitial pneumonia, including idiopathic pulmonary fibrosis (IPF) and non-IPF.
**Analysis could not be done.*
The bold values means statistically different.

there were 10 patients confirmed with EGFR mutations receiving EGFR-TKIs in first-line treatment. The median OS of the 9 patients with advanced-stage LC was 16.2 months, and 4 (44.4%) of them experienced more than one stage treatments. Besides, preliminary evidence suggests that TKIs can be continued after TKI-induced ILD in the case of steroid coverage and/or dose reduction (Shah, 2016). Considering the long-term survival of ILD-LC patients with driver genes and mutations, TKIs should be administered at the first stage treatments.

The application of immune checkpoint inhibitors (ICIs) is a milestone in lung cancer, and the occurrence of immune-related adverse events (irAEs) such as checkpoint inhibitor-related pneumonitis (CIPs) is inevitable (Jain et al., 2018). The high mortality rate was observed in severe grade CIPs in NSCLC (Suresh et al., 2018; Tone et al., 2019), and pre-existing ILD is a risk factor for developing CIPs (Kanai et al., 2018). Therefore, CIPs maybe a serious threat to patients with ILD-LC though there was no report of AE-ILD induced by ICIs. However, compared with TKIs-related pneumonia, CIPs have a higher response rate to corticosteroid therapy and a lower mortality rate (Beom et al., 2016; Kato et al., 2017). For inoperable patients with mild IIP receiving nivolumab, a pilot study conducted by Fujimoto et al. (2017, 2019)showed no AE-ILD, while a phase II showed that 2 of 18 patients developed grade 2 pneumonitis, which could be treated using corticosteroid therapy. There was no AE-ILD or CIP observed in our advanced stage LC patients receiving immunotherapy with a median OS of 8.6 months, while 1 of them died of tumor progression within 1 month. This suggests that immunotherapy may be a good choice for these patients, but more clinical studies are needed to confirm it.

For advanced LC with ILD, the most appropriate anti-cancer regimens should bring the fewest AEs rather than the best anti-tumor effect. However, it is still necessary to look for prognostic factors that affect OS. We conducted a prognosis analysis in the advanced anti-cancer cohort and found the IIP was associated with poor prognosis, while anti-angiogenic therapy was an independent protective factor that improves the prognosis of advanced LC with ILD. There was in line with expectations that IIP is a prognostic risk factor of ILD-LC, because IIP, especially IPF, has a worse prognosis compared to CTD-ILD (Lim et al., 2019). Vascular endothelial growth factor (VEGF), a potent stimulator of vascular permeability and angiogenesis, plays an important role in lung diseases, including injury, fibrosis and cancer, as well as AE of IPF (Simler et al., 2004; Weis and Cheresh, 2005; McKeown et al., 2009). Nintedanib, an anti-angiogenic agent targeting VEGF, has been proven to have anti-cancer and anti-pulmonary fibrosis effects and reduce AE-ILD in patients with IPF (Reck et al., 2014; Richeldi et al., 2014; Hilberg et al., 2018; Fabre and Nicholson, 2020). Besides, nintedanib and bevacizumab have been shown to reduce the risk of chemotherapy-related AE-ILD in patients with lung cancer (Shimizu et al., 2014; Enomoto et al., 2015; Hamada et al., 2019). Anlotinib, a new anti-angiogenesis agent approved globally in 2018, has been proven attenuating bleomycin-induced pulmonary fibrosis in mice via the TGF-β1 signaling pathway (Ruan et al., 2020). Recombinant human endostatin and apatinib have not been evaluated to reduce AE in patients with ILD. In our study, anti-angiogenic agents mentioned above were included in the analysis. Although we failed to confirm whether anti-angiogenesis can reduce the acute exacerbation of ILD, we found that patients with advanced-stage LC receiving systematic therapy benefited from anti-angiogenic therapy. The possible reasons for anti-angiogenic therapy as an independent protective factor are as follows: 1. exerting the anti-tumor effect directly; 2. reducing AE-ILD and enabling patients to receive more anti-tumor treatments. Therefore, anti-angiogenic agents may be a good choice for patients with ILD-LC.

ILD-LC is a rare disease with poor prognosis, which is a part of severe lung cancer (Xie et al., 2019). These patients often face challenges in anti-cancer treatment because of poor PS scores or lung function caused by the progression of ILD. Furthermore, they may fail to receive anti-cancer treatment due to the slow progression or treatment-related AE-ILD. However, our research shows that patients with ILD-LC benefit from anti-cancer treatment. Our research shows that patients with ILD-LC benefit from anti-cancer treatment. In particular, these patients can live longer after using anti-angiogenic drugs, which suggests that anti-angiogenic therapy may be an important part of ILD-LC anti-cancer therapy.

Several limitations need to be noted regarding this real-world study. First, this is a retrospective study conducted over a long time. This study failed to reflect the current treatment status of ILD-LC due to the anti-cancer therapy of lung cancer has undergone great changes. Second, the lack of acute exacerbation and lung function data in most patients makes it impossible for us to analyze the toxicity and true efficacy of anti-cancer treatments. Our interpretation of survival data is inadequate. Third, the present study involves a variety of anti-angiogenic drugs and cannot be analyzed separately due to the limited sample size. Further investigations and larger patient groups are needed to confirm the protective effect of anti-angiogenic agents in patients with ILD-LC treated with anti-cancer therapy.

CONCLUSION

Patients with ILD-LC have very poor prognosis. Appropriate anti-tumor treatment can prolong the survival time of patients who can tolerate it. Targeted therapy and immunotherapy are alternative treatments for LC patients with mild ILD. For ILD patients with advanced LC, anti-angiogenic regimens significantly improve their prognosis.

was not required for this study in accordance with the national legislation and the institutional requirements.

AUTHOR CONTRIBUTIONS

XX, WL, and ZC: conception and design. QY, LMi, OM, HQ, LQ, LS, LC, WX, YS, HW, LMe, WP, and ZC: provision of study materials or patients. LW and LN: collection and assembly of data. XX, LW, LN, LX, LC, WX, YS, and HW: data analysis and interpretation. XX, WL, and LN: manuscript writing. All authors: final approval of the manuscript.

ACKNOWLEDGMENTS

We appreciate the patients and their families for their contributions to this study.

REFERENCES

Amundson, W. H., Racila, E., Allen, T., Dincer, H. E., Tomic, R., et al. (2019). Acute exacerbation of interstitial lung disease after procedures. *Respir. Med.* 150, 30–37. doi: 10.1016/j.rmed.2019.02.012

Asahina, H., Oizumi, S., Takamura, K., Harada, T., Harada, M., et al. (2019). A prospective phase II study of carboplatin and nab-paclitaxel in patients with advanced non-small cell lung cancer and concomitant interstitial lung disease (HOT1302). *Lung Cancer* 138, 65–71. doi: 10.1016/j.lungcan.2019.09.020

ATS and ERS (2002). American Thoracic Society/European Respiratory Society International Multidisciplinary Consensus Classification of the Idiopathic Interstitial Pneumonias. This joint statement of the American Thoracic Society (ATS), and the European Respiratory Society (ERS) was adopted by the ATS board of directors, June 2001 and by the ERS Executive Committee, June 2001. *Am. J. Respir. Crit. Care Med.* 165, 277–304. doi: 10.1164/ajrccm.165.2.ats01

Beom, S. H., Kim, D. W., Sim, S. H., Keam, B., Park, J. H., et al. (2016). Gefitinib-Induced interstitial lung disease in korean lung cancer patients. *Cancer Res. Treat.* 48, 88–97. doi: 10.4143/crt.2014.201

Cottin, V., Crestani, B., Cadranel, J., Cordier, J. F., Marchand-Adam, S., et al. (2017). French practical guidelines for the diagnosis and management of idiopathic pulmonary fibrosis - 2017 update. Full-length version. *Rev. Mal. Respir.* 34, 900–968. doi: 10.1016/j.rmr.2017.07.017

Enomoto, Y., Inui, N., Yoshimura, K., Nishimoto, K., Mori, K., et al. (2016). Lung cancer development in patients with connective tissue disease-related interstitial lung disease: A retrospective observational study. *Medicine* 95:e5716. doi: 10.1097/MD.0000000000005716

Enomoto, Y., Kenmotsu, H., Watanabe, N., Baba, T., Murakami, H., et al. (2015). Efficacy and safety of combined carboplatin, paclitaxel, and bevacizumab for patients with advanced non-squamous non-small cell lung cancer with pre-existing interstitial lung disease: A retrospective multi-institutional study. *Anticancer Res.* 35, 4259–4263.

Fabre, A., and Nicholson, A. G. (2020). Nintedanib in progressive fibrosing interstitial lung diseases. *N. Engl. J. Med.* 382:780.

Fujimoto, D., Morimoto, T., Ito, J., Sato, Y., Ito, M., et al. (2017). A pilot trial of nivolumab treatment for advanced non-small cell lung cancer patients with mild idiopathic interstitial pneumonia. *Lung Cancer* 111, 1–5. doi: 10.1016/j.lungcan.2017.06.008

Fujimoto, D., Yomota, M., Sekine, A., Morita, M., Morimoto, T., et al. (2019). Nivolumab for advanced non-small cell lung cancer patients with mild idiopathic interstitial pneumonia: A multicenter, open-label single-arm phase II trial. *Lung Cancer* 134, 274–278. doi: 10.1016/j.lungcan.2019.06.001

Gemma, A., Kusumoto, M., Kurihara, Y., Masuda, N., Banno, S., et al. (2019). Interstitial lung disease onset and its risk factors in japanese patients with ALK-Positive NSCLC after treatment with crizotinib. *J. Thorac. Oncol.* 14, 672–682. doi: 10.1016/j.jtho.2018.11.022

Glick, D., Lyen, S., Kandel, S., Shapera, S., Le, L. W., et al. (2018). Impact of pretreatment interstitial lung disease on radiation pneumonitis and survival in patients treated with lung stereotactic body radiation therapy (SBRT). *Clin. Lung Cancer* 19, 219–226. doi: 10.1016/j.cllc.2017.06.021

Hagiwara, Y., Nakayama, Y., Kudo, S., Hayakawa, T., Nakamura, N., et al. (2020). Nationwide survey of radiation therapy in Japan for lung cancer complicated with interstitial lung disease. *J. Radiat. Res.* 61, 563–574. doi: 10.1093/jrr/rraa018

Hamada, S., Ichiyasu, H., Ikeda, T., Inaba, M., Kashiwabara, K., et al. (2019). Protective effect of bevacizumab on chemotherapy-related acute exacerbation of interstitial lung disease in patients with advanced non-squamous non-small cell lung cancer. *BMC Pulmonary Med.* 19:72. doi: 10.1186/s12890-019-0838-2

Hanibuchi, M., Kakiuchi, S., Atagi, S., Ogushi, F., Shimizu, E., et al. (2018). A multicenter, open-label, phase II trial of S-1 plus carboplatin in advanced non-small cell lung cancer patients with interstitial lung disease. *Lung Cancer* 125, 93–99. doi: 10.1016/j.lungcan.2018.09.007

Hilberg, F., Tontsch-Grunt, U., Baum, A., Le, A. T., Doebele, R. C., et al. (2018). Triple angiokinase inhibitor nintedanib directly inhibits tumor cell growth and induces tumor shrinkage via blocking oncogenic receptor tyrosine kinases. *J. Pharmacol. Exp. Ther.* 364, 494–503. doi: 10.1124/jpet.117.244129

Homma, S., Bando, M., Azuma, A., Sakamoto, S., Sugino, K., et al. (2018). Japanese guideline for the treatment of idiopathic pulmonary fibrosis. *Respir. Investig.* 56, 268–291. doi: 10.1016/j.resinv.2018.03.003

Jain, A., Shannon, V. R., and Sheshadri, A. (2018). Immune-Related adverse events: Pneumonitis. *Adv. Exp. Med. Biol.* 995, 131–149. doi: 10.1007/978-3-030-02505-2_6

Jung, H. I., Park, J. S., Lee, M., Park, B., Kim, H. J., et al. (2018). Prevalence of lung cancer in patients with interstitial lung disease is higher than in those with chronic obstructive pulmonary disease. *Medicine* 97:e71. doi: 10.1097/MD.0000000000010071

Kanai, O., Kim, Y. H., Demura, Y., Kanai, M., Ito, T., et al. (2018). Efficacy and safety of nivolumab in non-small cell lung cancer with preexisting interstitial lung disease. *Thorac. Cancer* 9, 847–855. doi: 10.1111/1759-7714.12759

Kato, T., Masuda, N., Nakanishi, Y., Takahashi, M., Hida, T., et al. (2017). Nivolumab-induced interstitial lung disease analysis of two phase II studies patients with recurrent or advanced non-small-cell lung cancer. *Lung Cancer* 104, 111–118. doi: 10.1016/j.lungcan.2016.12.016

Kawahara, T., Sakashita, H., Suzuki, T., Tateishi, T., and Miyazaki, Y. (2019). Real world data of combined lung cancer and interstitial lung disease. *J. Thorac. Dis.* 11, 4144–4151. doi: 10.21037/jtd.2019.10.01

Kenmotsu, H., Naito, T., Mori, K., Ko, R., Ono, A., et al. (2015). Effect of platinum-based chemotherapy for non-small cell lung cancer patients with interstitial lung disease. *Cancer Chemother. Pharmacol.* 75, 521–526. doi: 10.1007/s00280-014-2670-y

Kenmotsu, H., Yoh, K., Mori, K., Ono, A., Baba, T., et al. (2019). Phase II study of nab-paclitaxel + carboplatin for patients with non-small-cell lung cancer and interstitial lung disease. *Cancer Sci.* 110, 3738–3745. doi: 10.1111/cas.14217

Kobayashi, H., Naito, T., Omae, K., Omori, S., Nakashima, K., et al. (2018). Impact of interstitial lung disease classification on the development of acute exacerbation of interstitial lung disease and prognosis in patients with stage III Non-Small-Cell lung cancer and interstitial lung disease treated with chemoradiotherapy. *J. Cancer* 9, 2054–2060. doi: 10.7150/jca.24936

Lim, J. U., Gil, B. M., Kang, H. S., Oh, J., Kim, Y. H., et al. (2019). Interstitial pneumonia with autoimmune features show better survival and less exacerbations compared to idiopathic pulmonary fibrosis. *BMC Pulm. Med.* 19:120. doi: 10.1186/s12890-019-0868-9

McKeown, S., Richter, A. G., O'Kane, C., McAuley, D. F., and Thickett, D. R. (2009). MMP expression and abnormal lung permeability are important determinants of outcome in IPF. *Eur. Respir. J.* 33, 77–84. doi: 10.1183/09031936.00060708

Minegishi, Y., Kuribayashi, H., Kitamura, K., Mizutani, H., Kosaihira, S., et al. (2011a). The feasibility study of Carboplatin plus Etoposide for advanced small cell lung cancer with idiopathic interstitial pneumonias. *J. Thorac. Oncol.* 6, 801–807. doi: 10.1097/JTO.0b013e3182103d3c

Minegishi, Y., Sudoh, J., Kuribayasi, H., Mizutani, H., Seike, M., et al. (2011b). The safety and efficacy of weekly paclitaxel in combination with carboplatin for advanced non-small cell lung cancer with idiopathic interstitial pneumonias. *Lung Cancer* 71, 70–74. doi: 10.1016/j.lungcan.2010.04.014

Minegishi, Y., Takenaka, K., Mizutani, H., Sudoh, J., Noro, R., et al. (2009). Exacerbation of idiopathic interstitial pneumonias associated with lung cancer therapy. *Intern. Med.* 48, 665–672. doi: 10.2169/internalmedicine.48.1650

Naccache, J. M., Gibiot, Q., Monnet, I., Antoine, M., Wislez, M., et al. (2018). Lung cancer and interstitial lung disease: A literature review. *J. Thorac. Dis.* 10, 3829–3844. doi: 10.21037/jtd.2018.05.75

Omori, T., Tajiri, M., Baba, T., Ogura, T., Iwasawa, T., et al. (2015). Pulmonary resection for lung cancer in patients with idiopathic interstitial pneumonia. *Ann. Thorac. Surg.* 100, 954–960. doi: 10.1016/j.athoracsur.2015.03.094

Raghu, G., Nyberg, F., and Morgan, G. (2004). The epidemiology of interstitial lung disease and its association with lung cancer. *Br. J. Cancer* 91(Suppl. 2), S3–S10. doi: 10.1038/sj.bjc.6602061

Reck, M., Kaiser, R., Mellemgaard, A., Douillard, J. Y., Orlov, S., et al. (2014). Docetaxel plus nintedanib versus docetaxel plus placebo in patients with previously treated non-small-cell lung cancer (LUME-Lung 1): A phase 3, double-blind, randomised controlled trial. *Lancet Oncol.* 15, 143–155. doi: 10.1016/S1470-2045(13)70586-2

Richeldi, L., du Bois, R. M., Raghu, G., Azuma, A., Brown, K. K., et al. (2014). Efficacy and safety of nintedanib in idiopathic pulmonary fibrosis. *N. Engl. J. Med.* 370, 2071–2082. doi: 10.1056/NEJMoa1402584

Ruan, H., Lv, Z., Liu, S., Zhang, L., Huang, K., et al. (2020). Anlotinib attenuated bleomycin-induced pulmonary fibrosis via the TGF-beta1 signalling pathway. *J. Pharm. Pharmacol.* 72, 44–55. doi: 10.1111/jphp.13183

Saijo, A., Hanibuchi, M., Goto, H., Toyoda, Y., Tezuka, T., et al. (2017). An analysis of the clinical features of lung cancer in patients with connective tissue diseases. *Respir. Investig.* 55, 153–160. doi: 10.1016/j.resinv.2016.11.003

Sato, T., Teramukai, S., Kondo, H., Watanabe, A., Ebina, M., et al. (2014). Impact and predictors of acute exacerbation of interstitial lung diseases after pulmonary resection for lung cancer. *J. Thorac. Cardiovasc. Surg.* 147, 1604–1611. doi: 10.1016/j.jtcvs.2013.09.050

Sato, T., Watanabe, A., Kondo, H., Kanzaki, M., Okubo, K., et al. (2015). Long-term results and predictors of survival after surgical resection of patients with lung cancer and interstitial lung diseases. *J. Thorac. Cardiovasc. Surg.* 149, 70–71. doi: 10.1016/j.jtcvs.2014.08.086

Sekine, A., Satoh, H., Baba, T., Ikeda, S., Okuda, R., et al. (2016). Safety and efficacy of S-1 in combination with carboplatin in non-small cell lung cancer patients with interstitial lung disease: A pilot study. *Cancer Chemother. Pharmacol.* 77, 1245–1252. doi: 10.1007/s00280-016-3040-8

Shah, R. R. (2016). Tyrosine kinase Inhibitor-Induced interstitial lung disease: Clinical features, diagnostic challenges, and therapeutic dilemmas. *Drug Saf.* 39, 1073–1091. doi: 10.1007/s40264-016-0450-9

Shi, L., Tang, J., Tong, L., and Liu, Z. (2014). Risk of interstitial lung disease with gefitinib and erlotinib in advanced non-small cell lung cancer: A systematic review and meta-analysis of clinical trials. *Lung Cancer* 83, 231–239. doi: 10.1016/j.lungcan.2013.11.016

Shimizu, R., Fujimoto, D., Kato, R., Otoshi, T., Kawamura, T., et al. (2014). The safety and efficacy of paclitaxel and carboplatin with or without bevacizumab for treating patients with advanced nonsquamous non-small cell lung cancer with interstitial lung disease. *Cancer Chemother. Pharmacol.* 74, 1159–1166. doi: 10.1007/s00280-014-2590-x

Shintani, Y., Ohta, M., Iwasaki, T., Ikeda, N., Tomita, E., et al. (2010). Predictive factors for postoperative acute exacerbation of interstitial pneumonia combined with lung cancer. *Gen. Thorac. Cardiovasc. Surg.* 58, 182–185. doi: 10.1007/s11748-009-0569-z

Simler, N. R., Brenchley, P. E., Horrocks, A. W., Greaves, S. M., Hasleton, P. S., et al. (2004). Angiogenic cytokines in patients with idiopathic interstitial pneumonia. *Thorax* 59, 581–585. doi: 10.1136/thx.2003.009860

Suresh, K., Voong, K. R., Shankar, B., Forde, P. M., Ettinger, D. S., et al. (2018). Pneumonitis in Non-Small cell lung cancer patients receiving immune checkpoint immunotherapy: Incidence and risk factors. *J. Thorac. Oncol.* 13, 1930–1939. doi: 10.1016/j.jtho.2018.08.2035

Tomassetti, S., Gurioli, C., Ryu, J. H., Decker, P. A., Ravaglia, C., et al. (2015). The impact of lung cancer on survival of idiopathic pulmonary fibrosis. *Chest* 147, 157–164. doi: 10.1378/chest.14-0359

Tone, M., Izumo, T., Awano, N., Kuse, N., Inomata, M., et al. (2019). High mortality and poor treatment efficacy of immune checkpoint inhibitors in patients with severe grade checkpoint inhibitor pneumonitis in non-small cell lung cancer. *Thorac. Cancer* 10, 2006–2012. doi: 10.1111/1759-7714.13187

Usui, K., Tanai, C., Tanaka, Y., Noda, H., and Ishihara, T. (2011). The prevalence of pulmonary fibrosis combined with emphysema in patients with lung cancer. *Respirology* 16, 326–331. doi: 10.1111/j.1440-1843.2010.01907.x

Watanabe, N., Taniguchi, H., Kondoh, Y., Kimura, T., Kataoka, K., et al. (2013). Efficacy of chemotherapy for advanced non-small cell lung cancer with idiopathic pulmonary fibrosis. *Respiration* 85, 326–331. doi: 10.1159/000342046

Watanabe, S., Saeki, K., Waseda, Y., Murata, A., Takato, H., et al. (2018). Lung cancer in connective tissue disease-associated interstitial lung disease: Clinical features and impact on outcomes. *J. Thoracic Dis.* 10, 799–807. doi: 10.21037/jtd.2017.12.134

Weis, S. M., and Cheresh, D. A. (2005). Pathophysiological consequences of VEGF-induced vascular permeability. *Nature* 437, 497–504. doi: 10.1038/nature03987

Xie, Z., Zhou, C., Qin, Y., Ouyang, M., Li, S., et al. (2019). [Diagnosis and treatment strategy for advanced severe lung cancer]. *Chin. J. Pract. Internal Med.* 39, 416–419. doi: 10.19538/j.nk2019050106

Yamaguchi, S., Ohguri, T., Ide, S., Aoki, T., Imada, H., et al. (2013). Stereotactic body radiotherapy for lung tumors in patients with subclinical interstitial lung disease: The potential risk of extensive radiation pneumonitis. *Lung Cancer* 82, 260–265. doi: 10.1016/j.lungcan.2013.08.024

Yoo, H., Jeong, B. H., Chung, M. J., Lee, K. S., Kwon, O. J., et al. (2019). Risk factors and clinical characteristics of lung cancer in idiopathic pulmonary fibrosis: A retrospective cohort study. *BMC Pulm. Med.* 19:149. doi: 10.1186/s12890-019-0905-8

9

ECMO Rescues Patients with Acute Respiratory Failure Related to GPA

Rongjun Wan [1,2], Wenzhe Yang [1], Xinhua Ma [3], Wei Yang [1], Pinhua Pan [1], Chengping Hu [1], Qiong Chen [2], Yaou Zhou [4], Rongli Lu [1], Yimin Fang [1] and Yuanyuan Li [1]*

[1] Department of Respiratory Medicine (Department of Respiratory and Critical Care Medicine), Xiangya Hospital, Central South University, Changsha, China, [2] National Clinical Research Center for Geriatric Disorders, Xiangya Hospital, Central South University, Changsha, China, [3] Department of Critical Care Medicine, Xiangya Hospital, Central South University, Changsha, China, [4] Department of Rheumatology and Immunology, Xiangya Hospital, Central South University, Changsha, China

***Correspondence:**
Yuanyuan Li
leeround@csu.edu.cn

Granulomatosis with polyangiitis (GPA) is a subtype of anti-neutrophil cytoplasmic antibody-associated vasculitis with a wide range of clinical symptoms related to the systemic involvement of small blood vessels. The respiratory system is one of the most frequently involved, and life-threatening acute respiratory failure could occur due to diffusive alveolar hemorrhage and tracheal stenosis. When maximum mechanical ventilation is unable to maintain oxygenation, extracorporeal membrane oxygenation (ECMO) should be considered as the final respiratory supportive method, if available. Here we present a 32-year-old male patient with acute respiratory failure (ARF) related to GPA, who was rescued by winning time for accurate diagnosis and appropriate treatment. Additionally, we reviewed more than 60 GPA-related ARF cases on multiple online databases, summarized the clinical manifestations of these patients, and concluded that ECMO plays an important role in further respiratory support for ARF patients with GPA and assists in accurate and timely diagnosis and appropriate treatment, thus helping them recuperate.

Keywords: diffuse alveolar hemorrhage, ANCA-associated vasculitis, extracorporeal membrane oxygenation, acute respiratory failure, granulomatosis with polyangiitis

INTRODUCTION

Granulomatosis with polyangiitis (GPA), formerly termed Wegener's granulomatosis, is the most common pathogenesis of anti-neutrophil cytoplasmic antibody (ANCA)-associated vasculitis (AAV) and highly relate to PR3-ANCA (1). The diversiform characteristics of GPA can refer to almost all body systems, particularly the lungs and kidneys (2). Pulmonary hemorrhagic nephritis syndrome is the most frequent cause of acute respiratory failure (ARF), and intensive care unit (ICU) supervision with advanced respiratory support and renal replacement treatment is necessary to help those patients recuperate (3, 4).

Extracorporeal membrane oxygenation (ECMO) is the final respiratory support technique for severe acute respiratory distress syndrome (ARDS) after maximum mechanical ventilation fails to provide optimal oxygen levels in the blood (5, 6). Although systemic anticoagulation is required during ECMO, with the advancement of technology, diffuse alveolar hemorrhage (DAH) has become a potential indication of ECMO as well.

According to a literature review, only the respiratory system is involved in patients with GPA, and ARF at the onset of symptoms is rare (7). Here we report a case of GPA with ARF at the onset of the disease. The disease progressed from shortness of breath to severe respiratory failure in 3 weeks, and maximum mechanical ventilation could not maintain oxygenation. The patient eventually recovered after venovenous extracorporeal membrane oxygenation (VV-ECMO), plasmapheresis, and immunosuppressive treatment (**Figure 1**). Within 2 years of follow-up, the patient showed a great prognosis.

In this study, we also reviewed 60 cases of ARF caused by GPA as published in academic journals; among this series, 22 patients recovered successfully after ECMO support.

CASE REPORT

On March 13, 2018, a 32-year-old male patient was admitted to the respiratory acute ICU (RICU) at our hospital owing to cough, expectoration, dyspnea for 3 weeks, and fever for 1 week. At 3 weeks before admission, he developed a dry cough and fever sequentially, and the fever was irregular with the highest temperature of 38.0°C, and it was difficult to get a reduction through centrifugation. In a local hospital, a computed tomography (CT) scan showed multiple shadows, and physicians prescribed demethylvancomycin, meropenem, and oseltamivir based on an empirical diagnosis of community-acquired pneumonia (CAP). However, the anti-microorganism treatment was ineffective, and the patient progressed into expectorating blood-stained sputum and dyspnea. For improved treatment, the patient was transferred to the emergency department on March 9. Before he became ill, he worked as a metal mechanical processing engineer for 8 years and had a history of metallic dust and chemical aerosol inhalation. He also had a smoking history of 1.25 pack-years.

After admission to our hospital, the patient reported aggravation of dyspnea with white mucus sputum. Physical examination showed that his body temperature was between 38.0 and 39.0°C without downtrend; the respiratory rate was 30 times/min, auscultation demonstrated only a reduction of breath sound at both sides of the lung, and no rales were revealed. There were no hemorrhagic spots or rashes on the skin. Laboratory examinations showed elevated procalcitonin, C-reactive protein, and erythrocyte sedimentation rate. On CT re-scan in this patient, multiple cavities emerged in his right lung. An empirical diagnosis of severe CAP was established. On estimation, methicillin-resistant *Staphylococcus aureus* or fungus was the most probable pathogen; thus, the patient was treated using linezolid, voriconazole, and levofloxacin. However, the patient continued to develop dyspnea and hyperpyrexia, indicating the probability of incorrect diagnosis. Simultaneously, the patient's blood gas analysis revealed a type I respiratory failure, with an oxygenation index of approximately 100. Although high-flow mask oxygen inhalation and non-invasive positive pressure ventilation (NIPPV) were administered sequentially, the blood oxygenation worsened, and the patient was transferred to our RICU on March 8. Considering that NIPPV did not improve oxygenation, a bedside chest film revealed consolidation in the lungs bilaterally, and the oxygenation index dropped to 60. Hence, bedside bronchoscope-guided intubation and invasive ventilation were performed. Although maximum ventilatory support was provided under sedation and analgesia, the oxygenation index did not show any improvement at 5 h later. Based on the small amount of hemorrhagic secretion in the trachea under bronchoscopy and consolidation of the gravity areas of the lower lungs by critical ultrasonic imaging, DAH was suspected, and more advanced life support systems were planned. Thus, our team performed VV-ECMO through the internal jugular and femoral veins. The ventilator was changed to synchronized intermittent mandatory ventilation sequentially, and blood gas analysis improved immediately (**Table 1**). Thus, the diagnosis of potential connective tissue diseases such as pulmonary vasculitis was made.

On the day after ECMO was established, the patient's immune disorder-related test results were back, with negative anti-nucleic antibody and anti-dsDNA antibody and positive cytoplasmic anti-neutrophil cytoplasmic antibody (c-ANCA) and proteinase3 (PR3) antibodies; we confirmed the patient's diagnosis as GPA. Considering medical images, airway hemorrhagic secretion, and results of positive autoantibodies, the ARF of this patient was suspected to be due to DAH. Immunosuppressive therapy immediately replaced the antibiotics. Methylprednisolone impact therapy (March 16–18, 500 mg Qd) and maintenance therapy (March 20 and later, 40 mg Qd), cyclophosphamide (0.2 g, Qod), and plasmapheresis (March 19, 21, and 27; three times in total) were administered. Subsequently, the oxygenation and lung conditions of this patient gradually improved (**Figure 1**, **Table 1**). On the 12th day after ECMO, the latter was removed after interrupting the oxygen source of ECMO for 4 h. At 1 day later, intubation was removed after evaluation. High-flow nasal cannula oxygen therapy (HFNC) was observed to be sufficient to maintain oxygenation. On April 3, the patient was transferred to the rheumatology department and treated for another 4 days. On April 6, the patient was discharged in a good respiratory condition.

During follow-up, methylprednisolone and cyclophos phamide were maintained, and the dosages were gradually reduced, and the patient showed a stable condition. Multiple CT scans showed diminishing cavities; however, fibrosis persisted (**Figure 2**).

METHODS

Data Collection

A literature search was performed in MEDLINE/PUBMED, Embase, and Scopus databases using the terms, "respiratory failure," "Wegener's granulomatosis," and "granulomatosis with polyangiitis." The article type was limited to case reports when eligible literature was collected from Embase. Furthermore, wild retrieval was performed through Google Scholar. All conference papers and reports that were not in English were excluded, owing to a lack of medical details. By reading the abstract and full text, we collected data on patients with respiratory failure related to GPA, and the inclusion criteria were as follows: (1)

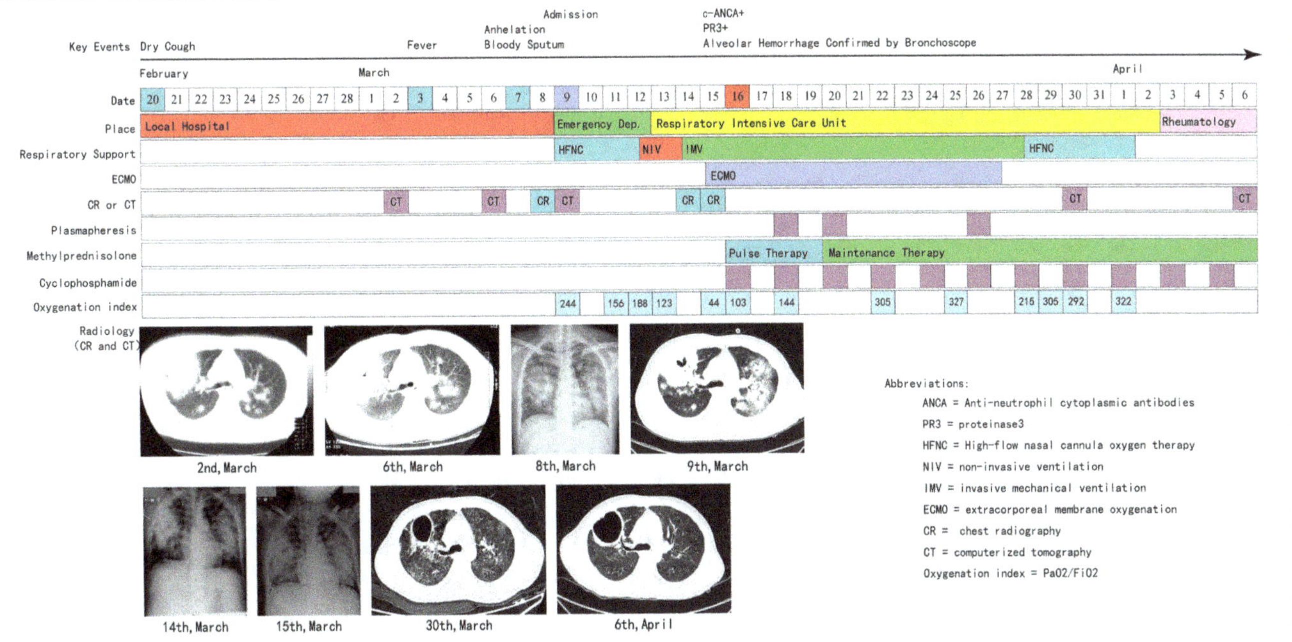

FIGURE 1 | Time-line of courses and treatments.

diagnosed with GPA, (2) acute respiratory failure and mechanical ventilation, and (3) the patient's medical history was described in detail. We reviewed the basic information, clinical characteristics, laboratory results, radiology characteristics, ECMO application and type, treatment, and prognosis among these patients.

Statistical Analysis

We used the Wilcoxon rank-sum test to assess the statistical difference in the age between patients who were administered ECMO or not. We also used Fisher's exact test to examine differences of other clinical characteristics between the two groups. Patients who lacked specific items were excluded when performing statistical analyses on relative items. $P < 0.05$ was considered significant. All the analyses were performed in R software (version 3.6.3).

RESULTS

The overall schematic general information and clinical manifestations are presented in **Table 2**. Among the 61 cases in this review (including our case), 32 were women (32/61). The mean age was 35.0 years (interquartile range, IQR: 32.0–57.0). However, the mean age of patients who received ECMO was 27.0 years (IQR, 20.8–33.8), those who did not receive ECMO was 51.0, and their IQR was 30.0–61.5, much higher than that of patients who received ECMO treatment (**Table 3**).

In this series, 41 patients had respiratory symptoms at the onset of their disorders (41/61); among them, patients who received ECMO treatment had a higher proportion (18/22 vs. 23/39), but without statistical significance. Except for our patients and the patient reported by Falk et al. (58), all patients in this series presented with symptoms of extrapulmonary involvement (59/61). Regarding respiratory failure, DAH was the main reason for GPA patients developing ARF (59/61), while in the other two cases, airway stenosis-related ventilation dysfunction was considered to be the etiology. There were three cases infected with cytomegalovirus, one with pneumocystis jirovecii pneumonia, and one with mucormycosis after immunosuppressive treatment.

By examining imaging manifestations, after excluding patients without radiological information, we found that the extent of involvement was related to the severity of the respiratory failure. Patients with DAH mainly displaying infiltration (45/58) and other imaging findings such as cavities (9/58), consolidation (13/58), and nodules (15/58) were relatively rare. Comparing patients who received and did not receive ECMO (**Table 3**), the infiltration proportion was much higher in those who received ECMO treatment (15/18 vs. 30/39), while the number of nodules was much lower (3/19 vs. 12/39). Among the two cases of airway stenosis, stenosis was detected in the radiological image directly in one patient, while another displayed pneumothorax and emphysema, which indirectly indicated airway stenosis. However, there were no statistical differences between the two groups in terms of radiological manifestations.

Except for cases not mentioned, tested, or classified, most of the patients in the series had a positive c-ANCA (42/46), and the most frequent antigen type was PR3 (35/38). P-ANCA (2/46) and MPO (2/38) were positive in only two patients, while c/p-ANCA double-positive and PR3/MPO double-positive were found in one patient each.

About ECMO, 22 patients received ECMO support in this series (22/61). Among those ECMO patients, 17 received

TABLE 1 | Extracorporeal membrane oxygenation (ECMO) and SIMV parameters and results of arterial blood gas analysis.

Time	ECMO				SIMV					Blood gas analysis			
	Pump (rpm)	Blood flow (L/min)	Air flow (L/min)	Air FiO_2 (%)	RR (/min)	TV (ml)	Pressure (cmH_2O)	PEEP (cmH_2O)	Air FiO_2 (%)	pH	pCO_2	pO_2	OI (pO_2/FiO_2)
1st day (before ECMO)	-	–	–	–	44–54 (SPONT)	–	12	8–20	100	7.29	59	44	44
1st day (after ECMO)	3,485	3.8	5	100	14	380	10	12	60	7.43	36	65	65
2nd day	3,510	4.34	7	100	14	240	10	12	50	7.45	41	62	103
3rd day	3,555	4.33	6	100	–	–	–	–	–	–	–	–	–
4th day	–	–	–	–	14	223	10	12	50	7.41	48	72	144
6th day	3,555	4.32	8	100	–	–	–	–	50	–	–	–	–
7th day	3,555	4.23	7.5	100	–	–	–	–	50	–	–	–	–
8th day	3,500	4.02	8	100	–	–	–	–	50	7.49	43	120	305
9th day	–	–	–	–	14	244	10	10	40	–	–	–	–
10th day	3,480	4	8	100	–	–	–	–	40	–	–	–	–
11th day	3,480	3.64	8	100	14	240	10	10	40	7.46	44	131	327
12th day (removal of ECMO)	3,480	4	6.5	40	14	380	10	14	60	7.51	40	129	215
13th day (HFNC)	–	–	–	–	–	–	–	–	–	7.47	38	146	292
15th day	–	–	–	–	–	–	–	–	–	7.48	38	129	322

SIMV, synchronized intermittent mandatory ventilation; RR, respiratory rate; TV, tide volume; OI, oxygenation index; PEEP, positive end-expiratory pressure; SPONT, continuous spontaneous ventilation; HFNC, high-flow nasal cannula oxygen therapy; –, not applicable or no data or not changed.

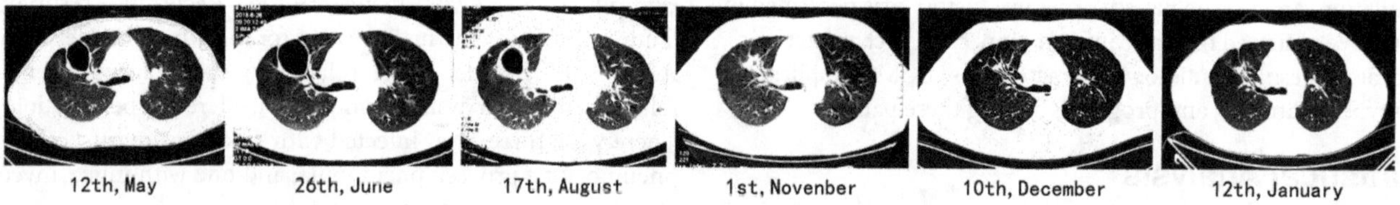

FIGURE 2 | Chest CT scans at follow up.

VV-ECMO (20/22), one received VA-ECMO (1/22), and one received VA-ECMO and VV-ECMO (1/22) sequentially. All patients, except the one who died before diagnosis, were administered glucocorticoids (60/61); cyclophosphamide was another important immunosuppressive drug for combinational utilization (52/61), while other immunosuppressive drugs such as methotrexate (1/61) and mycophenolate mofetil (1/61) were seldom used. Ten patients in this series received rituximab, a drug developed in recent years. Additionally, plasma exchange was also widely used in this series (34/61), and the proportion of patients receiving ECMO was 16/22, while that in non-ECMO was 18/39 (**Table 3**).

Finally, 14 patients died in this series due to ARF (14/61); none of them received ECMO support (**Table 3**), and the results showed a higher survival rate of patients in the ECMO group.

DISCUSSION

GPA is a type of AAV; 85% of the patients with GPA show positive ANCA, mainly PR3-ANCA, and only a few demonstrate MPO-ANCAs (62). GPA is a multisystem vasculitis syndrome characterized by granulomatous lesions and necrotizing vasculitis, and all small blood vessels could be involved. The clinical symptoms of GPA vary and cover a wide range of symptoms, including fever, fatigue, weight loss, poor appetite, anorexia, arteritis, night sweats, cough, and dyspnea (63). Treatment strategies generally involve 3–6 months of remission induction plus more than 24 months of maintenance treatment using glucocorticoids in combination with immunosuppressors; sometimes, rituximab is added during the induction, and maintenance period (7).

More than 90% of patients with GPA have upper or lower respiratory tract involvement; however, the clinical manifestations can be asymptomatic to life-threatening respiratory failure. Among them, DAH and subglottic stenosis are the most common characteristics of GPA respiratory tract involvement (64, 65). Including the case, we reported that the main cause of respiratory failure was DAH in our series, and subglottic stenosis was relatively rare. It is noteworthy that patients with GPA may be

TABLE 2 | Case reports of respiratory failure due to granulomatosis with polyangiitis.

Case	Author	Publication year	Age	Gender	Respiratory onset	Extrapulmonary involvement	Reason of respiratory failure	ANCA		Radiology	ECMO		Immune-suppression	Plasma pheresis	Rituximab	Outcome
								Type	Antigen		Use and type	Duration (days)				
1	Leak et al. (8)	1967	61	Female	No	Yes	DAH	–	–	Infiltration, nodule	Not used	–	GC	No	No	Death
2	Leak et al. (8)	1967	45	Female	Yes	Yes	DAH	–	–	Cavity, infiltration	Not used	–	GC	No	No	Discharged
3	Hensley et al. (9)	1979	57	Female	No	Yes	DAH	–	–	Infiltration	Not used	–	GC, Cyc	No	No	Discharged
4	Feinstein et al. (10)	1985	22	Male	No	Yes	DAH	–	–	Cavity, infiltration	Not used	–	GC, Cyc	Yes	No	Discharged
5	Grupe and Colvin (11)	1986	15	Male	No	Yes	DAH	–	–	Infiltration	Not used	–	GC, Cyc	Yes	No	Death
6	Lenclud et al. (12)	1989	69	Female	Yes	Yes	DAH	p	–	Infiltration	Not used	–	GC, Cyc	No	No	Death
7	Lenclud et al. (12)	1989	70	Male	Yes	Yes	DAH	Positive	–	Infiltration	Not used	–	GC, Cyc	No	No	Discharged
8	Coggins et al. (13)	1989	56	Male	Yes	Yes	DAH	p/c	PR3/MPO	Infiltration	Not used	–	GC, Cyc	Yes	No	Death
9	Sanchez et al. (14)	1989	82	Female	Yes	Yes	DAH	–	–	Infiltration	Not used	–	GC, Cyc	No	No	Death
10	Misset et al. (15)	1991	35	Female	Yes	Yes	DAH	Negative	–	Infiltration	Not used	–	GC, Cyc	No	No	Discharged
11	Yoshimura et al. (16)	1992	58	Male	No	Yes	DAH	c	–	Nodule	Not used	–	GC, Cyc	No	No	Death
12	Odeh, M. et al. (17)	1993	75	Female	No	Yes	DAH	–	–	Consolidation	Not used	–	GC, Cyc	No	No	Death
13	Pradhan et al. (18)	2000	15	Female	Yes	Yes	DAH	p	MPO	Nodule	Not used	–	GC, Cyc	No	No	Discharged
14	Ullmer et al. (19)	2000	62	Male	Yes	Yes	DAH/PCP	c	–	Nodule, infiltration	Not used	–	GC, Cyc	No	No	Discharged
15	Hermon et al. (20)	2003	17	Female	No	Yes	DAH	c	PR3	Infiltration	Not used	–	GC, Cyc	No	No	Discharged
16	Senf et al. (21)	2003	35	Male	No	Yes	DAH/ hydro thorax	c	PR3	Nodule, infiltration	Not used	–	GC, Cyc	Yes	Yes	Discharged
17	Prutkin et al. (22)	2003	56	Male	Yes	Yes	DAH	c	PR3	Infiltration, consolidation	Not used	–	GC, Cyc	No	No	Discharged

(Continued)

TABLE 2 | Continued

Case	Author	Publication year	Age	Gender	Respiratory onset	Extrapulmonary involvement	Reason of respiratory failure	ANCA		Radiology	ECMO		Immune-suppression	Plasma pheresis	Rituximab	Outcome
								Type	Antigen		Use and type	Duration (days)				
18	Griffith et al. (23)	2003	28	Male	Yes	Yes	DAH	c	PR3	Infiltration	Not used	–	GC, Cyc	Yes	No	Discharged
19	Steinau et al. (24)	2003	19	Male	Yes	Yes	DAH	c	PR3	Infiltration	Not used	–	GC, Cyc	No	No	Discharged
20	Nguyen et al. (25)	2005	20	Male	No	Yes	DAH	c	–	Infiltration	Not used	–	GC, Cyc	Yes	No	Discharged
21	Mera et al. (26)	2007	19	Male	Yes	Yes	DAH	c	PR3	Cavity, nodule	Not used	–	GC, Cyc	No	No	Discharged
22	Mukhopadhyay et al. (27)	2010	37	Male	Yes	Yes	DAH	c	PR3	Consolidation	Not used	–	(Death)	No	No	Death
23	Esposito et al. (28)	2010	7	Female	Yes	Yes	DAH	c	PR3	Infiltration, consolidation	Not used	–	GC, Cyc	No	No	Discharged
24	Berthoux et al. (29)	2011	54	Male	No	Yes	DAH	c	PR3	Consolidation	Not used	–	GC, Cyc	Yes	Yes	Discharged
25	Mahajan et al. (30)	2011	35	Male	Yes	Yes	DAH	c	–	Infiltration	Not used	–	GC, Cyc	No	No	Discharged
26	Marina et al. (31)	2011	64	Female	Yes	Yes	DAH/ mucormy cosis	c	PR3	Infiltration, nodule	Not used	–	GC, Cyc	Yes	No	Death
27	Cardenas–Garcia et al. (32)	2012	51	Female	Yes	Yes	DAH	c	–	Infiltration	Not used	–	GC, Cyc	Yes	No	Discharged
28	Ishiguro et al. (33)	2012	73	Female	No	Yes	DAH/CMV	Positive	PR3	Infiltration, nodule	Not used	–	GC, Cyc	No	No	Death
29	Kaya et al. (34)	2013	48	Male	No	Yes	DAH	c	PR3	Infiltration, nodule	Not used	–	GC, Cyc	Yes	No	Death
30	Powers et al. (35)	2013	32	Male	Yes	Yes	DAH	c	PR3	Infiltration, consolidation, nodule	Not used	–	GC, Cyc	Yes	Yes	Discharged
31	Haupt et al. (36)	2013	14	Female	Yes	Yes	DAH	c	PR3	Infiltration	Not used	–	GC	Yes	No	Discharged
32	Pinto et al. (37)	2014	65	Female	Yes	Yes	DAH/ pneumo thorax	c	PR3	Cavity	Not used	–	GC, Cyc	No	No	Death
33	Kaya et al. (34)	2014	60	Male	No	Yes	DAH	c	PR3	Infiltration	Not used	–	GC, Cyc	Yes	No	Discharged
34	Moreno-González et al. (38)	2014	42	Male	Yes	Yes	DAH/PTE	Positive	PR3	Infiltration, nodule	Not used	–	GC, Cyc	Yes	Yes	Discharged

(Continued)

TABLE 2 | Continued

Case	Author	Publication year	Age	Gender	Respiratory onset	Extrapulmonary involvement	Reason of respiratory failure	ANCA		Radiology	ECMO		Immune-suppression	Plasma pheresis	Rituximab	Outcome
								Type	Antigen		Use and type	Duration (days)				
35	Hilal et al. (39)	2015	55	Female	Yes	Yes	DAH/CMV	c	PR3	Infiltration	Not used	–	GC	Yes	Yes	Death
36	Fukui et al. (40)	2015	69	Male	No	Yes	DAH/CMV	c	MPO	Consolidation	Not used	–	GC, Cyc	Yes	No	Death
37	Tajarernmuang et al. (41)	2016	48	Female	No	Yes	Airway stenosis	c	PR3	Stenosis	Not used	–	GC, Cyc	No	No	Discharged
38	Ning et al. (42)	2018	70	Female	Yes	Yes	DAH	c	PR3	Nodule, infiltration, cavity	Not used	–	GC, MMF	Yes	No	Discharged
39	Sattar et al. (43)	2019	60	Female	No	Yes	DAH	c	PR3	Cavity, infiltration	Not used	–	GC, Cyc	Yes	No	Discharged
40	Hartmann et al. (44)	1994	20	Female	No	Yes	DAH	c	–	Infiltration	VV	6	GC, Cyc	Yes	No	Discharged
41	Loscar et al. (45)	1997	19	Female	No	Yes	DAH	c	PR3	–	VV	10	GC, Cyc	No	No	Discharged
42	Matsumoto et al. (46)	2000	29	Female	Yes	Yes	DAH	c	–	Nodule, infiltration	VA	3.4	GC, Cyc	No	No	Discharged
43	Rosengarten et al. (47)	2002	27	Female	Yes	Yes	DAH	c	PR3	Infiltration	VV	15	GC, Cyc	No	No	Discharged
44	Hernandez et al. (48)	2002	13	Male	Yes	Yes	DAH	c	–	Infiltration	VV	9	GC, Cyc	Yes	No	Discharged
45	Ahmed et al. (49)	2004	26	Female	Yes	Yes	DAH	c	–	Cavity, infiltration	VV	14	GC, Cyc	Yes	No	Discharged
46	Gay et al. (50)	2005	26	Female	Yes	Yes	DAH	c	–	Cavity, infiltration	VV	10	GC, Cyc	Yes	No	Discharged
47	Balasubramanian et al. (51)	2005	53	Male	No	Yes	DAH	c	PR3	Infiltration	VV	NA	GC, Cyc	Yes	No	Discharged
48	Joseph et al. (52)	2011	13	Male	Yes	Yes	DAH	Positive	PR3	Infiltration	VV	7	GC	Yes	No	Discharged
49	Barnes et al. (53)	2012	50	Female	Yes	Yes	DAH	c	PR3	Consolidation	VV	1.5	GC, Cyc	Yes	No	Discharged
50	Hohenforst et al. (54)	2013	65	Female	Yes	Yes	DAH	Positive	PR3	Infiltration	VV	10	GC, Cyc	Yes	No	Discharged
51	Yusuff et al. (55)	2015	23	Female	Yes	Yes	DAH	c	PR3	–	VV	13	GC, Cyc	No	No	Discharged

(Continued)

TABLE 2 | Continued

Case	Author	Publication year	Age	Gender	Respiratory onset	Extrapulmonary involvement	Reason of respiratory failure	ANCA		Radiology	ECMO		Immune-suppression	Plasma pheresis	Rituximab	Outcome
								Type	Antigen		Use and type	Duration (days)				
52	Yusuff et al. (55)	2015	27	Male	Yes	Yes	DAH	c	–	Infiltration	VV	21	GC, Cyc	Yes	Yes	Discharged
53	Rawal et al. (56)	2016	28	Male	Yes	Yes	DAH	Positive	PR3	Infiltration	VV	21	GC, Cyc	Yes	No	Discharged
54	Vanoli et al. (57)	2017	33	Male	Yes	Yes	DAH	c	PR3	Consolidation, infiltration	VV	NA	GC, Cyc	Yes	Yes	Discharged
55	Falk et al. (58)	2017	17	Female	Yes	No	Airway stenosis	c	PR3	Emphysema	VA and VV	21	GC, Cyc	Yes	Yes	Discharged
56	Delvino et al. (59)	2019	45	Male	Yes	Yes	DAH	c	PR3	Infiltration	VV	6	GC, Cyc	Yes	No	Discharged
57	Delvino et al. (59)	2019	45	Male	No	Yes	DAH	c	PR3	Nodule, consolidation	VV	14	GC, MTX	No	Yes	Discharged
58	Goel et al. (60)	2020	34	Female	Yes	Yes	DAH	c	PR3	Nodule, consolidation	VV	7	GC, Cyc	Yes	No	Discharged
59	Yin et al. (61)	2020	25	Female	Yes	Yes	DAH	Positive	–	Infiltration, consolidation	VV	52	GC, Cyc	No	No	Discharged
60	Yin et al. (61)	2020	18	Female	Yes	Yes	DAH	Positive	–	–	VV	123	GC	Yes	Yes	Lung transplant
61	This case	2020	32	Male	Yes	No	DAH	c	PR3	Cavity, infiltration, consolidation	VV	12	GC, Cyc	Yes	No	Discharged

PTE, pulmonary thromboembolism.

TABLE 3 | Summary of cases of respiratory failure due to GPA.

	Total (IQR/%) ($n = 61$)	ECMO (IQR/%) ($n = 22$)	Non-ECMO (IQR/%) ($n = 39$)	*P*-value
Publication time				0.08
Before 2000	17 (27.87)	3 (13.64)	14 (35.90)	–
After 2000	44 (72.13)	19 (86.36)	25 (64.10)	–
Age	35.00 (23.00–57.00)	27.00 (20.75–33.75)	51.00 (30.00–61.50)	<0.01
Female	32 (52.45)	13 (52.63)	19 (53.13)	0.59
Respiratory onset	41 (67.21)	18 (81.82)	23 (58.97)	0.09
ANCA				0.80
No information	7 (11.48)	0	7 (17.95)	–
Negative	1 (1.64)	0	1 (2.56)	–
Unknown type	8 (13.11)	5 (22.72)	3 (7.69)	–
c-ANCA	42 (68.85)	17 (77.27)	25 (64.10)	–
p-ANCA	2 (3.28)	0	2 (5.13)	–
p + c-ANCA	1 (1.64)	0	1 (2.56)	–
ANCA antigen				0.69
No information	23 (37.70)	8 (36.36)	15 (38.46)	–
PR3	35 (57.38)	14 (63.64)	21 (53.85)	–
MPO	2 (3.28)	0	2 (5.13)	–
PR3 + MPO	1 (1.64)	0	1 (2.56)	–
Radiology				
No information	3 (4.92)	3 (13.64)	0	–
Infiltration	45 (73.77)	15 (68.18)	30 (76.92)	0.55
Consolidation	13 (21.31)	6 (27.27)	7 (17.95)	0.07
Cavity	9 (14.75)	3 (13.64)	6 (15.38)	1
Nodule	15 (24.59)	3 (13.64)	12 (30.77)	0.22
Stenosis	1 (1.64)	0	1 (2.56)	1
Emphysema	1 (1.64)	1 (4.55)	0	0.36
Treatment				
GC	60 (98.36)	22 (100.00)	38 (97.44)	1
CYC	52 (85.25)	19 (86.36)	33 (84.62)	1
MTX	1 (1.64)	1 (4.54)	0	0.34
MMF	1 (1.64)	0	1 (2.56)	1
Plasmapheresis	34 (55.74)	16 (72.73)	18 (46.15)	0.06
Rituximab	10 (16.39)	5 (22.73)	5 (12.82)	0.47
Death				<0.01 (total death)
Before 2000	7 (11.48)	0	7 (17.95)	0.55
After 2000	7 (11.48)	0	7 (17.95)	0.03

–, not applicable.

associated with opportunistic infections of the lungs due to immunosuppressive therapy.

GPA-related DAH occurs in 7–45% of patients with GPA (65, 66). Fewer than 10% of cases with DAH are serious with life-threatening conditions (29); most of them are GPA patients with alveolar hemorrhage, and their mortality rate is six times that of those without alveolar hemorrhage (67). Among patients with GPA, 60% are caused by DAH (43). Any degree of DAH should be considered a serious manifestation of the disease as it can quickly progress to respiratory failure (62). The underlying pathophysiological mechanism of GPA-related DAH is linked to antibodies related to ANCA, which interact with inflammatory cells (neutrophils, monocytes, and lymphocytes) and cytokines (particularly Th1 cytokines, namely, tumor necrosis factor and interferon-γ) and then initiate and perpetuate vasculitis (68, 69). The basement membrane of capillaries is destroyed during these processes, and erythrocytes are allowed to enter the alveolar space with fluid (69). These processes damage the gas exchange of the affected lung area. However, the symptoms of DAH, including dyspnea, hypoxia, anemia, and lack of imaging findings of diffuse alveolar filling, are not specific; however, hemoptysis is relatively rare in DAH. In clinical practice, when a case with imaging findings indicates extensive infiltration but is refractory to anti-infective treatment, bronchial alveolar lavage under bronchoscopy is recommended to ascertain the occurrence of DAH (62), and immunological examination should also be conducted to obtain a definitive diagnosis that can help clinicians arrange immunosuppressive treatment earlier.

Moreover, similar to DAH, the symptoms of subglottic stenosis lack specificity, ranging from coughing and dyspnea to life-threatening stridor (65). Unlike DAH, subglottic stenosis generally does not show any positive findings on radiology, bronchoscopy is needed to confirm the diagnosis, and the severity of respiratory involvement is related to the location, length, and degree of stenosis (65). In addition, rapid progress to respiratory failure may occur among these patients soon after admission (41, 58).

Our patient has a severe case of the disease that progressed rapidly to respiratory failure within 3 days of admission, and respiratory support was upgraded from HFNC and NIPPV to intermittent mandatory ventilation (IMV) and ECMO in a short period. Additionally, the patient had no extrapulmonary manifestations, and severe infective pneumonia was the first clinical diagnosis. GPA was not diagnosed until a positive ANCA result was reported. At this time, ECMO was used for approximately 12 h. This case showed that GPA may present with unspecified clinical symptoms and radiological manifestations with rapid progress into respiratory failure, which leads to difficulties in early diagnosis and proper treatment.

Therefore, when respiratory symptoms occur in patients with GPA, etiological treatment and powerful respiratory support should be provided as soon as possible. Glucocorticoids and cyclophosphamide are the first-line drugs for impact and maintenance treatment. Rituximab and plasmapheresis should be considered when feasible (7). Respiratory support should be chosen based on oxygenation conditions, and HFNC should be upgraded early to IMV or ECMO when necessary and available (5) to further timely diagnose and treat. In this case series, all patients received ECMO as they were unable to maintain oxygenation through basic respiratory support; among them, one patient received VV-ECMO and VA-ECMO sequentially due to circulatory dysfunction related to mediastinal emphysema.

ARF is one of the indications for ECMO support. Since the first patient with ARDS was rescued using ECMO in 1972 (70), it has been increasingly used in ARF (71). Without ECMO support, our patient would not have survived. In our series, none of the patients could maintain oxygenation under mechanical ventilation before ECMO, indicating that ECMO can improve the prognosis of respiratory failure caused by GPA (59) and provide the possibility of later recovery. In other studies, such as the conventional ventilatory support vs. extracorporeal membrane oxygenation for severe acute respiratory failure in 2009, ECMO significantly improved the disability-free survival rate of patients with severe ARF (72). ECMO to rescue lung injury in severe ARDS (EOLIA) in 2008 showed that ECMO can significantly reduce the probability of 60-day treatment failure in patients with severe ARDS and increase the days of improved oxygenation, and no renal failure has occurred (73). However, whether ECMO can improve the prognosis of ARF remains controversial. There was no statistical significance in terms of prognosis between ECMO and non-ECMO users among patients with ARDS in the EOLIA study (73). Among patients with immune-related DAH, ECMO did not improve the survival rates (20 vs. 38%, $p = 0.323$) (74). Although these studies showed negative results, we should note that the early termination of the EOLIA study and the high proportion of patients who received remedial treatments from the traditional treatment group transferred to the ECMO group may lead to no statistically significant difference in mortality between the two groups. In studies of patients with ARDS owing to DAH (74), those who required ECMO generally had a lower oxygenation index (87 vs. 62, $p = 0.017$), more days of mechanical ventilation (21 vs. 9.5, $p < 0.001$), and higher alveolar–arterial gradient (450 vs. 586, $p = 0.017$), which indicates that even if these two groups of patients are included in the study under the same criteria, the oxygenation index may be much worse in patients who used ECMO, which may generate negative results.

Hence, regardless of the conclusions of future clinical studies on whether ECMO can improve the prognosis of patients with GAP-related respiratory failure, we recommend ECMO as a transitional method for those with respiratory failure caused by GPA who cannot maintain oxygenation through mechanical ventilation. Moreover, ECMO could win some time for these patients to be correctly diagnosed and treated later (74).

CONCLUSION

ECMO provides the final respiratory support for GPA-related critical respiratory failure and assists patients who cannot maintain oxygenation using mechanical ventilation for further definitive diagnosis and treatment. However, whether it can improve the clinical outcomes of GPA-related respiratory failure remains to be further studied.

AUTHOR CONTRIBUTIONS

RW and YL reviewed the lectures and wrote the manuscript. WenY, XM, WeiY, YZ, RL, and YF collected and arranged the materials. CH, QC, and PP viewed the complete manuscript. All authors contributed to the article and approved the submitted version.

ACKNOWLEDGMENTS

We would like to thank Editage (www.editage.cn) for English language editing.

REFERENCES

Nasser M, Cottin V. Alveolar hemorrhage in vasculitis (Primary and Secondary). *Semin Respir Crit Care Med.* (2018) 39:482– 93. doi: 10.1055/s-0038-1668533

Lamprecht P, Kerstein A, Klapa S, Schinke S, Karsten CM, Yu X, et al. Pathogenetic and clinical aspects of anti-neutrophil cytoplasmic autoantibody-associated vasculitides. *Front Immunol.* (2018) 9:680. doi: 10.3389/fimmu.2018.00680

Geri G, Terrier B, Heshmati F, Moussaoui H, Massot J, Mira JP, et al. Effect of plasma exchange in acute respiratory failure due to Anti- neutrophil cytoplasmic antibody-associated vasculitis. *Critic Care.* (2018) 22:328. doi: 10.1186/s13054-018-2264-x

Demiselle J, Auchabie J, Beloncle F, Gatault P, Grange S, Du Cheyron D, et al. Patients with ANCA-associated vasculitis admitted to the intensive care unit with acute vasculitis manifestations: a retrospective and comparative multicentric study. *Ann Intensive Care.* (2017) 7:39. doi: 10.1186/s13613-017-0262-9

Goligher EC, Ferguson ND, Brochard LJ. Clinical challenges in mechanical ventilation. *Lancet.* (2016) 387:1856–66. doi: 10.1016/S0140-6736(16)30176-3

Combes A, Pesenti A, Ranieri VM. Fifty years of research in ARDS. Is extracorporeal circulation the future of acute respiratory distress syndrome management? *Am J Respir Crit Care Med.* (2017) 195:1161– 70. doi: 10.1164/rccm.201701-0217CP

Salvador F. ANCA associated vasculitis. *Eur J Intern Med.* (2020) 74:18– 28. doi: 10.1016/j.ejim.2020.01.011

Leak D, Clein GP. Acute Wegener's granulomatosis. *Thorax.* (1967) 22:437– 43. doi: 10.1136/thx.22.5.437

Hensley MJ, Feldman NT, Lazarus JM, Galvanek EG. Diffuse pulmonary hemorrhage and rapidly progressive renal failure. an uncommon presentation of Wegener's granulomatosis. *Am J Med.* (1979) 66:894–8. doi: 10.1016/0002-9343(79)91149-5

Feinstein EI, Kitt D, Collins JF, Boylen T, Koss M. Hemoptysis and acute renal failure in a young man. *Am J Nephrol.* (1985) 5:64–70. doi: 10.1159/000166908

Grupe WE, Colvin RB. Case records of the Massachusetts General Hospital. Weekly clinicopathological exercises. Case 12-1986. A 15-year-old boy with hemoptysis and occult blood in the urine. *N Engl J Med.* (1986) 314:834– 44. doi: 10.1056/NEJM198603273141307

Lenclud C, De Vuyst P, Dupont E, Depierreux M, Ketelbant P, Goldman M. Wegener's granulomatosis presenting as acute respiratory failure with anti-neutrophil-cytoplasm antibodies. *Chest.* (1989) 96:345–7. doi: 10.1378/chest.96.2.345

Coggins CH, Niles JL, Fienberg R. Case records of the Massachusetts General Hospital. Weekly clinicopathological exercises. Case 25-1989. A 56-year-old man with hemoptysis and microscopic hematuria. *N Engl J Med.* (1989) 320:1677–86. doi: 10.1056/NEJM198906223202508

Sanchez-Masiques J, Ettensohn DB. Alveolar hemorrhage in Wegener's granulomatosis. *Am J Med Sci.* (1989) 297:390– 3. doi: 10.1097/00000441-198906000-00013

Misset B, Glotz D, Escudier B, Nochy D, Bosq J, Gilles E, et al. Wegener's granulomatosis presenting as diffuse pulmonary hemorrhage. *Intensive Care Med.* (1991) 17:118–20. doi: 10.1007/BF01691435

Yoshimura N, Matsubara O, Tamura A, Kasuga T, Mark EJ. Wegener's granulomatosis. associated with diffuse pulmonary hemorrhage. *Acta Pathol Jpn.* (1992) 42:657–61. doi: 10.1111/j.1440-1827.1992.tb03047.x

Odeh M, Best LA, Kerner H, Bassan H, Oliven A. Localized Wegener's granulomatosis relapsing as diffuse massive intra-alveolar hemorrhage. *Chest.* (1993) 104:955–6. doi: 10.1378/chest.104.3.955

Pradhan M, Meyers KE, Guttenberg M, Kaplan BS. Wegener granulomatosis– an atypical case. *Pediatr Nephrol.* (2000) 14:862–71. doi: 10.1007/PL00013445

Ullmer E, Mayr M, Binet I, Ebnother-Staub C, Dalquen P, Soler M, et al. Granulomatous Pneumocystis carinii pneumonia in Wegener's granulomatosis. *Eur Respir J.* (2000) 15:213– 6. doi: 10.1183/09031936.00.15121300

Hermon MM, Golej J, Emminger W, Puig S, Szepfalusi Z, Trittenwein G. Acute hemorrhagic respiratory failure caused by Wegener's granulomatosis successfully treated by bronchoalveolar lavage with diluted surfactant. *Wien Klin Wochenschr.* (2003) 115:793–6. doi: 10.1007/BF03040505

Senf R, Jürgensen JS, Teichgräber U, Kampf D, Schindler R. Ruptured arterial aneurysm of the kidney in a patient with Wegener's granulomatosis. *Nephrol Dialysis Transp.* (2003) 18:2671–3. doi: 10.1093/ndt/gfg380

Prutkin JM, Barry P, Zaas D. Cases from the osler medical service at Johns Hopkins University. *Am J Med.* (2003) 115:150– 3. doi: 10.1016/S0002-9343(03)00356-5

Griffith M, Brett S. The pulmonary physician in critical care illustrative case 3: pulmonary vasculitis. *Thorax.* (2003) 58:543–6. doi: 10.1136/thorax.58.6.543

Steinau F, Deja M, Weber-Carstens S, Busch T, Kaisers U. Onset of acute respiratory distress syndrome following severe pulmonary hemorrhage in a patient with anti-neutrophil cytoplasmic antibody associated vasculitis. *Intensive Care Med.* (2003) 29:504. doi: 10.1007/s00134-003-1647-9

Nguyen T, Martin MK, Indrikovs AJ. Plasmapheresis for diffuse alveolar hemorrhage in a patient with Wegener's granulomatosis: case report and review of the literature. *J Clin Apher.* (2005) 20:230–4. doi: 10.1002/jca.20069

Mera A, Wada M, Miyajima M. [A case of Wegener's granulomatosis presenting as severe acute respiratory failure]. *Nihon Kokyuki Gakkai Zasshi.* (2007) 45:262–6.

Mukhopadhyay S, Hensley RG, Tazelaar HD. Cardiac involvement in Wegener granulomatosis diagnosed at autopsy. *Cardiovasc Pathol.* (2010) 19:312–5. doi: 10.1016/j.carpath.2009.06.011

Esposito S, Corona F, Defilippi A, Petaccia A, Chidini G, Dell'Era L, et al. Wegener's granulomatosis presenting with life-threatening lung hemorrhage in a 7-year-old child. *Rheumatol Int.* (2010) 30:1665– 8. doi: 10.1007/s00296-009-1132-z

Berthoux E, Padilla M, Chavez L, Colombe B, Bosseray A, Massot C. Unusual evolution in Wegener's granulomatosis: recovery of pulmonary involvement while renal disease progressed to end-stage. *Ren Fail.* (2011) 33:1032–6. doi: 10.3109/0886022X.2011.610547

Mahajan V, Whig J, Kashyap A, Gupta S. Diffuse alveolar hemorrhage in Wegener's granulomatosis. *Lung India.* (2011) 28:52–5. doi: 10.4103/0970-2113.76302

Marina M, Maria A. A fatal case of treatment-related adverse effects in granulomatosis with polyangiitis (Wegener's Granulomatosis). *Open J Rheumatol Autoimmune Dis.* (2011) 1:5–9. doi: 10.4236/ojra.2011.12002

Cardenas-Garcia J, Farmakiotis D, Baldovino BP, Kim P. Wegener's granulomatosis in a middle-aged woman presenting with dyspnea, rash, hemoptysis and recurrent eye complaints: a case report. *J Med Case Rep.* (2012) 6:335. doi: 10.1186/1752-1947-6-335

Ishiguro T, Takayanagi N, Yamaguchi S, Shimizu Y, Yanagisawa T, Sugita Y, et al. Pulmonary capillaritis in Wegener's granulomatosis detected via transbronchial lung biopsy. *Intern Med.* (2012) 51:905– 9. doi: 10.2169/internalmedicine.51.6518

Kaya H, Yilmaz S, Sezgi C, Abakay O, Taylan M, Sen H, et al. Two cases of extrapulmonary onset granulomatosis with polyangiitis which caused diffuse alveolar haemorrhage. *Respir Med Case Rep.* (2014) 13:32– 6. doi: 10.1016/j.rmcr.2014.09.002

Powers B, Uppalapati A, Gogineni S, Jamkhana ZA. Rituximab-a drug with many facets and cures: a treatment for acute refractory hypoxemic respiratory failure secondary to severe granulomatosis with polyangiitis. *Case Rep Crit Care.* (2013) 2013:123134. doi: 10.1155/2013/123134

Haupt ME, Pires-Ervoes J, Brannen ML, Klein-Gitelman MS, Prestridge AL, Nevin MA. Successful use of plasmapheresis for granulomatosis with polyangiitis presenting as diffuse alveolar hemorrhage. *Pediatr Pulmonol.* (2013) 48:614–6. doi: 10.1002/ppul.22666

Pinto B, Dhir V, Singh PK, Gowda KK, Sharma A. Granulomatosis with polyangiitis and severe respiratory involvement. *J Emerg Med.* (2014) 47:e79– 81. doi: 10.1016/j.jemermed.2014.01.037

Moreno-González G, Corral-Ansa L, Sabater-Riera J, Solanich-Moreno X, Mañez-Mendiluce R. Pulmonary thromboembolism and diffuse alveolar hemorrhage in granulomatosis with polyangiitis vasculitis. *Respiratory Care.* (2014) 59:e206–e9. doi: 10.4187/respcare.03162

Hilal T. Fatal cytomegalovirus disease after combination therapy with corticosteroids and rituximab for granulomatosis with polyangiitis. *Case Rep Rheumatol.* (2015) 2015:538137. doi: 10.1155/2015/538137

Fukui S, Iwamoto N, Tsuji S, Umeda M, Nishino A, Nakashima Y, et al. Diffuse alveolar hemorrhage emerging one week after starting high- dose corticosteroid therapy for granulomatosis with polyangiitis (GPA) with systemic lupus erythematosus (SLE). *Intern Med.* (2015) 54:2681– 6. doi: 10.2169/internalmedicine.54.5299

Tajarernmuang P, Limsukon A, Liwsrisakun C, Wannasopha Y. Severe bilateral bronchial stenosis with acute respiratory failure from granulomatosis with polyangiitis. *Respirol Case Rep.* (2016) 4:e00189. doi: 10.1002/rcr2.189

Ning S, Zhang X, Xu C, Dang X, Cheng H, Zhu K, et al. Methylprednisolone and plasmapheresis are effective for life-threatening diffuse alveolar hemorrhage and gastrointestinal hemorrhage in granulomatosis with polyangiitis: a case report and literature review. *Medicine.* (2018) 97:e0592. doi: 10.1097/MD.0000000000010592

Sattar Y, Susheela AT, Ullah W, Usman N, Zafrullah F. Use of plasmapheresis and immunosuppressants to treat diffuse alveolar hemorrhage in a patient with granulomatosis with polyangiitis. *Medicina.* (2019) 55:378. doi: 10.3390/medicina55070378

Hartmann A, Nordal KP, Svennevig J, Noddeland H, Pedersen T, Skarbovik AJ, et al. Successful use of artificial lung (ECMO) and kidney in the treatment of a 20-year-old female with Wegener's syndrome. *Nephrol Dial Transplant.* (1994) 9:316–9.

Loscar M, Hummel T, Haller M, Briegel J, Wiebecke B, Samtleben W, et al. [ARDS and Wegener granulomatosis]. *Anaesthesist.* (1997) 46:969- 73. doi: 10.1007/s001010050494

Matsumoto T, Ueki K, Tamura S, Ideura H, Tsukada Y, Maezawa A, et al. Extracorporeal membrane oxygenation for the management of respiratory failure due to ANCA-associated vasculitis. *Scand J Rheumatol.* (2000) 29:195- 7. doi: 10.1080/030097400750002111

Rosengarten A, Elmore P, Epstein J. Long distance road transport of a patient with Wegener's Granulomatosis and respiratory failure using extracorporeal membrane oxygenation. *Emerg Med.* (2002) 14:181- 7. doi: 10.1046/j.1442-2026.2002.00315.x

Hernandez ME, Lovrekovic G, Schears G, Helfaer M, Friedman D, Stafford P, et al. Acute onset of Wegener's granulomatosis and diffuse alveolar hemorrhage treated successfully by extracorporeal membrane oxygenation. *Pediatric Criti Care Med.* (2002) 3:63–6. doi: 10.1097/00130478-200201000-00014

Ahmed SH, Aziz T, Cochran J, Highland K. Use of extracorporeal membrane oxygenation in a patient with diffuse alveolar hemorrhage. *Chest.* (2004) 126:305–9. doi: 10.1378/chest.126.1.305

Gay SE, Ankney N, Cochran JB, Highland KB. Critical care challenges in the adult ECMO patient. *Dimens Crit Care Nurs.* (2005) 24:157–62; quiz 63–4. doi: 10.1097/00003465-200507000-00001

Balasubramanian SK, Tiruvoipati R, Chatterjee S, Sosnowski A, Firmin RK. Extracorporeal membrane oxygenation with lepirudin anticoagulation for Wegener's granulomatosis with heparin-induced thrombocytopenia. *Asaio J.* (2005) 51:477–9. doi: 10.1097/01.mat.0000169123.21946.31

Joseph M, Charles AG. Early extracorporeal life support as rescue for Wegener granulomatosis with diffuse alveolar hemorrhage and acute respiratory distress syndrome: a case report and literature review. *Pediatr Emerg Care.* (2011) 27:1163–6. doi: 10.1097/PEC.0b013e31823b01a2

Barnes SL, Naughton M, Douglass J, Murphy D. Extracorporeal membrane oxygenation with plasma exchange in a patient with alveolar haemorrhage secondary to Wegener's granulomatosis. *Intern Med J.* (2012) 42:341- 2. doi: 10.1111/j.1445-5994.2012.02720.x

Hohenforst-Schmidt W, Petermann A, Visouli A, Zarogoulidis P, Darwiche K, Kougioumtzi I, et al. Successful application of extracorporeal membrane oxygenation due to pulmonary hemorrhage secondary to granulomatosis with polyangiitis. *Drug Des Devel Ther.* (2013) 7:627–33. doi: 10.2147/DDDT.S47156

Yusuff H, Malagon I, Robson K, Parmar J, Hamilton P, Falter F. Extracorporeal membrane oxygenation for Life-threatening ANCA-positive pulmonary capillaritis. a review of UK experience. *Heart Lung Vessel.* (2015) 7:159–67.

Rawal G, Kumar R, Yadav S. ECMO rescue therapy in diffuse alveolar haemorrhage: a case report with review of literature. *J Clin Diagn Res.* (2016) 10:Od10–1. doi: 10.7860/JCDR/2016/20649.7969

Vanoli J, Riva M, Vergnano B, D'Andrea G, L'Imperio V, Pozzi MR, et al. Granulomatosis with polyangiitis presenting with diffuse alveolar hemorrhage requiring extracorporeal membrane oxygenation with rapid multiorgan relapse: A case report. *Medicine.* (2017) 96:e6024. doi: 10.1097/MD.0000000000006024

Falk L, Broman LM. Extracorporeal membrane oxygenation rescue in adolescent with bronchiolitis obliterans-organizing pneumonia like Wegener's granulomatosis. *Clin Case Rep.* (2017) 5:29–34. doi: 10.1002/ccr3.752

Delvino P, Monti S, Balduzzi S, Belliato M, Montecucco C, Caporali R. The role of extra-corporeal membrane oxygenation (ECMO) in the treatment of diffuse alveolar haemorrhage secondary to ANCA-associated vasculitis: report of two cases and review of the literature. *Rheumatol Int.* (2019) 39:367–75. doi: 10.1007/s00296-018-4116-z

Goel MK, Chauhan M, Kumar A, Wadwa P, Maitra G, Talegaonkkar M, et al. A case of refractory hypoxemic respiratory failure due to antineutrophil cytoplasmic antibodies-associated diffuse alveolar hemorrhage rescued by extracorporeal membrane oxygenation. *Indian J Crit Care Med.* (2020) 24:879–81. doi: 10.5005/jp-journals-10071-23585

Yin K, March RJ, Hoopes CW, Balk RA, Raman J, Lateef OB, et al. Extracorporeal membrane oxygenation in the management of granulomatosis with polyangiitis. *J Cardiac Surg.* (2021) 36:743–7. doi: 10.1111/jocs.15252

Thompson GE, Specks U. Update on the management of respiratory manifestations of the antineutrophil cytoplasmic antibodies-associated vasculitides. *Clin Chest Med.* (2019) 40:573–82. doi: 10.1016/j.ccm.2019.05.012

Almouhawis HA, Leao JC, Fedele S, Porter SR. Wegener's granulomatosis: a review of clinical features and an update in diagnosis and treatment. *J Oral Pathol Med.* (2013) 42:507–16. doi: 10.1111/jop.12030

Wick MR. Pulmonary disorders that are potentially associated with anti-neutrophilic cytoplasmic antibodies: a brief review. *Semin Diagn Pathol.* (2018) 35:304–14. doi: 10.1053/j.semdp.2018. 08.005

Thickett DR, Richter AG, Nathani N, Perkins GD, Harper L. Pulmonary manifestations of anti-neutrophil cytoplasmic antibody (ANCA)-positive vasculitis. *Rheumatology.* (2006) 45:261–8. doi: 10.1093/rheumatology/kei217

Quartuccio L, Bond M, Isola M, Monti S, Felicetti M, Furini F, et al. Alveolar haemorrhage in ANCA-associated vasculitis: long- term outcome and mortality predictors. *J Autoimmun.* (2020) 108:102397. doi: 10.1016/j.jaut.2019.102397

Caetano J, Fernandes das Neves M, Oliveira S, Delgado Alves J. Refractory Wegener's granulomatosis presenting with alveolar haemorrhage, treated with rituximab. *BMJ Case Rep.* (2014) 2014:bcr2014208510. doi: 10.1136/bcr-2014-208510

Scapa JV, Fishbein GA, Wallace WD, Fishbein MC. Diffuse alveolar hemorrhage and pulmonary vasculitides: histopathologic findings. *Semin Respir Crit Care Med.* (2018) 39:425–33. doi: 10.1055/s-0038-1669412

Martinez-Martinez MU, Oostdam DAH, Abud-Mendoza C. Diffuse alveolar hemorrhage in autoimmune diseases. *Curr Rheumatol Rep.* (2017) 19:27. doi: 10.1007/s11926-017-0651-y

Hill JD, O'Brien TG, Murray JJ, Dontigny L, Bramson ML, Osborn JJ, et al. Prolonged extracorporeal oxygenation for acute post-traumatic respiratory failure (shock-lung syndrome). use of the Bramson membrane lung. *N Engl J Med.* (1972) 286:629–34. doi: 10.1056/NEJM1972032328 61204

Parekh M, Abrams D, Brodie D, Yip NH. Extracorporeal membrane oxygenation for ARDS: optimization of lung protective ventilation. *Respir Care.* (2018) 63:1180–8. doi: 10.4187/respcare.06262

Peek GJ, Mugford M, Tiruvoipati R, Wilson A, Allen E, Thalanany MM, et al. Efficacy and economic assessment of conventional ventilatory support versus extracorporeal membrane oxygenation for severe adult respiratory failure (CESAR): a multicentre randomised controlled trial. *Lancet.* (2009) 374:1351–63. doi: 10.1016/S0140-6736(09)61069-2

Combes A, Hajage D, Capellier G, Demoule A, Lavoue S, Guervilly C, et al. Extracorporeal membrane oxygenation for severe acute respiratory distress syndrome. *N Engl J Med.* (2018) 378:1965–75. doi: 10.1056/NEJMoa1800385

Seeliger B, Stahl K, Schenk H, Schmidt JJ, Wiesner O, Welte T, et al. Extracorporeal membrane oxygenation for severe ARDS due to immune diffuse alveolar hemorrhage: a retrospective observational study. *Chest.* (2020) 157:744–7. doi: 10.1016/j.chest.2019.10.021

10

Biomarkers in the Diagnosis and Prognosis of Sarcoidosis: Current Use and Future Prospects

Raisa Kraaijvanger [1†], *Montse Janssen Bonás* [1†], *Adriane D. M. Vorselaars* [1] *and Marcel Veltkamp* [1,2*]

[1] Department of Pulmonology, ILD Center of Excellence, St. Antonius Hospital, Nieuwegein, Netherlands, [2] Department of Pulmonology, University Medical Center, Utrecht, Netherlands

***Correspondence:**
Marcel Veltkamp
m.veltkamp@antoniusziekenhuis.nl

[†] *These authors have contributed equally to this work*

Sarcoidosis is a heterogeneous disease in terms of presentation, duration, and severity. Due to this heterogeneity, it is difficult to align treatment decisions. Biomarkers have proved to be useful for the diagnosis and prognosis of many diseases, and over the years, many biomarkers have been proposed to facilitate diagnosis, prognosis, and treatment decisions. Unfortunately, the ideal biomarker for sarcoidosis has not yet been discovered. The most commonly used biomarkers are serum and bronchoalveolar lavage biomarkers, but these lack the necessary specificity and sensitivity. In sarcoidosis, therefore, a combination of these biomarkers is often used to establish a proper diagnosis or detect possible progression. Other potential biomarkers include imaging tools and cell signaling pathways. Fluor-18-deoxyglucose positron emission tomography and high-resolution computed tomography have been proven to be more sensitive for the diagnosis and prognosis of both pulmonary and cardiac sarcoidosis than the serum biomarkers ACE and sIL-2R. There is an upcoming role for exploration of signaling pathways in sarcoidosis pathogenesis. The JAK/STAT and mTOR pathways in particular have been investigated because of their role in granuloma formation. The activation of these signaling pathways also proved to be a specific biomarker for the prognosis of sarcoidosis. Furthermore, both imaging and cell signaling biomarkers also enable patients who might benefit from a particular type of treatment to be distinguished from those who will not. In conclusion, the diagnostic and prognostic path of sarcoidosis involves many different types of existing and new biomarker. Research addressing biomarkers and disease pathology is ongoing in order to find the ideal sensitive and specific biomarker for this disease.

Keywords: biomarkers, serum, bronchoalveolar lavage, imaging biomarkers, future biomarkers, sarcoidosis

INTRODUCTION

Sarcoidosis is a systemic inflammatory disorder of unknown cause which can lead to a variety of clinical symptoms. It commonly affects the lungs and intrathoracic lymph nodes, and is characterized by the formation of non-caseating epithelioid cell granulomas (1). In case of pulmonary involvement, granuloma formation can result in a decreased lung volume and diffusing capacity, with further shortness of breath (2). In most cases, the inflammation of sarcoidosis resolves within 2–3 years. In about 10–30% of the patients, however, the inflammation persists, leading to a chronic, sometimes progressive and even fibrotic disease for which treatment is required (3, 4). Mortality attributable to sarcoidosis is estimated between 0.5 and 5%, which is clinically relevant for a disease affecting relatively young people (5).

The diagnostic trajectory of sarcoidosis is long and complicated; it requires invasive methods like bronchoalveolar lavage and evidence of granuloma in lung or other tissue through a biopsy (6, 7). The diagnosis of sarcoidosis is then established by excluding other diseases with similar clinical or histopathological features (8).

The discovery of a specific biomarker for this disease would help diagnose sarcoidosis. According to the National Institutes of Health Biomarker Definitions Working Group, a biomarker is "a characteristic that can be objectively measured and evaluated as an indicator of normal biological processes, pathogenic processes, or pharmacologic responses to a therapeutic intervention" (9). Such predicative biomarkers are already widely used to detect the presence and severity of a variety of inflammatory diseases. However, no specific biomarker for sarcoidosis has so far been identified (2). A predictive biomarker would also be useful for treatment decisions. Because of the heterogeneity of sarcoidosis, it currently remains unclear who will benefit from a specific type of treatment (10).

The ideal biomarker should not be related to other diseases and should be highly sensitive. Moreover, it should not be invasive, and should be reproducible. Also, the ideal biomarker should be inexpensive (11). A combination of measurable biomarkers and cytology would help to understand the changes within the body that are caused by sarcoidosis, as well as the occurrence and progression of the disease, and would enable personalized treatment (2).

In this review, we address current and possible future biomarkers in sarcoidosis. Serum and bronchoalveolar lavage biomarkers are discussed in terms of antigen presentation, granuloma formation, and T-cell activation. As regards imaging, we focus on the value of chest X-ray, fluor-18-deoxyglucose positron emission tomography (^{18}F-FDG PET) and high-resolution computed tomography (HRCT) as diagnostic and prognostic tools in sarcoidosis.

SERUM BIOMARKERS

Most serum biomarkers found in sarcoidosis are produced by inflammatory cells involved in granuloma formation (**Figure 1**). In this overview, biomarkers are discussed for each of the cell types associated with the biomarkers (**Table S1**).

Macrophages

Monocyte-derived macrophages are known to be key players in granuloma formation. In order to regulate granuloma formation, monocytes, and macrophages produce a number of cytokines, chemokines and other signaling proteins. Many of these have been previously described as potential serum biomarkers in sarcoidosis and normally correlate with granuloma burden (12).

Serum Angiotensin-Converting Enzyme

The most well-known serum biomarker in sarcoidosis is serum angiotensin-converting enzyme (sACE). sACE is an acid glycoprotein which converts angiotensin I into angiotensin II. It is mainly produced by activated alveolar macrophages and correlates with granuloma burden and radiological stages II and III (13). Elevated serum levels of ACE have been intensively studied since 1975 and this is currently the most frequently used laboratory test in sarcoidosis (14). Roughly 30–80% of sarcoidosis patients have increased sACE levels, and sensitivity ranges between 22 and 86% and specificity between 54 and 95% (8). Due to the low sensitivity of sACE levels, their value as a diagnostic or prognostic tool remains a matter of debate. The low sensitivity of elevated sACE levels in sarcoidosis patients is partly due to the fact that sACE levels have been found to be increased in several other inflammatory diseases, like tuberculosis, berylliosis, histoplasmosis, Gaucher's disease and many others (15–18).

Furthermore, ACE levels in the normal range could in fact be elevated in specific patients. This is based on the influence of an insertion (I) or deletion (D) polymorphism in the ACE gene on sACE levels (19). In healthy controls, subjects with an II genotype had a significantly lower serum ACE concentration compared to subjects with a DD genotype. In clinical practice, a Z-score has been developed that corrects the ACE activity for the I/D polymorphism (19, 20). Using the correction for this I/D polymorphism results in a different interpretation in 8.5% of measurements (19).

ACE could also have a role in predicting treatment outcome. High serum levels of ACE before treatment correlate significantly with lung function improvement after 6 months of methotrexate treatment (21). What has to be kept in mind is the use of ACE inhibitors in patients with sarcoidosis (22). If patients with sarcoidosis use ACE inhibitors, serum ACE levels cannot be used in diagnosis or disease monitoring, and should be interpreted carefully (23).

Lysozyme

Lysozyme is a bacteriolytic enzyme that hydrolyses glycosidic bonds in order to degrade peptidoglycans in bacterial cell walls. At the site of infection lysozyme activity limits the cause of inflammation by rapidly degrading peptidoglycans (24). In sarcoidosis, lysozyme is produced by monocyte-macrophage systems and epithelioid cells, and is involved in granuloma formation. Increased concentration of lysozyme is mainly observed at onset of disease and has low sensitivity for sarcoidosis. Hence, lysozyme is more suitable as a prognostic rather than a diagnostic tool (25, 26).

Neopterin

Neopterin is a non-specific marker of inflammation produced by activated monocytes, macrophages, dendritic cells, and endothelial cells upon stimulation mainly by interferon gamma (IFN-γ) (27). Neopterin is released in response to cytokines mostly produced by T-cells and natural killer cells. The interaction between T-cells, macrophages, and dendritic cells in the process of granuloma formation could be due to the higher neopterin levels which have been found in sarcoidosis patients with active disease (28, 29). Although serum neopterin levels seem to be increased in sarcoidosis patients, the specificity of neopterin for sarcoidosis is low; therefore, it has little value as a diagnostic biomarker. Nevertheless, it could be a potential marker for disease activity and predictor of progression, but further research is required (30).

YKL40

The human cartilage glycoprotein-39 or YKL-40 is a growth factor for fibroblasts and vascular endothelial cells and is secreted by macrophages and neutrophils. Increased serum YKL-40 levels have been found in patients with diseases characterized by inflammation, tissue remodeling and ongoing fibrosis (31). In sarcoidosis patients, serum YKL-40 levels have been found to be elevated and to inversely correlate with diffusing capacity of the lung for carbon monoxide (DLCO) at presentation. In addition, serum YKL-40 levels are higher in patients with active sarcoidosis than in patients with inactive sarcoidosis (32, 33). A correlation has been found between YKL-40 levels and both sIL-2R levels and sACE levels in patients with active sarcoidosis, suggesting YKL-40 to be a marker for granuloma burden (33). At this moment, however, little is known about the value of serum YKL-40 levels, and more research is required to determine the value of YKL-40 as a diagnostic or prognostic biomarker in sarcoidosis (28).

sCD163

CD163 is a transmembrane hemoglobin-haptoglobin scavenger receptor expressed selectively on most macrophages in human tissues and on at least 10–30% of monocytes. Expression of CD163 is increased by IL-6, IL-10, glucocorticoids, and most immunomodulatory factors. Expression of CD163 decreases under the influence of tumor necrosis factor (TNF), interferon gamma (IFN-γ), and transforming growth factor beta (TGF-β). These are all cytokines involved in granuloma formation and disease activity. This may suggest a correlation between the expression of CD163 and inflammatory status in sarcoidosis patients. Shortly after activation of the toll-like receptors-2,4, and 5 (TLR), CD163 is shed into the environment as soluble CD163 (sCD163) (34). This quick release of sCD163 into the environment after TLR activation implies a role in inflammation, but no specific function of sCD163 has yet been identified (35). sCD163 may inhibit T-cell proliferation and activation, although the exact mechanism for this effect remains unclear. Nevertheless, the increase of sCD163 levels after stimulation of TLR suggests that sCD163 may play a role in inflammatory disorders mediated by monocyte-macrophage lineage cells. In sarcoidosis patients sCD163 was found to be significantly increased in comparison to healthy controls and correlated with sIL-2R and sACE levels (36). Although little is known about the role of sCD163 in sarcoidosis, it may be a useful biomarker with potentially high sensitivity but low specificity. In other diseases like RA, MS and Crohn's disease, sCD163 has been associated with disease activity and suggested as a useful predictor of progression (35, 37).

CC Chemokine Ligand 18

C-C motive chemokine ligand 18 (CCL18) is a CC chemokine produced primarily by antigen-presenting cells such as macrophages, dendritic cells, and peripheral blood monocytes. CCL18 is chemotactic for both naive and activated T-lymphocytes. Elevated levels of CCL18 have been detected in serum of patients with T-cell helper 2 (Th2) predominant diseases like idiopathic pulmonary fibrosis, bronchial asthma and scleroderma (38). CCL18 can stimulate the mRNA and protein production of collagen, possibly stimulating fibrosis. In sarcoidosis patients, elevated levels of CCL18 have been found in patients with active disease (39). Unfortunately, CCL18 is elevated in most interstitial lung diseases, and also in Gaucher's disease, so it is not suitable as a diagnostic biomarker for sarcoidosis. However, CCL18 has potential to be used as a marker to monitor disease and predict progression (39), as was already suggested by Prasse et al. (40), who demonstrated that CCL18 levels in bronchoalveolar lavage (BAL) correlate with the scadding stage.

Serum Amyloid A

Serum amyloid A (SAA) is produced by the liver during an acute phase reaction. In inflammatory conditions, macrophages produce high levels of SAA, which indicates that elevated levels of SAA are a clinical marker of inflammation. Elevated levels of SAA are found in several inflammatory diseases like RA and Crohn's disease (41). Elevated levels of SAA have also been found in sarcoidosis, and appear to correlate with a decline in lung function (42). Sarcoidosis has been suggested as a heterogeneous disease, with multiple potential triggers such as metals or micro-organisms (43). If in the future patients could be distinguished based on possible triggers, it would be interesting to study SAA as a biomarker in a specific subgroup of sarcoidosis patients with micro-organisms such as mycobacteria or propionic bacteria as suspected triggers (44).

Chitotriosidase

Chitotriosidase (CTO) is an enzyme of the chitinase family. It degrades chitin, a polymer found in cell walls of fungi and the exoskeletons of insects and crustaceans. Pulmonary neutrophils and macrophages can secrete CTO upon stimulation of toll-like receptors (TLRs) by IFN-γ, TNF, and granulocyte/macrophage colony-stimulating factor (GM-CSF). CTO serum levels directly correlate with sACE levels (45). Highest serum levels were found in patients with progressive disease and were found to decrease upon treatment with prednisone or other immunosuppressant therapy. As a diagnostic marker, CTO is less useful due to low specificity. CTO serum levels have been found to be elevated in other diseases like Gaucher's disease, malaria, multiple sclerosis, atherosclerosis, Alzheimer's disease, and tuberculosis (20). However, CTO sensitivity and specificity are higher than those of other serum biomarkers, making CTO a potentially useful biomarker in sarcoidosis. CTO serum levels have prognostic value in sarcoidosis and can be used to monitor disease activity, with the potential to be used as a diagnostic tool for this disease (45, 46).

Monocytes

As mentioned above, macrophages are key players in granuloma formation. However, macrophages are difficult to study or use as diagnostic/prognostic biomarkers, since they are predominantly found in tissue and granuloma. Monocytes are precursors of macrophages and are found in the bloodstream, making them accessible and interesting as biomarkers in sarcoidosis. There are three subtypes of monocytes, classical monocytes (CD14++/CD16–), intermediate monocytes (CD14+/CD16+) and non-classical monocytes (CD14–/CD16++). Intermediate and non-classical monocytes are more inflammatory type monocytes, and have been found to be elevated in sarcoidosis (47). In addition, treatments with prednisone and infliximab have been shown to have a downregulating effect on intermediate and non-classical monocytes, suggesting a role in disease activity and prognostic value for response to treatment (48, 49). In addition to the CD14 and CD16 surface markers, many different monocyte surface markers have been studied, with promising results (50, 51). However, circulating intermediate and non-classical monocytes have also been found to be elevated in other diseases, like cardiovascular diseases and other interstitial diseases, thus decreasing its specificity (52, 53). Circulating subtypes of monocytes are potentially interesting prognostic biomarkers, but further research is required.

T-Cells

T-cells play an important role in the development of granulomas. Antigen presenting cells like macrophages present peptides to T-helper (Th) cells via MHC class II molecules. This activates T-cells and leads to greater proliferation and recruitment of neutrophils and monocytes (54). Based on T-cell activation, many T-cell cytokines and chemokines have been described as potential biomarkers for sarcoidosis. The activation of T-cells can be seen as a crucial step in the perpetuation of granuloma formation.

Serum Soluble Interleukin 2 Receptor

Serum soluble interleukin 2 receptor (sIL-2R) is the circulating form of the membrane IL-2R, a proposed marker of disease activity in sarcoidosis. Upon activation, Th1 cells upregulate the expression of IL-2R on the cell surface, and are able to shed sIL-2R into circulation (55). Increased sIL-2R levels are therefore considered to be a marker of Th1 cell activation in the formation and perpetuation of granuloma (56). Increased levels of sIL-2R in sarcoidosis patients have been described since 1983 (57). Unfortunately, elevated sIL-2R levels are not specific for sarcoidosis, as elevated serum levels of sIL-2R are found in other granulomatous diseases, hematological malignancies, and various autoimmune disorders (10). Even though the use of sIL-2R as a diagnostic marker for sarcoidosis remains a matter of debate, a recent study performed in patients suspected of sarcoidosis has shown a sensitivity of 88% and a specificity of 85% (58). This indicates that sIL-2R can be a useful tool in the diagnosis of sarcoidosis when combined with other (imaging) biomarkers and clinical features in the process of diagnosis.

sIL-2R seems to correlate with active disease and multiple organ involvement, and can possibly predict progression and relapse after discontinuation of therapy (59–61) Furthermore, sIL-2R can be used as a prognostic tool to determine if therapy is needed and/or to predict relapse after discontinuation of therapy (21, 59). Moreover, sIL-2R can be used in serial measurements during therapy or in follow-up to evaluate treatment effect (11).

It is important to state that patients with impaired renal function have elevated sIL-2R. This can result in high sIL-2R levels in the absence of active disease. Since renal impairment can occur in sarcoidosis patients, this effect has to be kept in mind when sIL-2R is used as a marker to monitor disease activity (59).

B-Cells

Although the innate immune system and T-cell immunity are known to be involved in the pathogenesis of sarcoidosis, it is becoming increasingly evident that B-cells are involved in granuloma formation as well. B-cell accumulation has been shown in granuloma and pulmonary lesions, and a positive effect of B-cell depletion has been reported (62, 63).

B-Cell Activating Factor

B-cell activating factor (BAFF) is a cytokine of the TNF family with a critical role in B-cell development and function. *In vivo* and *in vitro* studies have shown that blocking of BAFF results in reduced follicular and marginal zone B-cell numbers, while overexpression of BAFF in mice resulted in an increase in activated B-cells, activated T-cells, autoantibody production, and hypergammaglobulinemia. In sarcoidosis patients, higher levels of BAFF have been found in serum in comparison to healthy controls (64–66). However, elevated BAFF levels are not specific for sarcoidosis, as these have also been found in other immunomodulatory diseases like systemic lupus erythematosus (SLE) and rheumatoid arthritis (RA) (67). In addition to elevated serum levels being found in sarcoidosis patients, a correlation between BAFF levels and disease severity has been shown. Highest levels of BAFF in sarcoidosis patients are associated with multiple organ involvement, decline in pulmonary function, and more advanced chest radiographic stages (II/III) (64). In a different study, higher serum levels of BAFF were associated with a higher frequency of eye and skin involvement and with increased levels of sACE, lysozyme, and IFN-γ (66). Although much is still unknown about the mechanisms of BAFF in sarcoidosis patients, results reported so far seem promising enough to further explore the value of BAFF as a prognostic or even diagnostic biomarker in sarcoidosis.

Naïve and Memory B-Cells

The B-cell ablative rituximab targets CD20, a marker expressed on the surface of naïve and memory B-cells, and has been shown to yield clinical improvement in some sarcoidosis patients (63, 68). This observation suggests a role for naïve and memory B-cells in sarcoidosis pathophysiology. When phenotyping B-cells, subpopulations are distributed differently in sarcoidosis patients in comparison to healthy controls (62, 69, 70). Naïve B-cell populations have been found to be elevated in sarcoidosis patients, and memory B-cells have been found to be downregulated in sarcoidosis patients (62). However, not all studies found the memory B-cells to be downregulated (69). When comparing sarcoidosis patients with and without pulmonary involvement, only the naïve mature B-cells are different between the two groups: sarcoidosis patients without pulmonary involvement do not have increased numbers of naïve mature B-cells.

Not only are numbers of naïve and memory B-cells altered, but sarcoid B-cells were found to be anergic in chronic sarcoidosis. This anergy could be partly due to the reduced levels of NF-κB/p65 found in sarcoid B-cells. B-cells with reduced NF-κB have an impaired response to antigens (69, 71). Furthermore, when memory B-cells are reduced, this may lead to a defective antibody response that is not able to eliminate the antigens responsible for granuloma formation. These findings suggest an important and possibly pathogenic role for B-cells in sarcoidosis, but the involvement of the different B-cell populations in granuloma formation remains unclear (62).

Regulatory B-Cells

Regulatory B-cells (Bregs) are IL-10 producing B-cells. This type of B-cell has been found to reduce inflammation through cytoplasmic IL-10 expression (72). Phenotyping B-cell populations in sarcoidosis patients revealed that circulating numbers of IL-10 producing B-cells were elevated in patients

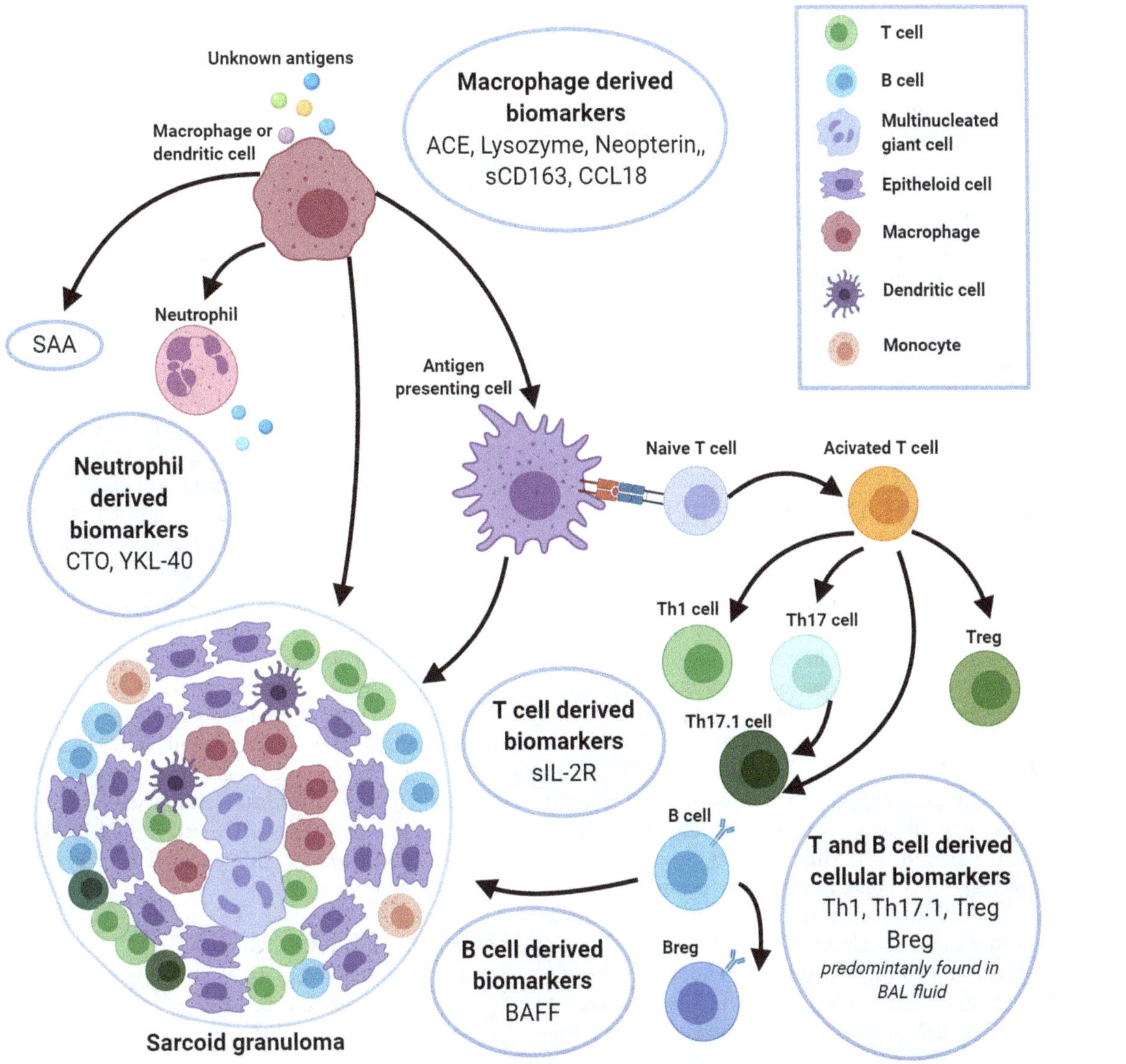

FIGURE 1 | An integrated overview of serum and bronchoalveolar lavage fluid biomarkers produced by cells of the innate and adaptive immune system, involved in the formation of granulomas in sarcoidosis. The sarcoidosis granuloma consists of a tightly formed core of epithelioid and multinucleated-giant cells (MGCs) encircled especially by T helper (Th) cells, but also by B cells, macrophages and dendritic cells (DCs). During this granuloma formation a variety of biomarkers is released by these inflammatory cells. Macrophages are key players in granuloma formation and produce a number of inflammatory biomarkers [e.g., serum angiotensin-converting enzyme (sACE), lysozyme, neopterin, CD163, C-C motive chemokine ligand 18 (CCL18), serum amyloid A (SAA)]. Macrophages activate T-cells by presenting a triggering antigen, which results in an upregulated expression of soluble interleukin 2 receptor (sIL-2R). Apart from T-cells, B-cells also have shown to play a role in granuloma formation. Crucial for the B-cell maturation and function is the biomarker B-cell activating factor (BAFF). All these biomarkers may be useful for the diagnosis and prognosis of sarcoidosis. Figure created with Biorender.com.

with active sarcoidosis. Both the frequency and absolute numbers were significantly higher in active sarcoidosis. Although current knowledge of IL-10 producing B-cells is insufficient to draw any conclusion on the role of Bregs, it seems that there is an altered B-cell homeostasis in active sarcoidosis.

This observation does appear to be in line with findings in other inflammatory diseases like SLE, RA, and multiple sclerosis. Furthermore, since IL-10 is important in the development of fibrosis, this association could justify further research into this population of B-cells (62, 65).

In conclusion, B-cells are relatively new and somewhat unknown cells in sarcoidosis. However, since B-cells seem to be involved in several processes in sarcoidosis pathogenesis, the expectation would be that BAFF levels and memory, naïve, and regulatory B-cell counts could be used to assess disease activity and could possibly be used in the diagnosis of sarcoidosis. However, further research is required before B-cell counts and BAFF levels can be used as biomarkers in sarcoidosis.

Combining Serum Biomarkers

All biomarkers mentioned above as serum biomarkers appear to have the same limitations, namely, insufficient sensitivity and specificity. Since many biomarkers have shown a mutual positive correlation (25, 28, 73), different combinations are being explored. Using a combination of different biomarkers, various studies have already demonstrated an increase of both sensitivity and specificity (74–76).

BRONCHOALVEOLAR LAVAGE FLUID

The diagnosis of sarcoidosis is often confirmed by analyzing bronchoalveolar lavage fluid (BALF) (77). Various cells and soluble components in BALF, such as proteins and cytokines, have been addressed in different immunological studies. These studies have considerably increased our understanding of the immunopathogenesis of sarcoidosis (29, 77) (**Table S2**).

CD4/CD8 Ratio

In sarcoidosis, the percentage of lymphocytes in BALF is often increased. Sensitivity of lymphocytosis was found to range between 68 and 95% (78, 79). This variation is related to the fact that an increase in lymphocytes in BALF is nonspecific for sarcoidosis, as it is also observed in other granulomatous and lung diseases (10, 29, 80). The observation that CD4+ T-cells play an important role in the development of sarcoidosis has helped distinguish sarcoidosis from other diseases (81). Measurement of the ratio of CD4/CD8 T-cells has been used to differentiate sarcoidosis from other diseases since the 1980s (29, 80). Increased CD4/CD8 ratio was observed in sarcoidosis patients, with a sensitivity of between 54 and 80% and a specificity of between 59 and 80% (10, 29, 78, 79). In the clinic, the diagnosis of sarcoidosis is supported by a CD4/CD8 ratio >3.5 and lymphocytosis > 15%. However, BALF lymphocytosis is not a universal finding in sarcoidosis (81). A recent study by Darlington et al. (82) showed that the measurement of the proportion of T-cell receptor (TCR) CD4+ Va2.3+ T-cells in BALF could also be a biomarker in addition to the CD4/CD8 ratio, to support a sarcoidosis diagnosis. TCR Va2.3 gene segments were found to be increased in BALF, especially in patients with an HLA-DRB1*03 genotype, which is usually found in patients with Löfgren's syndrome (LS). This biomarker therefore proved to be more useful for the diagnosis of LS, while the CD4/CD8 ratio is useful for the diagnosis of any type of sarcoidosis. On the other hand, specificity proved to be higher for CD4+ Va2.3+ T-cells compared to the CD4/CD8 ratio in BALF (97 vs. 92%), which will help with the diagnosis of sarcoidosis (82). Despite the frequent use of the CD4/CD8 ratio for the diagnosis of sarcoidosis, this ratio does not reflect the severity of the disease (29).

CD103+CD4+/CD4+ Ratio

While the CD4/CD8 ratio is useful for the diagnosis of sarcoidosis, sensitivity and specificity of this biomarker are low. Therefore the expression of other cellular markers in this subset of T-cells have been explored.

Expression of the aEβ7/CD103β7 integrin (CD103) has been related to the retention of intraepithelial lymphocytes (IEL) in mucosal tissue of the lung. CD103 is expressed by lymphocytes within the bronchial epithelium, some alveolar wall lymphocytes and CD4+ T-cells in the BAL. Expression of CD103 on CD4+ T-cells in BAL fluid is found to be different in ILD patients, depending on the type of disease (83). In patients with sarcoidosis, numbers of CD103 CD4+ T-cells in BAL fluid are significantly lower than in other lung diseases (83). Therefore, differential expression of CD103 on CD4+ T-cells could serve as a diagnostic marker for sarcoidosis. However, there is some controversy on the use of the CD103+CD4+/CD4+ ratio as a diagnostic tool for sarcoidosis. The sensitivity and specificity seems to depend strongly on the population used in the study. Heron et al. (84) and Bretagne et al. (85) show a significant decrease in the CD103+CD4+/CD4+ ratio in sarcoidosis patients in comparison to other ILD while a study by Hyldgaard et al. (79) does not show a similar decrease. The difference in outcome might be explained by the inclusion of patients without alveolar lymphocytosis by Hyldgaard et al. (79).

While the CD103+CD4+/CD4+ appears to be a useful diagnostic tool in sarcoidosis caution should be taken with the interpretation of this ratio. Therefore, a CD103+CD4+/CD4+ ratio 0.2 can be seen as additional evidence pointing towards a diagnosis of sarcoidosis.

T-Helper 17.1 Cells

For a long time, sarcoidosis was seen as a Th1-driven disease, because of the variety of type 1 specific cytokines present in BALF and serum of sarcoidosis patients, including IFN-γ, IL-12, and IL-18. However, nowadays it is accepted that sarcoidosis is driven by a combination of Th1- and Th17-associated factors (86). Th17 cells normally produce IL-17A and IL-17F, but in sarcoidosis Th17 cells were also observed to produce IFN-γ (12, 87). These cells are referred to as Th17.1 cells and are thought to derive from classically polarized Th17 cells. Th17 cells have a high plasticity and were found to be able to differentiate into a Th1-like phenotype, in which the majority mainly produce IFN-γ (87, 88). Both Th17 and

Th17.1 cells were identified in sarcoidosis patients, and these Th-cells were found to express different chemokine receptors, and demonstrated different cytokine effector functions. The number of Th17.1 cells proved to be significantly higher in the BALF, but not the blood, of sarcoidosis patients, compared to healthy controls (88). Th17.1 cells are promising immunological markers in the diagnosis of sarcoidosis, but results are based on small cohorts, so further research is required to determine the diagnostic value. Additionally, it was seen that there is a significant association between the number of Th17.1 cells in BALF and the development of chronic sarcoidosis, making these cells an interesting prognostic marker for the development of (chronic) pulmonary sarcoidosis (87).

Regulatory T-Cells

Regulatory T-cells or Treg cells may also play an important role in the development of sarcoidosis. Treg cells normally suppress immune responses by the host immune system against self and foreign antigens. In the case of sarcoidosis, it is hypothesized that Tregs are functionally defective or exhausted, making them unable to fully suppress the immune responses (89). The dysfunction of Tregs in sarcoidosis, resulting in impaired self-tolerance and failed immune homeostasis, could be an important element in the pathogenesis of sarcoidosis (90). A Polish study showed that the dysfunction of Tregs resulted in an exaggerated Th1 response in sarcoidosis patients (91). The diagnostic value of Tregs in sarcoidosis remains to be determined. A number of possible correlations between Tregs and disease activity have been described, with prognostic values. A Scandinavian study showed that a low Treg level in BALF was associated with a favorable prognosis (92). On the other hand, a German study reported that a decreased Treg level in BALF corresponded with the development of chronic disease (93).

Although there are thus conflicting results on the presence and effect of Tregs in active sarcoidosis, what is clear is that an imbalance exists between Th17 and Tregs. Th17 cells are elevated in the blood of sarcoidosis patients, while the number of Tregs is decreased (90). The Treg/Th17 ratio proved to be inversely related to disease activity, decreasing in those with relapsing pulmonary sarcoidosis and increasing in those with chronic active disease (12, 94).

Neutrophils

Neutrophils are important players in the innate immune system, but their role in sarcoidosis is still little understood. Neutrophils are attracted by chemokines, such as IL-8, which are released by monocytes and macrophages (12). Patients in an advanced radiological stage of sarcoidosis (stage II or III), or with an unfavorable evolution, were reported to have an elevated percentage of neutrophils in BALF compared to healthy controls. Furthermore, BALF neutrophil levels were significantly higher in patients with progressive disease compared to those with stable disease. Therefore, neutrophils may be useful markers of progressive disease (29, 95). A possible origin of this correlation could be the large number of proteases, like collagenase or gelatinase, which may initiate collagen destruction and remodeling, leading to the development of pulmonary fibrosis (12).

Natural Killer (NK) Cells

Other immune cells in BALF which are associated with poor outcome and an advanced radiological stage are natural killer (NK) cells (95). NK cells (CD3–CD16/56+) are part of the first-line defense of the immune system (96). They are suspected to play a role in several inflammatory pulmonary diseases because of their ability to produce cytokines (95). IFN-γ is released by active NK cells and stimulates TNF-α secretion from alveolar macrophages, which is associated with progressive and corticosteroid resistant disease (95). An impaired lung function was shown to be associated with a high level of NK cells in the lungs. Furthermore, sarcoidosis patients requiring steroid treatment also had a higher percentage of these cells in BALF (95).

Natural Killer T (NKT) Cells

Natural killer T (NKT) cells (CD3+CD16/56+) are a regulatory T cell lineage which both express T cell (CD3) and NK (CD16/56+) receptors on their surface membranes, thereby influencing both Th1 and Th2 cytokine systems and stimulating cell-mediated immunity or suppressing autoimmune responses (96, 97). NK cells are able to release a various cytokines determined by antigen signal strength, including IFN-γ, TNF-α, and a variety of interleukins (IL-4, IL-10, IL-13, IL-17, IL-21) (97). In sarcoidosis patients reduced numbers of NKT cells were found in blood and BALF (98–100). However, there are also reports on the accumulation of NKT cell in granulomatous lesions of sarcoidosis patients (99). Deficiency and/or impaired function of NKT cells results in loss of the immunoregulation, which might contribute to the prolonged T-cell activity characteristic for sarcoidosis (101).

CXCL9, CXCL10, and CXCL11

The monocyte-macrophage cell lineage is the origin of the expression of a variety of cytokines and chemokines that play many different roles in the inflammatory phenotype of sarcoidosis, including T-cell attraction and promotion of Th1/Th17 differentiation (8). Some interesting chemokines were found to be elevated in the BALF and serum of sarcoidosis patients. These included chemokines that are part of the CXC chemokine subfamily; CXCL9, CXCL10, and CXCL11 (102, 103). These chemokines bind to the CXCR3 receptor and thereby recruit CD4+ T-cells, monocytes and other inflammatory cells to the site of inflammation (103). Although these chemokines share common functions, there are differences in their biological properties (103, 104). One major difference is the fact that CXCL9 and CXCL11 can solely be induced by IFN-γ, while CXCL10 can also be induced by TNF-α, IFN-α, and LPS (103, 104). These differences may influence the clinical outcomes of these chemokines (104). In tuberculosis, this chemokine subfamily was already found to represent useful biomarkers for the prediction of disease progression and therapy response (105, 106).

In the case of sarcoidosis, a recent study by Arger et al. (103) showed that CXCL10 correlates negatively with lung function, and that elevated CXCL10 also correlates with higher dyspnea scores in longitudinal analyses. These correlations could not be found for CXCL9. However, CXCL9 proved to be positively associated with the total number of organs involved in sarcoidosis. CXCL11 proved to be negatively associated lung function and correlated positively with the number of organs involved (103). It was speculated that each of these chemokines could be used to help predict the clinical outcome of a sarcoidosis patient, as well as acting as biomarkers for both pulmonary outcomes and response to therapy (103).

Krebs von den Lungen-6

Krebs von den Lungen-6 (KL6) is a human high molecular weight MUC1 mucin protein derived from type II pneumocytes and respiratory bronchiolar epithelial cells (107). An increased level of KL-6 reflects damaged or regenerating type II pneumocytes (108).

Elevated levels of KL-6 have been found in BALF and serum in patients with idiopathic pulmonary fibrosis, sarcoidosis, and other ILDs (109–112).

The fact that it is not a disease specific marker indicates that it has no major role in diagnosing sarcoidosis. However, in sarcoidosis patients both serum and BALF levels of KL-6 correlate with higher serum ACE levels and CD4+/CD8+ ratio (25, 112). Suggesting usefulness as a disease monitoring tool. It is demonstrated that the highest level of KL-6 can be found in patients with radiological stage IV pulmonary sarcoidosis (25, 76, 111) suggesting a potential role as a marker of severity of pulmonary sarcoidosis.

Combining BALF Biomarkers

The biomarkers mentioned above give limited information about pulmonary sarcoidosis as individual biomarkers. However, combining some of these biomarkers may be helpful in the diagnosis and prognosis of pulmonary sarcoidosis. CD4/CD8 ratio and CD103+CD4+/CD4+ ratio appear to be useful diagnostic biomarkers to support the diagnosis of sarcoidosis, while disease severity can be predicted and monitored by a correlation between KL-6 and CD4+/CD8+ ratio. Furthermore, disease progression can be monitored trough the percentage of neutrophils, NK cells, and NKT cells in BALF. In addition, Th17.1 cells and Treg cells are promising prognostic biomarkers, however, further research is required to determine the diagnostic value. The BALF chemokines CXCL9-11 in their turn may be useful biomarkers for treatment decisions.

IMAGING BIOMARKERS

Clinical manifestations of sarcoidosis are highly variable and any organ can be affected. For pulmonary sarcoidosis, chest X-ray, and high-resolution computed tomography (HRCT) are frequently used. However, in sarcoidosis patients with extrapulmonary manifestations, such as cardiac sarcoidosis or neurosarcoidosis, other imaging modalities are warranted. For these patients, magnetic resonance imaging (MRI) and fluor-18-deoxyglucose positron emission tomography (^{18}F-FDG PET) scanning are increasingly recognized as essential imaging techniques for adequately identifying sarcoidosis localization and determining disease management (113).

TABLE 1 | Radiographic staging of sarcoidosis patients at presentation according to the scadding criteria.

Radiographic stage	Chest X-ray	Frequency (%)	Resolution (%)
0	Normal	5–15	
I	BHL	25–65	60–90
II	BHL and pulmonary infiltrates	20–40	40–70
III	Pulmonary infiltrates without BHL	10–15	10–20
1V	Advanced pulmonary fibrosis	5	0

The estimated frequency at presentation is given as well as the probability of spontaneous resolution during disease course (BHL, bilateral hilar lymphadenopathy) (1, 114, 116).

Chest X-ray

Conventional chest radiography is performed in most patients with sarcoidosis and is abnormal in over 90% of cases (114). Sarcoidosis is commonly staged according to its appearance on chest X-ray. This staging system was introduced by Scadding almost six decades ago (115), but still holds a prominent position in assessment of sarcoidosis. Scadding classified chest radiography findings in sarcoidosis into five stages, shown in **Table 1**.

An interesting feature of the abovementioned Scadding stages is the fact that it gives prognostic information both on resolution of disease as well as mortality (1, 114, 116, 117). Spontaneous resolution varies from 60 to 90% in stage I disease to no resolution in stage IV fibrotic disease. Furthermore, Kirkil et al. (117) demonstrated that mortality rates were correlated to Scadding stages with the highest mortality in patients presenting with stage IV disease.

Shortcomings of conventional chest X-ray is the fact that in absence of pathological confirmation, clinical features together with chest X-ray can be diagnostic in stage I and II disease but are less accurate in stage 0, II, and IV disease (1). Furthermore, only moderate agreement on Scadding stages is reported in literature (118). Finally, Judson et al. (119) demonstrated that chest X-ray was inadequate to reliably detect acute exacerbations of pulmonary sarcoidosis. These are some reasons why the HRCT now has a prominent place in the diagnosis and monitoring of sarcoidosis.

High-Resolution Computed Tomography

HRCT has a solid position in the diagnostic approach and follow-up of sarcoidosis, as it provides high-resolution slides of the pulmonary parenchyma. Although widely used, quantification of HRCT results remains a difficult task even for experienced radiologists and pulmonologists. A reliable inter- and intra-patient comparison of results requires standardized quantification of HRCT findings.

In a pioneering approach to objectively quantifying HRCT results, Oberstein et al. developed a scoring system based on the sum of typical patterns of parenchymal involvement, combined with lymph node enlargement and pleural involvement. The

Oberstein score yielded high correlation coefficients with BAL total cell count and sIL-2R (120).

Drent et al., who also found a good interobserver agreement in a retrospective cohort of 80 sarcoidosis patients, later replicated the Oberstein score. They also found a correlation between pulmonary function and HRCT abnormality scores for all subgroups except lymph node enlargement (121). When used together with serum sIL-2R values, the HRCT scoring system can predict disease activity and could replace ^{18}F-FDG PET (122). Although this finding was not replicated, it could be an important finding especially with regard to cost-effectiveness and the fact that ^{18}F-FDG PET is not universally available.

In order to objectively quantify HRCT results regarding the extent and activity of sarcoidosis, Benamore et al. more recently developed the CT activity score (CTAS), which consists of CT extent scores for nodularity, ground-glass opacification, interlobular septal thickening and consolidation. The total CTAS was found to predict response to treatment in FVC after 1 year in their cohort of 100 patients. Furthermore, CTAS had a high degree of interobserver agreement (123).

A retrospective study of a cohort of 57 patient reproduced these results and found significant correlations with lung function changes after six months of therapy (Change in %VC: $r = 0.543$, $P < 0.001$). Furthermore, higher CTAS scores were seen in patients with high sACE levels (124). Even though the results of these HRCT scoring systems are promising, they are still not widely implemented in standard patient care.

Fluor-18-Deoxyglucose Positron Emission Tomography

Over the past decade, ^{18}F-FDG PET has gained territory as an important and reliable imaging biomarker in severe sarcoidosis (125).

Prior to ^{18}F-FDG PET, gallium-67 (^{67}Ga) scintigraphy was the most frequently used form of nuclear imaging in sarcoidosis, but ^{18}F-FDG PET has replaced it, as it was shown to be more accurate in depicting extrathoracic lesions (126) and yields high quality images with superior contrast and spatial resolution compared to ^{67}Ga scintigraphy (127). ^{18}F-FDG PET can be used as a diagnostic marker, but also to predict treatment response and prognosis.

^{18}F-FDG PET as a Diagnostic Marker in Pulmonary Sarcoidosis

Although it is not necessary to obtain an ^{18}F-FDG PET scan of every new sarcoidosis patient, it sometimes provides valuable information for the diagnostic process. In patients in whom the diagnosis of sarcoidosis is suspected, the extent of organ involvement and disease activity can be visualized using ^{18}F-FDG PET. A prospective study of 36 newly diagnosed untreated sarcoidosis patients showed visual activity on ^{18}F-FDG PET in 34 patients (94%). Furthermore, ^{18}F-FDG PET was far more sensitive than ACE and sIL2R in this study (128).

In a small retrospective study of 23 biopsy-proven sarcoidosis patients with an indication to receive corticosteroid therapy, 91.7% had ^{18}F-FDG PET positive findings. Sensitivity improved to 100% after skin involvement was excluded (129).

In a large retrospective study of 158 sarcoidosis patients, 75% had ^{18}F-FDG PET positive findings (130). In some patients, new occult organ localizations such as cardiac or ossal sarcoidosis can be detected with ^{18}F-FDG PET (131). As ^{18}F-FDG PET can reveal occult localizations, it can also be used to determine the most suitable biopsy site (7). In a study of 89 patients with unexplained disabling symptoms, 73% had signs of disease activity on ^{18}F-FDG PET, which were mostly extrathoracic (132).

^{18}F-FDG PET as a Marker of Therapeutic Response and Prognosis in Pulmonary Sarcoidosis

The natural disease course of sarcoidosis is very unpredictable, with not all patients being in need of systemic therapy. It is highly important, but very difficult, to distinguish patients who might benefit from treatment from those who will not.

A reasonable number of reports objectifying ^{18}F-FDG PET as a predictor of treatment response have been published over the past few years. Keijsers et al. studied 43 newly-diagnosed sarcoidosis patients and found that patients with increased lung parenchymal activity on ^{18}F-FDG PET had significantly lower DLCO. Moreover, high parenchymal activity was a predictor of improvement in pulmonary function upon treatment with corticosteroids. Patients without parenchymal activity assessed by ^{18}F-FDG PET did not show decreasing pulmonary function when untreated (133). A prospective study included 56 severe sarcoidosis patients, refractory to first- and second-line treatment, who were treated with the anti-TNF drug infliximab. High ^{18}F-FDG PET activity of the pulmonary parenchyma (SUVmax) at baseline was able to predict lung function improvement after 6 months of treatment ($R = 0.62$, $p = 0.0004$) (134) (**Figure 2**). As anti-TNF therapy is costly and known to cause side-effects, ^{18}F-FDG PET can be very useful in therapeutic decision making, especially for this group of refractory patients.

In a study of 90 sarcoidosis patients with persistent symptoms, 72% had signs of activity on ^{18}F-FDG PET. Furthermore, 38 patients (51%) with positive ^{18}F-FDG PET results had normal ACE levels, suggesting an added value of ^{18}F-FDG PET as an adjunct to serum biomarkers (135).

To date it is unknown what the optimal duration of systemic therapy should be. ^{18}F-FDG PET is a potential tool to determine which patients are at risk for relapse of disease activity and symptoms. In a retrospective study, Vorselaars et al. (59) assessed the risk of relapse after discontinuation of infliximab therapy in severe sarcoidosis patients, and found that high activity ($SUV_{max} > 6$) of mediastinal lymphnodes on ^{18}F-FDG PET is a predictor of relapse after discontinuation of infliximab therapy, with a hazard ratio of 4.33 ($p < 0.001$). This suggests that high activity on ^{18}F-FDG PET reflects the burden of inflammation and therefore the need for prolonged therapy. A small retrospective study of 23 newly diagnosed sarcoidosis patients showed that persistent disease activity on ^{18}F-FDG PET during the first months of corticosteroid treatment is a predictor of relapse (129).

Most studies have used the maximum standard uptake value (SUV_{max}) to quantify disease activity. Recently, a new tool for the quantification of disease activity of the pulmonary parenchyma was proposed. Volumetric ^{18}F-FDG PET analysis of global lung

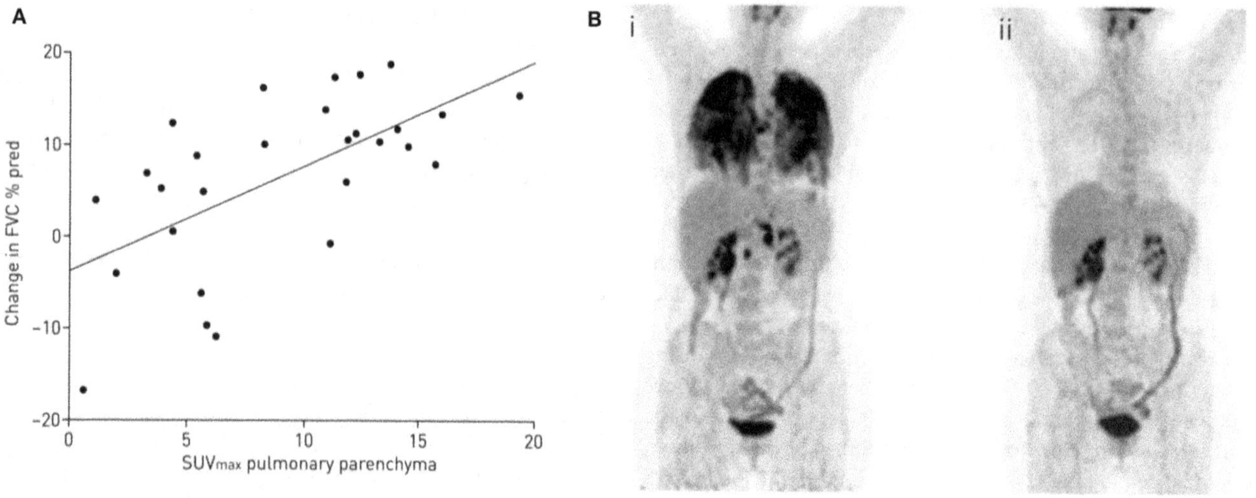

FIGURE 2 | (A) ^{18}F-fluorodeoxyglucose (FDG) by positron emission tomography (PET) activity and improvement in pulmonary function. Correlation between high activity of pulmonary parenchyma on ^{18}F-FDG PET (maximum standardized uptake value [SUV_{max}]) at baseline and improvement in forced vital capacity (FVC) in patients with a pulmonary treatment indication ($R = 0.62$, $p = 0.0004$). Reproduced and modified from (134) with permission. **(B)** Example of a PET-CT scan of a sarcoidosis patient with pulmonary involvement, before (i) and after (ii) 6 months of infliximab therapy.

inflammation was proposed by Adams et al. (136) and possibly correlates better with conventional serum biomarkers ACE and sIL-2R than SUV_{max}. TluG (Total Lung Glycolysis) measures the total activity of the pulmonary parenchyma, and although this derivative from the total lesion glycolysis in oncology studies looks promising, it was not superior to SUV_{max} in predicting lung function change during infliximab therapy (137).

Cardiac Imaging Biomarkers

Current improved imaging techniques are leading to higher rates of incidence and recognition of cardiac sarcoidosis than previously reported (138). Approximately 5% of all sarcoidosis patients will have clinically relevant cardiac involvement (139).

Magnetic Resonance Imaging in Cardiac Sarcoidosis

The diagnosis of cardiac sarcoidosis can be challenging, as the diagnostic yield of endomyocardial biopsy is low and this procedure also has potential hazards (138). Cardiac Magnetic Resonance Imaging (CMR) is acknowledged in the diagnostic guidelines for cardiac sarcoidosis (140). Late gadolinium enhancement (LGE) on CMR (in a pattern consistent with cardiac sarcoidosis) in patients with known biopsy-proven sarcoidosis and no other explanation for cardiac disease can be used as a criterion to diagnose sarcoidosis (140).

Formation of edema or scar tissue in the myocardium or pericardium shows late gadolinium enhancement on CMR, as gadolinium is an extracellular contrast agent. Late gadolinium enhancement can potentially be optimized with the use of T1/T2 mapping, which can potentially discriminate between fibrosis (T1 mapping) and extracellular water/edema (T2 mapping) (141). T1/T2 mapping for this use needs further evaluation.

A large number of studies have found LGE on CMR to be an independent prognostic biomarker (142, 143). A large prospective cohort study of 321 sarcoidosis patients by Kouranos et al. (144) showed that LGE was an independent predictor of the primary endpoint (composite of death, life-threatening arrhythmias, admission for heart failure, and heart transplantation) with a hazard ratio of 5.7 ($P < 0.004$). Moreover, a large meta-analysis including 10 studies and a total of 760 patients concluded that patients with LGE on CMR were at increased risk of events, compared to patients without LGE (11.9 vs. 1.1%; $P < 0.001$), even if they had preserved left ventricle systolic function (11.6 vs. 0.7%; $P < 0.0011$) (145). A study investigating both LGE on CMR and uptake on ^{18}F-FDG PET in 56 sarcoidosis patients with high clinical suspicion of cardiac sarcoidosis showed that LGE alone was the primary risk factor for events (arrhythmia/death). The authors suggest that future events may be driven by the presence of myocardial fibrosis instead of inflammation (146).

^{18}F-FDG PET in Cardiac Sarcoidosis

^{18}F-FDG PET has an important role as a diagnostic marker for cardiac involvement and is included in the Hearth Rhythm Society Guideline for diagnosis of cardiac sarcoidosis. "Patchy uptake on dedicated cardiac PET (in a pattern consistent with Cardiac Sarcoidosis)" in the right context can point towards the diagnosis (140).

Due to the high rate of glucose metabolism in the human heart, cardiac assessment on ^{18}F-FDG PET can be challenging. In a randomized trial of 82 patients, an 18-h fast with low carbohydrate diet preparation significantly reduced diffuse cardiac left ventricle uptake (147). A large meta-review including 559 patients revealed that the diagnostic sensitivity and specificity were significantly improved by increased fasting time and heparin administration before scanning ($P = 0.01, 0.02$) (148).

The added value of ^{18}F-FDG PET in combination with CMR in the diagnostic process was studied in a cohort of 107 patients suspected of cardiac sarcoidosis. Added value was found in 45% of patients, as they were reclassified as likely to have cardiac sarcoidosis, most of them (80%) being correctly reclassified when compared with the final diagnosis (149).

Combining cardiac ^{18}F-FDG PET with rubidium-82 to evaluate perfusion defects can increase the prognostic value. In a study including 118 consecutive cardiac sarcoidosis patients, the presence of both perfusion defects and increased FDG uptake identified patients at higher risk for VT or death HR 3.9 ($p < 0.01$) (150).

Newer PET/CMR scans are now available offering the possibility to perform cardiac ^{18}F-FDG PET and CMR together, depicting both the pattern of injury and disease activity in a single scan (151).

Furthermore, ^{18}F-FDG PET can be used to replace cardiac MRI in patients in whom the latter is contraindicated (e.g., devices, severe claustrophobia) (138).

Neuroimaging Biomarkers

Neurosarcoidosis (NS) refers to the involvement of the central nervous system (CNS) and is seen in approximately 5% of all sarcoidosis patients. It is a serious and devastating complication which is difficult to diagnose because of the many different ways in which this disease can present itself (152, 153).

Magnetic Resonance Imaging in Neurosarcoidosis

The Zajicek criteria are commonly used to define the diagnosis of NS. In the Zajicek critera the diagnosis of NS is considered definite if there is biopsy confirmation of neural tissue, probable if there is evidence of neurological inflammation together with biopsy proven systemic sarcoidosis and possible when the presentation is typical and other potential causes have been excluded (154). In addition to histopathological tissue confirmation, imaging is used for the diagnosis of NS. Positive gallium-67 scintigraphy, MRI, ^{18}F-FDG PET, and HRCT are used in different steps of the diagnostic process (155).

The gold standard to evaluate involvement of the CNS is the use of contrast enhanced MRI. The most common abnormalities seen in neurosarcoidosis patients at MRI are periventricular white matter lesions, meningitis or meningoencephalitis, solid parenchymal enhancing lesions, cranial neuritis, and hydrocephalus (156).

Unfortunately, NS is very hard to diagnose, especially in the absence of systemic sarcoidosis. In addition to a number of imaging methods the analysis of cerebrospinal fluid and blood are performed, despite the low sensitivity of these tests (157).

^{18}F-FDG PET in Neurosarcoidosis

As mentioned previously, MRI is the gold standard to evaluate CNS involvement in sarcoidosis. However, ^{18}F-FDG PET can occasionally be helpful in demonstrating neurologic involvement not visualized on MRI (158). Furthermore, PET can help in detecting systemic manifestations of sarcoidosis other than neurological involvement (159) or assess disease activity during treatment of NS (160).

FUTURE BIOMARKERS

JAK/STAT Signaling

The accumulation and activation of macrophages that form granulomas in sarcoidosis are driven by IFN-γ secretion. IFN-γ signaling is partly dependent on a specific signaling pathway named the Janus kinase/signaling transducer and activator of transcription (JAK/STAT) pathway (161). This pathway can activate a total of 6 STATs. Gene expression studies showed that the JAK/STAT signaling pathway is differentially expressed in most sarcoidosis patients, and that this pathway is more activated compared to healthy controls. Genes regulated by STAT1 in particular showed to be elevated in the blood of sarcoidosis patients (4, 162, 163). In addition to STAT1, STAT3 was also found to play a role in the granuloma formation. While STAT1 is primarily activated within granuloma macrophages, STAT3 is activated in between the granulomas in lymphocytes (162, 164).

Recently, various case reports have been published in which JAK/STAT inhibitors like tofacitinib and ruxolitinib were successfully used to treat patients with therapy-refractory sarcoidosis (165, 166).

It may be useful in the future to further unravel this pathway and focus on which specific patients may benefit from this therapy and whether JAK/STAT activation markers can act as biomarkers.

mTOR Signaling

The mechanistic target of rapamycin (mTOR) signaling pathway is involved in cellular metabolism as well as proliferation and has been implicated in an increasing number of pathological conditions (167).

It has been demonstrated in a mouse model that granuloma can be formed spontaneously when the mTORC1-inhibitor TSC2 is depleted. It was also found that sarcoid granulomas from patients with active and progressive disease showed active mTORC1 signaling (168). A decreased expression of TSC1 was observed in 33% of the sarcoidosis patients studied, leading to increased mTORC1 activation (168). Interestingly, whole exome sequencing (WES) suggested that the mTOR signaling pathway could be involved in the development of familial sarcoidosis (169). In terms of clinical relevance, successful treatment of a sarcoidosis patient with the mTOR inhibitor rapamycin has been reported (133). As with JAK/STAT inhibition, it may also be useful in the future to further unravel the mTORC1 pathway in sarcoidosis, to see whether markers of mTORC1 activation can be used as therapeutic biomarkers in sarcoidosis. A focus of interest could be whether absence of mTORC1 activation can predict treatment response with rapamycin. Rapamycin has been successfully used to treat a patient suffering from sarcoidosis (89).

Hair Cortisol

In sarcoidosis, 50–70% of the patients experience fatigue, some even experience chronic fatigue. Fatigue can still be present when sarcoidosis has clinically resolved, causing an impaired quality of life (170). One of the factors which is suspected to play a role in fatigue is stress. When the body is under psychological or physical stress, the hormone cortisol is released. Cortisol levels are commonly measured in serum, saliva, or urine, only acute changes are represented in this way. This could be overcome by measuring multiple samples during the day, but this would be labor-intensive and invasive, which in itself would increase cortisol release (171, 172). An emerging alternative technique is the analysis of scalp hair samples. Hair analysis has been done for decades, mostly to detect drugs of abuse. Hair samples are easy to collect in a non-invasive way and can be stored at room temperature.

The average scalp hair grows by 1 cm/month, so this method can retrospectively measure the production of these hormones over months (171, 172). The first study measuring cortisol levels of sarcoidosis patients in hair samples was performed by Van Manen et al. (171). This study showed that hair cortisol and cortisone levels were significantly higher in sarcoidosis patients compared to healthy controls, and that these increased levels related positively to the reported psychological distress, assessed by questionnaires. However, no differences in hair cortisol levels were found between sarcoidosis patients with and without fatigue.

Hair cortisol levels could be a future long-term biomarker for the measurement of chronic stress in sarcoidosis. A great advantage of this biomarker is that it is non-invasive and easily available, and can be used in a retrospective way. Using only one or a few hair strings, it may be possible to screen for fatigue and physical distress as well as to measure it in follow-up measurements. This can be used as an alternative to the currently used questionnaires, preventing variations in scores as to when patients fill in multiple questionnaires over time (171).

Labeled PET-Tracers

A PET-traceable biomarker specific for sarcoid granulomas would expand the possibilities to diagnose this disease as well as response to treatment (127). ^{18}F-FDG has been shown to be a useful PET-tracer in severe sarcoidosis. Other tracers, such as somatostatin receptors (SSTRs) like ^{68}Ga-DOTA-NaI-octreotide (DOTANOC) or ^{68}GA-DOTA-D-Phe-Tyr-octreotide (DOTATOC), would appear to be reliable alternatives to ^{18}F-FDG. Multiple inflammatory cells that are found in granulomas, including epithelioid cells and macrophages, have SSTRs on their surface, while normal monocytes have not. In the case of cardiac sarcoidosis, DOTANOC is taken up by sarcoid lesions but not by normal myocardium (173). More research is needed to determine the clinical value of these different PET tracers.

Although PET is a useful technique, it might not be able to function as a diagnostic biomarker of sarcoidosis on its own. Nevertheless, this technique provides evidence supporting or refuting the diagnosis and gives additional information about active disease in specific organs.

Another interesting application is specific labeling of the target drug used in sarcoidosis treatment with PET tracers. Radioactively labeling infliximab with technetium-99 m (99mTC) allows responders to infliximab therapy to be distinguished from non-responders. This imaging method is already being used in several TNF-α mediated diseases, such as RA, inflammatory bowel disease (IBD) and spondyloarthropathy (174). In sarcoidosis, Vis et al. (174) quantified serum TNF-α levels with ^{99m}TC-infliximab to evaluate disease activity and to identify responders, partial responders or non-responder priors to infliximab therapy. They showed that ^{99m}TC-infliximab accumulation was highest in patients with an indication for systemic treatment (174). ^{99m}TC-infliximab has not yet found its way into clinical practice for sarcoidosis.

OMICS

Sarcoidosis is a complex systemic disease reflecting immunological responses to different antigens in patients with certain genetic susceptibility (8, 175). Omics is an emerging field of research that encompasses genomics, epigenomics, transcriptomics, proteomics as well as metabolomics and is already widely used to understand polygenic and phenotypically diverse diseases and may also help identify more effective disease biomarkers in sarcoidosis (8, 175, 176).

In sarcoidosis, multiple diagnostic and prognostic biomarkers are already being identified by using single nucleotide polymorphism (SNP) technology, RNA sequencing and pathway analysis (175). Strong associations were found between sarcoidosis and various polymorphisms of the HLA allele and IL-1α. Various SNPs were also found to play a role in sarcoidosis pathogenesis, such as BTNL2, annexin A11, and NOTCH4, but the biological significance of several identified SNPs is unclear (noncoding) (175). A greater understanding of sarcoidosis may be obtained by moving beyond specific biomarkers to unbiased genome-wide analytic approaches. A study comparing lung tissue of sarcoidosis patients with that of healthy controls found that genes regulating macrophage-derived proteases and Th1 immune responses were differentially upregulated in sarcoidosis. Furthermore, IL23 and IL23R of the Th17 pathway and IL21 of STAT3 were also upregulated in sarcoidosis skin lesions compared to normal skin. Analyzing gene expression in peripheral blood proved to be a reliable surrogate for the use of tissue specimens, as it was able to reliably distinguish sarcoidosis patients from healthy controls, making this a useful approach to diagnosing and monitoring sarcoidosis (175). Based on current research, it is to be expected that the field of omics will further identify new promising biomarkers in sarcoidosis in the near future.

CONCLUSION

Although numerous biomarkers have been evaluated for patients with sarcoidosis in recent decades, no gold standard has been set for their use in diagnosis or predicting disease course. Combinations of several serum biomarkers have been explored, with promising results, but the Holy Grail remains to be discovered. Future research should focus on combining serum or BALF biomarkers and further refined imaging techniques such as CT, MRI, and PET. Data on successful treatment of sarcoidosis patients with JAK/STAT and mTORC1 inhibitors suggests that these new immunological pathways should also be explored for new prognostic biomarkers in the near future.

AUTHOR CONTRIBUTIONS

RK, MJ, and AV wrote the manuscript, contributed to the concept, and designing of the work. AV and MV revised the work critically for important intellectual content. RK and MJ set up the reference database. All authors contributed to the article and approved the submitted version.

REFERENCES

Statement on Sarcoidosis. Joint Statement of the American Thoracic Society (ATS), the European Respiratory Society (ERS) and the World Association of Sarcoidosis and Other Granulomatous Disorders (WASOG) Adopted by the ATS Board of Directors and by the ERS Executive Committee, February 1999. *Am J Respir Crit Care Med.* (1999) 160:736– 55. doi: 10.1164/ajrccm.160.2.ats4-99

Tarasidis A, Arce S. Immune response biomarkers as indicators of sarcoidosis presence, prognosis, and possible treatment: an Immunopathogenic perspective. *Autoimmun Rev.* (2020) 19:102462. doi: 10.1016/j.autrev.2020.102462

Broos CE, Koth LL, Van Nimwegen M, In'T Veen JCCM, Paulissen SMJ, Van Hamburg JP, et al. Increased T-helper 17.1 cells in sarcoidosis mediastinal lymph nodes. *Eur Respir J.* (2018) 51:1701124. doi: 10.1183/13993003.01124-2017

Zhou T, Casanova N, Pouladi N, Wang T, Lussier Y, Knox KS, et al. Identification of Jak-STAT signaling involvement in sarcoidosis severity via a novel microRNA-regulated peripheral blood mononuclear cell gene signature. *Sci Rep.* (2017) 7:4237. doi: 10.1038/s41598-017-04109-6

Reich JM. Mortality of intrathoracic sarcoidosis in referral vs population- based settings: Influence of stage, ethnicity, and corticosteroid therapy. *Chest.* (2002) 121:32–9. doi: 10.1378/chest.121.1.32

Prasse A. The diagnosis, differential diagnosis, and treatment of sarcoidosis. *Dtsch Aerzteblatt Online.* (2016) 113:565–73. doi: 10.3238/arztebl.2016.0565

Valeyre D, Prasse A, Nunes H, Uzunhan Y, Brillet PY, Müller-Quernheim J. Sarcoidosis. *Lancet.* (2014) 383:1155- 67. doi: 10.1016/S0140-6736(13)60680-7

Ramos-Casals M, Retamozo S, Sisó-Almirall A, Pérez-Alvarez R, Pallarés L, Brito-Zerón P. Clinically-useful serum biomarkers for diagnosis and prognosis of sarcoidosis. *Expert Rev Clin Immunol.* (2019) 15:391- 405. doi: 10.1080/1744666X.2019.1568240

Atkinson AJ, Colburn WA, DeGruttola VG, DeMets DL, Downing GJ, Hoth DF, et al. Biomarkers and surrogate endpoints: preferred definitions and conceptual framework. *Clin Pharmacol Ther.* (2001) 68:89- 95. doi: 10.1067/mcp.2001.113989

Chopra A, Kalkanis A, Judson MA. Biomarkers in sarcoidosis. *Expert Rev Clin Immunol.* (2016) 12:1191–208. doi: 10.1080/1744666X.2016.11 96135

Schimmelpennink MC, Vorselaars ADM, Grutters JC. Biomarkers in sarcoidosis. In: Baughman RP, editor. *Sarcoidosis A Clinician's Guide.* Elsevier - Health Sciences Division. (2019). pp. 219–238.

Zissel G, Müller-Quernheim J. Cellular players in the immunopathogenesis of sarcoidosis. *Clin Chest Med.* (2015) 36:549–60. doi: 10.1016/j.ccm.2015.08.016

Kahkouee S, Samadi K, Alai A, Abedini A, Rezaiian L. Serum ACE level in sarcoidosis patients with typical and atypical HRCT manifestation. *Polish J Radiol.* (2016) 81:458–61. doi: 10.12659/PJR.897708

Lieberman J. Elevation of serum angiotension-converting- enzyme (ACE) level in sarcoidosis. *Am J Med.* (1975) 59:356- 72. doi: 10.1016/0002-9343(75)90395-2

Brice EAW, Friedlander W, Bateman ED, Kirsch RE. Serum angiotensin- converting enzyme activity, concentration, and specific activity in granulomatous interstitial lung disease, tuberculosis, and COPD. *Chest.* (1995) 107:706–10. doi: 10.1378/chest.107.3.706

Maier LA, Raynolds MV, Young DA, Barker EA, Newman LS. Angiotensin-1 converting enzyme polymorphisms in chronic beryllium disease. *Am J Respir Crit Care Med.* (1999) 159:1342–50. doi: 10.1164/ajrccm.159.4.9806106

Studdy P, Bird, James DG, Sherlock S. Serum angiotensin-converting enzyme (SACE) in sarcoidosis and other granulomatous disorders. *Trans Med Soc Lond.* (1978) 95:54–9.

Ryder KW, Jay SJ, Kiblawi SO, Hull MT. Serum Angiotensin Converting Enzyme Activity in Patients With Histoplasmosis. *JAMA J Am Med Assoc.* (1983) 249:1888–9. doi: 10.1001/jama.249.14.1888

Kruit A, Grutters JC, Gerritsen WBM, Kos S, Wodzig WKWH, van den Bosch JMM, et al. ACE I/D-corrected Z-scores to identify normal and elevated ACE activity in sarcoidosis. *Respir Med.* (2007) 101:510– 5. doi: 10.1016/j.rmed.2006.06.025

Lopes MC, Amadeu TP, Ribeiro-Alves M, da Costa CH, Rodrigues LS, Bessa EJC, et al. Identification of active sarcoidosis using chitotriosidase and angiotensin-converting enzyme. *Lung.* (2019) 197:295–302. doi: 10.1007/s00408-019-00219-2

Vorselaars ADM, van Moorsel CHM, Zanen P, Ruven HJT, Claessen AME, van Velzen-Blad H, et al. ACE and sIL-2R correlate with lung function improvement in sarcoidosis during methotrexate therapy. *Respir Med.* (2015) 109:279–85. doi: 10.1016/j.rmed.2014.11.009

Kandolin R, Lehtonen J, Airaksinen J, Vihinen T, Miettinen H, Ylitalo K, et al. Cardiac sarcoidosis: Epidemiology, characteristics, and outcome over 25 years in a nationwide study. *Circulation.* (2015) 131:624– 32. doi: 10.1161/CIRCULATIONAHA.114.011522

Krasowski MD, Savage J, Ehlers A, Maakestad J, Schmidt GA, La'Ulu SL, et al. Ordering of the serum angiotensin-converting enzyme test in patients receiving angiotensin-converting enzyme inhibitor th erapy an avoidable but common error. *Chest.* (2015) 148:1447–53. doi: 10.1378/chest. 15-1061

Majcherczyk PA, Langen H, Heumann D, Fountoulakis M, Glauser MP, Moreillon P. Digestion of Streptococcus pneumoniae cell walls with its major peptidoglycan hydrolase releases branched stem peptides carrying proinflammatory activity. *J Biol Chem.* (1999) 274:12537– 43. doi: 10.1074/jbc.274.18.12537

Bergantini L, Bianchi F, Cameli P, Mazzei MA, Fui A, Sestini P, et al. Prognostic biomarkers of sarcoidosis: a comparative study of serum chitotriosidase, ACE, lysozyme, and KL-6. *Dis Markers.* (2019) 2019:1– 7. doi: 10.1155/2019/8565423

Tomita H, Sato S, Matsuda R, Sugiura Y, Kawaguchi H, Niimi T, et al. Serum lysozyme levels and clinical features of sarcoidosis. *Lung.* (1999) 177:161–7. doi: 10.1007/PL00007637

Hoffmann G, Wirleitner B, Fuchs D. Potential role of immune system activation-associated production of neopterin derivatives in humans. *Inflamm Res.* (2003) 52:313–21. doi: 10.1007/s00011-003-1181-9

Gelisgen R, Seyhan E, Simsek G, Durmus S, Uysal P, Sozer V, et al. YKL- 40, soluble IL-2 receptor, angiotensin converting enzyme and C-reactive protein: comparison of markers of sarcoidosis activity. *Biomolecules.* (2018) 8:84. doi: 10.3390/biom8030084

Ziegenhagen MW, Rothe ME, Schlaak M, Müller-Quernheim J. Bronchoalveolar and serological parameters reflecting the severity of sarcoidosis. *Eur Respir J.* (2003) 21:407– 413. doi: 10.1183/09031936.03.00010403

Hoffmann G, Rieder J, Smolny M, Seibel M, Wirleitner B, Fuchs D, et al. Neopterin-induced expression of intercellular adhesion molecule-1 (ICAM-in type II-like alveolar epithelial cells. *Clin Exp Immunol.* (1999) 118:434– 40. doi: 10.1046/j.1365-2249.1999.01071.x

Korthagen NM, van Moorsel CHM, Zanen P, Ruven HJ, Grutters JC. Evaluation of circulating YKL-40 levels in idiopathic interstitial pneumonias. *Lung.* (2014) 192:975–80. doi: 10.1007/s00408-014-9647-9

Kruit A, Grutters JC, Ruven HJT, van Moorsel CCM, van den Bosch JMM. A CHI3L1 gene polymorphism is associated with serum levels of YKL-40, a novel sarcoidosis marker. *Respir Med.* (2007) 101:1563– 71. doi: 10.1016/j.rmed.2006.12.006

Johansen JS, Milman N, Hansen M, Garbarsch C, Price PA, Graudal N. Increased serum YKL-40 in patients with pulmonary sarcoidosis - a potential marker of disease activity? *Respir Med.* (2005) 99:396– 402. doi: 10.1016/j.rmed.2004.09.016

Weaver LK, Pioli PA, Wardwell K, Vogel SN, Guyre PM. Up-regulation of human monocyte CD163 upon activation of cell-surface Toll-like receptors. *J Leukoc Biol.* (2007) 81:663–71. doi: 10.1189/jlb.0706428

Møller HJ. Soluble CD163. *Scand J Clin Lab Invest.* (2012) 72:1– 3. doi: 10.3109/00365513.2011.626868

Tanimura H, Mizuno K, Okamoto H. Serum levels of soluble CD163 as a useful marker of macrophage/monocyte activity in sarcoidosis patients. *Sarcoidosis Vasc Diffus Lung Dis.* (2015) 32:99–105. Available online at: https://mattioli1885journals.com/index.php/sarcoidosis/article/view/3544

Etzerodt A, Moestrup SK. CD163 and inflammation: biological, diagnostic, and therapeutic aspects. *Antioxidants Redox Signal.* (2013) 18:2352– 63. doi: 10.1089/ars.2012.4834

Boot RG, Hollak CEM, Verhoek M, Alberts C, Jonkers RE, Aerts JM. Plasma chitotriosidase and CCL18 as surrogate markers for granulomatous macrophages in sarcoidosis. *Clin Chim Acta.* (2010) 411:31–6. doi: 10.1016/j.cca.2009.09.034

Sixt SU, Guzman J, Cai M, Costabel U, Sarria R, Bonella F, et al. CCL18 in serum, BAL fluid and alveolar macrophage culture supernatant in interstitial lung diseases. *Respir Med.* (2013) 107:1444–52. doi: 10.1016/j.rmed.2013.06.004

Prasse A, Pechkovsky D V., Toews GB, Jungraithmayr W, Kollert F, Goldmann T, et al. A vicious circle of alveolar macrophages and fibroblasts perpetuates pulmonary fibrosis via CCL18. *Am J Respir Crit Care Med.* (2006) 173:781–92. doi: 10.1164/rccm.200509-1518OC

Eklund KK, Niemi K, Kovanen PT. Immune functions of serum amyloid A. *Crit Rev Immunol.* (2012) 32:335–48. doi: 10.1615/CritRevImmunol.v32.i4.40

Bargagli E, Magi B, Olivieri C, Bianchi N, Landi C, Rottoli P. Analysis of serum amyloid A in sarcoidosis patients. *Respir Med.* (2011) 105:775– 80. doi: 10.1016/j.rmed.2010.12.010

Beijer E, Veltkamp M, Meek B, Moller DR. Etiology and immunopathogenesis of sarcoidosis: novel insights. *Semin Respir Crit Care Med.* (2017) 38:404–16. doi: 10.1055/s-0037-1603087

Jiang TT, Shi LY, Wei LL, Li X, Yang S, Wang C, et al. Serum amyloid A, protein Z, and C4b-binding protein β chain as new potential biomarkers for pulmonary tuberculosis. *PLoS One.* (2017) 12:e0173304. doi: 10.1371/journal.pone.0173304

Popevic´ S, Šumarac Z, Jovanovic´ D, Babic´ D, Stjepanovic´ M, Jovic˘ic´ S, Šobic´-Šaranovic´ D, Filipovic´ S, et al. Verifying sarcoidosis activity: chitotriosidase versus ACE in sarcoidosis - a case-control study. *J Med Biochem.* (2016) 35:390–400. doi: 10.1515/jomb-2016-0017

Bargagli E, Bennett D, Maggiorelli C, Di Sipio P, Margollicci M, Bianchi N, et al. Human chitotriosidase: a sensitive biomarker of sarcoidosis. *J Clin Immunol.* (2013) 33:264–70. doi: 10.1007/s10875-012-9754-4

Okamoto H, Mizuno K, Horio T. Circulating $CD14^+$ $CD16^+$ monocytes are expanded in sarcoidosis patients. *J Dermatol.* (2003) 30:503–9. doi: 10.1111/j.1346-8138.2003.tb00424.x

Hijdra D, Vorselaars ADM, Crommelin HA, van Moorsel CHM, Meek B, Claessen AME, et al. Can intermediate monocytes predict response to infliximab therapy in sarcoidosis? *Eur Respir J.* (2016) 48:1242– 5. doi: 10.1183/13993003.00709-2016

Fingerle-Rowson G, Angstwurm M, Andreesen R, Ziegler-Heitbrock HWL. Selective depletion of $CD14^+$ $CD16^+$ monocytes by glucocorticoid therapy. *Clin Exp Immunol.* (1998) 112:501–6. doi: 10.1046/j.1365-2249.1998.00617.x

Heron M, Grutters JC, Van Velzen-Blad H, Veltkamp M, Claessen AME, Van Den Bosch JMM. Increased expression of CD16, CD69, and very late antigen-1 on blood monocytes in active sarcoidosis. *Chest.* (2008) 134:1001– 8. doi: 10.1378/chest.08-0443

Davis BH, Zarev PV. Human monocyte CD163 expression inversely correlates with soluble CD163 plasma levels. *Cytom Part B Clin Cytom.* (2005) 63:16–22. doi: 10.1002/cyto.b.20031

Berg KE, Ljungcrantz I, Andersson L, Bryngelsson C, Hedblad B, Fredrikson GN, et al. Elevated $CD14^{++}$ CD16-monocytes predict cardiovascular events. *Circ Cardiovasc Genet.* (2012) 5:121–32. doi: 10.1161/CIRCGENETICS.111.960385

Hou J, Zhang M, Ding Y, Wang X, Li T, Gao P, et al. Circulating $CD14^+$ $CD163^+$ $CD206^+$ M2 monocytes are increased in patients with early stage of idiopathic membranous nephropathy. *Mediators Inflamm.* (2018) 2018:1–10. doi: 10.1155/2018/5270657

Iannuzzi MC, Fontana JR. Sarcoidosis: clinical presentation, immunopathogenesis, and therapeutics. *JAMA.* (2011) 167:1225–31. doi: 10.1001/jama.2011.10

Rubin LA, Nelson DL. The soluble interleukin-2 receptor: biology, function, and clinical application. *Ann Intern Med.* (1990) 113:619. doi: 10.7326/0003-4819-113-8-619

Sakthivel P, Bruder D. Mechanism of granuloma formation in sarcoidosis. *Curr Opin Hematol.* (2017) 24:59–5. doi: 10.1097/MOH.0000000000000301

Hunninghake GW, Bedell GN, Zavala DC, Monick M, Brady M. Role of interleukin-2 release by lung T-cells in active pulmonary sarcoidosis. *Am Rev Respir Dis.* (1983) 218:634–8.

Eurelings LEM, Miedema JR, Dalm VASH, Van Daele PLA, Van Hagen PM, Van Laar JAM, et al. Sensitivity and specificity of serum soluble interleukin-2 receptor for diagnosing sarcoidosis in a population of patients suspected of sarcoidosis. *PLoS One.* (2019) 14:e0223897. doi: 10.1371/journal.pone.0223897

Vorselaars ADM, Verwoerd A, Van Moorsel CHM, Keijsers RGM, Rijkers GT, Grutters JC. Prediction of relapse after discontinuation of infliximab therapy in severe sarcoidosis. *Eur Respir J.* (2014) 43:602– 9. doi: 10.1183/09031936.00055213

Ogata-Suetsugu S, Hamada N, Takayama K, Tsubouchi K, Arimura-Omori M, Nakanishi Y. The clinical value of serum soluble interleukin-2 receptor in pulmonary sarcoidosis. *Sarcoidosis Vasc Diffus Lung Dis.* (2017) 34:41– 7. doi: 10.36141/svdld.v34i1.5045

Grutters JC, Fellrath JM, Mulder L, Janssen R, Van Den Bosch JMM, Van Velzen-Blad H. Serum soluble interleukin-2 receptor measurement in patients with sarcoidosis: a clinical evaluation. *Chest.* (2003) 124:186– 95. doi: 10.1378/chest.124.1.186

Kudryavtsev I, Serebriakova M, Starshinova A, Zinchenko Y, Basantsova N, Malkova A, et al. Imbalance in B cell and T follicular helper cell subsets in pulmonary sarcoidosis. *Sci Rep.* (2020) 10:1059. doi: 10.1038/s41598-020-57741-0

Cinetto F, Compagno N, Scarpa R, Malipiero G, Agostini C. Rituximab in refractory sarcoidosis: a single centre experience. *Clin Mol Allergy.* (2015) 13:19. doi: 10.1186/s12948-015-0025-9

Ando M, Goto A, Takeno Y, Yamasue M, Komiya K, Umeki K, et al. Significant elevation of the levels of B-cell activating factor (BAFF) in patients with sarcoidosis. *Clin Rheumatol.* (2018) 37:2833– 8. doi: 10.1007/s10067-018-4183-2

Saussine A, Tazi A, Feuillet S, Rybojad M, Juillard C, Bergeron A, et al. Active chronic sarcoidosis is characterized by increased transitional blood B cells, increased IL-10-producing regulatory B cells and high BAFF levels. *PLoS One.* (2012) 7:e43588. doi: 10.1371/journal.pone.00 43588

Ueda-Hayakawa I, Tanimura H, Osawa M, Iwasaka H, Ohe S, Yamazaki F, et al. Elevated serum BAFF levels in patients with sarcoidosis: association with disease activity. *Rheumatology.* (2013) 52:1658–66. doi: 10.1093/rheumatology/ket186

Becker-Merok A, Nikolaisen C, Nossent HC. B-lymphocyte activating factor in systemic lupus erythematosus and rheumatoid arthritis in relation to autoantibody levels, disease measures and time. *Lupus.* (2006) 15:570– 6. doi: 10.1177/0961203306071871

Belkhou A, Younsi R, El Bouchti I, El Hassani S. Rituximab as a treatment alternative in sarcoidosis. *Jt Bone Spine.* (2008) 75:511– 2. doi: 10.1016/j.jbspin.2008.01.025

Lee NS, Barber L, Akula SM, Sigounas G, Kataria YP, Arce S. Disturbed homeostasis and multiple signaling defects in the peripheral blood B- cell compartment of patients with severe chronic sarcoidosis. *Clin Vaccine Immunol.* (2011) 18:1306–11. doi: 10.1128/CVI.05118-11

Kamphuis LS, Van Zelm MC, Lam KH, Rimmelzwaan GF, Baarsma GS, Dik WA, et al. Perigranuloma localization and abnormal maturation of B cells emerging key players in sarcoidosis? *Am J Respir Crit Care Med.* (2013) 187:406–16. doi: 10.1164/rccm.201206-1024OC

Doi TS, Takahashi T, Taguchi O, Azuma T, Obata Y. NF-κB RelA- deficient lymphocytes: Normal development of T cells and B cells, impaired production of IgA and IgG1 and reduced proliferative responses. *J Exp Med.* (1997) 185:953–61. doi: 10.1084/jem.185.5.953

Fillatreau S, Sweenie CH, McGeachy MJ, Gray D, Anderton SM. B cells regulate autoimmunity by provision of IL-10. *Nat Immunol.* (2002) 3:944– 50. doi: 10.1038/ni833

Thi Hong Nguyen C, Kambe N, Kishimoto I, Ueda-Hayakawa I, Okamoto H. Serum soluble interleukin-2 receptor level is more sensitive than angiotensin-converting enzyme or lysozyme for diagnosis of sarcoidosis and may be a marker of multiple organ involvement. *J Dermatol.* (2017) 44:789–97. doi: 10.1111/1346-8138.13792

Enyedi A, Csongrádi A, Altorjay IT, Beke GL, Váradi C, Enyedi EE, et al. Combined application of angiotensin converting enzyme and chitotriosidase analysis improves the laboratory diagnosis of sarcoidosis. *Clin Chim Acta.* (2020) 500:155–62. doi: 10.1016/j.cca.2019.10.010

Bargagli E, Bianchi N, Margollicci M, Olivieri C, Luddi A, Coviello G, et al. Chitotriosidase and soluble IL-2 receptor: comparison of two markers of sarcoidosis severity. *Scand J Clin Lab Invest.* (2008) 68:479– 83. doi: 10.1080/00365510701854975

Miyoshi S, Hamada H, Kadowaki T, Hamaguchi N, Ito R, Irifune K, et al. Comparative evaluation of serum markers in pulmonary sarcoidosis. *Chest.* (2010) 137:1391–7. doi: 10.1378/chest.09-1975

Hamsten C, Wiklundh E, Grönlund H, Schwenk JM, Uhlén M, Eklund A, et al. Elevated levels of FN1 and CCL2 in bronchoalveolar lavage fluid from sarcoidosis patients. *Respir Res.* (2016) 17:69. doi: 10.1186/s12931-016-0381-0

Tanriverdi H, Erboy F, Altinsoy B, Uygur F, Arasli M, Ozel Tekin I, et al. Bronchoalveolar lavage fluid characteristics of patients with sarcoidosis and nonsarcoidosis interstitial lung diseases: ten-year experience of a single center in turkey. *Iran Red Crescent Med J.* (2015) 17:e31103. doi: 10.5812/ircmj.31103

Hyldgaard C, Kaae S, Riddervold M, Hoffmann HJ, Hilberg O. Value of s-ACE, BAL lymphocytosis, and $CD4^{+}/CD8^{+}$ and $CD103^{+}$ $CD4^{+}/CD4^{+}$ T-cell ratios in diagnosis of sarcoidosis. *Eur Respir J.* (2012) 39:1037– 1039. doi: 10.1183/09031936.00144311

Costabel U. CD4/CD8 ratios in bronchoalveolar lavage fluid: of value for diagnosing sarcoidosis? *Eur Respir J.* (1997) 10:2699–700. doi: 10.1183/09031936.97.10122699

Kantrow SP, Meyer KC, Kidd P, Raghu G. The CD4/CD8 ratio in BAL fluid is highly variable in sarcoidosis. *Eur Respir J.* (1997) 10:2716– 21. doi: 10.1183/09031936.97.10122716

Darlington P, Kullberg S, Eklund A, Grunewald J. Lung $CD4^{+}$ $V\alpha2.3^{+}$ T-cells in sarcoidosis cohorts with Löfgren's syndrome. *Respir Res.* (2020) 21:61. doi: 10.1186/s12931-020-1327-0

Kolopp-Sarda MN, Kohler C, De March AK, Béné MC, Faure G. Discriminative immunophenotype of bronchoalveolar lavage CD4 lymphocytes in sarcoidosis. *Lab Investig.* (2000) 80:1065–9. doi: 10.1038/labinvest.3780111

Heron M, Slieker WAT, Zanen P, van Lochem EG, Hooijkaas H, van den Bosch JMM, et al. Evaluation of CD103 as a cellular marker for the diagnosis of pulmonary sarcoidosis. *Clin Immunol.* (2008) 126:338– 44. doi: 10.1016/j.clim.2007.11.005

Bretagne L, Diatta ID, Faouzi M, Nobile A, Bongiovanni M, Nicod LP, et al. Diagnostic value of the $CD103^{+}$ $CD4^{+}/CD4^{+}$ ratio to differentiate sarcoidosis from other causes of lymphocytic alveolitis. *Respiration.* (2016) 91:486–96. doi: 10.1159/000446606

Facco M, Cabrelle A, Teramo A, Olivieri V, Gnoato M, Teolato S, et al. Sarcoidosis is a Th1/Th17 multisystem disorder. *Thorax.* (2011) 66:144– 50. doi: 10.1136/thx.2010.140319

Broos CE, Hendriks RW, Kool M. T-cell immunology in sarcoidosis: Disruption of a delicate balance between helper and regulatory T-cells. *Curr Opin Pulm Med.* (2016) 22:476–83. doi: 10.1097/MCP.0000000000000303

Ramstein J, Broos CE, Simpson LJ, Mark Ansel K, Sun SA, Ho ME, et al. IFN-γproducing t-helper 17.1 cells are increased in sarcoidosis and are more prevalent than t-helper type 1 cells. *Am J Respir Crit Care Med.* (2016) 193:1281–91. doi: 10.1164/rccm.201507-1499OC

Bennett D, Bargagli E, Refini RM, Rottoli P. New concepts in the pathogenesis of sarcoidosis. *Expert Rev Respir Med.* (2019) 13:981– 91. doi: 10.1080/17476348.2019.1655401

Zhang B, Dai Q, Jin X, Liang D, Li X, Lu H, et al. Phosphoinositide 3-kinase/protein kinase B inhibition restores regulatory T cell's function in pulmonary sarcoidosis. *J Cell Physiol.* (2019) 234:19911–20. doi: 10.1002/jcp.28589

Kachamakova-Trojanowska N, Jazwa-Kusior A, Szade K, Kasper L, Soja J, Andrychiewicz A, et al. Molecular profiling of regulatory T cells in pulmonary sarcoidosis. *J Autoimmun.* (2018) 94:56–69. doi: 10.1016/j.jaut.2018.07.012

Wikén M, Grunewald J, Eklund A, Wahlström J. Higher monocyte expression of TLR2 and TLR4, and enhanced pro-inflammatory synergy of TLR2 with NOD2 stimulation in sarcoidosis. *J Clin Immunol.* (2009) 29:78–89. doi: 10.1007/s10875-008-9225-0

Prasse A, Zissel G, Lützen N, Schupp J, Schmiedlin R, Gonzalez-Rey E, et al. Inhaled vasoactive intestinal peptide exerts immunoregulatory effects in sarcoidosis. *Am J Respir Crit Care Med.* (2010) 182:540– 8. doi: 10.1164/rccm.200909-1451OC

Patterson KC, Chen ES. The pathogenesis of pulmonary sarcoidosis and implications for treatment. *Chest.* (2018) 153:1432–42. doi: 10.1016/j.chest.2017.11.030

Tutor-Ureta P, Citores MJ, Castejón R, Mellor-Pita S, Yebra-Bango M, Romero Y, et al. Prognostic value of neutrophils and NK cells in bronchoalveolar lavage of sarcoidosis. *Cytom Part B Clin Cytom.* (2006) 70:416–22. doi: 10.1002/cyto.b.20120

Bergantini L, Cameli P, d'Alessandro M, Vagaggini C, Refini R, Landi C, et al. NK and NKT-like cells in granulomatous and fibrotic lung diseases. *Clin Exp Med.* (2019) 19:487–94. doi: 10.1007/s10238-019-00578-3

Berzins SP, Ritchie DS. Natural killer T cells: Drivers or passengers in preventing human disease? *Nat Rev Immunol.* (2014) 14:640–6. doi: 10.1038/nri3725

Morgenthau AS, Iannuzzi MC. Recent advances in sarcoidosis. *Chest.* (2011) 139:174–82. doi: 10.1378/chest.10-0188

Kobayashi S, Kaneko Y, Seino KI, Yamada Y, Motohashi S, Koike J, et al. Impaired IFN-γ production of Vα24 NKT cells in non-remitting sarcoidosis. *Int Immunol.* (2004) 16:215–22. doi: 10.1093/intimm/dxh020

Korosec P, Rijavec M, Silar M, Kern I, Kosnik M, Osolnik K. Deficiency of pulmonary Vα24 Vβ11 natural killer T cells in corticosteroid-naïve sarcoidosis patients. *Respir Med.* (2010) 104:571–7. doi: 10.1016/j.rmed.2009.11.008

Ho L-P, Urban BC, Thickett DR, Davies RJ, McMichael AJ. Deficiency of a subset of T-cells with immunoregulatory properties in sarcoidosis. *Lancet.* (2005) 365:1062–72. doi: 10.1016/S0140-6736(05)71143-0

Busuttil A, Weigt SS, Keane MP, Xue YY, Palchevskiy V, Burdick MD, et al. CXCR3 ligands are augmented during the pathogenesis of pulmonary sarcoidosis. *Eur Respir J.* (2009) 34:676–86. doi: 10.1183/09031936.001 57508

Arger NK, Ho ME, Allen IE, Benn BS, Woodruff PG, Koth LL. CXCL9 and CXCL10 are differentially associated with systemic organ involvement and pulmonary disease severity in sarcoidosis. *Respir Med.* (2020) 161:105822. doi: 10.1016/j.rmed.2019.105822

Arger NK, Ho M, Woodruff PG, Koth LL. Serum CXCL11 correlates with pulmonary outcomes and disease burden in sarcoidosis. *Respir Med.* (2019) 152:89–96. doi: 10.1016/j.rmed.2019.04.005

Lee K, Chung W, Jung Y, Kim Y, Park J, Sheen S, et al. CXCR3 ligands as clinical markers for pulmonary tuberculosis. *Int J Tuberc Lung Dis.* (2015) 19:191–9. doi: 10.5588/ijtld.14.0525

Chung W, Lee K, Jung Y, Kim Y, Park J, Sheen S, et al. Serum CXCR3 ligands as biomarkers for the diagnosis and treatment monitoring of tuberculosis. *Int J Tuberc Lung Dis.* (2015) 19:1476–84. doi: 10.5588/ijtld. 15.0325

Kohno N, Kyoizumi S, Awaya Y, Fukuhara H, Yamakido M, Akiyama M. New serum indicator of interstitial pneumonitis activity. Sialylated carbohydrate antigen KL-6. *Chest.* (1989) 96:68–73. doi: 10.1378/chest.96.1.68

Menon B, Tiwari M, Gopi A, Raj P, Panwar K. Serum krebs von den lungen- 6 (KL-6): a promising biomarker in sarcoidosis. *MOJ Curr Res Rev.* (2018) 1:45–7. doi: 10.15406/mojcrr.2018.01.00009

Kohno N, Awaya Y, Oyama T, Yamakido M, Akiyama M, Inoue Y, et al. KL-6, a mucin-like glycoprotein, in bronchoalveolar lavage fluid from patients with interstitial lung disease. *Am Rev Respir Dis.* (1993) 148:637– 42. doi: 10.1164/ajrccm/148.3.637

Kunitake R, Kuwano K, Yoshida K, Maeyama T, Kawasaki M, Hagimoto N, et al. KL-6, surfactant protein A and D in bronchoalveolar lavage fluid from patients with pulmonary sarcoidosis. *Respiration.* (2001) 68:488– 95. doi: 10.1159/000050556

Janssen R, Sato H, Grutters JC, Bernard A, Van Velzen-Blad H, Du Bois RM, et al. Study of clara cell 16, KL-6, and surfactant protein-D in serum as disease markers in pulmonary sarcoidosis. *Chest.* (2003) 124:2119– 25. doi: 10.1378/chest.124.6.2119

D'Alessandro M, Carleo A, Cameli P, Bergantini L, Perrone A, Vietri L, et al. BAL biomarkers' panel for differential diagnosis of interstitial lung diseases. *Clin Exp Med.* (2020) 20:207–16. doi: 10.1007/s10238-020-00608-5

Keijsers RG, Veltkamp M, Grutters JC. Chest imaging. *Clin Chest Med.* (2015) 36:603–19. doi: 10.1016/j.ccm.2015.08.004

Baughman RP, Teirstein AS, Judson MA, Rossman MD, Yeager H, Bresnitz EA, et al. Clinical characteristics of patients in a case control study of sarcoidosis. *Am J Respir Crit Care Med.* (2001) 164:1885– 9. doi: 10.1164/ajrccm.164.10.2104046

Scadding JG. Prognosis of intrathoracic sarcoidosis in England. A review of 136 cases after five years' observation. *Br Med J.* (1961) 2:1165– 72. doi: 10.1136/bmj.2.5261.1165

Silva M, Nunes H, Valeyre D, Sverzellati N. Imaging of sarcoidosis. *Clin Rev Allergy Immunol.* (2015) 49:45–53. doi: 10.1007/s12016-015-8478-7

Kirkil G, Lower EE, Baughman RP. Predictors of mortality in pulmonary sarcoidosis. *Chest.* (2018) 153:105–13. doi: 10.1016/j.chest.2017.07.008

Baughman RP, Shipley R, Desai S, Drent M, Judson MA, Costabel U, et al. Changes in chest roentgenogram of sarcoidosis patients during a clinical trial of infliximab therapy: comparison of different methods of evaluation. *Chest.* (2009) 136:526–35. doi: 10.1378/chest.08-1876

Judson MA, Gilbert GE, Rodgers JK, Greer CF, Schabel SI. The utility of the chest radiograph in diagnosing exacerbations of pulmonary sarcoidosis. *Respirology.* (2008) 13:97–102. doi: 10.1111/j.1440-1843.2007.01206.x

Oberstein A, Von Zitzewitz H, Schweden F, Müller-Quernheim J. Non invasive evaluation of the inflammatory activity in sarcoidosis with high-resolution computed tomography. *Sarcoidosis Vasc Diffus Lung Dis.* (1997) 14:65-72

Drent M, De Vries J, Lenters M, Lamers RJS, Rothkranz-Kos S, Wouters EFM, et al. Sarcoidosis: assessment of disease severity using HRCT. *Eur Radiol.* (2003) 13:2462–71. doi: 10.1007/s00330-003-1965-x

Mostard RLM, Kuijk SMJV, Verschakelen JA, van Kroonenburgh MJPG, Nelemans PJ, Wijnen PAHM, et al. A predictive tool for an effective use of 18F-FDG PET in assessing activity of sarcoidosis. *BMC Pulm Med.* (2012) 12:57. doi: 10.1186/1471-2466-12-57

Benamore R, Kendrick YR, Repapi E, Helm E, Cole SL, Taylor S, et al. CTAS: A CT score to quantify disease activity in pulmonary sarcoidosis. *Thorax.* (2016) 71:1161–3. doi: 10.1136/thoraxjnl-2016-208833

Duan J, Xu Y, Zhu H, Zhang H, Sun S, Sun H, et al. Relationship between CT activity score with lung function and the serum angiotensin converting enzyme in pulmonary sarcoidosis on chest HRCT. *Medicine (Baltimore).* (2018) 97:15–9. doi: 10.1097/MD.00000000000 12205

Adams H, Keijsers RG, Korenromp IHE, Grutters JC. FDG PET for gauging of sarcoid disease activity. *Semin Respir Crit Care Med.* (2014) 35:352– 61. doi: 10.1055/s-0034-1376866

Nishiyama Y, Yamamoto Y, Fukunaga K, Takinami H, Iwado Y, Satoh K, et al. Comparative evaluation of ^{18} F-FDG PET and ^{67} Ga scintigraphy in patients with sarcoidosis. *J Nucl Med.* (2006) 47:1571–6. Available online at: http:// jnm. snmjournals.org/content/47/10/1571

Treglia G, Taralli S, Giordano A. Emerging role of whole-body 18F-fluorodeoxyglucose positron emission tomography as a marker of disease activity in patients with sarcoidosis: A systematic review. *Sarcoidosis Vasc Diffus Lung Dis.* (2011) 28:87–94 doi: 10.4081/itjm.2012.21

Keijsers RG, Verzijlbergen FJ, Oyen WJ, Van Den Bosch JM, Ruven HJ, Van Velzen-Blad H, et al. 18F-FDG PET, genotype-corrected ACE and sIL- 2R in newly diagnosed sarcoidosis. *Eur J Nucl Med Mol Imaging.* (2009) 36:1131–7. doi: 10.1007/s00259-009-1097-x

Chen H, Jin R, Wang Y, Li L, Li K, He Y. The utility of 18F-FDG PET/CT for monitoring response and predicting prognosis after glucocorticoids therapy for sarcoidosis. *Biomed Res Int.* (2018) 2018:6. doi: 10.1155/2018/1823710

Cremers JP, Van Kroonenburgh MJ, Mostard RLM, Vöö SA, Wijnen PA, Koek GH, et al. Extent of disease activity assessed by ^{18} F-FDG PET/CT in a Dutch sarcoidosis population. *Sarcoidosis Vasc Diffus Lung Dis.* (2014) 31:37–45. Available online at: https://mattioli1885journals.com/ index.php/sarcoidosis/article/view/2948

Teirstein AS, Machac J, Almeida O, Lu P, Padilla ML, Iannuzzi MC. Results of 188 whole-body fluorodeoxyglucose positron emission tomography scans in 137 patients with sarcoidosis. *Chest.* (2007) 132:1949– 53. doi: 10.1378/chest.07-1178

Mostard RLM, Vöö S, Van Kroonenburgh MJPG, Verschakelen JA, Wijnen PAHM, Nelemans PJ, et al. Inflammatory activity assessment by F18 FDG-PET/CT in persistent symptomatic sarcoidosis. *Respir Med.* (2011) 105:1917–24. doi: 10.1016/j.rmed.2011.08.012

Keijsers RG, Verzijlbergen FJ, Van Den Bosch JM, Zanen P, Van De Garde EM, Oyen WJ, et al. 18F-FDG PET as a predictor of pulmonary function in sarcoidosis. *Sarcoidosis Vasc Diffus Lung Dis.* (2011) 28:123–9. Available online at: https://mattioli1885journals.com/index.php/sarcoidosis/ article/view/2542

Vorselaars ADM, Crommelin HA, Deneer VHM, Meek B, Claessen AME, Keijsers RGM, et al. Effectiveness of infliximab in refractory FDG PET-positive sarcoidosis. *Eur Respir J.* (2015) 46:175–85. doi: 10.1183/09031936.00227014

Sobic-Saranovic D, Grozdic I, Videnovic-Ivanov J, Vucinic-Mihailovic V, Artiko V, Saranovic D, et al. The utility of 18F-FDG PET/CT for diagnosis and adjustment of therapy in patients with active chronic sarcoidosis. *J Nucl Med.* (2012) 53:1543–9. doi: 10.2967/jnumed.112.104380

Adams H, van Rooij R, van Moorsel CHM, Spee-Dropkova M, Grutters JC, Keijsers RG. Volumetric FDG PET analysis of global lung inflammation: new tool for precision medicine in pulmonary sarcoidosis? *Sarcoidosis Vasc Diffus Lung Dis.* (2018) 35:44–54. doi: 10.36141/svdld.v35i1.5807

Schimmelpennink MC, Vorselaars ADM, Veltkamp M, Keijsers RGM. Quantification of pulmonary disease activity in sarcoidosis measured with 18F-FDG PET/CT: SUVmax versus total lung glycolysis. *EJNMMI Res.* (2019) 9:54. doi: 10.1186/s13550-019-0505-x

Bakker AL, Grutters JC, Keijsers RG, Post MC. Cardiac sarcoidosis: challenges in clinical practice. *Curr Opin Pulm Med.* (2017) 23:468– 75. doi: 10.1097/MCP.0000000000000410

Birnie DH, Kandolin R, Nery PB, Kupari M. Cardiac manifestations of sarcoidosis: diagnosis and management. *Eur Heart J.* (2017) 38:2663–70. doi: 10.1093/eurheartj/ehw328

Birnie DH, Sauer WH, Bogun F, Cooper JM, Culver DA, Duvernoy CS, et al. HRS expert consensus statement on the diagnosis and management of arrhythmias associated with cardiac sarcoidosis. *Hear Rhythm.* (2014) 11:1304–23. doi: 10.1016/j.hrthm.2014.03.043

Greulich S, Kitterer D, Latus J, Aguor E, Steubing H, Kaesemann P, et al. Comprehensive cardiovascular magnetic resonance assessment in patients with sarcoidosis and preserved left ventricular ejection fraction. *Circ Cardiovasc Imaging.* (2016) 9:e005022. doi: 10.1161/CIRCIMAGING.116.005022

Greulich S, Deluigi CC, Gloekler S, Wahl A, Zürn C, Kramer U, et al. CMR imaging predicts death and other adverse events in suspected cardiac sarcoidosis. *JACC Cardiovasc Imaging.* (2013) 6:501– 511. doi: 10.1016/j.jcmg.2012.10.021

Nadel J, Lancefield T, Voskoboinik A, Taylor AJ. Late gadolinium enhancement identified with cardiac magnetic resonance imaging in sarcoidosis patients is associated with long-term ventricular arrhythmia and sudden cardiac death. *Eur Hear J Cardiovasc Imaging.* (2015) 16:634– 41. doi: 10.1093/ehjci/jeu294

Kouranos V, Tzelepis GE, Rapti A, Mavrogeni S, Aggeli K, Douskou M, et al. Complementary role of CMR to conventional screening in the diagnosis and prognosis of cardiac sarcoidosis. *JACC Cardiovasc Imaging.* (2017) 10:1437–47. doi: 10.1016/j.jcmg.2016.11.019

Coleman GC, Shaw PW, Balfour PC, Gonzalez JA, Kramer CM, Patel AR, et al. Prognostic value of myocardial scarring on CMR in patients with cardiac sarcoidosis. *JACC Cardiovasc Imaging.* (2017) 10:411– 20. doi: 10.1016/j.jcmg.2016.05.009

Bravo PE, Raghu G, Rosenthal DG, Elman S, Petek BJ, Soine LA, et al. Risk assessment of patients with clinical manifestations of cardiac sarcoidosis with positron emission tomography and magnetic resonance imaging. *Int J Cardiol.* (2017) 241:457–62. doi: 10.1016/j.ijcard.2017.03.033

Manabe O, Yoshinaga K, Ohira H, Masuda A, Sato T, Tsujino I, et al. The effects of 18-h fasting with low-carbohydrate diet preparation on suppressed physiological myocardial 18F-fluorodeoxyglucose (FDG) uptake and possible minimal effects of unfractionated heparin use in patients with suspected cardiac involvement sarcoid. *J Nucl Cardiol.* (2016) 23:244– 52. doi: 10.1007/s12350-015-0226-0

Tang R, Wang JTY, Wang L, Le K, Huang Y, Hickey AJ, et al. Impact of patient preparation on the diagnostic performance of 18F-FDG PET in cardiac sarcoidosis a systematic review and meta-analysis. *Clin Nucl Med.* (2016) 41:e327–e39. doi: 10.1097/RLU.0000000000001063

Vita T, Okada DR, Veillet-Chowdhury M, Bravo PE, Mullins E, Hulten E, et al. Complementary value of cardiac magnetic resonance imaging and positron emission tomography/computed tomography in the assessment of cardiac sarcoidosis. *Circ Cardiovasc Imaging.* (2018) 11:e007030. doi: 10.1161/CIRCIMAGING.117.007030

Blankstein R, Osborne M, Naya M, Waller A, Kim CK, Murthy VL, et al. Cardiac positron emission tomography enhances prognostic assessments of patients with suspected cardiac sarcoidosis. *J Am Coll Cardiol.* (2014) 63:329–36. doi: 10.1016/j.jacc.2013.09.022

Dweck MR, Abgral R, Trivieri MG, Robson PM, Karakatsanis N, Mani V, et al. Hybrid magnetic resonance imaging and positron emission tomography with fluorodeoxyglucose to diagnose active cardiac sarcoidosis. *JACC Cardiovasc Imaging.* (2018) 11:94–107. doi: 10.1016/j.jcmg.2017.02.021

Hoitsma E, Faber CG, Drent M, Sharma OP. Neurosarcoidosis: a clinical dilemma. *Lancet Neurol.* (2004) 3:397– 407. doi: 10.1016/S1474-4422(04)00805-1

Marangoni S, Argentiero V, Tavolato B. Neurosarcoidosis: clinical description of 7 cases with a proposal for a new diagnostic strategy. *J Neurol.* (2006) 253:488–95. doi: 10.1007/s00415-005-0043-5

Zajicek JP, Scolding NJ, Foster O, Rovaris M, Evanson J, Moseley IF, et al. Central nervous system sarcoidosis-diagnosis and management. *QJM Mon J Assoc Physicians.* (1999) 92:103–17. doi: 10.1093/qjmed/92.2.103

Bathla G, Singh AK, Policeni B, Agarwal A, Case B. Imaging of neurosarcoidosis: common, uncommon, and rare. *Clin Radiol.* (2016) 71:96– 106. doi: 10.1016/j.crad.2015.09.007

Voortman M, Hendriks CMR, Elfferich MDP, Bonella F, Møller J, De Vries J, et al. The burden of sarcoidosis symptoms from a patient perspective. *Lung.* (2019) 197:155–61 doi: 10.1007/s00408-019-00206-7

Vargas DL, Stern BJ. Neurosarcoidosis: diagnosis and management. *Semin Respir Crit Care Med.* (2010) 31:419–27. doi: 10.1055/s-0030-1262210

Huang JF, Aksamit AJ, Staff NP. MRI and PET imaging discordance in neurosarcoidosis. *Neurology.* (2012) 79:1070. doi: 10.1212/WNL.0b013e3182684672

Sammarra I, Barbagallo G, Labate A, Mondello B, Albonico G, Maisano M, et al. Value of multimodal imaging approach to diagnosis of neurosarcoidosis. *Brain Sci.* (2019) 9:243. doi: 10.3390/brainsci9100243

Rivière E, Schwartz P, MacHelart I, Greib C, Pellegrin JL, Viallard JF, et al. Neurosarcoidosis and infliximab therapy monitored by 18FDG PET/CT. *QJM.* (2019) 112:695–7. doi: 10.1093/qjmed/hcz148

Shuai K, Liu B. Regulation of JAK-STAT signalling in the immune system. *Nat Rev Immunol.* (2003) 3:900–11 doi: 10.1038/nri1226

Rosenbaum JT, Pasadhika S, Crouser ED, Choi D, Harrington CA, Lewis JA, et al. Hypothesis: Sarcoidosis is a STAT1-mediated disease. *Clin Immunol.* (2009) 132:174–83. doi: 10.1016/j.clim.2009. 04.010

Wei JJ, Kallenbach LR, Kreider M, Leung TH, Rosenbach M. Resolution of cutaneous sarcoidosis after Janus kinase inhibitor therapy for concomitant polycythemia vera. *JAAD Case Rep.* (2019) 5:360–1. doi: 10.1016/j.jdcr.2019.02.006

Damsky W, Thakral D, McGeary MK, Leventhal J, Galan A, King B. Janus kinase inhibition induces disease remission in cutaneous sarcoidosis and granuloma annulare. *J Am Acad Dermatol.* (2020) 82:612– 21. doi: 10.1016/j.jaad.2019.05.098

Damsky W, Thakral D, Emeagwali N, Galan A, King B. Tofacitinib treatment and molecular analysis of cutaneous sarcoidosis. *N Engl J Med.* (2018) 379:2540–6. doi: 10.1056/NEJMoa1805958

Rotenberg C, Besnard V, Brillet PY, Giraudier S, Nunes H, Valeyre D. Dramatic response of refractory sarcoidosis under ruxolitinib in a patient with associated JAK2-mutated polycythemia. *Eur Respir J.* (2018) 52:1801482. doi: 10.1183/13993003.01482-2018

Laplante M, Sabatini DM. MTOR signaling in growth control and disease. *Cell.* (2012) 149:274–93. doi: 10.1016/j.cell.2012.03.017

Linke M, Pham HTT, Katholnig K, Schnöller T, Miller A, Demel F, et al. Chronic signaling via the metabolic checkpoint kinase mTORC1 induces macrophage granuloma formation and marks sarcoidosis progression. *Nat Immunol.* (2017) 18:293–302. doi: 10.1038/ ni.3655

Calender A, Lim CX, Weichhart T, Buisson A, Besnard V, Rollat-Farnier PA, et al. Exome sequencing and pathogenicity-network analysis of five French families implicate mTOR signalling and autophagy in familial sarcoidosis. *Eur Respir J.* (2019) 54:1900430. doi: 10.1183/13993003.004 30-2019

Korenromp IHE, Heijnen CJ, Vogels OJM, Van Den Bosch JMM, Grutters JC. Characterization of chronic fatigue in patients with sarcoidosis in clinical remission. *Chest.* (2011) 140:441–7. doi: 10.1378/chest.10-2629

Van Manen MJG, Wester VL, Van Rossum EFC, Van Den Toorn LM, Dorst KY, De Rijke YB, et al. Scalp hair cortisol and testosterone levels in patients with sarcoidosis. *PLoS One.* (2019) 14:1–15. doi: 10.1371/journal.pone.0215763

Russell E, Koren G, Rieder M, Van Uum S. Hair cortisol as a biological marker of chronic stress: Current status, future directions and unanswered questions. *Psychoneuroendocrinology.* (2012) 37:589– 601. doi: 10.1016/j.psyneuen.2011.09.009

Gormsen LC, Haraldsen A, Kramer S, Dias AH, Kim WY, Borghammer P. A dual tracer 68Ga-DOTANOC PET/CT and 18F-FDG PET/CT pilot study for detection of cardiac sarcoidosis. *EJNMMI Res.* (2016) 6:52. doi: 10.1186/s13550-016-0207-6

Vis R, Malviya G, Signore A, Grutters JC, Meek B, Van De Garde EMW, et al. 99mTc-anti-TNF-α antibody for the imaging of disease activity in pulmonary sarcoidosis. *Eur Respir J.* (2016) 47:1198–207. doi: 10.1183/13993003.01352-2015

Culver DA, Judson MA. New advances in the management of pulmonary sarcoidosis. *BMJ.* (2019) 367:l5553. doi: 10.1136/bmj.l5553

Futami Y, Takeda Y, Koba T, Kida H, Kumanogoh A, Ueda K. Proteomic profiling of serum exosomes to find novel biomarkers in sarcoidosis. *Am J Respir Crit Care Med.* (2020) 201:A4489. doi: 10.1164/ajrccm-conference.2019.199.1_MeetingAbstracts.A4489

11

Management and Thinking on the Treatment of Cancer Patients during the COVID-19

Shuangyue Pan[1,2], Jiahong Jiang[2], Zheling Chen[2] and Liu Yang[2*]*

[1] The Second Clinical Medical College, Zhejiang Chinese Medical University, Hangzhou, China, [2] Center of Oncology, Department of Medical Oncology, Zhejiang Provincial People's Hospital, People's Hospital of Hangzhou Medical College, Hangzhou, China

***Correspondence:**
Liu Yang
yangliuqq2003@163.com;
yangliu@hmc.edu.cn
Zheling Chen
383974903@qq.com*

Coronavirus disease-2019 (COVID-19) has spread rapidly around the world and has become a public health emergency of international concern. The weekly epidemiological report issued by the WHO pointed out that new coronavirus variants have appeared in 131 countries and regions, which demonstrates that the current epidemic situation is still severe. As of now, the severe acute respiratory syndrome coronavirus (SARS-CoV-2) has been widespread worldwide for more than one year and poses a serious threat to the health of vulnerable groups such as those with malignancies, the elderly, and the immunocompromised. Compared with the general population, cancer patients with COVID-19 infection are more likely to have serious clinical adverse events, leading to higher mortality. There is no doubt that during the COVID-19 epidemic, whether it is with regards to how to prevent infection or how to continue anti-tumor treatment, cancer patients are in a difficult situation. Meanwhile, an international patient with malignant Hodgkin's lymphoma who was cured after being infected with the new coronavirus surprised us, and it inspires more scientists to explore the relationship between infection, immunity, and tumors. Relevantly, through multi-disciplinary discussion, scientists put forward more new perspectives on the treatment of future tumors and the management of SARS-CoV-2 diseases. In this review, the impact of COVID-19 on cancer patients is discussed in detail and the recommendations for the diagnosis, treatment and management of cancer patients will be put forward under the challenge of the COVID-19 epidemic. Furthermore, the safety and effectiveness of the SARS-CoV-2 vaccine will be discussed, and we will also put forward our insights on cancer immunity.

Keywords: COVID-19, SARS-CoV-2, management, cancer patients, vaccine, cancer immunity

INTRODUCTION

The novel coronavirus disease 2019 (COVID-19) caused by the severe acute respiratory syndrome coronavirus named SARS-CoV-2 occurred in Wuhan, Hubei in December 2019 and has now spread globally (Yu et al., 2020). SARS-CoV-2 virus is an enveloped positive single-stranded RNA virus that can infect both humans and animals (Velavan and Meyer, 2020). Human-to-human transmission has been proven by the infection of 15 medical staff in a Wuhan hospital (Paules et al., 2020). As of Feb 7, 2021, the total number of confirmed cases was 106,277,685 worldwide, and the total number of deaths was 2,316,660 (Real-Time Tracking of New Coronavirus Pneumonia Epidemic, 2021). In a clinical study from China, 81% of the cases were classified as mild pneumonia; 14% of the cases had serious diseases such as dyspnea and decreased blood oxygen saturation and 5% of the cases had respiratory failure, septic shock, or multiple organ failure.

Among them, the overall case fatality rate was 2.3% (1,023 of 44,672 confirmed cases). However, the case fatality rate of patients aged 80 and over has increased to 14.8% (The Novel Coronavirus Pneumonia Emergency Response Epidemiology Team, 2020).

Cancer patients are commonly in a state of systemic immunosuppression due to anti-tumor therapies (such as chemotherapy or radiotherapy), so they are more susceptible to be infected with the SARS-CoV-2 virus (Liang et al., 2020). Nevertheless, anti-tumor therapy is essential for cancer patients to control their condition. Therefore, it is challenging to strengthen the management of anti-tumor treatment while preventing infection. Recently, the vaccination of the SARS-CoV-2 virus has given us full confidence in defeating COVID-19, and the case of a tumor patient cured after being infected with the SARS-CoV-2 virus has triggered our thinking.

This review aims to discuss approaches of management for cancer patients during the pandemic and provide our insights on the cure of tumor patient infected with the SARS-CoV-2 virus.

CANCER PATIENTS DURING THE COVID-19

Morbidity and Mortality of Cancer Patients

On the one hand, cancer patients are generally malnourished and have lower ability to fight SARS-CoV-2 virus; on the other hand, cancer patients have immunodeficiency due to the systematic treatment. These factors make cancer patients more susceptible to SARS-CoV-2 virus, and the mortality rate will be higher than normal (Wang and Zhang, 2020). A retrospective study in Zhongnan Hospital of Wuhan University showed that the infection rate of SARS-CoV-2 in cancer patients is 0.79% (12 of 1,524 patients; 95%CI; 0.3–1.2%). However, the cumulative incidence of all COVID-19 cases reported in Wuhan is 0.37% (41,152 of 11,081,000 cases; data cut off on February 17, 2020) (Yu et al., 2020). Cancer patients infected with the SARS-CoV-2 virus have more risk factors than patients without cancer (Heathcote et al., 2020). A study collected and analyzed 2007 confirmed cases of COVID-19 in 575 hospitals in China, of which 1,590 cases of infection are valid data. The study found that patients with cancer are older than patients without cancer (average age 63.1 years old [SD 12.1] vs 48.7 years old [16.2]), more likely to have a history of smoking (four [22%] of 18 patients vs 107 [7%] of 1,572 patients), had more polypnea (eight [47%] of 17 patients vs 323 [23%] of 1,377 patients), and more severe baseline CT manifestation (17 [94%] of 18 patients vs 1,113 [71%] of 1,572 patients) (Liang et al., 2020). These risk factors directly cause the mortality of cancer patients infected with the SARS-CoV-2 virus to be higher than that of the healthy population. A multi-centural study including 105 cancer patients and 536 age-matched non-cancer patients confirmed with COVID-19 showed that compared with COVID-19 patients without cancer, cancer patients have higher observed mortality (OR 2.34, 95% CI [1.15, 4.77]; $p = 0.03$), and a higher ICU hospitalization rate (OR 2.84, 95%) CI [1.59, 5.08]; $p < 0.01$) (Dai et al., 2020).

Differentiation of Cancer Patients and COVID-19

Cancer patients have complex conditions, with many non-specific clinical symptoms and signs. For example, lung cancer patients' own lung manifestations, tumor fever, immune-related pneumonia, and other manifestations. During this special period, it is necessary to actively differentiate from COVID-19. Multiple studies have shown that the main clinical manifestations of COVID-19 are fever, cough, and dyspnea (Huang et al., 2020; Jiang et al., 2020; Zhang L. et al., 2020). Although non-cancer and cancer patients with COVID-19 have similar clinical manifestations, a study screened 13,077 SARS-CoV-2 patients and finally compared the clinical characteristics of 232 cancer patients and 519 matched cancer-free patients. Studies have shown that cancer patients infected with the SARS-CoV-2 virus were more likely to have dyspnea and CT scans showed that ground-glass opacity and patchy opacity were more common. Furthermore, the pro-inflammatory cytokines of cancer patients including TNF-α, IL-6, and IL-2R were higher than those of patients without cancer. The lymphocytes, CD4+ T cells, CD8+ T cell counts, and the ratio of CD4+ T cells to CD8+ T cells in cancer patients decreased more significantly (Tian et al., 2020). Special attention should be paid to the appearance of any of these characteristics to minimize the risk of underdiagnosing cancer patients with COVID-19 infection.

In general, the fever of tumor patients can be divided into tumor fever, drug fever, and infection. Tumor fever refers to the response of the immune system to tumor necrosis and stress factors produced by tumors which is generally ≤38.5°C with no inducement and lasts for a long time. Experimental treatment with antibiotics is ineffective (Pasikhova et al., 2017). Drug fever means that fever occurs during medication and stops after drug withdrawal. The median time of fever caused by antineoplastic drugs is about 0.5 days after administration (Patel and Gallagher, 2010). Fever caused by infection usually has a higher temperature and can be reflected by blood routine tests.

All patients diagnosed with COVID-19 have varying degrees of lung abnormalities, which can be seen in chest computed tomography (CT) imaging (Huang et al., 2020; **Figure 1**). Most cases of COVID-19 showed bilateral parenchymal ground-glass opacity (GGO) or consolidative pulmonary opacity on CT scans, and the enlargement and consolidation of GGO usually indicate the progression of COVID-19 (Chung et al., 2020). The characteristics of COVID-19 also include reticular pattern, linear subpleural opacity, bronchial dilatation, centrilobular nodules and tree-in-bud (Zhang Y. J. et al., 2020). Through the imaging performance of CT, we can distinguish lung cancer from COVID-19 through the following points. First of all, most COVID-19 patients have bilateral lesions while most cancer patients have unilateral lung lesions. Secondly, most COVID-19 patients have more than one type of lung lesion, while lung cancer patients tend to have either pure GGO or mixed GGO. What is more, COVID-19 shows more patchy lesions, while lung cancer shows more

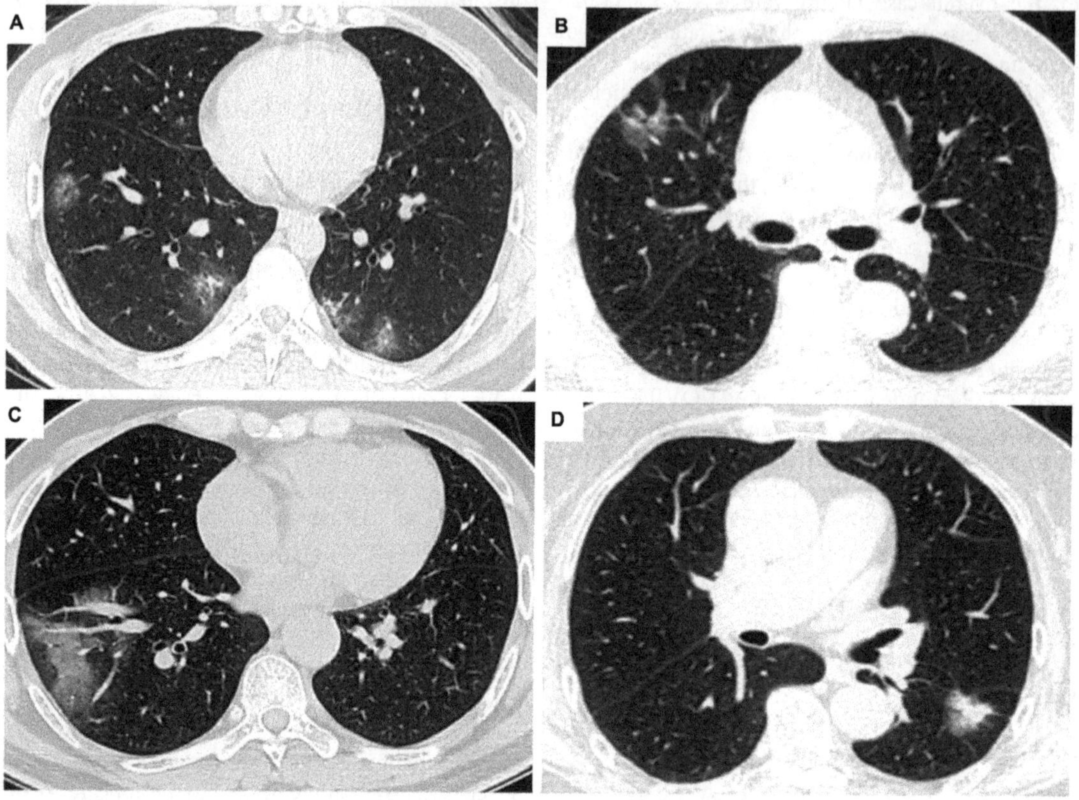

FIGURE 1 | CT images of lung cancer patients and COVID-19 (Transl Lung Cancer Res.2020 Aug;9(4):1516-1527.doi: 10.21037/tlcr-20-892). **(A)** CT scan of a patient diagnosed with COVID-19: The lesion is GGO, and there is no sign of pleural retraction or vascular convergence. **(B)** CT scan of a patient diagnosed with lung cancer, with pleural retraction and cystic change. **(C)** CT scan of a patient diagnosed with COVID-19, the lesion showed patchy turbidity, irregular shape, and no pleural retraction. **(D)** CT scan of a patient diagnosed with lung cancer, with pleural retraction, lobulated sign, and spiculate protuberance.

oval lesions (Zhang Y. J. et al., 2020; **Table 1**). There are many types of lung cancer that various imaging manifestations may reveal, therefore, we need to use RT-PCR and next-generation sequencing methods applied to respiratory tract specimens to assist identification when necessary.

Is Anti-tumor Treatment a Contraindication During the COVID-19?

Cancer patients are at increased risk of death and serious clinical events due to COVID-19 infection. However, risk of adverse events does not seem to be increased by cancer therapies (Heathcote et al., 2020). Between April 15 and 26, 2020, a total of 1,227 tumor patients were tested for SARS-CoV-2 using RT-qPCR in the tumor clinic, and 78 (6.4%) were positive. Among them, 75 (96.2%) were asymptomatic infections. Fourteen cancer patients out of 75 asymptomatic infections received chemotherapy or immunotherapy (±4 weeks of SARS-CoV-2 test), 48 (61.5%) of 78 patients who tested positive received glucocorticoid combination therapy. None of the patients with asymptomatic infection had unexpected complications caused by SARS-CoV-2 infection. These data indicate that the incidence of symptoms due to COVID-19 is relatively low among patients treated with chemotherapy and other immunosuppressive agents (such as glucocorticoids). Therefore, whether anti-tumor therapy is a contraindication during the epidemic is still inconclusive (Hempel et al., 2020).

Studies have shown that the risk of death in patients infected with COVID-19 is significantly related to the increase in patient age (odds ratio 9.42 [95% CI 6.56–10.02]; $p < 0.0001$) and significant correlation with other comorbidities, such as hypertension (1.95 [1.36–2.80]; $p < 0.001$) and cardiovascular disease (2.32 [1.47–3.64]). Anti-tumor treatment does not increase the risk of death from new coronary pneumonia in cancer patients (Lee et al., 2020). Therefore, for cancer patients,

TABLE 1 | CT differentiation of lung cancer and COVID-19.

	Lung cancer	COVID-19
Lesion(in most cases)	Unilateral	Bilateral
Lesion form	Oval lesions	Patchy lesions
Involved lobes	Less	More
Types of lung disease	Pure GGO or mixed GGO	More than one
Characteristic performance	lobulated signs, pleural retraction, cystic changes and signs of vascular convergence	Air bronchography, reticular pattern, subpleural linear opacity, bronchiectasis, lobular nodules and tree-in-bud

risk-benefit assessment must be carried out. If the benefits outweigh the risks, cancer treatment should continue (Gosain et al., 2020; Zhao Q. et al., 2020; **Figure 2**).

Patients at the priority level 1 do not need to go to the hospital for treatment unless necessary, and can communicate with doctors through telemedicine and other methods; Patients at the priority level 2 can delay treatment appropriately; patients at the priority level 3 should go to the hospital for treatment with protective measures.

Cancer Patients With Different Treatment Modalities

Cancer Patients Undergoing Surgery

During the COVID-19 pandemic, patients with tumors requiring surgery should be strictly screened for infection with the SARS-CoV-2 Virus, and a comprehensive assessment should be made based on the patient's overall condition as to whether surgery can be performed to avoid serious adverse events. An international study conducted in 235 hospitals in 24 countries/regions included all surgical patients who were confirmed to have SARS-CoV-2 infection. The primary outcome measure was the 30-day mortality rate after surgery, and the secondary outcome measure was pneumonia, acute respiratory distress syndrome, or accidental ventilation after surgery. Among 1,128 patients undergoing surgery, 294 patients (26.1%) were confirmed to have SARS-CoV-2 infection before surgery, their 30-day mortality rate was 23.8% (268 out of 1,128). Pulmonary complications occurred in 577 (51.2%) of 1,128 patients. The 30-day mortality rate of these patients was 38% (219 of 577), accounting for 82.6% of all deaths (219 of 265) (Nepogodiev et al., 2020). Therefore, it is necessary to carefully consider the surgical operation of cancer patients during the epidemic.

If cancer patients do not receive surgery in time, how long will the extension affect the survival rate or the probability of complete resection? Studies have shown that for cancers treated with surgery first, the median safe postponement period (SPP) is 3 weeks which is 6 weeks from diagnosis. For 48% of cancer types, the SPP was at least 4 weeks. For patients who received neoadjuvant therapy such as chemotherapy or radiotherapy, the median SPP was 8 weeks which is 26 weeks from diagnosis. For 76% of cancer types, the SPP is at least 6 weeks (Kiran and Turaga, 2020). Through this study, we can find that most cancer operations can be postponed for at least 4 weeks without significantly affecting the survival of the patient. The tumor will not progress significantly, and there is no significant difference in the probability of complete tumor resection.

Cancer Patients Undergoing Routine Chemotherapy

During the COVID-19 pandemic, the main concern of patients receiving chemotherapy was the decrease in anti-tumor efficacy due to the interruption of chemotherapy. While we pay attention to the adverse effects of the epidemic on the delay of chemotherapy for tumor patients, we should also treat the adjustment of chemotherapy regimens rationally (Zhao Z. et al., 2020). Based on the fact that anti-cancer therapy may bring greater risks, some patients may voluntarily choose treatments with lower potential efficacy but a lower degree of myelosuppression (Battershill, 2006). Patients who receive conventional chemotherapy can consider switching from intravenous chemotherapy to oral anticancer drugs, which can reduce the number of visits to the hospital and thus reduce the risk of infection (Gosain et al., 2020). In addition, with the advent of elastic pumps, chemotherapy at home has become more and more common (Shereen and Salman, 2019). In order to reduce the duration of exposure in the hospital, the hospital pharmacy department can deliver medicine to patients by express delivery (Willan et al., 2020). The treatment of lung cancer patients during the COVID-19 pandemic can give us some suggestions: some scholars have proposed that multiple variables should be considered when formulating a diagnosis and treatment plan for lung cancer patients, including virus prevalence, capacity of

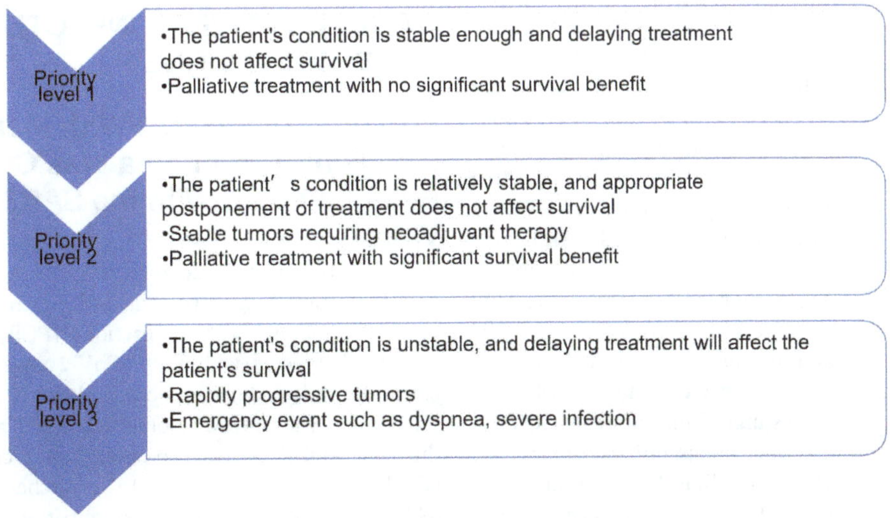

FIGURE 2 | Classified treatment management according to the actual situation of cancer patients.

local medical institutions, patient infection risk, cancer status, patient comorbidities, age, etc. After considering these factors, the treatment of lung cancer patients is divided into five groups "Should be started when Possible," "Should not be stopped without justification," "Can be given preferentially," "Can be withheld or delayed after careful consideration," "Should not be started without justification" (Banna et al., 2020). Under the guidance of oncologists, the treatment strategy should be adjusted appropriately according to the progress of tumor patients, the stage and effect of anti-tumor therapy, local epidemic situation, and so on (Zhao Z. et al., 2020).

Cancer Patients With Radiotherapy

Studies have shown that delayed radiotherapy and interruption of radiotherapy may contribute to inferior local control and overall survival of cancer patients (Yao et al., 2018). Radiotherapy requires specific equipment, and community hospitals have no extra resources to reserve linear accelerators, simulators or mold rooms for patients, the radiotherapy center cannot disperse patients, therefore it will be in a high-risk area (Mukherjee et al., 2003). During the outbreak of COVID-19 in Wuhan, the department of radiotherapy center has taken the following measures: divide the radiotherapy center into different infection control areas and provide different levels of protection; implement daily symptom testing standards for patients receiving treatment; design and implement a revised radiotherapy workflow, special treatment area cleaning and disinfection policies and procedures (Wei et al., 2020).

Cancer Patients Receiving Immunotherapy

Immune checkpoint inhibitors play an anti-tumor effect by regulating the body's own immune response. Checkpoint antibody inhibitors, such as anti-PD-1/PD-L1, are novel inhibitors that function as tumor suppressors by regulating immune cell-tumor cell interaction (Alsaab et al., 2017). The research team analyzed a total of 800 patients with COVID-19 diagnosed with cancer and symptoms. Among them, 412 (52%) patients had mild COVID-19 symptoms; eventually 226 patients (28%) died. The research team found that in the past 4 weeks, patients using immunotherapy, hormone therapy, targeted therapy, and radiation therapy had no significant impact on mortality (Lee et al., 2020). However, research results published by the famous Memorial Sloan-Kettering Cancer Center (MSKCC) in New York, United States revealed that cancer patients who use immunotherapy (mainly PD-1/PD-L1 inhibitors) were more dangerous after infection with SARS-CoV-2 virus and required a higher proportion of hospitalization, the rate of severe pneumonia was also higher (Robilotti et al., 2020). Cancer immunotherapy can effectively prolong the survival period of cancer patients but also cause some adverse reactions such as organ inflammation, the most common of which is immune-related pneumonia. Distinguishing between COVID-19 pneumonia and immune-related pneumonia is a diagnostic challenge (Suresh et al., 2018). The clinical manifestations of immune-related pneumonia and COVID-19 are similar and they can both show symmetrical patchy GGO and consolidation area in CT imaging. Therefore, a diagnostic algorithm is proposed to distinguish immune-related pneumonia and COVID-19. The first step is RT-PCR screening. Secondly, laboratory examination and CT imaging features are helpful for identification. There is no obvious specificity in the hemogram of immune-related pneumonia, just CRP and ESR are often increased. In the early stage of COVID-19 patients, peripheral blood leukocytes were normal or decreased, lymphocyte count decreased, CRP and ESR increased in most patients, D-dimer and liver enzymes, LDH, muscle enzymes, myoglobin, and troponin increased in severe patients (Kattan et al., 2020; Wu et al., 2020). Besides, further bronchoscopy is needed if necessary (Dumoulin et al., 2020).

Cancer Patients Participating in Clinical Trials

During the COVID-19 period, individualized management of clinical trials should be carried out to maximize the protection of patients' interests. Effectively guard against COVID-19 and ensure the scientific nature of clinical experiments at the same time. The Food and Drug Administration (FDA) has issued guidelines for institutions to protect trial participants and administer investigational products by changing monitoring methods (FDA, 2020). The progress of clinical trials may be slowed down due to the impact of the epidemic, because clinical trial subjects have strict standards and time limits for drug administration, efficacy evaluation, safety evaluation, follow-up, and so on. It requires the cooperation of subjects, researchers, sponsors, clinical research coordinators, and other relevant participants under the supervision of ethics. The clinical trial activities during the COVID-19 period should be tailored to the changing epidemic situation. Suspension of some non-therapeutic intervention trials could be considered, and clinical trials that continue after discussion will continue to obtain all the tests and data points needed for the study (Gosain et al., 2020). The researchers can manage according to the different dosage forms used by the subjects, subjects taking oral drugs can be followed up remotely by telephone or Internet, and the researchers can send the drugs to the subjects by express delivery.

CANCER PATIENTS INFECTED WITH SARS-COV-2 VIRUS

A Patient Diagnosed With Malignant Hodgkin's Lymphoma Was Cured After Being Infected With the SARS-CoV-2 Virus

Recently, two British doctors reported a special case: a 61-year-old man diagnosed with Hodgkin's lymphoma [EBV viral polymerase chain reaction (PCR) 4,800 copies/ml; log^{10}3.68] infected with SARS-CoV-2 virus and was not given corticosteroids and immunochemotherapy. After 4 months, PET CT showed widespread resolution of the lymphadenopathy and the EBV viral PCR had also fallen to 413 copies/ml (log^{10}2.62) (Challenor and Tucker, 2021). Researchers suspected that the SARS-CoV-2 virus stimulated an anti-tumor immune response, killing the virus while also killing cancer cells. This is not the only case that the tumor is cured after infection. The case in 2012 reported that a 67-year-old woman with lymphoma infected with pneumonia and colitis and the tumor also disappeared completely (Buckner et al., 2012). Although lymphoma does not represent all tumors, it does give us a great inspiration. In fact, there have been similar records dating back hundreds of years. Some doctors even tried to inject pathogens into cancer patients to induce fever to treat cancer. This is actually the original form of immunotherapy. In recent years, PD-1 inhibitors, CTLA-4 inhibitors, CAR-T therapy, CAR-NK therapy, and other modern immunotherapies have been successful, bringing hope to many cancer patients. The idea that activating the immune system can fight cancer has been widely accepted.

The Contradiction Between the Treatment of Infectious Diseases and Anti-tumor Treatment

Infection is one of the most common complications of anti-tumor therapy. Anti-tumor treatment destroys the patients' immune system, resulting in neutropenia which can lead to more severe infection. The use of antiviral therapy in cancer patients infected with COVID-19 remains controversial. Among cancer patients infected with COVID-19 in a case report, 20 patients (71.4%) were treated with antiviral drugs empirically; 9 patients (32.1%) received a combination of antiviral drugs, 15 patients (53.6%) received systemic corticosteroid therapy, 12 patients (35.7%) received intravenous immunoglobulin. The data from the case did not report that the patient population had benefited from it. Instead, of the 6 cancer patients who received anti-tumor treatment within 14 days of being diagnosed with COVID-19, 5 (83%) had serious incidents (Zhang L. et al., 2020). Although the available information is very limited, it is not recommended to use anticancer drugs and antiviral treatments at the same time outside of clinical trials to avoid unexpected pharmacokinetic interactions and toxicity (Raymond et al., 2020).

The Impact of Infection on Tumor Prognosis

As mentioned above, a patient with lymphoma had tumor regression after being infected with the SARS-CoV-2 virus. The case of cancer patients whose tumor disappeared after infection has been reported many times. A review of past reports found that self-healing was usually related to acute infections such as bacteria and viruses, fever, and immune stimulation (Buckner et al., 2012; Challenor and Tucker, 2021). The idea of stimulating the human immune response to treat cancer and other diseases has been proven in trials.

Vaccines are a typical example of preventing the invasion of microorganisms by stimulating the human immune response. Bacille Calmette-Guerin (BCG), a live attenuated strain of Mycobacterium bovis, is the first live-attenuated vaccines used in humans. BCG provides 80% protection against severe and disseminated tuberculosis in children and can also reduce the risk of adult tuberculosis (Ritz et al., 2008). In the 1980s, BCG became the first choice for the treatment of early *in situ* bladder cancer. As long as the patient's immune system is normal, the tumor burden is small, the BCG vaccine can directly contact the tumor, and the dosage of the drug is sufficient, the BCG vaccine can eliminate the tumor in 70% of patients (Babaian, 2021). Researchers have found that urothelial cells and immune system cells both play a crucial role in the anti-tumor treatment of BCG. BCG vaccine can stimulate the body's immune response through its internalization, bladder cancer cells up-regulate the expression of MHC class II and ICAM-1 and secrete various cytokines, including IL-6. In addition to bladder cancer cells, dendritic cells may also play a role in the recruitment of immune cells, initially granulocytes, then macrophages and lymphocytes (Redelman-Sidi et al., 2014).

In addition to BCG, oncolytic viruses can achieve anti-tumor effects through the dual mechanism of selective killing of tumor cells and inducing systemic anti-tumor immunity. Oncolytic viruses are attenuated viruses that infect tumor cells to enhance the body's natural immune response. Oncolytic viruses have direct and indirect toxic effects on tumor cells, such as autolysis, honing of immune cells, destruction of vascular supply, and enhancement of other auxiliary anti-cancer therapies (Russell et al., 2012). Currently, the oncolytic virus treatment drug talimogene laherparepvec (T-Vec or Imlygic) for metastatic melanoma has been approved by the FDA.

Therefore, the pathogenic bacterium is not completely harmful to cancer patients, and there are many clinical applications that use the properties of pathogenic bacterium to bring cancer patients benefits such as the use of inactivated pathogenic bacterium to prepare vaccines; the use of genetically engineered viruses as carriers for gene therapy; using viruses to target cancer, etc.

CANCER PATIENTS AND SARS-COV-2 VACCINES

In order to control the spread of the SARS-CoV-2 virus in a timely and effective manner, researchers have made efforts to develop vaccines (Hodgson et al., 2021). On November 9, 2020, Pfizer and BioNTech announced that the vaccine BNT162b2 against COVID-19 had succeeded in the Phase 3 study. Interim analysis showed that compared with placebo, two vaccination of the mRNA vaccine at 21 days intervals can reduce the infection rate of the symptomatic new coronavirus SARS-CoV-2 by 90% (Pfizer, 2020). The other clinical trial in the United States showed that the effective rate of mRNA-1273 vaccine in preventing COVID-19 diseases was 94.1% (Baden et al., 2021). At present, five COVID-19 vaccines have been approved for marketing or emergency use in China, including three inactivated vaccines and one adenovirus vector vaccine. Vaccines are essential to prevent COVID-19 and to protect patients with high-risk complications. As of April 1, 2021, more than 590 million people have been vaccinated worldwide (Caixin, 2021).

Cancer patients and their families are very concerned about a question: Can cancer patients get the COVID-19 vaccine? Due to the low immune function of cancer patients, the live microorganisms in the live attenuated vaccines will increase the risk; the live vaccines may cause excessive immunity in patients receiving immunotherapy due to the activation of immunity in the body. Therefore, according to the latest NCCN guidelines, live attenuated vaccines cannot be used for tumor patients with weakened immune function (NCPGI, 2020). However, despite the fact that the vaccines marketed in China are inactivated, patients with malignant tumors are still listed as one of the contraindications due to lack of clinical data. Therefore, it is still necessary to strengthen the management of cancer patients for hospital departments and cancer patients should also pay attention to personal management.

COVID-19 PREVENTION AND CONTROL MANAGEMENT IN HOSPITAL DEPARTMENTS

All departments of the hospital must provide patients with preventive and control measures, and each department must establish a COVID-19 prevention program within the department, which is composed of the core team of the department and the supervisors of each work link. It is essential to provide infection prevention training and education to all medical staff in the department and develop a clear process that everyone can strictly follow and implement (The Healthcare Infection Control Practices Advisory Committee [HICPAC], 2018). For outpatients, first of all, the number of outpatients should be controlled to the least level for reducing exposure to infection. Secondly, necessary temperature tests, emphasizing the importance of wearing masks and hand hygiene are effective measures to reduce infections (Al-Shamsi et al., 2020). It is recommended that qualified hospitals actively develop telehealth strategies to provide health care and reduce personnel gathering and unnecessary cross-infection (Centers for Disease Control and Prevention, 2020; Zhao Q. et al., 2020). For hospitalized cancer patients, strict screening must be carried out before anti-cancer treatment (**Figure 3**). Data from China shows that chest CT is more sensitive than RT-PCR for diagnosing COVID-19,therefore, the screening of the cancer patients for infection requires two examinations of chest CT scan and RT-PCR to consolidate the diagnosis (Ai et al., 2020).

PERSONAL MANAGEMENT AND SOCIAL ASSISTANCE FOR CANCER PATIENTS

Cancer patients should try to avoid going in and out of public places which is more likely to be exposed to SARS-CoV-2 virus, and ideally wear a mask when in close contact with others to prevent spread of respiratory secretions when they are coughing, sneezing, or talking (Centers for Disease Control and Prevention, 2020). Enhancing immunity and reducing the

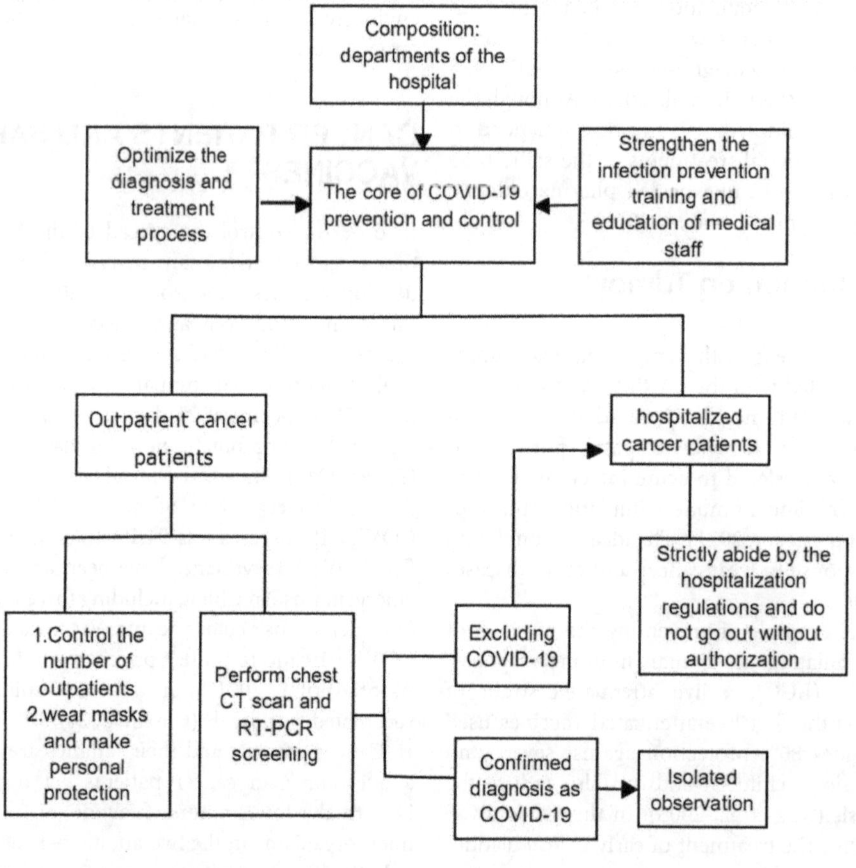

FIGURE 3 | COVID-19 prevention and control management in hospital departments.

risk of exposure are important principles for cancer patients to prevent SARS-CoV-2 infections. Supplementation with some of dietary components such as dietary protein, omega-3 fatty acids, vitamin A can improve the conditions of cancer patients and enhance immunity (BourBour et al., 2020). Besides, the psychological bearing capacity of cancer patients is lower than that of normal people, coupled with social distance measures, isolation measures, and visitor restrictions, which limit the mental strength of cancer patients from family support (Al-Shamsi et al., 2020). We believe that while doing a good job in the prevention and control of the epidemic situation, we also need to pay attention to the mental health of tumor patients, and the research and application of related assessment, intervention and treatment measures is extremely urgent. Therefore, hospitals and medical workers should provide mental support to patients, and psychosocial workers should make maximum use of available resources to intervene patients to meet the continuous needs of patients and their families (Wang et al., 2020).

USE TELEMEDICINE TO ACHIEVE FULL MANAGEMENT OF CANCER PATIENTS

Telemedicine has been shown to reduce medical costs and provide health care to populations with limited access to medical care (Sirintrapun and Lopez, 2020; Tashkandi et al., 2020). Examples of successful telemedicine in oncology include chemotherapy monitoring, symptom management, survival care, palliative care, and clinical trials (Sirintrapun and Lopez, 2020). It has been confirmed in several clinical trials that the outcome of telemedicine is similar to that of face-to-face care (Sirintrapun and Lopez, 2020). We can reduce the number of hospital visits during the COVID-19 pandemic by replacing some clinics with virtual clinics (via videoconferencing or telephone calls) (Tashkandi et al., 2020). In addition, we can also use store-and-forward methods, such as the short message service (SMS), email consultation, or regularly collect and upload data through networked devices to monitor symptoms and signs (McLean et al., 2013). Patients who do not have access to active treatment during the COVID-19 pandemic are particularly suitable for telemedicine. However, virtual telemedicine management is a developing tool to provide medical services to cancer patients under specific conditions. The main limitations of telemedicine include the jurisdiction of medical practice, restrictions on physical examination, and problems related to telemedicine reimbursement, etc. (Sirintrapun and Lopez, 2020).

CONCLUSION

The COVID-19 pandemic has caused a huge public health crisis, which has brought tremendous pressure to medical staff and also brought unprecedented challenges to the treatment and management of cancer patients. This review provides detailed suggestions for dealing with COVID-19 from different aspects to help cancer patients affected by the epidemic. The development of the epidemic is very rapid, far beyond our imagination. Therefore, clinicians and medical personnel must strictly follow the epidemic prevention and control measures and modify or adjust the recommendations provided here as needed.

AUTHOR CONTRIBUTIONS

ZC and LY contributed to the conception and design of the work and data processing and analysis. ZC and SP performed the studies. ZC and SP prepared the majority of the manuscript and LY revised it critically. All authors have given final approvals to the version to be published.

REFERENCES

Ai, T., Yang, Z., Hou, H., Zhan, C., Chen, C., Lv, W., et al. (2020). Correlation of chest CT and RT-PCR testing in Coronavirus. Disease 2019 (COVID-19) in China: a report of 1014 cases. *Radiology* 296:642.

Alsaab, H. O., Sau, S., Alzhrani, R., Tatiparti, K., Bhise, K., Kashaw, S. K., et al. (2017). PD-1 and PD-L1 checkpoint signaling inhibition for cancer immunotherapy: mechanism, combinations, and clinical outcome. *Front. Pharmacol.* 8:561. doi: 10.3389/fphar.2017.00561

Al-Shamsi, H. O., Alhazzani, W., Alhuraiji, A., Coomes, E. A., Chemaly, R. F., Almuhanna, M., et al. (2020). A practical approach to the management of cancer patients during the novel Coronavirus disease 2019 (COVID-19) pandemic: an international collaborative group. *Oncologist* 25:e0936-45.

Babaian, K. N. (2021). *Bacillus Calmette-Guérin Immunotherapy for Bladder Cancer Overview of BCG Immunotherapy.* Cham: Springer.

Baden, L. R., El Sahly, H. M., Essink, B., Kotloff, K., Frey, S., Novak, R., et al. (2021). Efficacy and safety of the mRNA-1273 SARS-CoV-2 vaccine. *N. Engl. J. Med.* 384, 403–416.

Banna, G., Curioni-Fontecedro, A., Friedlaender, A., and Addeo, A. (2020). How we treat patients with lung cancer during the SARS-CoV-2 pandemic: primum non nocere. *ESMO Open* 4:e000785. doi: 10.1136/esmoopen-2020-000785

Battershill, P. M. (2006). Influenza pandemic planningfor cancer patients. *Curr. Oncol.* 13, 119–120. doi: 10.3390/curroncol13040012

BourBour, F., Mirzaei Dahka, S., Gholamalizadeh, M., Akbari, M. E., Shadnoush, M., Haghighi, M., et al. (2020). Nutrients in prevention, treatment, and management of viral infections; special focus on Coronavirus. *Arch. Physiol. Biochem.* 9, 1–10. doi: 10.1080/13813455.2020.1791188

Buckner, T. W., Dunphy, C., Fedoriw, Y. D., van Deventer, H. W., Foster, M. C., Richards, K. L., et al. (2012). Complete spontaneous remission of diffuse large B-cell lymphoma of the maxillary sinus after concurrent infections. *Clin. Lymphoma Myeloma Leuk.* 12, 455–458. doi: 10.1016/j.clml.2012.06.007

Caixin (2021). Available online at: https://opinion.caixin.com/2021-04-02/101685017.html. (accessed April 2, 2021).

Centers for Disease Control and Prevention (2020). *Interim Infection Prevention and Control Recommendations for Healthcare Personnel during the Coronavirus Disease 2019 (COVID-19) Pandemic.* Atlanta, GE: Centers for Disease Control and Prevention.

Challenor, S., and Tucker, D. (2021). SARS-CoV-2-induced remission of Hodgkin lymphoma. *Haematology* 192:415. doi: 10.1111/bjh.17116

Chung, M., Bernheim, A., Mei, X., Zhang, N., Huang, M., Zeng, X., et al. (2020). CT imaging features of 2019 novel Coronavirus (2019-nCoV). *Radiology* 295, 202–207.

Dai, M., Liu, D., Liu, M., Zhou, F., Li, G., Chen, Z., et al. (2020). Patients with Cancer appear more vulnerable to SARS-CoV-2: a multicenter study during the COVID-19 Outbreak. *Cancer Discov.* 10, 783–791.

Dumoulin, D. W., Gietema, H. A., Paats, M. S., Hendriks, L. E. L., and Cornelissen, R. (2020). Differentiation of COVID-19 pneumonitis and ICI induced pneumonitis. *Front. Oncol.* 10:577696. doi: 10.3389/fonc.2020.577696

FDA (2020). *FDA Guidance on Conduct of Clinical Trials of Medical Products During COVID-19 Pandemic*. Silver Spring: FDA.

Gosain, R., Abdou, Y., Singh, A., Rana, N., Puzanov, I., and Ernstoff, M. S. (2020). COVID-19 and cancer: a comprehensive review. *Curr. Oncol. Rep.* 22:53.

Heathcote, L. C., Zion, S. R., and Crum, A. J. (2020). Cancer survivorship-considering mindsets. *JAMA Oncol.* 6, 1468–1469. doi: 10.1001/jamaoncol.2020.2482

Hempel, L., Piehler, A., Pfaffl, M. W., Molnar, J., Kirchner, B., Robert, S., et al. (2020). SARS-CoV-2 infections in cancer outpatients—Most infected patients are asymptomatic carriers without impact on chemotherapy. *Cancer Med.* 9, 8020–8028. doi: 10.1002/cam4.3435

Hodgson, S. H., Mansatta, K., Mallett, G., Harris, V., Emary, K. R. W., and Pollard, A. J. (2021). What defines an efficacious COVID-19 vaccine? A review of the challenges assessing the clinical efficacy of vaccines against SARS-CoV-2. *Lancet Infect. Dis.* 21:e0026-35.

Huang, C., Wang, Y., Li, X., Ren, L., Zhao, J., Hu, Y., et al. (2020). Clinical features of patients infected with 2019 novel coronavirus in Wuhan, China. *Lancet* 395, 497–506.

Jiang, F., Deng, L., Zhang, L., Cai, Y., Cheung, C. W., and Xia, Z. (2020). Review of the clinical characteristics of Coronavirus disease 2019 (COVID-19). *J. Gen. Intern. Med.* 35, 1545–1549.

Kattan, J., Kattan, C., and Assi, T. (2020). Do checkpoint inhibitors compromise the cancer patients' immunity and increase the vulnerability to COVID-19 infection? *Immunotherapy* 12, 351–354. doi: 10.2217/imt-2020-0077

Kiran, S. G., and Turaga, K. (2020). Are we harming cancer patients by delaying their cancer surgery during the COVID-19 pandemic? *Ann. Surg.* doi: 10.1097/SLA.0000000000003967

Lee, L. Y. W., Cazier, J.-B., Angelis, V., Arnold, R., Bisht, V., Campton, N. A., et al. (2020). COVID-19 mortality in patients with cancer on chemotherapy or other anticancer treatments: a prospective cohort study. *Lancet* 395, 1919–1926.

Liang, W., Guan, W., Chen, R., Wang, W., Li, J., Xu, K., et al. (2020). Cancer patients in SARS-CoV-2 infection: a nationwide analysis in China. *Lancet Oncol.* 21, 335–337. doi: 10.1016/s1470-2045(20)30096-6

McLean, S., Sheikh, A., Cresswell, K., Nurmatov, U., Mukherjee, M., Hemmi, A., et al. (2013) The impact of telehealthcare on the quality and safety of care: a systematic overview. *PLoS One* 8:e71238. doi: 10.1371/journal.pone.0071238

Mukherjee, R. K., Back, M. F., Lu, J. J., Shakespeare, T. P., and Wynne, C. J. (2003). Hiding in the Bunker: challenges for a radiation oncology department operating in the Severe Acute Respiratory Syndrome outbreak. *Austr. Radiol.* 47, 143–145.

NCPGI (2020). Oncology, Prevention and Treatment of Cancer-Related Infections. NCCN clinical guidelines. doi: 10.1046/j.0004-8461.2003.01165.x

Nepogodiev, D., Bhangu, A., Glasbey, J. C., Li, E., Omar, O. M., Simoes, J. F. F., et al. (2020). Mortality and pulmonary complications in patients undergoing surgery with perioperative SARS-CoV-2 infection: an international cohort study. *Lancet* 396, 27–38.

Pasikhova, Y., Ludlow, S., and Baluch, A. (2017). Fever in patients with cancer. *Cancer Control.* 24, 193–197. doi: 10.1177/107327481702400212

Patel, R. A., and Gallagher, J. (2010). Drug fever. *Pharmacotherapy* 30, 57–69.

Paules, C. I., Marston, H. D., and Fauci, A. S. (2020). Coronavirus infections-more than just the common cold. *JAMA* 323, 707–708. doi: 10.1001/jama.2020.0757

Pfizer (2020). *Pfizer And Biontech Announce Vaccine Candidate Against Covid-19 Achieved Success In First Interim Analysis From Phase 3 Study*. Available online at: https://www.pfizer.com/news/press-release/press-release-detail/pfizer-and-biontechannounce-vaccine-candidate-against.

Raymond, E., Thieblemont, C., Alran, S., and Faivre, S. (2020). Impact of the COVID-19 outbreak on the management of patients with cancer. *Target Oncol.* 15, 249–259. doi: 10.1007/s11523-020-00721-1

Real-Time Tracking of New Coronavirus Pneumonia Epidemic (2021). *Real-Time Big Data Report on the Novel Coronavirus Pneumonia Outbreak*. News Broadcast.

Redelman-Sidi, G., Glickman, M. S., and Bochner, B. H. (2014). The mechanism of action of BCG therapy for bladder cancer–a current perspective. *Nat. Rev. Urol.* 11, 153–162. doi: 10.1038/nrurol.2014.15

Ritz, N., Hanekom, W. A., Robins-Browne, R., Britton, W. J., and Curtis, N. (2008). Influence of BCG vaccine strain on the immune response and protection against tuberculosis. *FEMS Microbiol. Rev.* 32, 821–841. doi: 10.1111/j.1574-6976.2008.00118.x

Robilotti, E. V., Babady, N. E., Mead, P. A., Rolling, T., Perez-Johnston, R., Bernardes, M., et al. (2020). Determinants of COVID-19 disease severity in patients with cancer. *Nat. Med.* 26, 1218–1223.

Russell, S. J., Peng, K. W., and Bell, J. C. (2012). Oncolytic virotherapy. *Nat. Biotechnol.* 30, 658–670.

Shereen, N. G., and Salman, D. (2019). Delivering chemotherapy at home: how much do we know? *Br. J. Commun. Nurs.* 24, 482–484. doi: 10.12968/bjcn.2019.24.10.482

Sirintrapun, S. J., and Lopez, A. M. (2020). Telemedicine in cancer care. *Am. Soc. Clin. Oncol. Educ. Book* 38, 125–126.

Suresh, K., Naidoo, J., Lin, C. T., and Danoff, S. (2018). Immune Checkpoint immunotherapy for non-small cell lung cancer: benefits and pulmonary toxicities. *Chest* 154, 1416–1423. doi: 10.1016/j.chest.2018.08.1048

Tashkandi, E., Zeeneldin, A., AlAbdulwahab, A., Elemam, O., Elsamany, S., Jastaniah, W., et al. (2020). Virtual management of patients with cancer during the COVID-19 pandemic: web-based questionnaire study. *J. Med. Internet Res.* 22:e19691. doi: 10.2196/19691

The Healthcare Infection Control Practices Advisory Committee [HICPAC] (2018). *Core Infection Prevention and Control Practices for Safe Healthcare Delivery in All Settings –Recommendations of the HICPAC*. Available online at: https://www.cdc.gov/hicpac/recommendations/core-practices.html.

The Novel Coronavirus Pneumonia Emergency Response Epidemiology Team (2020). Vital surveillances: the epidemiological characteristics of an outbreak of 2019 novel Coronavirus diseases (COVID-19) — China, 2020. *China CDC Weekly* 2, 113–122. doi: 10.46234/ccdcw2020.032

Tian, J., Yuan, X., Xiao, J., Zhong, Q., Yang, C., Liu, B., et al. (2020). Clinical characteristics and risk factors associated with COVID-19 disease severity in patients with cancer in Wuhan, China: a multicentre, retrospective, cohort study. *Lancet Oncol.* 21, 893–903.

Velavan, T. P., and Meyer, C. G. (2020). The COVID-19 epidemic. *Trop. Med. Int. Health* 25, 278–280.

Wang, C., Pan, R., Wan, X., Tan, Y., Xu, L., Ho, C. S., et al. (2020). Immediate psychological responses and associated factors during the initial stage of the 2019 coronavirus Disease (COVID-19) epidemic among the general population in China. *Int. J. Environ. Res. Public Health* 17:1729. doi: 10.3390/ijerph17051729

Wang, H., and Zhang, L. (2020). Risk of COVID-19 for patients with cancer. *Lancet Oncol.* 21:e180.

Wei, W., Zheng, D., Lei, Y., Wu, S., Verma, V., Liu, Y., et al. (2020). Radiotherapy workflow and protection procedures during the Coronavirus Disease 2019 (COVID-19) outbreak: experience of the Hubei Cancer hospital in Wuhan, China. *Radiother. Oncol.* 148, 203–210. doi: 10.1016/j.radonc.2020.03.029

Willan, J., King, A. J., Hayes, S., Collins, G. P., and Peniket, A. (2020). Care of haematology patients in a COVID-19 epidemic. *Br. J. Haematol.* 189, 241–243. doi: 10.1111/bjh.16620

Wu, Q., Chu, Q., Zhang, H., Yang, B., He, X., Zhong, Y., et al. (2020). Clinical outcomes of coronavirus disease 2019 (COVID-19) in cancer patients with prior exposure to immune checkpoint inhibitors. *Cancer Commun.* 40, 374–379. doi: 10.1002/cac2.12077

Yao, J. J., Jin, Y. N., Wang, S. Y., Zhang, F., Zhou, G. Q., Zhang, W. J., et al. (2018). The detrimental effects of radiotherapy interruption on local control after concurrent chemoradiotherapy for advanced T-stage nasopharyngeal carcinoma: an observational, prospective analysis. *BMC Cancer* 18:740. doi: 10.1186/s12885-018-4495-2

Yu, J., Ouyang, W., Chua, M. L. K., and Xie, C. (2020). SARS-CoV-2 transmission in patients with cancer at a tertiary care hospital in Wuhan, China. *JAMA Oncol.* 6, 1108–1110. doi: 10.1001/jamaoncol.2020.0980

Zhang, L., Zhu, F., Xie, L., Wang, C., Wang, J., Chen, R., et al. (2020). Clinical characteristics of COVID-19-infected cancer patients: a retrospective case study in three hospitals within Wuhan, China. *Ann. Oncol.* 31, 894–901. doi: 10.1016/j.annonc.2020.03.296

Zhang, Y. J., Yang, W. J., Liu, D., Cao, Y. Q., Zheng, Y. Y., Han, Y. C., et al. (2020). COVID-19 and early-stage lung cancer both featuring ground-glass opacities: a propensity score-matched study. *Transl. Lung Cancer Res.* 9, 1516–1527. doi: 10.21037/tlcr-20-892

Zhao, Q., Meng, M., Kumar, R., Wu, Y., Huang, J., Lian, N., et al. (2020). The impact of COPD and smoking history on the severity of COVID-19: a systemic review and meta-analysis. *J. Med. Virol.* 92, 1915–1921. doi: 10.1002/jmv.25889

Zhao, Z., Bai, H., Duan, J., and Wang, J. (2020). Recommendations of individualized medical treatment and common adverse events management for lung cancer patients during the outbreak of COVID-19 epidemic. *Thorac. Cancer* 11, 1752–1757. doi: 10.1111/1759-7714.13424

12

Pharmacological Mechanisms Underlying the Anti-Asthmatic Effects of Modified Guomin Decoction Determined by Network Pharmacology and Molecular Docking

Guishu Wang[1,2†], Bo Zhou[3†], Zheyi Wang[1†], Yufeng Meng[2], Yaqian Liu[1], Xiaoqin Yao[4,5] and Cuiling Feng[2,5*]*

[1] Dongzhimen Hospital Affiliated to Beijing University of Chinese Medicine, Beijing, China, [2] Department of TCM, Peking University People's Hospital, Beijing, China, [3] Xiyuan Hospital Affiliated to China Academy of Chinese Medical Sciences, Beijing, China, [4] Department of TCM, Peking University International Hospital, Beijing, China, [5] Department of Integration of Chinese and Western Medicine, School of Basic Medical Sciences, Peking University, Beijing, China

***Correspondence:**
Cuiling Feng
fengcuiling@sina.com
Xiaoqin Yao
yaoxiaoqin@pkuih.edu.cn

† These authors have contributed equally to this work

Background: Asthma is a chronic inflammatory disease characterized by Th2-predominant inflammation and airway remodeling. Modified Guo Min decoction (MGMD) has been an extensive practical strategy for allergic disorders in China. Although its potential anti-asthmatic activity has been reported, the exact mechanism of action of MGMD in asthma remains unexplored.

Methods: Network pharmacology approach was employed to predict the active components, potential targets, and molecular mechanism of MGMD for asthma treatment, including drug-likeness evaluation, oral bioavailability prediction, protein–protein interaction (PPI) network construction and analysis, Gene Ontology (GO) terms, and Reactome pathway annotation. Molecular docking was carried out to investigate interactions between active compounds and potential targets.

Results: A total of 92 active compounds and 72 anti-asthma targets of MGMD were selected for analysis. The GO enrichment analysis results indicated that the anti-asthmatic targets of MGMD mainly participate in inflammatory and in airway remolding processes. The Reactome pathway analysis showed that MGMD prevents asthma mainly through regulation of the IL-4 and IL-13 signaling and the specialized pro-resolving mediators (SPMs) biosynthesis. Molecular docking results suggest that each bioactive compounds (quercetin, wogonin, luteolin, naringenin, and kaempferol) is capable to bind with STAT3, PTGS2, JUN, VEGFA, EGFR, and ALOX5.

Conclusion: This study revealed the active ingredients and potential molecular mechanism by which MGMD treatment is effective against airway inflammation and remodeling in asthma through regulating IL-4 and IL-13 signaling and SPMs biosynthesis.

Keywords: asthma, airway inflammation, airway remodeling, Chinese medicine, network pharmacology

INTRODUCTION

Asthma is a globally prevalent chronic inflammatory pulmonary disease, with an estimated 358 million affected individuals (Soriano et al., 2017). Persistent airway inflammation is the hallmark of asthma, which is infiltrated eosinophils, T lymphocytes, mast cells, and release of pro-inflammatory cytokines and lipid mediators. Lipid mediators, such as specialized pro-resolving mediators (SPMs), play a decisive role in the resolution of inflammation in asthma (Schett and Neurath, 2018; Kytikova et al., 2019). Actions of SPMs generated from polyunsaturated fatty acids (PUFAs) include inhibition of eosinophil and neutrophil migration, and decrease of T helper 2 (Th2) cytokine production (e.g., IL-4, IL-5, and IL-13) (Barnig et al., 2018). SPMs are originated via lipoxygenase (LOX)–catalyzed reaction. SPMs include omega-6 PUFA arachidonic acid derived lipoxins, as well as omega-3 PUFA eicosapentaenoic acid (EPA) and docosahexaenoic acid (DHA) derived resolvins, protectins and maresins. Arachidonic acid also forms a range of pro-inflammatory mediators in asthma, such as prostaglandins via cyclooxygenase (COX)-2, and the leukotrienes via 5-LOX actions (Krishnamoorthy et al., 2018).

Airway remodeling is another key pathological features of asthma. It is characterized by thickening of basement membrane, goblet cell metaplasia, smooth muscle cell hyperplasia and hypertrophy, deposition of extracellular matrix proteins, vascular activation and angiogenesis (Jeffery, 2001; James and Wenzel, 2007). Synthesis of extracellular matrix components and collagen is promoted by epidermal growth factor (EGF) released by airway epithelial cells and TGF-β produced by myofibroblasts (Flood-Page et al., 2003; Le Cras et al., 2011). Under the influence of airway epithelial cells-derived endothelial growth factor (VEGF)-A, angiogenesis allow for extravasation of more inflammatory cells (Lambrecht and Hammad, 2012).

Traditional Chinese medicine (TCM) has been used to treat allergic diseases in Asia for hundreds of years (Liu L. et al., 2018). "Guo Min" means allergy in Chinese and Guo Min decoction (GMD) is a compound recipe composed by herbs, that raised by a well-known Chinese physician, Zhu Shenyu (Zhu and Liang, 1985). GMD has been widely used for allergic diseases treatment in China (Tao et al., 2018). The Modified Guo Min decoction (MGMD) comprises Fang Feng (*Radix Saposhnikoviae divaricate*, FF), Wu Mei (*Fructus Mume*, WM), Wu Wei Zi (*Schisandra chinensis*, WWZ), Yin Chai Hu (*Radix Stellariae*, YCH), Qian Hu (*radix Peucedani*, QH), and Jie Geng (*Radix Platycodi*, JG). Previous studies showed that prescriptions based on GMD increased the proportion of Th1 cells in the spleen tissue of asthmatic mice, reduced the Th2 subset of T cells, and balanced the number of Treg and Th17 cells (Qin et al., 2017). However, the therapeutic mechanisms of MGMD in asthma remain unclear. In this study, network pharmacology approach was used to explore the multi-components, multi-targets, and multi-pathways closely related to the anti-asthma effect of MGMD. The molecular docking method was also used to verify the binding of the active substance to the target of action to reveal and predict the efficacy of MGMD in asthma. The work scheme is shown in **Figure 1**.

Abbreviations: AD, anti-allergic decoction; ADME, absorption, distribution, metabolism, and excretion; ALOX5, arachidonate 5-lipoxygenase; BP, biological process; H-C-T, herb-compound-target; DHA, docosahexaenoic acid; DL, drug-likeness; FF, Fangfeng (*Saposhnikoviae Radix*); EPA, Eicosapentaenoic acid; GO, Gene ontology; HL, Half-life; JG, Jiegeng (*Platycodon grandiflorus*); JUN, c-Jun NH2-terminal kinase; MGMD, Modified Guo Min decoction; MF, molecular function; OB, oral bioavailability; PPI, Protein–protein interaction; PUFA, polyunsaturated fatty acid; QH, Qianhu (*Peucedanum praeruptorum*); SPM, Specialized pro-resolving mediator; TCM, traditional Chinese medicine; TCMSP, traditional Chinese medicine system pharmacology database; VEGFA, vascular endothelial growth factor A; WM, Wumei (*Prunus mume*); WWZ, Wuweizi (*Schisandra chinensis*); YCH, Yinchaihu (*Stellaria dichotoma L. var. lanceolata Bge*).

MATERIALS AND METHODS

Active Compounds Collection

The compounds of MGMD were extracted from the HERB database[1] (Fang et al., 2020) and the encyclopedia of traditional Chinese medicine (ETCM)[2] (Xu et al., 2019). HERB contains a comprehensive list of 7263 TCM herbs and 49258 ingredients by integrating multiple TCM databases included SymMap (Wu et al., 2019), TCMID 2.0 (Huang et al., 2018), TCMSP 2.3 (Ru et al., 2014), and TCM-ID (Chen et al., 2006). Oral bioavailability (OB) $\geq$ 30% and drug-likeness (DL) $\geq$ 0.18 were set as the thresholds to screen the active compounds from the TCMSP[3]. The properties of the other ingredients collected from the HERB were retrieved from the Swiss absorption, distribution, metabolism, and excretion (ADME) database[4]. The SMILES format files of the compounds were obtained from the PubChem[5] database (Kim et al., 2019). The screening criterion for gastrointestinal GI absorption was set as high, and DL was satisfied with both "yes" at the same time (Daina et al., 2017). Active ingredients from ETCM were retrieved as DL Grading "Good" (Xu et al., 2019).

Target Fishing

Identification of Predicted Targets of MGMD

The active ingredients in drugs exert their biological effects via molecular targets. The targets related to the active compounds presented in MGMD were searched from ETCM (Xu et al., 2019) and Similarity ensemble approach (SEA)[6] (Keiser et al., 2007). ETCM predicts targets by MedChem Studio and only outputs these targets with confidence score at least 0.8. The threshold of "human" and Tanimoto coefficients (Tc) > 0.57 were set to filter results predicted by SEA. The key targets corresponding to the compounds in such six herbs were obtained.

Building the Disease Target Database

Asthma-related targets were identified by integrating data from these databases: Comparative Toxicogenomics Database (CTD)[7]

[1]http://herb.ac.cn

[2]http://www.tcmip.cn/ETCM/index.php/Home/Index/

[3]http://tcmspw.com/tcmsp.php

[4]http://www.swissadme.ch/

[5]https://pubchem.ncbi.nlm.nih.gov/

[6]http://sea.bkslab.org

[7]http://ctdbase.org/

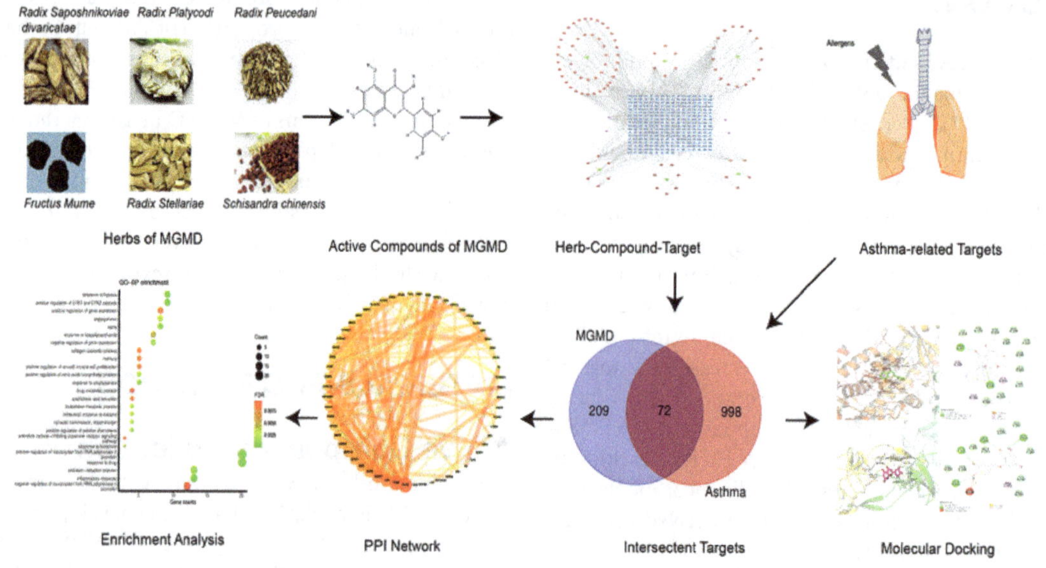

FIGURE 1 | Flowchart summarizing the work scheme of the study.

(Grondin et al., 2018), Online Mendelian Inheritance in Man (OMIM)[8] (Amberger and Hamosh, 2017), and the Human Gene Database (GeneCards)[9] (Safran et al., 2010). For filtering the targets, "asthma" was defined as the key word and results were restricted to human genes/proteins. Targets with a relevance score above the median were selected in GeneCards database. The overlapping targets between MGMD and asthma were likely to be potential action targets of MGMD in the treatment of asthma.

PPI Network Construction and Analysis

To obtain the data of protein–protein interaction (PPI), the candidate targets were inputted to STRING[10] with a minimum required interaction score > 0.7 and limited to "Homo sapiens" specie (von Mering et al., 2005). The visual network graphs were created by Cytoscape (version 3.7.1)[11], an open-source software platform for visualizing complex networks (Shannon et al., 2003). The target interaction network parameters were calculated by NetworkAnalyzer.

Molecular Complex Detection (MCODE) of Cytoscape was used to searching the highly connected sub-networks in the PPI network. In the illustrations depicting MCODE results, a vertex-weighting-based scheme was used to identify local high-density areas in the graph. Density was generally defined based on the connection level of the graph (Bader and Hogue, 2003).

Protein Functional Enrichment Analysis

To reveal the potential biological functions of MGMD in the treatment of asthma, functional enrichment analyses were performed by the Database for Annotation, Visualization and Integrated Discovery (DAVID, v6.8)[12] and Reactome[13] (Fabregat et al., 2018). The results for Gene ontology (GO) biological processes (BPs) and Reactome pathway enrichment were saved and sorted by the adjusted *P* value corrected by the false discovery rate (FDR) algorithm for each term.

Network Construction

To demonstrate the multi-compound therapeutic features of MGMD, network constructions were performed as follows: (1) herb-compound-target Network (H-C-T network) was constructed to explore the active compounds and their potential targets. The core compounds were obtained through the H-C-T network. (2) PPI networks were built to analyze the target interactions. Hub targets involved in MGMD treatment of asthma were selected from the PPI network. (3) BP sub-networks were established for classification analysis of BPs in MGMD treatment for asthma. (4) Target pathway network (T-P network) was constructed to show the functional pathways of MGMD for the therapy of asthma.

Molecular Docking

Molecular docking was conducted to validate if MGMD's compounds could bind to these targets. The 2D structures of the top five core compounds were downloaded from the TCMSP database (Ru et al., 2014). The structures were added charge and displayed rotatable keys by AutoDock Tools (version 1.5.6). The protein crystal structures corresponding to the core target genes were downloaded from the Protein Data Bank database (PDB)[14] (Burley et al., 2017). Water and hetero molecules of the proteins were removed by Pymol. Hydrogen atoms and charge operations

[8]https://omim.org/
[9]https://www.genecards.org/
[10]http://string-db.org
[11]http://www.cytoscape.org/
[12]https://david.ncifcrf.gov/
[13]https://reactome.org/
[14]http://www1.rcsb.org/

to the proteins was added by AutoDock Tools. The 3D Grid box for molecular docking simulation was also obtained by AutoDock tools was displayed by AutoDock Vina (version 1.1.2) (Trott and Olson, 2010). The results were analyzed and interpreted by PyMOL and Discovery Studio 2020.

RESULTS

Construction of Herb-Compound-Target Network

In this study, 96 active compounds were screened from the six herbs in MGMD. Among them, 51, 19, 7, 6, 8, and 5 compounds were from FF, QH, JG, WM, WWZ, and YCH, respectively. MGMD contains a complex mixture of ingredients, some of them overlapped across 2 herbs, including decursinol, deoxygomisin A, nodakenetin, and naringenin. A total of 92 active compounds were identified after eliminating redundant entries.

Five hundred and twenty-three targets were associated with the 92 components identified in MGMD, of which 149 were associated with FF, 151 with QH, 83 with JG, 77 with WM, 23 with WWZ, and 40 with YCH. After eliminating overlapping targets, there were 281 targets remaining.

The H-C-T network of MGMD was visualized in Cytoscape (**Figure 2**). The network contained 379 nodes and 1021 edges. Quercetin showed the highest degree of connectivity in the network with 76 targets, followed by wogonin with 57, luteolin with 55, naringenin with 51, and kaempferol with 40. The properties of the H-C-T network were suitable for displaying complex ingredients, multiple targets, and close interactions between ingredients and targets. Detailed information about the active compounds and targets identified in MGMD is shown in **Supplementary Table 1**.

Potential Asthma Targets

The targets for asthma were integrated from multi-source databases and a final list of 1,070 disease-related targets obtained after eliminating duplicates (**Supplementary Table 2**). 72 overlapping targets were identified as the key targets for studying the anti-asthmatic activity of the MGMD compounds (**Supplementary Table 3**).

Analysis of the Network of Overlapping Targets

Protein–Protein Interaction (PPI) Network

The STRING database was used to acquire PPI relationships of 72 potential protein targets of MGMD as related to the treatment of asthma. The visualized PPI network was constructed by Cystoscape 3.7.1, constructing by 72 nodes represented proteins and 205 edges represented the interactions between the proteins (**Figure 3A** and **Supplementary Table 4**). The average node degree value of the PPI network was 6.508. 28 protein targets had significantly higher node degree than the average in the PPI network, including STAT3, PTGS2,

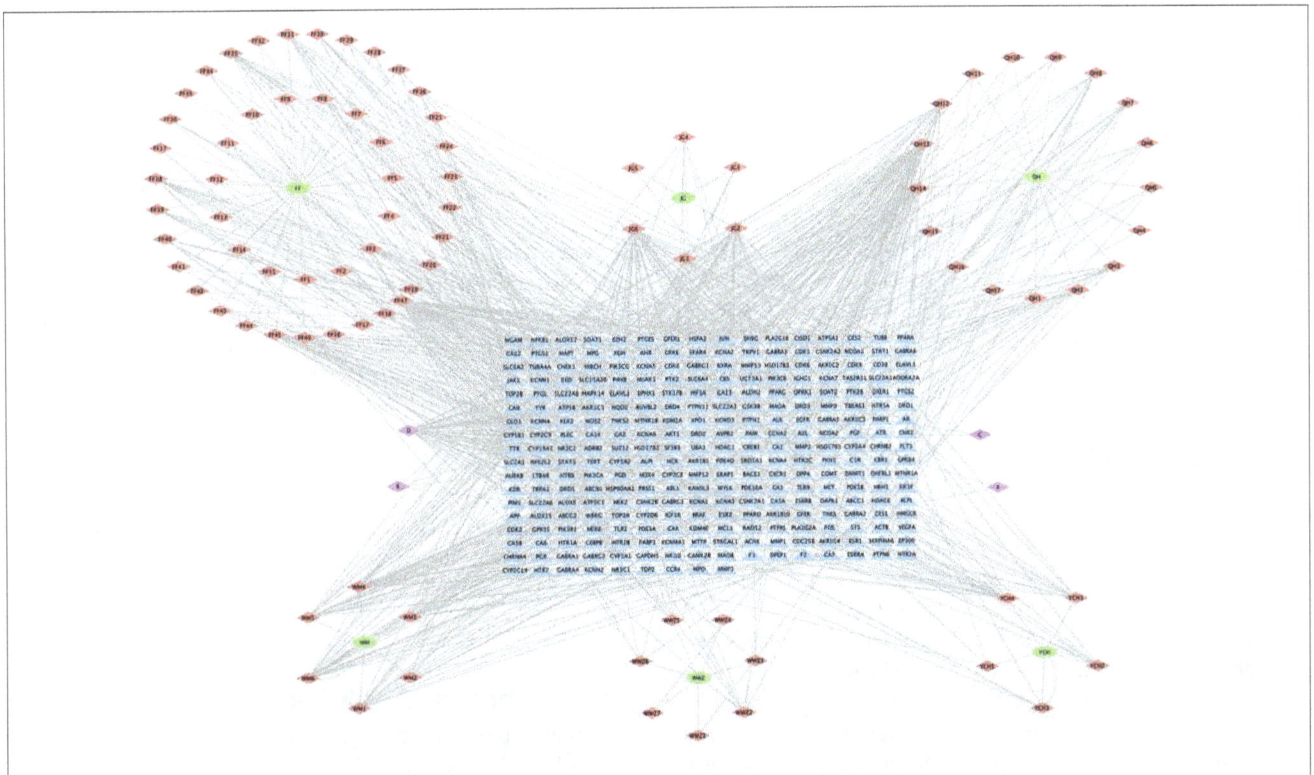

FIGURE 2 | Herb-Compound-Target network (H-C-T network) of MGMD. Green ellipses represent the herbs present in MGMD; pink diamonds represent active compounds in each herb; purple diamonds represent active compounds shared by two herbs, and blue triangles correspond to related targets (The IDs of the components are described in **Supplementary Table 1**).

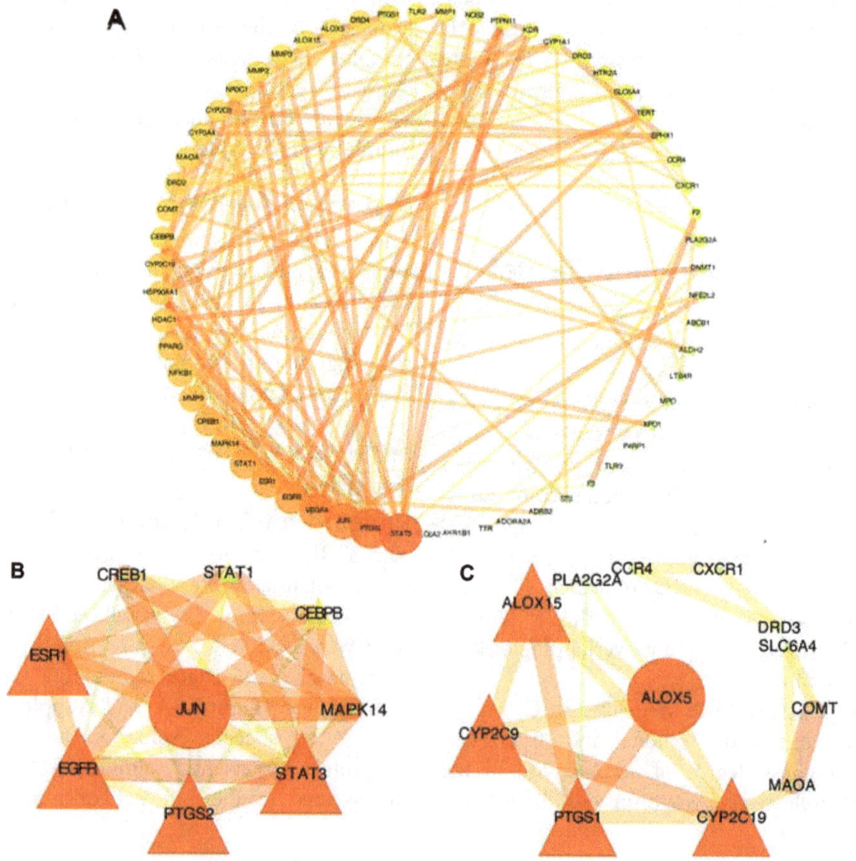

FIGURE 3 | PPI networks of MGMD for asthma treatment. Each node represents a protein target and each line represents the interaction between two nodes. Nodes in red are important and nodes in green are less important in the network. Panel **(A)** is the PPI network diagram arranged according to the df. Two clusters detected in the MGMD-asthma PPI network. Panels **(B,C)** show clusters 1 and 2, respectively. The ellipses are seed nodes of each cluster.

JUN, vascular endothelial growth factor A (VEGFA), EGFR, ESR1, STAT1, CREB1, MAPK14, MMP9, NFKB1, PPARG, CYP2C19, HDAC1, HSP90AA1, CYP3A4, COMT, MAOA, CYP2C9, DRD2, CEBPB, ALOX15, PTGS1, arachidonate 5-lipoxygenase (ALOX5), DRD4, NR3C1, MMP3, and MMP2. These 28 targets showed the preliminary relationships between active compound and potential protein targets of MGMD treatment in asthma.

Clustering Analysis of the PPI Network

Similar function clusters of the PPI network were selected by MCODE analysis based on topology to find densely interconnected regions using Cytoscape software. 2 clusters of functional modules were detected (K-core = 4) and the attribute values of the cluster were shown in **Figures 3B,C.**

Clusters in a PPI network are often protein complexes and parts of pathways, while clusters in a protein similarity network represent protein families. Cluster 1 comprised nine nodes and 33 edges with a score of 8.250 (**Figure 3B**). The seed node of this cluster was JUN (Jun proto-oncogene, also known as AP-1, cJUN, c-Jun), which involved in cell proliferation, differentiation, migration, transformation, and programmed cell death (Liu and Lin, 2007). Cluster 2 comprised 12 nodes and 21 sides with a score of 3.818 (**Figure 3C**). The seed node of this cluster was ALOX5 (arachidonate 5-lipoxygenase, also known as 5-LO, 5-LOX), an essential enzyme in the metabolism of arachidonic acid, which initiates the biosynthesis of leukotrienes (Bruno et al., 2018). Leukotrienes are powerful immune-regulating lipid mediators with established pathogenic roles in asthma. The connected proteins of ALOX5 in cluster 2 participating in the biosynthetic pathways of SPMs (Barnig et al., 2018; Kytikova et al., 2019), such as ALOX15 (15-LOX), cytochrome P450 proteins CYP2C9 and CYP2C19, are among the 28 protein targets which had higher node degree than the average in our PPI network. Thus, the constructed PPI network and the further functional clustering both indicate that MGMD intervene asthma by regulating SPMs biosynthesis.

GO Enrichment Analysis

To further explore the biological functions of the 72 potential targets of MGMD, GO enrichment analysis was constructed on DAVID website and obtained 76 terms (FDR < 0.05) of BPs. We found the top 25 most enriched BP terms represented in a bubble chart (**Figure 4A** and **Supplementary Table 5**). BP analysis

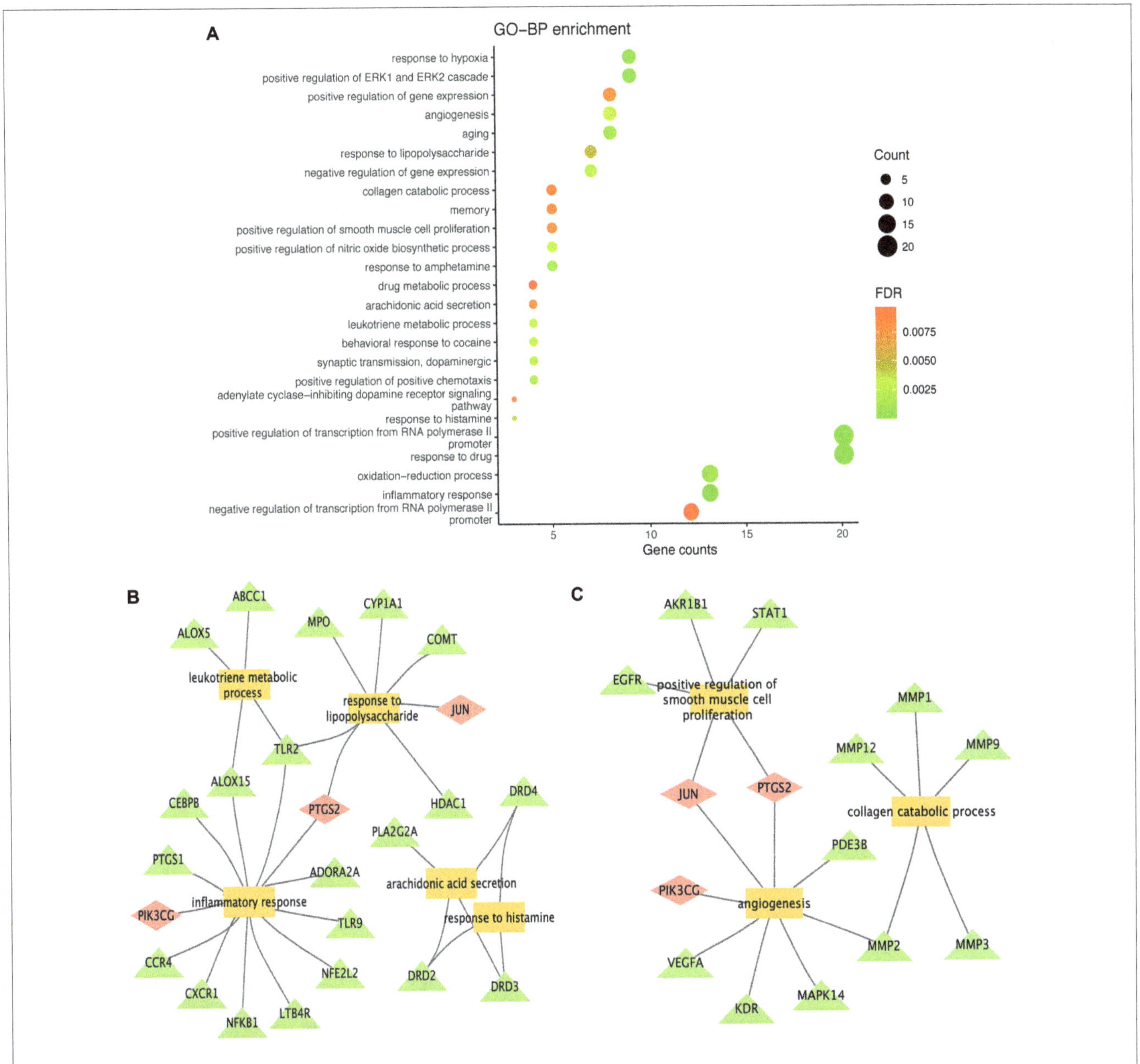

FIGURE 4 | Results of GO term enrichment analysis of targets. The GO bar plot represents the top 25 biological (BP) process **(A)**; inflammation and airway remodeling related to functional clusters represented by panels **(B,C)**, respectively. The yellow squares represent biological processes, the green triangles represent genes, and the pink diamonds represent genes common to both categories.

revealed that the potential targets of MGMD were remarkably enriched in inflammation and airway remodeling.

As shown in **Figure 4B**, the potential targets of MGMD were involved in inflammatory response (GO ID: 0006954), response to lipopolysaccharide (GO ID: 0032496), leukotriene metabolic process (GO ID: 0006691), arachidonic acid secretion (GO ID: 0050482) and positive regulation of nitric oxide biosynthetic process (GO ID: 0045429). In addition, the BPs of airway remodeling were mainly enriched in positive regulation of smooth muscle cell proliferation (GO ID: 0048661), angiogenesis (GO ID: 0001525) and collagen catabolic process (GO ID: 0030574) (**Figure 4C**).

Pathway Enrichment Analysis

Reactome pathway enrichment analysis obtained 123 items (FDR < 0.05) and the top 16 pathways at a significance threshold of FDR $< 10^{-5}$ were displayed (**Figure 5A** and **Table 1**). The pathways result was intensively enriched in SPMs biosynthesis and inflammatory and immune response, including arachidonic acid metabolism, metabolism of lipids, biosynthesis of EPA-derived SPMs, biosynthesis of DHA-derived SPMs, biosynthesis of DPAn-3 SPMs, interleukin-4 and interleukin-13 signaling, and signaling by interleukins and immune system.

The T-P network showed the associations of the top 16 pathways with 75 nodes and 187 edges (**Figure 5B**). The results

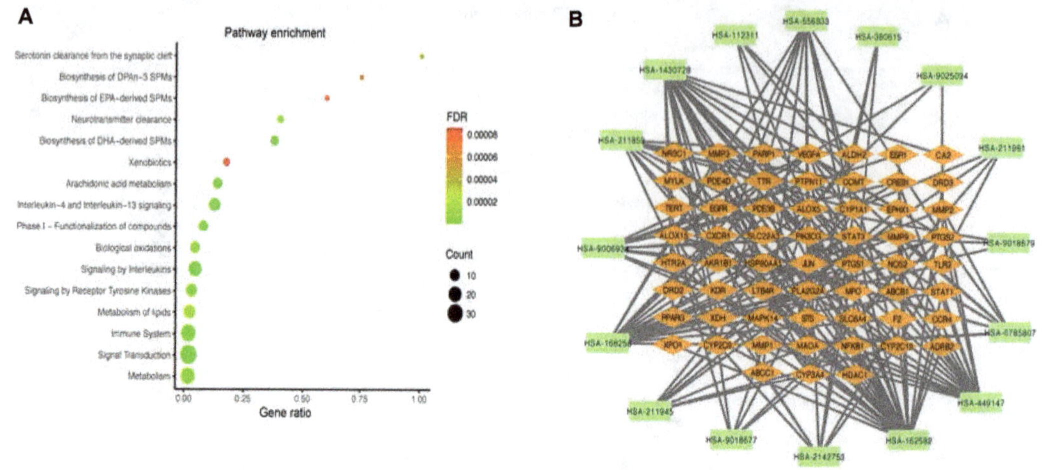

FIGURE 5 | Results of the pathway analysis of the top 16 pathways: Bubble diagram of pathway **(A)** and T-P network diagram **(B)**.

TABLE 1 | Information on enrichment analysis based on Reactome.

Term ID	Pathway	Counts	FDR	Genes
HSA-6785807	Interleukin-4 and Interleukin-13 signaling	13	2.47E-13	MMP2, STAT3, MMP3, MMP1, NOS2, HSP90AA1, MAOA, STAT1, PTGS2, MMP9, ALOX5, ALOX15, VEGFA
HSA-449147	Signaling by Interleukins	18	1.16E-11	MMP2, NFKB1, MAPK14, STAT3, MMP3, MMP1, NOS2, HSP90AA1, MAOA, PTPN11, STAT1, PTGS2, JUN, MMP9, ALOX5, CREB1, ALOX15, VEGFA
HSA-162582	Signal Transduction	33	4.72E-09	NFKB1, MAPK14, NR3C1, TTR, KDR, STAT3, EGFR, PDE3B, PPARG, CXCR1, MMP3, ADRB2, F2, TERT, CCR4, HSP90AA1, PTPN11, PDE4D, PIK3CG, MYLK, STAT1, DRD2, PARP1, JUN, MMP9, HDAC1, DRD3, LTB4R, XPO1, CREB1, ESR1, HTR2A, VEGFA
HSA-2142753	Arachidonic acid metabolism	8	1.49E-08	CYP2C9, PTGS1, PTGS2, CYP2C19, ALOX5, CYP1A1, ABCC1, ALOX15
HSA-9018677	Biosynthesis of DHA-derived SPMs	6	1.49E-08	CYP2C9, CYP3A4, PTGS2, ALOX5, CYP1A1, ALOX15
HSA-211945	Phase I - Functionalization of compounds	8	6.39E-07	CYP2C9, ALDH2, CYP3A4, MAOA, PTGS1, CYP2C19, CYP1A1, EPHX1
HSA-168256	Immune System	25	7.37E-07	MMP2, MPO, NFKB1, MAPK14, TTR, TLR2, STAT3, CXCR1, MMP3, F2, MMP1, NOS2, HSP90AA1, MAOA, PTPN11, STAT1, PTGS2, JUN, MMP9, ALOX5, XDH, PLA2G2A, CREB1, ALOX15, VEGFA
HSA-9006934	Signaling by Receptor Tyrosine Kinases	12	4.85E-06	MAPK14, KDR, STAT3, EGFR, PDE3B, HSP90AA1, PTPN11, STAT1, MMP9, CREB1, ESR1, VEGFA
HSA-211859	Biological oxidations	9	6.89E-06	CYP2C9, ALDH2, CYP3A4, MAOA, COMT, PTGS1, CYP2C19, CYP1A1, EPHX1
HSA-1430728	Metabolism	24	7.31E-06	STS, TTR, CYP2C9, ALDH2, SLC22A3, CA2, AKR1B1, PPARG, HSP90AA1, CYP3A4, MAOA, PIK3CG, COMT, PTGS1, PTGS2, CYP2C19, ALOX5, XDH, CYP1A1, ABCC1, PLA2G2A, ALOX15, ABCB1, EPHX1
HSA-112311	Neurotransmitter clearance	4	7.71E-06	SLC6A4, ALDH2, MAOA, COMT
HSA-556833	Metabolism of lipids	14	1.54E-05	STS, CYP2C9, AKR1B1, PPARG, CYP3A4, PIK3CG, PTGS1, PTGS2, CYP2C19, ALOX5, CYP1A1, ABCC1, PLA2G2A, ALOX15
HSA-380615	Serotonin clearance from the synaptic cleft	3	3.63E-05	SLC6A4, ALDH2, MAOA
HSA-9025094	Biosynthesis of DPAn-3 SPMs	3	5.97E-05	PTGS2, ALOX5, ALOX15
HSA-211981	Xenobiotics	4	8.52E-05	CYP2C9, CYP3A4, CYP2C19, CYP1A1
HSA-9018679	Biosynthesis of EPA-derived SPMs	3	8.52E-05	PTGS2, ALOX5, ALOX15

revealed that the active compounds of the MGMD had effects on asthma through regulating various pathways, in particular through improving airway inflammatory infiltration resulted from Th2 cytokine production and lipid mediators.

Molecular Docking Verification of Core Compounds and Core Protein Targets

Furthermore, we verified the binding affinity between core compounds and protein targets of MGMD by molecular docking. As screened in H-C-T network, quercetin, wogonin, luteolin, naringenin, and kaempferol were the core compounds of MGMD. The hub protein targets were identified by top 5 node degree of PPI network and seed node of clusters, included STAT3, PTGS2, JUN, VEGFA, EGFR, and ALOX5.

The results obtained by the molecular docking software were shown in **Table 2**. The Grid box was centered to cover the active binding site and all essential residues. For the STAT3, grid box (126Å × 60Å × 126Å) centered at (0.233, 28.877, 33.555) Å, for the PTGS2, grid box (76Å × 94Å × 90Å) centered at (33.269, −4.946, 7.759) Å, for the JUN, grid box (90Å × 72Å × 70Å) centered at (−16.564, 23.05, 26.225) Å, for the VEGFA, grid box (58Å × 40Å × 40Å) centered at (2.965, −4.946, 7.759) Å, for the EGFR, grid box (126Å × 126Å × 126Å) centered at (80.339, 11.821, 66.594) Å, for the ALOX5, grid box (70Å × 90Å × 96Å) centered at (4.01, 45.829, 3.32) Å. As seen from **Table 2**, the binding affinity for the five core compounds and protein crystal structures corresponding to the core target genes were all greater than −5 kcal/mol, indicating that the compound had a certain affinity for the protein crystal structure. Wogonin showed the high binding affinity of −8.8 kcal/mol in ALOX5, −6.2 kcal/mol in JUN and −6.2 kcal/mol in VEGFA. Luteolin showed the high binding affinity of −8.3 kcal/mol in EGFR, −9.3 kcal/mol in PTGS2 and −7.9 kcal/mol in STAT3. The small-molecule compounds were tightly bound to the protein residues via various interactions (**Figure 6** and **Table 2**).

TABLE 2 | The binding energy values of core compounds of MGMD and core targets.

Target	Compounds	binding affinity/(kcal/mol)
STAT3(6tlc)	Quercetin	−7.5
	Wogonin	−7.5
	Luteolin	−7.9
	Naringenin	−7.3
	Kaempferol	−7.7
PTGS2(5ikr)	Quercetin	−9.1
	Wogonin	−8.9
	Luteolin	−9.3
	Naringenin	−9
	Kaempferol	−9
JUN(5T01)	Quercetin	−5.9
	Wogonin	−6.2
	Luteolin	−5.9
	Naringenin	−5.8
	Kaempferol	−6.2
VEGRA(4kzn)	Quercetin	−5.8
	Wogonin	−6.2
	Luteolin	−5.8
	Naringenin	−5.7
	Kaempferol	−6
EGFR(5wb7)	Quercetin	−7.9
	Wogonin	−7.9
	Luteolin	−8.3
	Naringenin	−7.4
	Kaempferol	−7.9
ALOX5(3o8y)	Quercetin	−8.3
	Wogonin	−8.8
	Luteolin	−8.5
	Naringenin	−8.3
	Kaempferol	−8.2

DISCUSSION

Asthma is a major public health challenge in China that affecting 45.7 million adults aged 20 years or older (Huang et al., 2019). TCM has a long history of clinical practice with available records, which provides a considerable number of classical herbal formulas widely used for disease treatment and represents a unique resource for drug development (Chao et al., 2017). Among the complex mixtures of compounds present in herbal medicines, unique combinations in the traditional complex formulas may exert major efficacy by targeting specific nodes of cellular signaling to intervene a specific chronic disease (Stermitz et al., 2000). Network pharmacology is used to study the intervention mechanism of drugs on diseases by constructing a biological interaction network (Yang et al., 2013). It systematically reveals the therapeutic effects of drugs on diseases from the interaction relationship between drugs, targets, and disease (Liu J. et al., 2018; Zhang et al., 2018). In a previous clinical study, we have found that MGMD had significant efficacy on respiratory symptoms (Zhang, 2016). To provide further insight of underlying mechanisms, we used the systematic pharmacology method and molecular docking to explore the potential molecular mechanism of the bioactive compounds.

We obtained 92 active compounds of MGMD from HERB, ECTM, SEA databases. A total of 72 putative anti-asthmatic targets of MGMD were selected by overlapping the targets between the MGMD-associated targets and the predicted asthma targets. According the H-C-T network topological analysis, we found the core compounds contained quercetin, wogonin, luteolin, naringenin, and kaempferol. Intriguingly, these compounds have all been reported to have therapeutic effects on inflammatory disease in previous studies. It had been demonstrated that all of the five core ingredients can reduce the allergic airway inflammation, inhibit levels of Th2 cytokine, including IL-4, IL-5, and IL-13, in OVA-sensitized and-challenged animals (Park et al., 2009; Shi et al., 2014; Bui et al., 2017; Jang et al., 2017; Molitorisova et al., 2021). Moreover, quercetin can inhibit human neutrophil elastase-induced MUC5AC expression in human airway epithelial cells through PKC/EGFR/ERK signal transduction pathway (Li et al., 2012). Both wogonin and luteolin had effect on reduction of airway mucus production (Lucas et al., 2015; Wang et al., 2021),

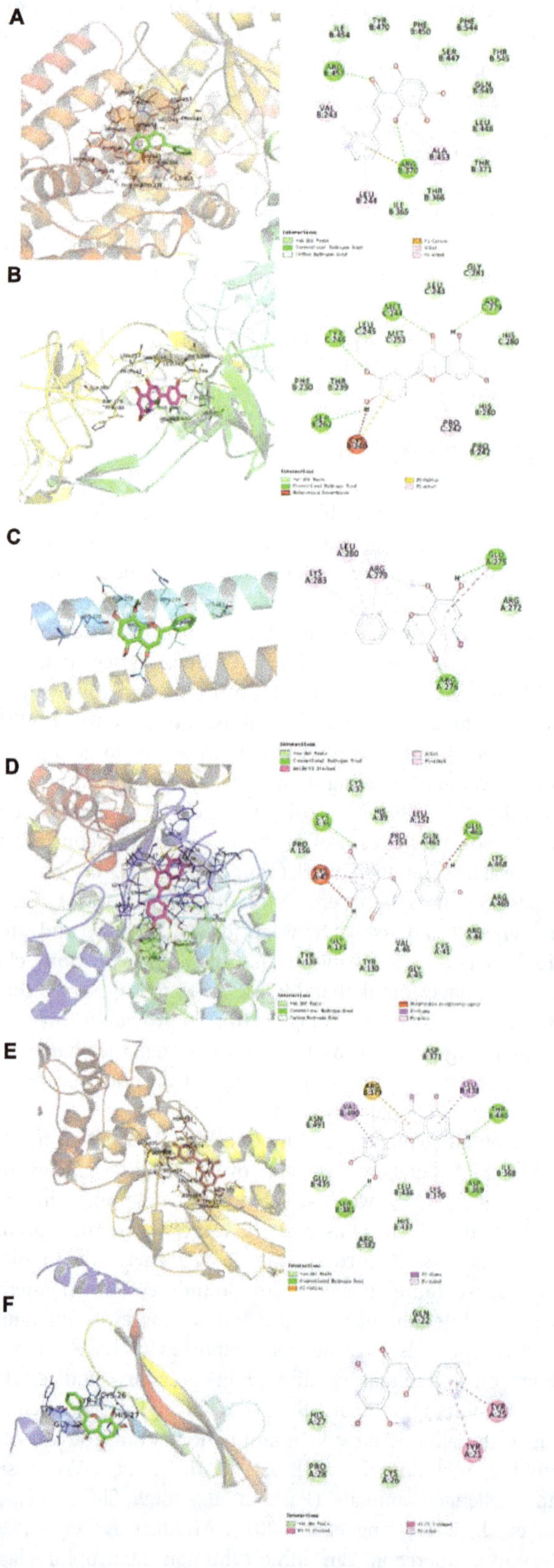

FIGURE 6 | Molecular docking diagram of ALOX5 **(A)**, JUN **(B)**, VEGFA **(C)** complexed with wogonin; EGFR **(D)**, PTGS2 **(E)**, and STAT3 **(F)** complexed with luteolin.

meanwhile luteolin can also decrease collagen deposition *in vovo* (Wang et al., 2021). In addition, it had reported that kaempferol alleviated airway inflammation through modulating Tyk2-STAT1/3 signaling responsive (Gong et al., 2013), and suppressed COX2 expression level in lung tissues in asthmatic mice (Kang et al., 2018). These previous studies suggest that MGMD is likely to decrease Th2 cytokine production in asthma mainly through compound of quercetin, wogonin, luteolin, naringenin, and kaempferol.

The PPI network was constructed by 72 potential targets of MGMD which were involved in asthma, and the network was further analyzed by MCODE clustering to explore the asthma related pathways. Our results suggested that the core potential targets of MGMD were intensively enriched in the pathways related to SPMs biosynthesis, including ALOX5 (5-LOX), ALOX15 (15-LOX), PTGS1 (COX1), PTGS2 (COX2), cytochrome P450 proteins CYP2C9 and CYP2C19, which paly pivotal role in the resolution of inflammation in asthma (Schett and Neurath, 2018; Kytikova et al., 2019). 5-LOX is a crucial enzyme which helps in the conversion of arachidonic acid to leukotrienes. With the increasing number of indications for anti-leukotriene drugs, the development of 5-LOX inhibitor agents for asthma becomes increasingly important (Bruno et al., 2018; Sinha et al., 2019). Our results argue a potential that MGMD is a 5-LOX inhibitor for the treatment of asthma, in turn suggest a promising mechanism by which MGMD intervene asthma.

Furthermore, STAT3, JUN, EGFR, and VEGFA were also the core potential targets in our PPI network results. STAT3 and JUN are closely related to the pathological process of asthma (Simeone-Penney et al., 2007; García-Menaya et al., 2019). STAT3 can induce gene expression of cytokines, chemokines, and adhesion molecules with an important role in directing the inflammatory response and act as a novel epithelial regulator of the allergic response by altering Th2 cell recruitment and effector function (Schumann et al., 1996; Simeone-Penney et al., 2007). JUN activation appears to be implicated in airway inflammation by contributing to regulate the expression of Th2 cytokines, chemokines, growth factors, and adhesion molecules, which is associated with several inflammation related disorders such as asthma and allergy (Haeggström and Funk, 2011). There are extensive studies focusing on the relation among EGFR, VEGFA and asthma pathophysiology, which describe airway remodeling, airway hypermucus secretion, as well as immunological responses of airway inflammation (Hoshino et al., 2001; Lee et al., 2004; Burgel and Nadel, 2008; Inoue et al., 2020). MGMD compounds may exert anti-inflammatory and anti-remodeling activity through regulating STAT3, JUN, EGFR, and VEGFA.

The GO enrichment results strengthen the evidence that candidate protein targets of MGMD are involved in airway inflammation and remodeling. The enriched BPs of anti-inflammatory in our results included inflammatory response, leukotriene metabolic process and arachidonic acid secretion, suggesting that MGMD could influenced the lipid mediators, both pro-inflammatory mediators and SPMs, to ameliorate the airway inflammation in asthma patients. Moreover, the typical airway remodeling processes, including positive regulation of

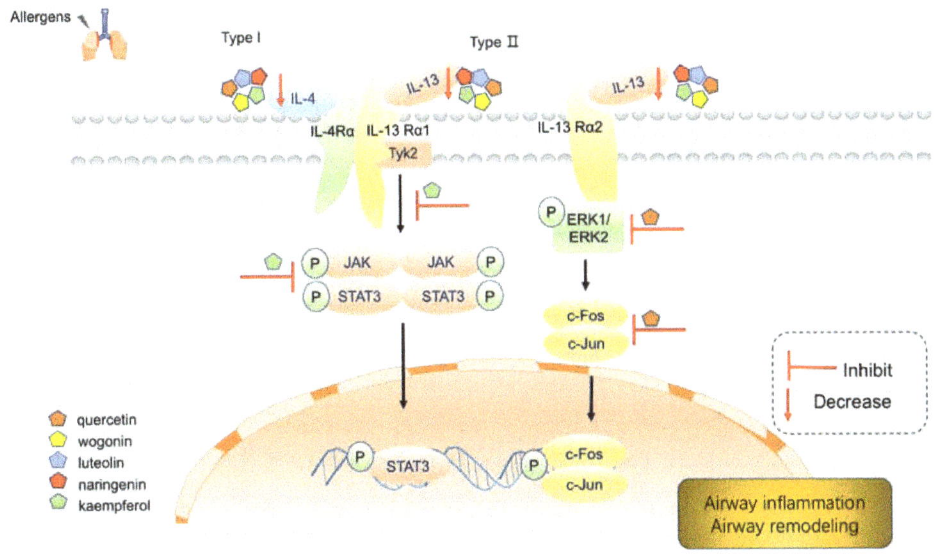

FIGURE 7 | Schematic diagram depicting main components of MGMD inhibits IL-4 and IL-13 to mitigate airway allergic responses.

smooth muscle cell proliferation, angiogenesis and collagen catabolic process, were also enriched by MGMD related targets. Combined with the PPI network results, we propose that MGMD regulates SPMs biosynthesis by ALOX5 to reduce airway inflammation and relieve airway remodeling process by suppressing the EGFR and VEGFA signaling.

Our Reactome pathway enrichment results consistently argue that MGMD reduces allergic airway inflammation through the biosynthetic pathways of SPMs. Arachidonic acid metabolism, metabolism of lipids, biosynthesis of EPA-derived SPMs, biosynthesis of DHA-derived SPMs and biosynthesis of DPAn-3 SPMs were all enriched in Reactome pathway enrichment analysis. Additionally, interleukin-4 and interleukin-13 signaling, signaling by interleukins and immune system pathways were also enriched in our results. IL-4 and IL-13 are principal regulatory cytokines mainly secreted by activated Th2 cells, crucially important during the immune response in allergy and asthma (Nelms et al., 1999; Hershey, 2003). The receptors of allergic cytokines, including IL-4, IL-5, and IL-13, trigger the JAK/STAT pathway (Hsieh et al., 2011; Howell et al., 2018). Therefore, we propose that MGMD compounds targets the IL-4 and IL-13 pathway, which in turn activate transcription factors to modulate clinical symptoms of asthma (**Figure 7**).

According to the compound-target interaction analysis, six targets with higher degrees on the PPI network (STAT3, PTGS2, JUN, VEGFA, EGFR, and ALOX5) were identified. In our molecular docking analysis, the binding mode with the best docking score was selected to analyze the interaction between the protein receptor and its predicted active compounds. The docking scores of all compound-target pairs are lower than −5 kcal/mol, indicating that each of the five core compounds (quercetin, wogonin, luteolin, naringenin, and kaempferol) has good binding affinity to all six targets. These results suggested that the core ingredients of MGMD could relieve airway inflammation and remodeling through binding STAT3, PTGS2, JUN, VEGFA, EGFR, and ALOX5.

CONCLUSION

On the ground of the above, network pharmacology strategy was presented to investigate the active compounds, potential anti-asthmatic targets and involved regulatory pathways in MGMD. Our results revealed the active ingredients and potential molecular mechanism by which MGMD treatment is effective against airway inflammation and remodeling in asthma through regulating IL-4 and IL-13 signaling and SPMs biosynthesis. These findings were partially validated previous studies. Our subsequent molecular docking showed that each bioactive compounds (quercetin, wogonin, luteolin, naringenin, and kaempferol) of MGMD has favorable binding abilities with STAT3, PTGS2, JUN, VEGFA, EGFR, and ALOX5, further arguing the potential molecular mechanism of action of MGMD in asthma. Our results will serve as a comprehensive reference for investigation of the mechanism by which MGMD intervene asthma.

AUTHOR CONTRIBUTIONS

GW, BZ, and ZW: conceptualization. GW and BZ: methodology and visualization. BZ: software. GW and ZW: writing–original draft preparation. BZ, YM, YL, and XY: writing–review and editing. XY and CF: supervision and project administration. All authors have read and agreed to the published version of the manuscript.

ACKNOWLEDGMENTS

We would like to thank Editage (www.editage.cn) for English language editing.

REFERENCES

Amberger, J. S., and Hamosh, A. (2017). Searching Online Mendelian Inheritance in Man (OMIM): a Knowledgebase of Human Genes and Genetic Phenotypes. *Curr. Protoc. Bioinformatics* 58, 1.2.1–1.2.12. doi: 10.1002/cpbi.27

Bader, G. D., and Hogue, C. W. V. (2003). An automated method for finding molecular complexes in large protein interaction networks. *BMC Bioinformatics* 4:2. doi: 10.1186/1471-2105-4-2

Barnig, C., Frossard, N., and Levy, B. D. (2018). Towards targeting resolution pathways of airway inflammation in asthma. *Pharmacol. Ther.* 186, 98–113. doi: 10.1016/j.pharmthera.2018.01.004

Bruno, F., Spaziano, G., Liparulo, A., Roviezzo, F., Nabavi, S. M., Sureda, A., et al. (2018). Recent advances in the search for novel 5-lipoxygenase inhibitors for the treatment of asthma. *Eur. J. Med. Chem.* 153, 65–72. doi: 10.1016/j.ejmech.2017.10.020

Bui, T. T., Piao, C. H., Song, C. H., Lee, C.-H., Shin, H. S., and Chai, O. H. (2017). Baicalein, wogonin, and Scutellaria baicalensis ethanol extract alleviate ovalbumin-induced allergic airway inflammation and mast cell-mediated anaphylactic shock by regulation of Th1/Th2 imbalance and histamine release. *Anat. Cell Biol.* 50, 124–134. doi: 10.5115/acb.2017.50.2.124

Burgel, P.-R., and Nadel, J. A. (2008). Epidermal growth factor receptor-mediated innate immune responses and their roles in airway diseases. *Eur. Respir. J.* 32, 1068–1081. doi: 10.1183/09031936.00172007

Burley, S. K., Berman, H. M., Kleywegt, G. J., Markley, J. L., Nakamura, H., and Velankar, S. (2017). Protein Data Bank (PDB): the Single Global Macromolecular Structure Archive. *Methods Mol. Biol.* 1607, 627–641. doi: 10.1007/978-1-4939-7000-1_26

Chao, J., Dai, Y., Verpoorte, R., Lam, W., Cheng, Y.-C., Pao, L.-H., et al. (2017). Major achievements of evidence-based traditional Chinese medicine in treating major diseases. *Biochem. Pharmacol.* 139, 94–104. doi: 10.1016/j.bcp.2017.06.123

Chen, X., Zhou, H., Liu, Y. B., Wang, J. F., Li, H., Ung, C. Y., et al. (2006). Database of traditional Chinese medicine and its application to studies of mechanism and to prescription validation. *Br. J. Pharmacol.* 149, 1092–1103. doi: 10.1038/sj.bjp.0706945

Daina, A., Michielin, O., and Zoete, V. (2017). SwissADME: a free web tool to evaluate pharmacokinetics, drug-likeness and medicinal chemistry friendliness of small molecules. *Sci. Rep.* 7:42717. doi: 10.1038/srep42717

Fabregat, A., Jupe, S., Matthews, L., Sidiropoulos, K., Gillespie, M., Garapati, P., et al. (2018). The Reactome Pathway Knowledgebase. *Nucleic Acids Res.* 46, D649–D655. doi: 10.1093/nar/gkx1132

Fang, S., Dong, L., Liu, L., Guo, J., Zhao, L., Zhang, J., et al. (2020). HERB: a high-throughput experiment- and reference-guided database of traditional Chinese medicine. *Nucleic Acids Res.* 49, D1197–D1206. doi: 10.1093/nar/gkaa1063

Flood-Page, P., Menzies-Gow, A., Phipps, S., Ying, S., Wangoo, A., Ludwig, M. S., et al. (2003). Anti-IL-5 treatment reduces deposition of ECM proteins in the bronchial subepithelial basement membrane of mild atopic asthmatics. *J. Clin. Invest.* 112, 1029–1036. doi: 10.1172/JCI17974

García-Menaya, J. M., Cordobés-Durán, C., García-Martín, E., and Agúndez, J. A. G. (2019). Pharmacogenetic Factors Affecting Asthma Treatment Response. Potential Implications for Drug Therapy. *Front. Pharmacol.* 10:520. doi: 10.3389/fphar.2019.00520

Gong, J.-H., Shin, D., Han, S.-Y., Park, S.-H., Kang, M.-K., Kim, J.-L., et al. (2013). Blockade of Airway Inflammation by Kaempferol via Disturbing Tyk-STAT Signaling in Airway Epithelial Cells and in Asthmatic Mice. *Evid. Based Complement. Alternat. Med.* 2013:250725. doi: 10.1155/2013/250725

Grondin, C. J., Davis, A. P., Wiegers, T. C., Wiegers, J. A., and Mattingly, C. J. (2018). Accessing an Expanded Exposure Science Module at the Comparative Toxicogenomics Database. *Environ. Health Perspect.* 126:014501. doi: 10.1289/EHP2873

Haeggström, J. Z., and Funk, C. D. (2011). Lipoxygenase and leukotriene pathways: biochemistry, biology, and roles in disease. *Chem. Rev.* 111, 5866–5898. doi: 10.1021/cr200246d

Hershey, G. K. K. (2003). IL-13 receptors and signaling pathways: an evolving web. *J. Allergy Clin. Immunol.* 111, 677–690. doi: 10.1067/mai.2003.1333

Hoshino, M., Takahashi, M., and Aoike, N. (2001). Expression of vascular endothelial growth factor, basic fibroblast growth factor, and angiogenin immunoreactivity in asthmatic airways and its relationship to angiogenesis. *J. Allergy Clin. Immunol.* 107, 295–301. doi: 10.1067/mai.2001.111928

Howell, M. D., Fitzsimons, C., and Smith, P. A. (2018). JAK/STAT inhibitors and other small molecule cytokine antagonists for the treatment of allergic disease. *Ann. Allergy Asthma Immunol.* 120, 367–375. doi: 10.1016/j.anai.2018.02.012

Hsieh, Y.-Y., Chang, C.-C., Hsu, C.-M., Wan, L., Chen, S.-Y., Lin, W.-H., et al. (2011). JAK-1 rs2780895 C-related genotype and allele but not JAK-1 rs10789166, rs4916008, rs2780885, rs17127114, and rs3806277 are associated with higher susceptibility to asthma. *Genet. Test. Mol. Biomarkers* 15, 841–847. doi: 10.1089/gtmb.2011.0002

Huang, K., Yang, T., Xu, J., Yang, L., Zhao, J., Zhang, X., et al. (2019). Prevalence, risk factors, and management of asthma in China: a national cross-sectional study. *Lancet* 394, 407–418. doi: 10.1016/S0140-6736(19)31147-X

Huang, L., Xie, D., Yu, Y., Liu, H., Shi, Y., Shi, T., et al. (2018). TCMID 2.0: a comprehensive resource for TCM. *Nucleic Acids Res.* 46, D1117–D1120. doi: 10.1093/nar/gkx1028

Inoue, H., Akimoto, K., Homma, T., Tanaka, A., and Sagara, H. (2020). Airway Epithelial Dysfunction in Asthma: relevant to Epidermal Growth Factor Receptors and Airway Epithelial Cells. *J. Clin. Med.* 9:3698. doi: 10.3390/jcm9113698

James, A. L., and Wenzel, S. (2007). Clinical relevance of airway remodelling in airway diseases. *Eur. Respir. J.* 30, 134–155. doi: 10.1183/09031936.00146905

Jang, T. Y., Jung, A.-Y., Kyung, T.-S., Kim, D.-Y., Hwang, J.-H., and Kim, Y. H. (2017). Anti-allergic effect of luteolin in mice with allergic asthma and rhinitis. *Cent. Eur. J. Immunol.* 42, 24–29. doi: 10.5114/ceji.2017.67315

Jeffery, P. K. (2001). Remodeling in Asthma and Chronic Obstructive Lung Disease. *Am. J. Respir. Crit. Care Med.* 164, S28–38. doi: 10.1164/ajrccm.164.supplement_2.2106061

Kang, D. R., Belal, S. A., Choe, H. S., Shin, D. K., and Shim, K. S. (2018). Effect of Kaempferol on Cyclooxygenase 2 (Cox2) and Cytosolic Phospholipase A2 (cPLA2) Protein Expression in BALB/c Mice. *Iran. J. Allergy Asthma Immunol.* 17, 428–435. doi: 10.18502/ijaai.v17i5.301

Keiser, M. J., Roth, B. L., Armbruster, B. N., Ernsberger, P., Irwin, J. J., and Shoichet, B. K. (2007). Relating protein pharmacology by ligand chemistry. *Nat. Biotechnol.* 25, 197–206. doi: 10.1038/nbt1284

Kim, S., Chen, J., Cheng, T., Gindulyte, A., He, J., He, S., et al. (2019). PubChem 2019 update: improved access to chemical data. *Nucleic Acids Res.* 47, D1102–D1109. doi: 10.1093/nar/gky1033

Krishnamoorthy, N., Abdulnour, R.-E. E., Walker, K. H., Engstrom, B. D., and Levy, B. D. (2018). Specialized Proresolving Mediators in Innate and Adaptive Immune Responses in Airway Diseases. *Physiol. Rev.* 98, 1335–1370. doi: 10.1152/physrev.00026.2017

Kytikova, O., Novgorodtseva, T., Denisenko, Y., Antonyuk, M., and Gvozdenko, T. (2019). Pro-Resolving Lipid Mediators in the Pathophysiology of Asthma. *Medicina* 55:284. doi: 10.3390/medicina55060284

Lambrecht, B. N., and Hammad, H. (2012). The airway epithelium in asthma. *Nat. Med.* 18, 684–692. doi: 10.1038/nm.2737

Le Cras, T. D., Acciani, T. H., Mushaben, E. M., Kramer, E. L., Pastura, P. A., Hardie, W. D., et al. (2011). Epithelial EGF receptor signaling mediates airway hyperreactivity and remodeling in a mouse model of chronic asthma. *Am. J. Physiol. Lung Cell. Mol. Physiol.* 300, L414–21. doi: 10.1152/ajplung.00346.2010

Lee, C. G., Link, H., Baluk, P., Homer, R. J., Chapoval, S., Bhandari, V., et al. (2004). Vascular endothelial growth factor (VEGF) induces remodeling and enhances TH2-mediated sensitization and inflammation in the lung. *Nat. Med.* 10, 1095–1103. doi: 10.1038/nm1105

Li, N., Li, Q., Zhou, X. D., Kolosov, V. P., and Perelman, J. M. (2012). The effect of quercetin on human neutrophil elastase-induced mucin5AC expression in human airway epithelial cells. *Int. Immunopharmacol.* 14, 195–201. doi: 10.1016/j.intimp.2012.07.008

Liu, J., and Lin, A. (2007). Wiring the cell signaling circuitry by the NF-κB and JNK1 crosstalk and its applications in human diseases. *Oncogene* 26, 3267–3278. doi: 10.1038/sj.onc.1210417

Liu, J., Liu, J., Shen, F., Qin, Z., Jiang, M., Zhu, J., et al. (2018). Systems pharmacology analysis of synergy of TCM: an example using saffron formula. *Sci. Rep.* 8:380. doi: 10.1038/s41598-017-18764-2

Liu, L., Wang, L., He, S., and Ma, Y. (2018). Immune Homeostasis: effects of Chinese Herbal Formulae and Herb-Derived Compounds on Allergic Asthma in Different Experimental Models. *Chin. J. Integr. Med.* 24, 390–398. doi: 10.1007/s11655-018-2836-2

Lucas, C. D., Dorward, D. A., Sharma, S., Rennie, J., Felton, J. M., Alessandri, A. L., et al. (2015). Wogonin Induces Eosinophil Apoptosis and Attenuates Allergic Airway Inflammation. *Am. J. Respir. Crit. Care Med.* 191, 626–636. doi: 10.1164/rccm.201408-1565OC

Molitorisova, M., Sutovska, M., Kazimierova, I., Barborikova, J., Joskova, M., Novakova, E., et al. (2021). The anti-asthmatic potential of flavonol kaempferol in an experimental model of allergic airway inflammation. *Eur. J. Pharmacol.* 891:173698. doi: 10.1016/j.ejphar.2020.173698

Nelms, K., Keegan, A. D., Zamorano, J., Ryan, J. J., and Paul, W. E. (1999). The IL-4 receptor: signaling mechanisms and biologic functions. *Annu. Rev. Immunol.* 17, 701–738. doi: 10.1146/annurev.immunol.17.1.701

Park, H., Lee, C.-M., Jung, I. D., Lee, J. S., Jeong, Y., Chang, J. H., et al. (2009). Quercetin regulates Th1/Th2 balance in a murine model of asthma. *Int. Immunopharmacol.* 9, 261–267. doi: 10.1016/j.intimp.2008.10.021

Qin, L., Lan, Y., and Ma, S. (2017). Effects of Modified Guomin Decoction on Treg Cell Specific Transcription Factor in Mice with Allergic Asthma. *Tradit. Chin. Drug Res. Clin. Pharmacol.* 28, 332–335.

Ru, J., Li, P., Wang, J., Zhou, W., Li, B., Huang, C., et al. (2014). TCMSP: a database of systems pharmacology for drug discovery from herbal medicines. *J. Cheminform.* 6:13. doi: 10.1186/1758-2946-6-13

Safran, M., Dalah, I., Alexander, J., Rosen, N., Iny Stein, T., Shmoish, M., et al. (2010). GeneCards Version 3: the human gene integrator. *Database* 2010:baq020. doi: 10.1093/database/baq020

Schett, G., and Neurath, M. F. (2018). Resolution of chronic inflammatory disease: universal and tissue-specific concepts. *Nat. Commun.* 9:3261. doi: 10.1038/s41467-018-05800-6

Schumann, R. R., Kirschning, C. J., Unbehaun, A., Aberle, H. P., Knope, H. P., Lamping, N., et al. (1996). The lipopolysaccharide-binding protein is a secretory class 1 acute-phase protein whose gene is transcriptionally activated by APRF/STAT/3 and other cytokine-inducible nuclear proteins. *Mol. Cell. Biol.* 16, 3490–3503. doi: 10.1128/mcb.16.7.3490

Shannon, P., Markiel, A., Ozier, O., Baliga, N. S., Wang, J. T., Ramage, D., et al. (2003). Cytoscape: a software environment for integrated models of biomolecular interaction networks. *Genome Res.* 13, 2498–2504. doi: 10.1101/gr.1239303

Shi, Y., Tan, Y., Mao, S., and Gu, W. (2014). Naringenin inhibits allergen-induced airway remodeling in a murine model of asthma. *Mol. Med. Rep.* 9, 1204–1208. doi: 10.3892/mmr.2014.1940

Simeone-Penney, M. C., Severgnini, M., Tu, P., Homer, R. J., Mariani, T. J., Cohn, L., et al. (2007). Airway epithelial STAT3 is required for allergic inflammation in a murine model of asthma. *J. Immunol.* 1950, 6191–6199. doi: 10.4049/jimmunol.178.10.6191

Sinha, S., Doble, M., and Manju, S. L. (2019). 5-Lipoxygenase as a drug target: a review on trends in inhibitors structural design, SAR and mechanism based approach. *Bioorg. Med. Chem.* 27, 3745–3759. doi: 10.1016/j.bmc.2019.06.040

Soriano, J. B., Abajobir, A. A., Abate, K. H., Abera, S. F., Agrawal, A., Ahmed, M. B., et al. (2017). Global, regional, and national deaths, prevalence, disability-adjusted life years, and years lived with disability for chronic obstructive pulmonary disease and asthma, 1990–2015: a systematic analysis for the Global Burden of Disease Study 2015. *Lancet Respir. Med.* 5, 691–706. doi: 10.1016/S2213-2600(17)30293-X

Stermitz, F. R., Lorenz, P., Tawara, J. N., Zenewicz, L. A., and Lewis, K. (2000). Synergy in a medicinal plant: antimicrobial action of berberine potentiated by 5′-methoxyhydnocarpin, a multidrug pump inhibitor. *Proc. Natl. Acad. Sci. U. S. A.* 97, 1433–1437. doi: 10.1073/pnas.030540597

Tao, T., Zhang, Y., Li, J., and Mei, C. (2018). Review of experiments and clinical application research on Guomin Decoction. *China J. Tradit. Chin. Med. Pharm.* 33, 242–244.

Trott, O., and Olson, A. J. (2010). AutoDock Vina: improving the speed and accuracy of docking with a new scoring function, efficient optimization, and multithreading. *J. Comput. Chem.* 31, 455–461. doi: 10.1002/jcc.21334

von Mering, C., Jensen, L. J., Snel, B., Hooper, S. D., Krupp, M., Foglierini, M., et al. (2005). STRING: known and predicted protein–protein associations, integrated and transferred across organisms. *Nucleic Acids Res.* 33, D433–7. doi: 10.1093/nar/gki005

Wang, S., Wuniqiemu, T., Tang, W., Teng, F., Bian, Q., Yi, L., et al. (2021). Luteolin inhibits autophagy in allergic asthma by activating PI3K/Akt/mTOR signaling and inhibiting Beclin-1-PI3KC3 complex. *Int. Immunopharmacol.* 94:107460. doi: 10.1016/j.intimp.2021.107460

Wu, Y., Zhang, F., Yang, K., Fang, S., Bu, D., Li, H., et al. (2019). SymMap: an integrative database of traditional Chinese medicine enhanced by symptom mapping. *Nucleic Acids Res.* 47, D1110–D1117. doi: 10.1093/nar/gky1021

Xu, H.-Y., Zhang, Y.-Q., Liu, Z.-M., Chen, T., Lv, C.-Y., Tang, S.-H., et al. (2019). ETCM: an encyclopaedia of traditional Chinese medicine. *Nucleic Acids Res.* 47, D976–D982. doi: 10.1093/nar/gky987

Yang, M., Chen, J.-L., Xu, L.-W., and Ji, G. (2013). Navigating traditional chinese medicine network pharmacology and computational tools. *Evid. Based Complement. Alternat. Med.* 2013:731969. doi: 10.1155/2013/731969

Zhang, G.-X., Zhang, Y.-Y., Zhang, X.-X., Wang, P.-Q., Liu, J., Liu, Q., et al. (2018). Different network pharmacology mechanisms of Danshen-based Fangjis in the treatment of stable angina. *Acta Pharmacol. Sin.* 39, 952–960. doi: 10.1038/aps.2017.191

Zhang, X. (2016). *Clinical And Animal Experimental Study Of Allergy Decoction Combined With Cough Suppressant To Interfere With Pm2.5.* Available online at: https://kns.cnki.net/kcms/detail/detail.aspx?dbcode=CMFD&dbname=CMFD201602&filename=1016071173.nh&v=THPQPTs5AmVKWk3lTRAFLU2OZN63qbJsXUW1RC1V3QQsD67MWJgqLm9VNc7mE1mF (accessed March 21, 2021).

Zhu, S., and Liang, X. (1985). Discussion on disease differentiation and medication based on syndrome differentiation from the application of Guomin Decoction. *Chin. J. Med.* 59:1985,

13

Sarcoidosis Epidemiology: Race Matters

*Kerry Maryse Hena**

Division of Pulmonary, Critical Care, and Sleep Medicine, Department of Medicine, New York University, New York, NY, United States

Correspondence:
Kerry Maryse Hena
kerry.hena@nyulangone.org

Rather than a single disease entity, sarcoidosis may be a constellation of "sarcoidoses" with a characteristic pattern of organ involvement and clinic course, depending upon the triggering exposure and underlying epidemiologic factors such as race. This review examines the racial disparities inherent to sarcoidosis disease course and mortality and discusses factors that may be responsible for these findings. In the United States, black patients with sarcoidosis experience more severe pulmonary disease, more multiorgan involvement, and an overall worse prognosis with higher rates of hospitalization and mortality. Beyond inherent genotype, ascertainment and access to medical care, physician implicit bias, and patient perceived discrimination likely play a role. Moving forward, epidemiologic concepts can be used to formulate strategies for control, treatment, and even prevention of disease in black Americans at risk for developing life-altering or life-threatening sarcoidosis phenotypes. Identification and rectification of modifiable risk factors such as socioeconomic status, lack of insurance, and financial barriers to care as well as the incorporation of implicit bias training for physician will likely lead to improvement in discordant outcomes.

Keywords: sarcoidosis, black race/ethnicity, sarcoidosis epidemiology, sarcoidosis mortality, implicit bias, health equity

INTRODUCTION

Sarcoidosis is a multisystem disease characterized by granulomatous inflammation. Although its etiology remains unknown, sarcoidosis is believed to represent a genetically primed abnormal immune response to an antigenic exposure (1). Rather than a single disease entity, sarcoidosis may be a constellation of "sarcoidoses" with a characteristic phenotype, depending upon the triggering exposure and underlying genotype. As such, race plays an important role in sarcoidosis epidemiology, disease presentation, and clinical outcomes (2).

In the United States, in particular, different phenotypic expressions are found between black and white subjects, likely resulting from genetics, environment, socioeconomics, implicit or racial biases, or a combination thereof. Given the current political climate and impetus for change in the United States, it is important to shed light on discordant clinical outcomes in vulnerable patient populations. This article examines the racial disparities inherent to sarcoidosis disease course and mortality and discusses factors that may be responsible for these findings.

INCIDENCE AND PREVALENCE

Consistently, black subjects are reported to be most affected by sarcoidosis, black females even more so. Studies reporting incidence and prevalence of sarcoidosis, broken down by race and sex if available, are presented in **Table 1**.

Dating back to the 1960's, researcher Andrew Z. Keller reported significantly different frequency distributions of sarcoidosis with black patients being more commonly diagnosed and treated than whites (12). In the 1990's, an analysis of race in patients from Detroit, Michigan suggested that the relative rates of sarcoidosis in black compared to white patients was as high as 4:1 (10.9/100,000 per year in whites and 35.5/100,000 in blacks) (10). In this study by Rybicki and colleagues, the highest annual age-specific incidence was found in black females aged 30–39 years (107/100,000) (10). A later analysis of sarcoidosis based on U.S. managed healthcare use from 2009 to 2013 showed that the incidence and prevalence of sarcoidosis was significantly higher for black (17.8 and 141.4 per 100,000) than for white individuals (8.1 and 49.8); the highest prevalence for sarcoidosis was again noted in black females (178.5) (4). Of note, additional minority populations, such as Hispanic and Asian patients, were significantly less likely to have sarcoidosis than black or white patients, consistent with what has been suggested in the past (4, 13). More recently, amongst participants in the Black Women's Health Study, incidence rates were observed as high as 71 per 100,000 per year in African American females (6).

In summary, sarcoidosis incidence and prevalence vary greatly based on race with a strong predilection for black populations in the United States, which may be the result of race-specific genetic associations and environmental socioeconomic factors.

GENETIC PREDISPOSITION

As stated previously, sarcoidosis likely results from an environmental insult in a genetically susceptible host. The high incidence and prevalence of sarcoidosis in black subjects suggests an inherent genetic susceptibility. In fact, first-degree relatives of black sarcoidosis cases have about a 3-fold disease risk increase (14).

Multiple sarcoidosis susceptibility loci have been explored in candidate gene and genome-wide association studies. These include the highly polymorphic human leukocyte antigen (HLA) genes, residing in the class II major histocompatibility complex (MHC) on chromosome 6, as well as other genes that influence antigen processing and presentation, T-cell activation and recruitment, and granulomatous inflammation at the core of sarcoidosis immunopathogenesis. A particular HLA allele, DQB1*0602, was shown to confer both increased susceptibility to sarcoidosis and a predilection for radiographic progression of disease in a family-based genetic association analysis of sarcoidosis in U.S. black families (15). Conversely, Butyrophilin-like 2 (BTNL2), which also resides in the class II MHC region on chromosome 6 and probably functions as a T-cell co-stimulatory molecule, has been shown to have a more modest association with sarcoidosis in black compared to white populations; this may be due to greater allelic diversity or an antagonistic effect of HLA class II risk alleles on BTNL2-associated risk in black samples (16). Amongst black siblings enrolled into the Sarcoidosis Genetic Analysis Consortium (SAGA), a genome scan found the strongest linkage signal on chromosome 5 (17). Subsequent fine mapping studies indicated a sarcoidosis susceptibility gene on chromosome 5q11.2 and a gene protective effect on 5p15.2 (18). Further stratification of black families by genetically determined ancestry revealed linkage differences by subpopulation, with previously reported linkage signals at 1p22, 3p21-14, 11p15, and 17q21 specific to ancestral heritage (19).

In all, given the identification of multiple candidate genes and suggestive regions for linkage, it is likely that more than one gene influences sarcoidosis susceptibility and disease presentation in black populations. This is further confounded by ancestral differences in admixed black communities residing in the United States.

DISEASE PRESENTATION

In sarcoidosis the granulomatous inflammation can affect virtually all organs and tissues. However, disease presentation, including extent and severity of disease, has been shown to vary based on demographic variables such as race. A Case-Control Etiologic Study of Sarcoidosis (ACCESS)—a prospective, multicenter study of sarcoidosis patients enrolled within 6 months of diagnosis—provided an opportunity to examine the association of demographic measures, socioeconomic status and barriers to care with severity of disease at presentation, as defined by extent of organ involvement, chest radiographic staging and basic spirometry (20, 21).

As far as organ involvement at presentation, ACCESS showed that black patients tend to experience more extrapulmonary sarcoidosis, affecting the skin (other than erythema nodosum), bone marrow, liver, extrathoracic lymph nodes and eyes (20). Calcium dysmetabolism, on the other hand, was more common in white patients (20). Only pulmonary involvement was independent of age, sex and race (20). Later ACCESS analyses demonstrated that lower income, the absence of private or Medicare health insurance, and other barriers to care were associated with sarcoidosis severity at presentation, as were black race and female sex (21). In comparison to ACCESS whites, ACCESS blacks were more likely to have more organs involved and lower FVC % predicted as well as family income of <US$20,000 and to have other public insurance such as Medicaid (21).

Therefore, in addition to a suspected genetic predisposition for more severe pulmonary and extrapulmonary disease, the association of black race with socioeconomic status (low income, public insurance) and severity of disease at presentation suggests that black patients are more likely to have financial barriers to care and resultant delay in seeking care than their white counterparts (21). Additionally, implicit bias—any unconsciously-held set of associations about a social group—impacts the behavior of both physicians and black patients, with physicians potentially discounting symptoms of sarcoidosis in

TABLE 1 | Sarcoidosis incidence estimates reported in the literature.

References	Country	Sex, race/ethnicity	Time period	Incidence per 100,000	Data source
Arkema et al. (3)	Sweden	Male and female, race not reported	2003–2013	11.5	National Patient Register
Baughman et al. (4)	USA	Male and female, multiracial	2010–2013	Black: 17.8 White: 8.1 Hispanic: 4.3 Asian: 3.2	Optum Health Care Database
Coquart et al. (5)	Guadeloupe, West Indies	Male and female, Afro Caribbean	2003–2010	2.3	Hospital and laboratory databases
Cozier et al. (6)	USA	Female, black	1995–2007	71	Black Women's Health Study, self-reported sarcoidosis
Duchemann et al. (7)	France, Greater Paris	Male and female, multiracial	2012	Overall: 4.9 Afro Caribbean: 16.9 North African: 9.7 Other: 6.4 European: 2.4	Hospitals in Seine-Saint-Denise County; social security
Dumas et al. (8)	USA	Female, multiracial	1989–2011	Overall: 11 Black: 43 White: 11	Nurses' Health Study II, self-reported
Hillerdal et al. (9)	Sweden, Uppsala County	Male and female, race not reported	1966–1980	Overall: 19 Male: 16.5 Female: 21.7	General Health Screening
Rybicki et al. (10)	USA, Detroit, MI	Male and female, multiracial	1990–1994	Black: 35.5 White: 10.9	Health Alliance Plan HMO
Ungprasert et al. (11)	USA, Olmsted County, MN	Male and female, 90% white	1976–2013	Male: 10.5 Female: 11	Rochester Epidemiology Project

black patients until more severe and/or black patients delaying care out of medical mistrust or perceived discrimination (22–25).

CLINICAL COURSE

While sarcoidosis tends to improve or remain stable in the majority of patients, longitudinal studies have shown worse outcomes are associated with black race and/or lower annual family income (26, 27). In the ACCESS 2 years follow-up study, black patients had a higher likelihood of decreasing FVC and developing new organ involvement over time (26). Similarly, clinical data from a large cohort of sarcoidosis patients followed at Medical University of South Carolina over a 12-years period, showed that black patients had more advanced radiographic stages of sarcoidosis, more organ involvement, and more frequently required anti-sarcoidosis medication compared to white patients (27).

Furthermore, black patients tend to have a higher rate of hospitalization for sarcoidosis. An analysis of the National Hospital Discharge Survey (NHDS) from 1979 to 2000 showed that mean rates of hospitalization were nine time higher for black patients (28). A retrospective study of the Nationwide Inpatient Sample supported this trend, demonstrating a near doubling of hospitalizations among sarcoidosis patients, with disproportionate rate increases in black, female, and older patients from 1998 to 2008 (29).

As such, black patients with sarcoidosis experience worse prognosis, more multiorgan involvement, and a higher rate of hospitalization. Beyond inherent genotype, ascertainment and access to preventative and primary care may also be playing a role in this disparity of outcomes for black individuals, as is implicit bias.

MORTALITY

Many patients with sarcoidosis have a benign clinical course, but for some, it is a chronic, life-altering, and even fatal disease. While overall mortality rates from sarcoidosis have been shown to be increasing, significant differences exist based on race. Data from the National Center for Health Statistics (NCHS), demonstrated a 3% average yearly increase in mortality rate for all-comers with sarcoidosis from 1988 to 2007 (30). However, the greatest absolute increase in sarcoidosis-related deaths was among black females (10 deaths per million) followed by black males (three deaths per million), in comparison to at most one death per million in white males or females (30). The most common cause of death was sarcoidosis itself; younger sarcoidosis decedents with pulmonary fibrosis were more likely to be black than white and have a cardiac involvement contribute to death. A later study using NCHS data from 1999 to 2010 with a focus on racial and sex disparities, showed a 12 times higher age-adjusted mortality rate for black patients compared with white patients

(16 vs. 1.3 per million, respectively) (31). Again, black sarcoidosis decedents died at an earlier age and more often had associated pulmonary hypertension (31). An early study by Gideon and Mannino reported a U.S. sarcoidosis mortality ratio, black: white, of 14:1 (32).

This race-specific trend of higher mortality from sarcoidosis at a younger age in black patients has multiple potential explanations, some more alarming than others. Hypotheses include increased incidence and severity of disease, a predilection for the lethal complications of pulmonary fibrosis and pulmonary hypertension, as well as long-standing systemic health and social inequities.

RACISM

As the Covid-19 pandemic has so powerfully illustrated, race plays a significant role as a determinant of health in the United States (33). Beyond socioeconomic factors, perceived discrimination has been linked to adverse health outcomes in mental and physical health domains (23–25). In addition to implicit or racial biases, the perception of discrimination or stigma of inferiority appears to induce physiological and psychological arousal with direct deleterious health consequences (34). While this has not been elucidated specifically in sarcoidosis, the association of perceived discrimination with poorer health outcomes has been explored across a broad range of outcomes, including cardiac disease, renal insufficiency and subclinical cerebrovascular disease (23–25).

FUTURE DIRECTIONS

Despite its nineteenth century origin and more than 100 years of inquiry, much about sarcoidosis is still unknown. Perhaps this is because of its many points of divergence—its variant epidemiology, varied triggering exposures and ultimately variable clinical phenotypes or "sarcoidoses." Regardless, its higher contraction and death rates in black Americans deserves further attention.

Ideally, future studies performed will improve our understating of the relationships among exposure, race and other epidemiologic factors, with current clinical phenotypes and outcomes. Such endeavors should include large, matched epidemiologic studies conducted in racially diverse populations, facilitated by large population data sets and disease registries. In addition to facilitating etiologic hypotheses of the exposure-host interaction at the core of sarcoidosis pathophysiology, epidemiologic concepts should be used to formulate strategies for control, treatment, and even prevention of disease in Black Americans who are at the greatest risk for developing life-altering or life-threatening disease. Identification and rectification of modifiable risk factors such as socioeconomic status, lack of insurance, and financial barriers to care will likely lead to improved outcomes. Making anti-racism or implicit bias training an essential professional competency would equip physicians with the tools needed to address racism and its adverse health effects (35).

Finally, these findings should influence research in the areas of health disparities and disease processes among various racial groups and between the sexes throughout the world. Achieving health equity requires valuing all individuals and populations equally, recognizing and rectifying historical injustices, and providing resources according to need. Health disparities will be eliminated *only* when health equity is achieved (36).

AUTHOR CONTRIBUTIONS

KH contributed a race-centered review of sarcoidosis epidemiology, highlighting racial disparities inherent to sarcoidosis disease course and mortality and discusses factors that may be responsible for these findings. She was the sole contributing author for this section.

REFERENCES

Valeyre D, Prasse A, Nunes H, Uzunhan Y, Brillet P-Y, Müller-Quernheim J. Sarcoidosis. *Lancet.* (2014) 383:1155–67. doi: 10.1016/S0140-6736(13)60680-7

Westney GE, Judson MA. Racial and ethnic disparities in sarcoidosis: from genetics to socioeconomics. *Clin Chest Med.* (2006) 27:453–62. doi: 10.1016/j.ccm.2006.04.002

Arkema EV, Grunewald J, Kullberg S, Eklund A, Askling J. Sarcoidosis incidence and prevalence: a nationwide register-based assessment in Sweden. *Eur Respiratory J.* (2016) 48:1690–9. doi: 10.1183/13993003.00477-2016

Baughman R, Field S, Costabel U, Crystal R, Culver D, Drent M, et al. Sarcoidosis in America: analysis based on health care use. *Ann Am Thorac Soc.* (2016) 13:1244–52. doi: 10.1513/AnnalsATS.201511-760OC

Coquart N, Cadelis G, Tressières B, Cordel N. Epidemiology of sarcoidosis in Afro-Caribbean people: a 7-year retrospective study in Guadeloupe. *Int J Dermatol.* (2014) 54:188–92. doi: 10.1111/ijd.12633

Cozier YC, Berman JS, Palmer JR, Boggs DA, Serlin DM, Rosenberg L. Sarcoidosis in black women in the United States: data from the Black Women's Health Study. *Chest.* (2011) 139:144–50. doi: 10.1378/chest.10-0413

Duchemann B, Annesi-Maesano I, Naurois CJD, Sanyal S, Brillet P-Y, Brauner M, et al. Prevalence and incidence of interstitial lung diseases in a multi-ethnic county of Greater Paris. *Eur Respiratory J.* (2017) 50:1602419. doi: 10.1183/13993003.02419-2016

Dumas O, Abramovitz L, Wiley AS, Cozier YC, Camargo CA. Epidemiology of sarcoidosis in a prospective cohort study of U.S. Women. *Ann Am Thoracic Soc.* (2016) 13:67–71. doi: 10.1513/AnnalsATS.201508-568BC

Hillerdal G, Nöu E, Osterman K, Schmekel B. Sarcoidosis: epidemiology and prognosis. A 15-year European study. *Am Rev Respir Dis.* (1984) 130:29–32.

Rybicki BA, Major M, Popovich J Jr, Maliarik MJ, Iannuzzi MC. Racial differences in sarcoidosis incidence: a 5-year study in a health maintenance organization. *Am J Epidemiol.* (1997) 145:234–41. doi: 10.1093/oxfordjournals.aje.a009096

Ungprasert P, Crowson CS, Matteson EL. Influence of gender on epidemiology and clinical manifestations of sarcoidosis: a population-based retrospective cohort study 1976–2013. *Lung.* (2017) 195:87–91. doi: 10.1007/s00408-016- 9952-6

Keller AZ. Hospital, age, racial, occupational, geographical, clinical and survivorship characteristics in the epidemiology of sarcoidosis. *Am J Epidemiol.* (1971) 94:222–30. doi: 10.1093/oxfordjournals.aje.a1 21316

Izumi T. Symposium: population differences in clinical features and prognosis of sarcoidosis throughout the world. *Sarcoidosis.* (1992) 9:S105–18.

Rybicki BA, Iannuzzi MC, Frederick MM, Thompson BW, Rossman MD, Bresnitz EA, et al. Familial aggregation of sarcoidosis. A case-control etiologic study of sarcoidosis (ACCESS). *Am J Respir Crit Care Med.* (2001) 164:2085- 91. doi: 10.1164/ajrccm.164.11.2106001

Iannuzzi MC, Maliarik MJ, Poisson LM, Rybicki BA. Sarcoidosis susceptibility and resistance HLA-DQB1 alleles in African Americans. *Am J Respir Crit Care Med.* (2003) 167:1225–31. doi: 10.1164/rccm.200209-1097OC

Rybicki BA, Walewski JL, Maliarik MJ, Kian H, Iannuzzi MC, ACCESS Research Group. The BTNL2 gene and sarcoidosis susceptibility in African Americans and Whites. *Am J Hum Genet.* (2005) 77:491– 9. doi: 10.1086/444435

Iannuzzi MC, Iyengar SK, Gray-McGuire C, Elston RC, Baughman RP, Donohue JF, et al. Genome-wide search for sarcoidosis susceptibility genes in African Americans. *Genes Immun.* (2005) 6:509–18. doi: 10.1038/sj.gene.6364235

Gray-McGuire C, Sinha R, Iyengar S, Millard C, Rybicki BA, Elston RC, et al. Genetic characterization and fine mapping of susceptibility loci for sarcoidosis in African Americans on chromosome 5. *Hum Genet.* (2006) 120:420–30. doi: 10.1007/s00439-006-0201-6

Thompson CL, Rybicki BA, Iannuzzi MC, Elston RC, Iyengar SK, Gray-McGuire C, et al. Reduction of sample heterogeneity through use of population substructure: an example from a population of African American families with sarcoidosis. *Am J Hum Genet.* (2006) 79:606– 13. doi: 10.1086/507847

Baughman RP, Teirstein AS, Judson MA, Rossman MD, Yeager Jr H, Bresnitz EA, et al. Clinical characteristics of patients in a case control study of sarcoidosis. *Am J Respir Crit Care Med.* (2001) 164:1885– 9. doi: 10.1164/ajrccm.164.10.2104046

Rabin DL, Thompson B, Brown KM, Judson MA, Huang X, Lackland DT, et al. Sarcoidosis: social predictors of severity at presentation. *Eur Respir J.* (2004) 24:601–8. doi: 10.1183/09031936.04.00070503

Blair IV, Steiner JF, Havranek EP. Unconscious (implicit) bias and health disparities: where do we go from here? *Perm J.* (2011) 15:71–78.

LaVeist TA, Nickerson KJ, Bowie JV. Attitudes about racism, medical mistrust, and satisfaction with care among African American and white cardiac patients. *Med Care Res Rev.* (2000) 57(Suppl.1):146–61. doi: 10.1177/1077558700057001S07

Beydoun MA, Poggi-Burke A, Zonderman AB, Rostant OS, Evans MK, Crews DC. Perceived discrimination and longitudinal change in kidney function among urban adults. *Psychosom Med.* (2017) 79:824– 34. doi: 10.1097/PSY.0000000000000478

Beatty Moody DL, Taylor AD, Leibel DK, Al-Najjar E, Katzel LI, Davatzikos C, et al. Lifetime discrimination burden, racial discrimination, and subclinical cerebrovascular disease among African Americans. *Health Psychol.* (2019) 38:63–74. doi: 10.1037/hea00 00638

Judson MA, Baughman RP, Thompson BW, Teirstein AS, Terrin ML, Rossman MD, et al. Two year prognosis of sarcoidosis: the ACCESS experience. *Sarcoidosis Vasc Diffuse Lung Dis.* (2003) 20:204–11.

Judson MA, Boan AD, Lackland DT. The clinical course of sarcoidosis: presentation, diagnosis, and treatment in a large white and black cohort in the United States. *Sarcoidosis Vasc Diffuse Lung Dis.* (2012) 29:119–27.

Foreman MG, Mannino DM, Kamugisha L, Westney GE. Hospitalization for patients with sarcoidosis:1979–2000. *Sarcoidosis Vasc Diffuse Lung Dis.* (2006) 23:124–129.

Gerke AK, Yang M, Tang F, Cavanaugh JE, Polgreen PM. Increased hospitalizations among sarcoidosis patients from 1998 to 2008: a population-based cohort study. *BMC Pulm Med.* (2012) 12:19. doi: 10.1186/1471-2466-12-19

Swigris JJ, Olson AL, Huie TJ, Fernandez-Perez ER, Solomon J, Sprunger D, et al. Sarcoidosis-related mortality in the United States from 1988 to 2007. *Am J Respir Crit Care Med.* (2011) 183:1524– 30. doi: 10.1164/rccm.201010-1679OC

Mirsaeidi M, Machado RF, Schraufnagel D, Sweiss NJ, Baughman RP. Racial difference in sarcoidosis mortality in the United States. *Chest.* (2015) 147:438–49. doi: 10.1378/chest.14-1120

Gideon NM, Mannino DM. Sarcoidosis mortality in the United States 1979– 1991: an analysis of multiple-cause mortality data. *Am J Med.* (1996) 100:423– 7. doi: 10.1016/S0002-9343(97)89518-6

Cyrus E, Clarke R, Hadley D, Bursac Z, Trepka MJ, Devieux JG, et al. The impact of COVID-19 on African American communities in the United States. *medRxiv [Preprint].* (2020). doi: 10.1101/2020.05.15.20096552

Williams DR, Neighbors HW, Jackson JS. Racial/ethnic discrimination and health: findings from community studies. *Am J Public Health.* (2008) 98(9Suppl.):S29–37. doi: 10.2105/AJPH.98.Supplement_1.S29

Hardeman RR, Medina EM, Boyd RW. Stolen breaths. *N Engl J Med.* (2020) 383:197–9. doi: 10.1056/NEJMp2021072

Jones CP. Systems of power, axes of inequity: parallels, intersections, braiding the strands. *Med Care.* (2014) 52(10Suppl.3):S71–5. doi: 10.1097/MLR.00000000000 00216

14

Mechanisms of Pulmonary Hypertension in Acute Respiratory Distress Syndrome (ARDS)

Lucy Revercomb[1,2†], *Ankit Hanmandlu*[2†], *Nancy Wareing*[2], *Bindu Akkanti*[3] *and Harry Karmouty-Quintana*[2,3*]

[1] Department of BioSciences, Rice University, Houston, TX, United States, [2] Department of Biochemistry and Molecular Biology, McGovern Medical School, University of Texas Health Science Center at Houston, Houston, TX, United States, [3] Divisions of Critical Care, Pulmonary and Sleep Medicine, McGovern Medical School, University of Texas Health Science Center at Houston, Houston, TX, United States

***Correspondence:**
Harry Karmouty-Quintana
harry.karmouty@uth.tmc.edu

† These authors have contributed equally to this work

Background: Acute respiratory distress syndrome (ARDS) is a severe and often fatal disease. The causes that lead to ARDS are multiple and include inhalation of salt water, smoke particles, or as a result of damage caused by respiratory viruses. ARDS can also arise due to systemic complications such as blood transfusions, sepsis, or pancreatitis. Unfortunately, despite a high mortality rate of 40%, there are limited treatment options available for ARDS outside of last resort options such as mechanical ventilation and extracorporeal support strategies.

Aim of review: A complication of ARDS is the development of pulmonary hypertension (PH); however, the mechanisms that lead to PH in ARDS are not fully understood. In this review, we summarize the known mechanisms that promote PH in ARDS.

Key scientific concepts of review: (1) Provide an overview of acute respiratory distress syndrome; (2) delineate the mechanisms that contribute to the development of PH in ARDS; (3) address the implications of PH in the setting of coronavirus disease 2019 (COVID-19).

Keywords: hyaluronan, renin angiotensin system, interleukin-6 (IL-6), vascular dysfunction and inflammation, acute lung injury, vasoconstriction, vascular remodelling

INTRODUCTION

Acute respiratory distress syndrome (ARDS) is a severe form of lung respiratory failure characterized by diffuse alveolar damage, inflammation, and acute onset of hypoxemia not explained by cardiac failure. Diagnostic criteria for ARDS include (1) presentation within 1 week of a known clinical insult, new, or worsening respiratory symptoms; (2) bilateral opacities consistent with pulmonary edema on chest imaging; (3) respiratory failure not fully explained by cardiac failure or fluid overload; and (4) physiologic values of arterial oxygen partial pressure to fractional inspired oxygen (PaO_2/FIO_2) $\leq$300 mmHg and positive end-expiratory pressure (PEEP) $\geq$5 cm H_2O (The ARDS Definition Task Force, 2012).

Several chronic disorders have been associated with the development of ARDS; however, the majority of ARDS develops from a pulmonary or non-pulmonary infection (Matthay and Zemans, 2011). ARDS can be triggered by many pathogenic conditions including sepsis, pancreatitis, and respiratory viruses such as the H5N1 avian influenza virus, the 1918 influenza pandemic, the severe acute respiratory syndrome-coronavirus (SARS-CoV), and most recently SARS-CoV-2 that causes coronavirus disease 2019 (COVID-19) (Imai et al., 2010; Rezoagli et al., 2017).

The pathogenesis of ARDS is typically divided into the acute, subacute, and chronic phases (Matthay and Zemans, 2011). The acute phase marks the first 1–6 days and is characterized by interstitial and alveolar edema, endothelial and epithelial injury, and the accumulation of neutrophils, macrophages, and red blood cells in the alveoli (Matthay and Zemans, 2011). The subacute phase marks the next 7–14 days and is characterized by some reabsorption of the edema, evidence of repair attempts by alveolar epithelial type II (AE2) cells, infiltration of fibroblasts, and collagen deposition (Matthay and Zemans, 2011). After 14 days, ARDS is considered to be in the chronic phase and there is often resolution of the acute neutrophilic infiltrate, accumulation of mononuclear cells and alveolar macrophages in the alveoli, and more fibrosis resulting from the alveolar epithelial repair (Matthay and Zemans, 2011).

ARDS is observed in 10–15% of admitted patients in intensive care units and more than 20% of patients undergoing invasive mechanical ventilation (Frutos-Vivar et al., 2004). In addition to this high prevalence and despite best measures, ARDS has a high mortality rate of up to 45% (Bellani et al., 2016). Treatment of ARDS is complex, involving ventilatory and non-ventilatory management strategies including conservative fluid management, low tidal volume ventilation, prone positioning, inhaled vasodilator therapy and in refractory cases, extra corporeal membrane oxygenation (Peek et al., 2009; Calcaianu et al., 2017).

ARDS is frequently complicated by pulmonary hypertension (PH), a pathologic condition involving a progressive increase in pulmonary vascular resistance (PVR) leading to right ventricular dysfunction (RVD) that ultimately results in RV failure (RVF) (Simonneau et al., 2019). PH is clinically defined as mean pulmonary arterial pressure (mPAP) > 20 mmHg measured by right heart catheterization (Simonneau et al., 2019). PH in the setting of ARDS falls under group 3 PH due to the presence of hypoxia and lung injury (Poor et al., 2012).

Potential underlying mechanisms of PH in ARDS include vessel obliteration, pulmonary vasoconstriction, and microthrombosis due to hypoxia, hypercapnia, and an imbalance in vasoactive mediators (Price and Wort, 2017). As an inflammatory condition, ARDS is characterized by endothelial cell injury and dysfunction (Price and Wort, 2017). Early in the pathogenesis of ARDS, thromboembolism, pulmonary vasoconstriction, and interstitial edema contribute to the development of PH by collectively elevating PVR (Moloney and Evans, 2003). Damage to the endothelium of the lung results in the accumulation and activation of neutrophils in the lung microvasculature, leading to degranulation and the release of toxic mediators including proteases, reactive oxygen species, proinflammatory cytokines, and procoagulant molecules, which promote vasoconstriction and an increase in PVR (Matthay and Zemans, 2011). The release of tissue factor (TF), an activator of the extrinsic clotting cascade, by endothelial cells elevates PVR through the local formation of microthrombi which obstruct blood flow (Ryan et al., 2014). Vascular remodeling and proliferation of smooth muscle cells through the release of endothelin-1 (ET-1) in the subacute and chronic phases of ARDS occludes the pulmonary vasculature, further increasing PVR and the accumulation of interstitial edema, contributing to the development of PH (Moloney and Evans, 2003). In addition, fibrocellular obliteration of the microvasculature in late phase ARDS disrupts blood flow and helps sustain the elevated PVR that leads to PH (Ryan et al., 2014).

Many of these mediators that are triggered after lung damage in ARDS are also central in the pathophysiology of PH, where injury to endothelial cells and increased levels of ET-1 and TF also contribute to increased vascular tone and remodeling in PH (Moloney and Evans, 2003; Tamosiuniene et al., 2011; Antoniak et al., 2014).

It has been proposed that the increase in inflammation characteristic of ARDS and secondary to ventilator-induced lung injury prompts the pulmonary vascular injury observed in PH (Meduri et al., 2009; Price and Wort, 2017). The incidence of RVD associated with ARDS has declined with the adoption of improvements in mechanical ventilation which lessen the intrathoracic airway pressure in ARDS patients (Vieillard-Baron et al., 2001). The ARDSnet trial has shown significant mortality benefit, with improvement of low tidal volume ventilation for RVD, and improvement of acute cor pulmonale, in severe cases of ARDS (Brower et al., 2000).

Despite advances in the management of ARDS, prevalence of PH in ARDS remains high. A 92% prevalence of PH was reported by Beiderlinden et al. (2006). Ñamendys-Silva et al. (2014), who used a strict selection criteria excluding any patients with clinical conditions that may have predisposed them to PH before the onset of ARDS, reported a prevalence of 46.6%. Villar et al. (1989) reported a similar prevalence of 54%. These findings are summarized in **Table 1** where mean pulmonary arterial pressure (mPAP) values determined by right-heart catheterization values ranged from 29 to 36 mmHg in patients with PH. The prevalence of acute cor pulmonale, the severest form of RV dysfunction in the setting of ARDS, is still reported to be as high as 20% (Dessap et al., 2016).

ARDS is a complex disease with multifactorial consequences; as such, in addition to elevated mPAP, other parameters have been strongly associated with mortality such as partial pressure of carbon dioxide ($PaCO_2$), partial pressure of oxygen (PaO_2), or PaO_2/fraction of inspired oxygen (FiO_2). Additionally, pulmonary vascular dysfunction, as measured by an increase in transpulmonary pressure gradient and PVR, was associated with increased mortality in ARDS patients (Monchi et al., 1998; Meduri et al., 2009; Bull et al., 2010; Calcaianu et al., 2017). In addition, the composite marker diastolic pulmonary gradient >7 mmHg and PVR >3 Wood Units (WU) seemed to provide a better description of hemodynamic and respiratory dysfunction than other measurements, correlating with a more severe illness and worse patient outcomes (Calcaianu et al., 2017). These findings are summarized in **Table 2** and underscore disruptions in the lung vasculature in ARDS as potential disease-amplifying effects that are not fully understood. Although a study showed no correlation between RVF and mortality in ARDS (Osman et al., 2009), other studies have reported an association between RVD and increased morbidity and mortality in ARDS (Monchi et al., 1998; Bull et al., 2010). Further, due to the effects on organ failure in severe ARDS, the severity of organ failure at admission is an

TABLE 1 | Prevalence of PH in ARDS.

mPAP (mmHg)					
All patients	**Without PH**	**PH**	**Method**	**Prevalence (%)**	**References**
35.4 ± 8.8			Right Heart Catheterization	92.2	Beiderlinden et al., 2006*
27.07 ± 10.29	19.19 ± 3.78	36.07 ± 7.50	Right Heart Catheterization	46.6	Ñamendys-Silva et al., 2014
	15 ± 3	29 ± 6	Right Heart Catheterization	54	Villar et al., 1989

individual mPAP values for patients with and without PH not provided.

TABLE 2 | Factors associated with mortality of PH in ARDS.

Variable	Survivors	Non-survivors	*P*-value	References
PaO_2 (mmHg)	75.95 ± 32.96	74.44 ± 16.47	0.888	Ñamendys-Silva et al., 2014
PaO_2/FiO_2 (mmHg)	144.64 ± 47.84	135.64 ± 44.81	0.616	
$PaCO_2$ (mmHg)	34.51 ± 5.15	40.59 ± 8.44	<0.001	
mPAP (mmHg)	28.32 ± 10.98	24.91 ± 9.08		
PaO_2/FiO_2	112 ± 39	93 ± 31	<0.05	Osman et al., 2009
$PaCO_2$	43 ± 7	48 ± 16	<0.05	
mPAP	27 ± 6	28 ± 8	<0.01	
PaO_2	88.7 ± 40.1	78.1 ± 38.5	0.002	Squara et al., 1998
PaO_2/FiO_2	149 ± 74	120 ± 59	0.0001	
$PaCO_2$	37.1 ± 8.2	38.8 ± 9.0	0.02	
mPAP	25.1 ± 7.3	26.8 ± 9.0	0.04	
mPAP	31.3 ± 8.3	32.4 ± 8.3	0.18	Bull et al., 2010
DPG	14.3 (11.3–18.3)	15.7 (12.3–22.3)	0.02	
PVRi	299.9 (199.4–416.1)	326.4 (206.4–518.7)	0.02	
$\Delta\ PaO_2/FiO_2 < 0$ (mmHg)			0.007	Calcaianu et al., 2017

important predictor of mortality (Ñamendys-Silva et al., 2014; Bellani et al., 2016).

Although PH is a frequent complication of ARDS, there is not a definitive correlation between the presence of PH and the severity and mortality of ARDS. Regardless, in instances of ARDS with or without PH, the mortality rate is very high. The toll of this mortality rate, and accordingly the need for novel therapies, has been demonstrated by the impact and death resulting from the pandemic of COVID-19 where pulmonary vascular abnormalities are present (Potus et al., 2020). A more comprehensive understanding of the role and mechanism of PH in ARDS is needed to improve therapies. In this review, we discuss the central pathways that contribute to PH in ARDS.

EXPERIMENTAL METHODOLOGY

We reviewed the current and past literature on ARDS to identify potential mechanisms that promote PH in ARDS.

RESULTS

The Renin–Angiotensin System

The renin–angiotensin system (RAS) is a primary cardiovascular regulatory system responsible for the regulation of blood pressure and electrolyte balance. RAS dysfunction has been proposed as a key pathogenic mechanism of inflammatory lung disease, including ARDS (Imai et al., 2010; Jia, 2016). Genetic variants in the RAS pathway have recently been implicated in the onset and severity of ARDS, specifically angiotensin-converting enzyme (ACE), and its derivatives (Imai et al., 2010). ACE is a peptidase that regulates RAS by cleaving angiotensin I (AngI) to generate angiotensin II (AngII). AngII subsequently binds to AngII receptor type 1 (AT1R) and AngII receptor type II (AT2R) to regulate RAS (Imai et al., 2010). It is primarily through AT1R that AngII causes growth and proliferation of pulmonary artery smooth muscle cells (PASMCs) correlated with pulmonary vascular remodeling (Morrell et al., 1999). This is attributed to AngII-mediated increases in expression of pro-inflammatory genes including interleukin-10 (IL-10), interleukin-6 (IL-6), tumor necrosis factor (TNF-α), and intracellular adhesion molecule-1 (ICAM-1) in fibroblasts and smooth muscle cells (Xianwei et al., 2012). Subsequent vascular remodeling and fibrotic changes contribute to the pathogenesis and progression of pulmonary fibrosis and PH (Kuba et al., 2006). Further, activation of AT1R by AngII promotes vasoconstriction (Iwai and Horiuchi, 2009), adding to the deleterious properties of AngII.

Angiotensin-converting enzyme 2 (ACE2) is an ACE homolog which regulates RAS through counterbalancing ACE activity. This homolog was termed ACE2 after it was identified and cloned from cDNA libraries by two independent groups (Donoghue et al., 2000; Tipnis et al., 2000). While ACE and ACE2 share 41.8% sequence identity, ACE2 negatively regulates RAS, opposing the role of ACE (Donoghue et al., 2000; Tipnis et al., 2000; Imai et al., 2010). ACE2 cleaves a single residue from AngI to yield angiotensin1–9 (Ang1–9) and removes a single residue from AngII to yield angiotensin1–7 (Ang1–7) (Donoghue et al., 2000; Tipnis et al., 2000), which downregulates AT1R-mediated actions by reducing AngII levels (Ferreira and Santos, 2005). In addition, Ang1–7 and Ang1–9 oppose AT1R through anti-inflammatory and antifibrotic actions, by binding the Mas receptor (MasR) and AT2R, respectively (Kreutz et al., 2020; South et al., 2020). In the pathogenesis of ARDS, ACE, AngII, and AT1R promote inflammation and PH, while ACE2, Ang1–7, and Ang1–9 serve to protect against ARDS and PH (Imai et al., 2005).

There is a polymorphism of ACE defined by the absence (deletion, D) or presence (insertion, I) of a 287-bp repeat in the coding sequence of intron 16 (Rigat et al., 1990). The human ACE D allele results in increased activity of ACE demonstrated by an increase in serum ACE levels. This polymorphism accounts for 47% of the variance in plasma ACE activity (Rigat et al., 1990). There also exists a pronounced correlation between the D allele and the development of ARDS, suggesting the role of RAS activation early in disease (Marshall et al., 2002). In addition, the ACE D/D allele correlates with increased mortality in ARDS especially in comparison with the ACE I/I allele which shows increased survival rate, marking the I/D polymorphism as a significant prognostic factor for ARDS outcome (Jerng et al., 2006). Thus, it is conceivable that the D allele may worsen PH in ARDS.

ACE2 expression has been located on lung alveolar epithelial cells (AECs) and enterocytes of the small intestine, and additionally on arterial smooth muscle cells and arterial and venous endothelial cells in all organs (Hamming et al., 2004). These areas of expression indicate an abundant presence of ACE2 in the lung and small intestine epithelia (Hamming et al., 2004). In addition, increased expression of ACE has been found in the muscularized intra-acinar pulmonary arteries of patients with PH, supporting the proposed role of ACE in PH (Orte et al., 2000), through the upregulation of AngII.

Many experiments have evaluated and found supporting evidence of the role of ACE in PH promoting inflammation and vascular dysfunction, with the activity of ACE2 serving as an important counterbalance. Experimental PH was associated with elevated ACE expression in the endothelial layer of small and elastic pulmonary arteries (Morrell et al., 1995; Orte et al., 2000; Schuster et al., 2012). While a significant decrease in ACE2 activity was observed in human pulmonary arterial hypertension (PAH) patients (Hemnes et al., 2018), ACE2 knockout mice display worsened lung function, increased vascular permeability, enhanced lung edema, and neutrophil accumulation, attributed to a downregulation of ACE2 (Imai et al., 2005). Later treatment of the ACE2-deficient mice with catalytically active recombinant ACE2 protein or ACE knockout resulted in improvement of severe lung failure as measured by lung elastance, edema formation, and histological changes associated with acute lung injury (ALI) (Imai et al., 2005). Administration of a single dose of recombinant human ACE2 (rhACE2) to PAH patients resulted in improvement of hemodynamic markers of PAH, including cardiac output and PVR (Hemnes et al., 2018). However, no improvement in clinical or physiological measures of ARDS were seen with the addition of exogenous ACE2 in patients with ARDS (Khan et al., 2017); however, these studies did not have the sufficient statistical power to identify potential clinical benefits. In other models of lung diseases, including bleomycin-induced lung fibrosis and moncrotaline-induced PH, it has been demonstrated that ACE2 plays a critical protective role (Ferreira and Santos, 2005; Yamazato et al., 2009; Zhang et al., 2009). The aforementioned findings support the conclusion that increasing ACE2 expression may present a novel approach for ARDS treatment and emphasize the need for a better understanding of the role of RAS in the pathogenesis of ARDS.

In contrast to the results of experimental ACE2 deletion, ACE knockout and AT1Ra-deficient mice showed marked improvement in ALI symptoms (Imai et al., 2005). Similarly, treatment of chronically hypoxic rats and mice with an AngII receptor antagonist or ACE blocker inhibited pulmonary vascular remodeling associated with the pathogenesis of PH (Nong et al., 1996). ACE-deficient mice with 34% of ACE activity exhibit the same remodeling as normal mice to their pulmonary arterioles, associating the presence of ACE with vascular remodeling (Suylen et al., 2001). In LPS and acid-induced ARDS with high-stretch ventilation, treatment with Ang1–7 reduced the acute inflammatory response and subsequent fibrosis and improved oxygenation (Asperen et al., 2011; Zambelli et al., 2015). Collectively, these studies implicate ACE in the pathogenesis of ARDS (Jerng et al., 2006).

In addition to its regulatory role, ACE2 acts as a functional receptor for SARS-CoV (Hamming et al., 2004). SARS-CoV-2 binds to the membrane-bound form of ACE2 leading to the host cell's internalization of the complex (South et al., 2020). Through this mechanism, SARS-CoV-2 and SARS-CoV-1 use ACE2 as a co-receptor for acquiring intracellular entry into the brain and lungs (Kuba et al., 2005; Hoffmann et al., 2020; Wrapp et al., 2020). This internalization of ACE2 results in a decrease of cell surface ACE2, preventing the degradation of disease-promoting AngII and generation of protective Ang1–7 (South et al., 2020). This reduction in pulmonary ACE2 may exacerbate systemic hypertension and PH, fibrosis post-viral infection, and respiratory distress (Imai et al., 2005; Kuba et al., 2005). Potential treatment of COVID-19, with the understanding of the role of ACE2 as a receptor for SARS-CoV-2, could include inhibition of the ACE2 receptor, spike protein-based vaccine, inhibition of transmembrane protease activity, or administration of soluble ACE2 (Cheng et al., 2020). Taken together, these findings support the role of RAS as an important modulator of PH in ARDS where it can modulate both vasoconstriction and vascular remodeling responses (**Figure 1**).

The Inflammatory Cascade

Protective mechanical ventilation strategies have improved outcomes of ARDS and PH together, but pulmonary vasculature dysfunction remains in 25% of affected patients and has been increasingly associated with sepsis (Bull et al., 2010; Boissier et al., 2013). Increased flow and ventilatory pressures result

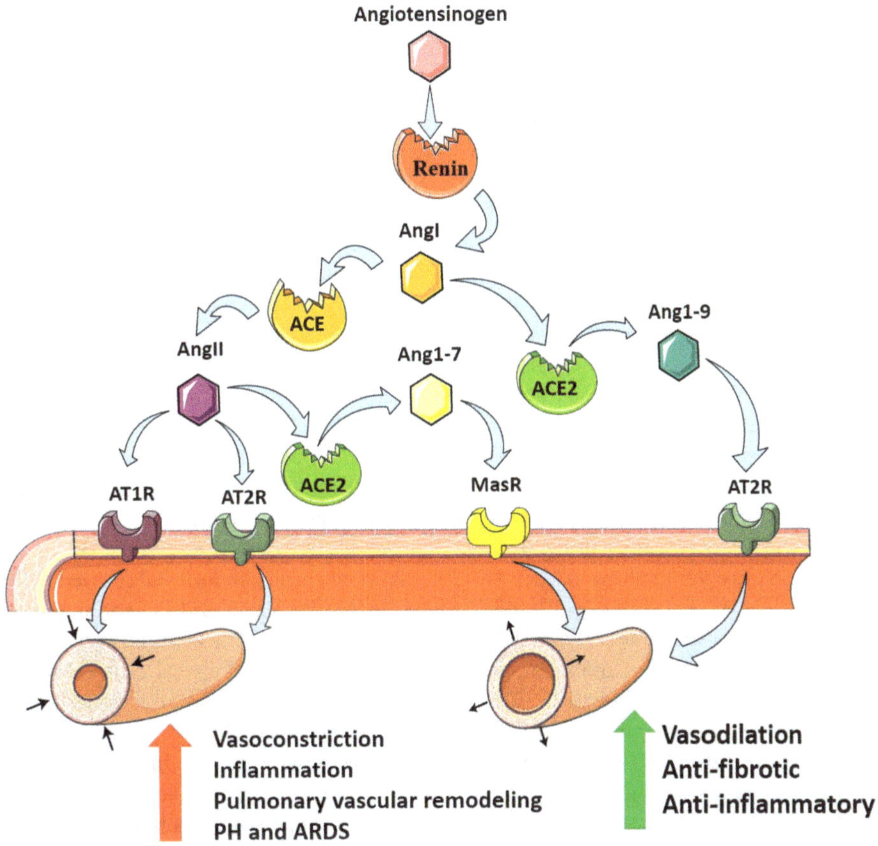

FIGURE 1 | The renin–angiotensin system and its contribution to PH in ARDS. Angiotensinogen (pink hexagon) is cleaved by renin (red circle) into angiotensin I (AngI, orange hexagon). Angiotensin-converting enzyme (ACE, orange circle) cleaves AngI producing angiotensin II (AngII, purple hexagon) which binds to angiotensin II receptor type 1 (AT1R, purple receptor) and angiotensin II receptor type 2 (AT2R, teal receptor), resulting in vasoconstriction, inflammation, and pulmonary vascular remodeling promoting PH in ARDS. Alternatively, angiotensin-converting enzyme 2 (ACE2, green circle) cleaves AngI producing angiotensin1–9 (Ang1–9, blue hexagon) which binds to AT2R, or AngII to produce angiotensin1–7 (Ang1–7, yellow hexagon) which binds to Mas receptor (MasR, yellow receptor). ACE2 counterbalances ACE, protecting against PH in ARDS through anti-fibrotic and anti-inflammatory actions and vasodilation.

in elevated cytokines, notably IL-6, which is attenuated with decreased flow (Ranieri et al., 1999; Samary et al., 2015). This is further highlighted by Pandolfi et al. who examined if IL-6 and acid sphingomyelinase (aSMase) contribute to PH in ARDS (Pandolfi et al., 2017). Through an LPS model of ARDS, they identified that the production of ceramide and IL-6 in rat PASMCs resulted in failed hypoxic vasoconstriction (HPV), endothelial dysfunction, and hyperresponsiveness to pulmonary vasoconstriction induced by serotonin (Pandolfi et al., 2017). Interestingly, blockade of aSMAse attenuated the progression of PH (Pandolfi et al., 2017). Taken together, it is evident that the upregulation of the inflammatory response after lung injury is a central mechanism in the development of PH in ARDS (Price and Wort, 2017).

There exist a multitude of cytokines that have been implicated in the inflammatory cascade in ALI including interleukins (ILs), interferons (IFNs), tumor necrosis factors (TNFs), chemokines, and colony-stimulating factors (CSFs) (Tisoncik et al., 2012). Many of the cytokines associated with the inflammatory cascade are also implicated in the pathogenesis of PH. The number of macrophages significantly increases in plexiform lesions of patients with severe PAH due to increased expression of chemokines in the lungs and chemokine receptors on monocytes (Gerasimovskaya et al., 2012; Florentin et al., 2018). Once activated, macrophages then induce the release of IL-6, IL-10, IL-1β, and TNF-α (Stow et al., 2009). This review will focus largely on IL-6, IL-10, and TNF-α.

IL-6 is an acute phase reactant that is produced as part of an inflammatory response perpetuated by the liver (Heinrich et al., 1990). Serum studies of patients with PAH show increased levels of IL-6 compared with healthy patients, and even demonstrate IL-6 levels as a more accurate prognostic marker than traditional clinical tests (Selimovic et al., 2009; Soon et al., 2010). IL-6 overexpression in mice led to increased muscularization of the proximal arterial tree and distal arteriolar vessels (Savale et al., 2009; Steiner et al., 2009). The muscularization presented with occlusive neointimal angioproliferative lesions that contained primarily endothelial and T cells (Savale et al., 2009; Steiner et al., 2009). This vascular remodeling resulted in an elevated right ventricular systolic pressure and increased right ventricular hypertrophy (Savale et al., 2009; Steiner et al., 2009). Furthermore, IL-6 has also been shown to be involved in the post-transcriptional mechanism of bone morphogenic protein receptor type 2 (BMPR2) downregulation through signal transducer and activator of transcription 3 (STAT3) and the microRNA cluster 17/92 (Brock et al., 2009). IL-6 has also been shown to participate in vascular remodeling by increasing the levels of matrix metallopeptidase 9 (MMP-9) and vascular endothelial growth factor receptor 2 (VEGFR2) that result in the proliferation of PASMCs and trigger the transdifferentiation of pulmonary endothelial cells to PASMCs (Steiner et al., 2009). Most studies have demonstrated that IL-6 exerts a protective effect in ARDS (Groth et al., 2014). This could suggest that the defensive IL-6 response in ARDS can inadvertently result in the development of PH. There are currently multiple clinical trials attempting to elucidate the role of anti-IL6 therapies to attenuate ARDS in COVID-19 (clinicaltrials.gov: NCT 00531856; NCT04363853; NCT04335071). Tocilizumab was used to attenuate the cytokine storm in select patients worldwide, but large randomized controlled trials are yet to show efficacy (Xu et al., 2020).

TNF-α is a pro-inflammatory cytokine secreted by macrophages that regulates cellular proliferation, differentiation, apoptosis, and survival (Parameswaran and Patial, 2010). Increased levels of TNF-α were found in patients suffering from PAH (Soon et al., 2010). TNF-α overexpression in experimental models results in the suppression of prostacyclin (PGI2: a potent vasodilator) mRNA and increased vascular reactivity (Stevens et al., 1992; Itoh et al., 2003). In addition, TNF-α overexpression in type II AECs led to increased septal destruction, bronchiolitis, pulmonary inflammation, and PH (Fujita et al., 2001). An association has been found between polymorphisms in the surfactant protein-B (SP-B) gene and an increased risk of developing ARDS (Gong et al., 2004). TNF expression has demonstrated potent inhibitory activity of SP B in a human lung adenocarcinoma cell line and decreased surfactant protein-A (SP-A) expression in lung epithelial cells through the p38/MAPK pathway (Berhane et al., 2000; Miakotina and Snyder, 2002). Therefore, this could imply that TNF-α upregulation in ARDS can co-present with PH by inducing atelectasis of alveoli through decreased surfactant production.

IL-10 is an important anti-inflammatory cytokine released by monocytes, macrophages, and several subsets of T cells including type 1 T helper (Th1) cells and regulatory T (Treg) cells (Sabat et al., 2010). Patients with PAH have elevated levels of IL-10, but interestingly increased levels of IL-10 were also observed in patients receiving PGI2 for the treatment of PAH (Groth et al., 2014). In a monocrotaline model of PAH in rats, the intramuscular injection of IL-10 prevented the development of PAH (Ito et al., 2007). Moreover, increased IL-10 production has been associated with the IL-10 promoter polymorphism at position −1082 (−1082GG) (Gong et al., 2006). In a study of 211 Caucasian ARDS patients, the −1082GG genotype resulted in decreased mortality and organ failure in comparison with controls (Gong et al., 2006). It is clear that IL-10 serves a protective role in ARDS and PH; to a greater extent in the −1082GG genotype. However, its efforts may be superseded by a more potent pro-inflammatory response despite persistently elevated IL-10.

Chemokines, or chemotactic cytokines, are a family of 40 low molecular weight proteins that stimulate leukocyte migration and function through their interactions with chemokine receptors (Luster, 1998; Mamazhakypov et al., 2021). There is an elevation in circulating chemokine levels in patients with varying forms of PH which include PH due to chronic obstructive pulmonary disease and lung fibrosis, PAH due to systemic sclerosis, idiopathic PAH, and chronic thromboembolic pulmonary hypertension (CTEPH) (Mamazhakypov et al., 2021). Apart from their roles as biomarkers and in inflammation, chemokines, and their receptors are also involved in pulmonary vascular dysfunction that contributes to PAH (Mamazhakypov et al., 2021). The CCL5–CCR5 axis has been implicated in PAH, most importantly as a mediator of PASMC proliferation *in vitro* (Amsellem et al., 2014). When the CCR5 antagonist maraviroc was administered, the proliferation was depleted (Amsellem et al., 2014). Moreover, CXCL10/CXCL4–CXCR3 axis dysregulation in pulmonary artery endothelial cells led to the loss of recanalization of blocked vessels in CTEPH and impaired angiogenesis (Zabini et al., 2012). CCL3 has also been shown to increase endothelin-1 expression in endothelial cells (Molet et al., 2000). In ARDS, chemokines are released by alveolar macrophages in response to bacterial products (Puneet et al., 2005). However, they can also be secreted by other cells in the local environment as part of an inflammatory cascade involving TNF and IL-1β (Puneet et al., 2005). This demonstrates that an initial inflammatory response in ARDS can be strengthened by an inflammatory cascade and potentiate pulmonary vascular dysfunction and eventual PH.

The importance of the inflammatory cascade in the pathogenesis of PH in ARDS is still not fully understood. Here, we present that a heightened pro-inflammatory response in ARDS can contribute to the development of PH through the involvement of TNF, IL-6, chemokines, and IL-10. These cytokines are implicated in a multitude of processes namely HPV failure, decreased surfactant production, imbalance of vasodilators and vasoconstrictors, PASMC proliferation, and loss of recanalization in blocked vessels. Conclusively, this can provide a new route for effective therapeutics.

Thrombosis

Thrombosis is a well-described phenomenon that presents in patients suffering from ARDS (Ryan et al., 2014). In a postmortem study of 22 ARDS patients, 19 patients (86%) exhibited macrothrombi in pulmonary arterial and capillary vessels and evidence of microthrombi (Tomashefski et al., 1983). This results from localized damage to the endothelial cell lining that causes the release of tissue factor (TF) in response to inflammation (Maniatis et al., 2008; Levi and Van Der Poll, 2010; Price et al., 2012). TF is a potent activator of the extrinsic coagulation cascade, and experimental models show inhibition of TF–Factor VIIa–Factor X complex reduces the extent of PH in ARDS (Welty-Wolf et al., 2001; MacKman, 2009). Furthermore, plasminogen activator inhibitor-I (PAI-1) levels are elevated in contrast with decreased levels of protein C and thrombin antithrombin (TAT) complexes in ARDS patients (Ware et al.,

2003, 2007). These markers suggest that ARDS promotes a hypercoagulable state while repressing fibrinolysis and is also associated with increased mortality (Ware et al., 2007).

Interactions between coagulation and an excessive inflammatory response are considered essential in the pathophysiology of ARDS (Frantzeskaki et al., 2017). Activation of coagulation pathways in ARDS results in the overproduction of thrombin that can further ameliorate inflammatory processes through proteinase-activated receptors (Frantzeskaki et al., 2017). Under non-pathological conditions, thrombin production is highly regulated by tissue factor pathway inhibitor, anti-thrombin III, and the protein C system (José et al., 2014). These feedback mechanisms can be diminished in inflammation due to increased consumption and decreased production of anticoagulants (José et al., 2014). It is evident that the formation of microthrombi is due to increased coagulability and can promote PH in ARDS patients through the pathological blockade of vessels.

More recently, ARDS secondary to SARS-CoV-2 infection (COVID-19) has been associated with an increase in the risk of thrombotic complications (mainly pulmonary embolisms) in comparison with non-ARDS SARS-CoV-2 infections (Helms et al., 2020). Longer prothrombin time (PT), increased levels of D-dimer and fibrin degradation products, longer activated partial thromboplastin time (aPTT), and decreased platelets were found in non-survivors of SARS-CoV-2 (Tang et al., 2020b; Xiaofang et al., 2020). These parameters are all related to a poor prognosis in infected patients (Tang et al., 2020b; Xiaofang et al., 2020). While experimental models of SARS-CoV-2 infections have not been widely studied, infection of SARS-CoV with ARDS results in increased fibrin deposition in mice (Gralinski et al., 2013). Furthermore, the use of low molecular weight heparin leads to reduced mortality in severe COVID-19 patients (Tang et al., 2020a). This suggests that a similar balance toward coagulation might exist in patients with ARDS-related SARS-CoV-2 and might provide significant prognostic value in severe infections. How the inflammatory and thrombotic pathways contribute to PH are represented diagrammatically in **Figure 2**.

Hypoxic Pulmonary Vasoconstriction

HPV is a unique and complex feature of the pulmonary circulation whereby hypoxic conditions lead to vasoconstriction, in contrast to the systemic circulation where hypoxia leads to vasodilation (Lumb and Slinger, 2015). HPV has an important physiological role; it acts to match perfusion to ventilation to optimize P_{O2} (McLoughlin, 2018). Thus, HPV shunts blood toward areas with high ventilation to maintain efficient gas exchange processes (Sylvester et al., 2012). In ALI settings, both clinically and experimentally, edema as a result of loss of barrier function leads to regional hypoxemia, activating HPV to shunt blood away from hypoxic areas of the lung to ventilated areas (Marshall et al., 1994; Fischer et al., 2004; Spöhr et al., 2007; Sylvester et al., 2012). This beneficial effect of HPV has been shown to be inhibited in experimental models of oleic acid, bleomycin, or endotoxin-induced ALI (Sylvester et al., 2012), underscoring the important role that HPV has in matching ventilation/perfusion. Herein, studies in mice have revealed that inhibition of ATP-regulated potassium channel Kir6.1, which is elevated after endotoxemia, was able to restore HPV in mice; however, the effects on lung inflammation were not assessed (Turzo et al., 2018). However, prolonged HPV can lead to the development of PH and high-altitude induced pulmonary edema (HAPE) which is characterized by patchy peripheral distribution of edema (Bartsch, 1999). Although this mechanism is distinct to the classic presentation of ARDS that has a strong inflammatory component, HAPE is characterized by the presence of pulmonary edema (Bartsch, 1999). Pulmonary edema is also a feature shared with ARDS that contributes to deficits in gas exchange and lung failure due to fluid accumulation in the alveolar spaces (The ARDS Definition Task Force, 2012). Thus, although distinct to ARDS, HAPE as a result of prolonged HPV represents a mechanism linking PH and the development of edema, a feature of ARDS.

An important downstream molecular consequence of hypoxia is the stabilization of hypoxia-inducible factor (HIF)-1A and HIF-2A. Under normoxic conditions, HIFs are degraded by prolylhydroxylases (PHDs); however, under hypoxia, the PHDs are inactivated allowing HIFs to stabilize (Eltzschig and Carmeliet, 2011). In ALI, the stabilization of HIF1A and HIF2A have been shown to limit injury (Karmouty-Quintana et al., 2013b; Gong et al., 2015; Huang et al., 2019). Deletion of endothelial cell HIF-1A expression inhibited endothelial proliferation and attenuated vascular repair processes in a model of sepsis-induced lung injury (Huang et al., 2019). Similarly, abrogation of endothelial HIF-2A resulted in defective adherens junction that was exacerbated after endotoxin challenge in mice, resulting in worsened lung injury (Gong et al., 2015). The downstream HIF-mediated mechanism is complex and includes many mediators; however, increased expression of ecto-nucleotidases CD39 and CD73 and the increased expression of the adenosine A2B receptor (ADORA2B) have been implicated in the accumulation of adenosine and subsequent protective effects of adenosine through activation of its receptors (Karmouty-Quintana et al., 2013b). Remarkably, these same mechanisms that are protective in acute lung injury settings have also been linked with the pathophysiology of PH. Genetic deletion of endothelial PHD2 and subsequent stabilization of HIF-2A has been linked with the spontaneous development of PH in mice associated with severe vascular remodeling (Dai Zhiyu et al., 2016). Several studies have also demonstrated an important role for HIF1A, adenosine, and ADORA2B activation as causative mediators in group 3 PH (Karmouty-Quintana et al., 2012, 2013a; Garcia-Morales et al., 2015; Rajagopal et al., 2021). Taken together, these studies illustrate the complexity of hypoxic–adenosinergic responses in the pathophysiology of ARDS and PH, whereas they are protective in ALI settings, they also promote features of PH and chronic lung injury. This duality is perhaps best highlighted by studies that determined the prevalence of HIF2A and PHD2 polymorphisms that are associated with improved adaptation to hypoxia in high-altitude residents in patients with ARDS. This study demonstrated that the PHD2 polymorphism *PHD2 RS516651-TT*, which is associated with increased adaptation to high altitude, was associated with a higher 30-days mortality

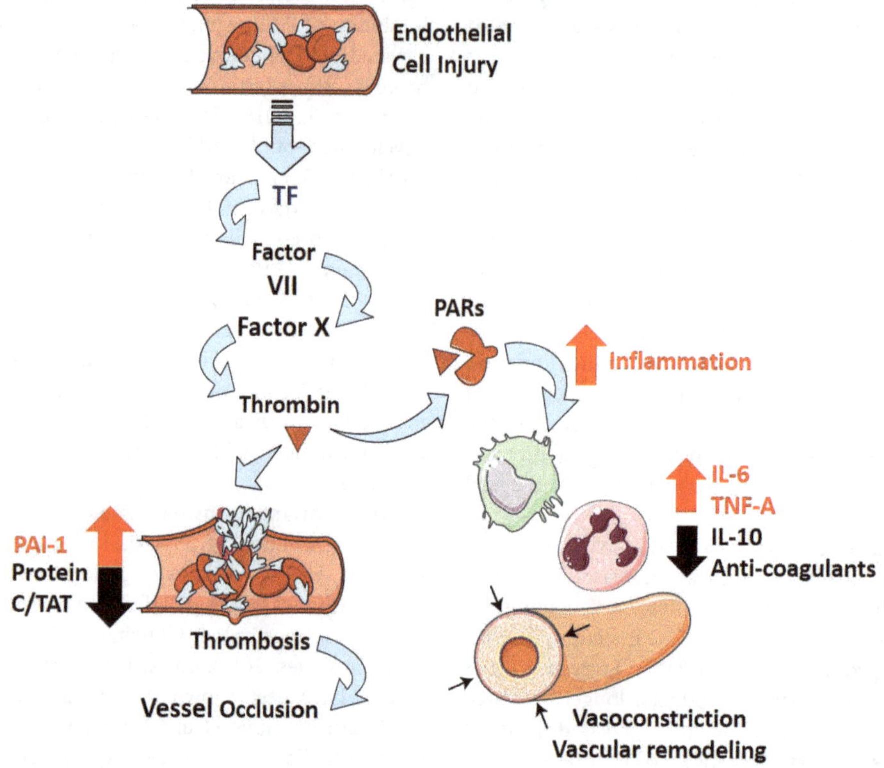

FIGURE 2 | Inflammation and thrombosis in ARDS and how they contribute to PH. Injury to the alveolar-capillary interface in ARDS leads to the release of tissue factor from the endothelial cells and induces coagulation through the extrinsic pathway. The penultimate mediator of coagulation, thrombin (dark red triangle), interacts with proteinase-associated receptors (PARs, dark red receptor) to promote inflammation (increase in IL-6, TNF-α, and IL-10) and suppress several negative regulatory elements of coagulation (decrease in Protein C, thrombin antithrombin complexes—TATs, anticoagulants; increase in plasminogen activator inhibitor 1—PAI-1). This leads to downstream effects of inflammatory cytokines (IL-6 and TNF-α) that include vascular remodeling and vasoconstriction, which overwhelm the protective effects of anti-inflammatory cytokine IL-10 and further incite thrombosis.

risk within 30 days of the onset of ARDS (Dötsch et al., 2017).

Endothelin

Increased levels of endothelin-1 (ET-1), a potent vasoconstriction agent (Davenport and Maguire, 1994), have been reported clinically in ARDS patients where they contribute not only to pulmonary vasoconstriction but also to promote lung edema (Druml et al., 1993; Sanai et al., 1996; Nakano et al., 2007). These observations are significant because inhibition of ET-1 is an important strategy in the treatment of PH (Clozel et al., 2013). Endothelin receptor antagonists (ERAs) have been used successfully in experimental models of ALI where they inhibited lung edema; unfortunately, pulmonary vascular pressures were not assessed in these studies (Guimarães et al., 2000; Araz et al., 2013). However, due to the effect of ERAs in modulating PH by promoting vasodilation and reducing inflammation in both PH and ALI (Guimarães et al., 2000; Araz et al., 2013; Clozel et al., 2013), its use in ARDS as a front-line therapy has been postulated (Araz, 2020).

Hyaluronan

PH in the setting of ARDS falls into WHO group 3 PH because it is strongly associated with hypoxia and the presence of lung injury (Poor et al., 2012). A recent review of mechanisms of group 3 PH associated with lung fibrosis has been recently published (Rajagopal et al., 2021). Interestingly, similar pathways are involved in both PH associated with ARDS and lung fibrosis such as inflammatory mediators, RAS, and endothelins (Rajagopal et al., 2021). In addition, the glycosaminoglycan hyaluronan has been implicated in PH associated with chronic lung diseases (Collum et al., 2017, 2019). Interestingly, hyaluronan is elevated in experimental lung injury (Ni et al., 2018; Bell et al., 2019), and its inhibition has been shown to be effective in models of ALI (McKallip et al., 2013, 2015). Thus, it is conceivable that in addition to promoting lung inflammation, excess hyaluronan in ARDS may also contribute to PH. In line with this, we hypothesize that the hypoxic environment in ARDS leads to increased expression or activity of CD73 and ADORA2B such as in PH in the setting of lung fibrosis (Garcia-Morales et al., 2015) that leads to accumulation of adenosine and subsequent activation of ADORA2B. Activation of this receptor has been shown to promote hyaluronan production through increased expression of hyaluronan synthases (HAS)-1 and 2 (Karmouty-Quintana et al., 2013a; Mertens et al., 2018). Interestingly, many recent publications have linked increased hyaluronan deposition in COVID-19 (Hellman et al., 2020; Kaber et al., 2020), a disease that is more and more associated with important cardiopulmonary complications (Karmouty-Quintana et al., 2020; Potus et al., 2020). Recent publications from our group have also demonstrated that inhibition of hyaluronan by 4-methylumbelliferone (4MU) attenuated PH by diminishing vascular remodeling (Collum et al., 2017, 2019). 4MU has also been postulated as a therapeutic for COVID-19–induced ARDS where it could not only attenuate the inflammatory effects but also dampen the cardiovascular complications (Karmouty-Quintana et al., 2020; Shi et al., 2020). The main pathways that contribute to PH after vascular injury are summarized in **Figure 3**.

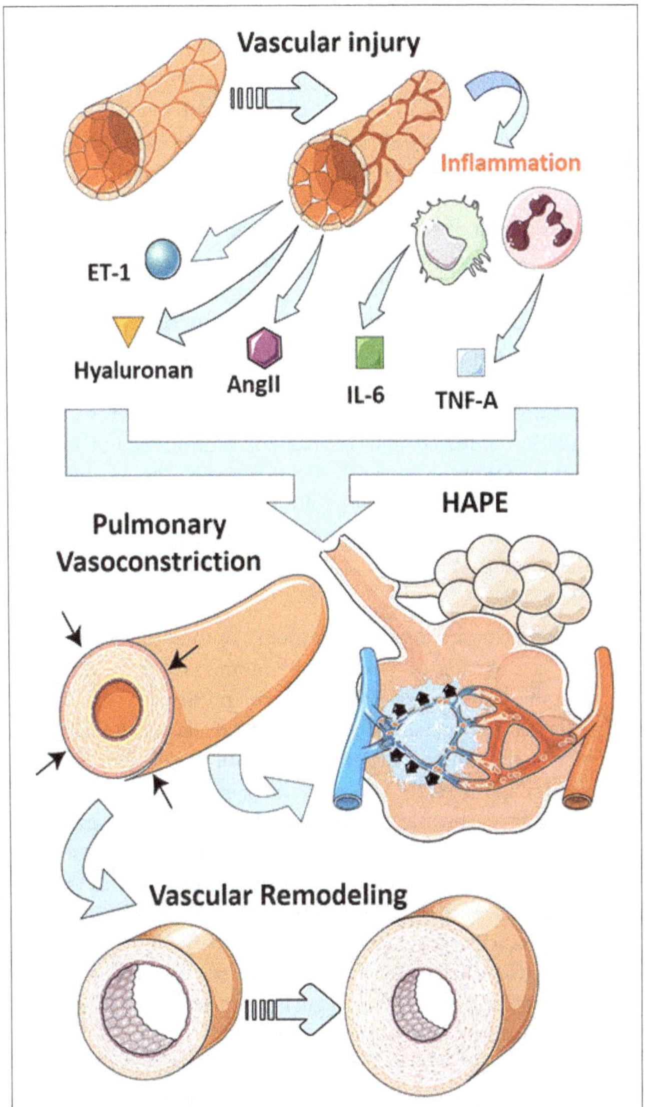

FIGURE 3 | Mechanisms that lead to PH in ARDS. Vascular injury in ARDS leads to the release of vasoactive mediators including endothelin-1 (ET-1-blue/green sphere), hyaluronan (golden triangle), and angiotensin II (AngII, purple hexagon). Further, vascular injury promotes inflammation that releases cytokines such as interleukin-6 (IL-6, green squares) and tumor necrosis factor (TNF)-α (blue squares). These vasoactive mediators and cytokines promote vascular remodeling and pulmonary vasoconstriction, hallmarks of pulmonary hypertension. Prolonged vasoconstriction can then lead to high-altitude pulmonary edema (HAPE), a form of lung injury similar to ARDS.

CONCLUSIONS

Mechanisms of PH in ARDS are complex and poorly understood. Evidence that PH increases the mortality in patients with ARDS is suggested by some studies, but definitive evidence is thwarted by inconsistent reports (Beiderlinden et al., 2006; Ñamendys-Silva et al., 2014; Calcaianu et al., 2017). However, it is clear that pulmonary vascular dysfunction is present in patients with ARDS and has indirect associations with mortality (Monchi et al., 1998; Bull et al., 2010). This review summarizes current understanding of the pathways that contribute to PH in ARDS, with specific commentary regarding the implications for the current COVID-19 pandemic.

The renin–angiotensin axis plays an important and multi-dimensional role in pulmonary vascular changes in both acute and chronic lung disease (Jia, 2016). A hyperactive form of ACE correlates with the development of and increased mortality in ARDS (Marshall et al., 2002; Jerng et al., 2006). Further, the increases in ACE and its specific catabolites have been shown to directly contribute to vascular remodeling in PH (Krege et al., 1995; Nong et al., 1996; Suylen et al., 2001). For example, activation of the AngII receptor AT1R directly promotes vasoconstriction and vascular remodeling, prominent drivers of PH (Iwai and Horiuchi, 2009). Conversely, the ACE homolog ACE2 is protective in PH, and increasing its expression would be a novel approach to PH-ARDS treatment (Imai et al., 2005). It is not surprising then that the loss of membrane-associated ACE2 in the lung caused by SARS-CoV has been proposed as a crucial mechanism for the rapidly progressive alveolar damage and vascular changes present in COVID-19 patients (Imai et al., 2005; Kuba et al., 2005). There are multiple clinical trials in the works investigating the prophylactic and therapeutic effect of angiotensin pathway–modulating drugs in preventing and treating patients with COVID-19–associated ARDS (clinicaltrials.gov; NCT04335786; NCT04337190).

Another critical contributing mechanism to ALI is a robust and exaggerated immune response, referred to here as the inflammatory cascade. Acute inflammation characterized by rapid and robust release of inflammatory cytokines such as IL-6, IL-10, and TNF is a central feature of ARDS (Tisoncik et al., 2012). These same mediators are also implicated in PH and may play key roles in the severe and acute inflammation observed in ARDS with PH. Of particular interest, the destructive IL-6 response in ARDS may contribute to the subsequent observations of PH in ARDS patients (Groth et al., 2014; Pandolfi et al., 2017). Therapeutics which target these inflammatory pathways are worth serious investigation. The inflammatory cascade, as a component of cytokine release syndrome, is thought to be involved in the development of ARDS in patients infected with SARS-CoV-2, where important changes to the pulmonary vasculature including features of PH have been reported (Potus et al., 2020; Sun et al., 2020). There are currently randomized controlled trials evaluating the efficacy of leronlimab, a CC chemokine receptor 5 (CCR5) modulator, in patients with mild to severe SARS-CoV-2–induced ARDS (clinicaltrials.gov, NCT04347239).

The ARDS-related inflammatory cascade has also been tied directly to another feature of ARDS: hypercoagulability and thrombosis. An altered thrombotic and fibrinolysis profile has been linked to PH in ARDS (Nieuwenhuizen et al., 2009). Inhibition of the coagulation cascade abrogates ARDS-related PH (Welty-Wolf et al., 2001; MacKman, 2009). In this review, we describe several molecular mechanisms that perpetuate this abnormal hemostatic state, and provide insight into novel diagnostic and therapeutic interventions that can increase positive outcomes in ARDS. The presence of underlying viral infections, in particular COVID-19 infection, in ARDS patients even further increases the risk of thrombotic events. While dysregulation of the coagulation cascade is observed in COVID-19 patients with either or both ARDS and PH, the mechanisms by which this occurs are not fully understood, thwarting the informed use of agents which interfere with hypercoagulability in these patients.

The unique vasoconstrictive response of the lungs to hypoxia presents a particularly complex phenomenon in ARDS and PH (Lumb and Slinger, 2015). Acute pulmonary edema in ALI activates the hypoxic response, which allows the lungs to maximize oxygenation efficiency (Marshall et al., 1994; Fischer et al., 2004; Spöhr et al., 2007; Sylvester et al., 2012). However, if HPV becomes chronic, it can result in the development of PH (Bartsch, 1999). As such, potential therapeutic enhancement of HPV in acute settings must be balanced by consideration of the long-term effects of HPV, which may increase the risk of PH. Viral infections are known to lead to hypoxia through pulmonary vascular and epithelial cell damage (Sun et al., 2020). As such, the role of disrupted vascular regulation in patients with severe COVID-19 warrants further investigation.

Two additional phenomena observed in ARDS are increased circulating ET-1 levels (Nakano et al., 2007) and exacerbated local deposition of hyaluronan in the lung parenchyma (McKallip et al., 2013, 2015; Ni et al., 2018; Bell et al., 2019). Interestingly, inhibition of both ET-1–mediated actions (Guimarães et al., 2000; Araz et al., 2013) and hyaluronan deposition (McKallip et al., 2013, 2015) are beneficial in models of ALI. While hyaluronan has been implicated in the pathogenesis of PH related to chronic lung disease (Collum et al., 2019; World Health Organization, 2020), neither ET-1 nor hyaluronan has been thoroughly investigated in ARDS-related PH.

An important aspect in the pathophysiology of PH in ARDS is the interplay between acute and chronic mediators that may promote features of PH. In the early stages of ALI, damage to the endothelium and subsequent increase of vasoactive mediators such as ET-1, IL-6, and TNF-A can promote pulmonary vasoconstriction leading to increased PVR. Similarly, loss of ACE2, such as after viral infections, leading to increased AngII and subsequent activation of AT2 receptors can also promote pulmonary vasoconstrictor responses. An important aspect of PH is vascular remodeling. Although it is unclear at what stage vascular remodeling is initiated in ARDS, it is conceivable that the protracted presence of mediators such as HIFs and the accumulation of adenosine initiate vascular remodeling processes that contribute further to the pathogenesis of PH in ARDS. In line with this, chronic phase of ARDS is known for its fibroproliferative milieu, where HIF (Delbrel et al., 2018), adenosine (Karmouty-Quintana et al., 2013b), and hyaluronan (Li et al., 2011) play central roles.

Given the ongoing COVID-19 global pandemic, it is crucial for the authors to address the implications of the aforementioned findings for patients with COVID-19. COVID-19 has infected over 64 million individuals and resulted in over 1.3 million deaths worldwide (https://coronavirus.jhu.edu/map.html accessed December 2, 2020). ARDS is the most common clinical course for patients with severe COVID-19 infections (Machhi et al., 2020). Prognosis for patients with ARDS is dismal, and some recent evidence suggests that the patients with COVID-19–related ARDS may face an even higher risk of death. As effective treatments for ARDS are lacking and a vaccine against COVID-19 has yet to be developed, it is critical that targetable mechanisms behind this devastating disease are discovered. A recent review has summarized the known mechanisms to date that promote pulmonary vascular dysfunction in SARS-CoV-2–induced ARDS and identified novel potential treatment options that target the vasculature (Karmouty-Quintana et al., 2020).

AUTHOR CONTRIBUTIONS

LR and AH contributed equally. All authors read and approved the manuscript.

REFERENCES

Amsellem, V., Lipskaia, L., Abid, S., Poupel, L., Houssaini, A., Quarck, R., et al. (2014). CCR5 as a treatment target in pulmonary arterial hypertension. *Circulation* 130, 880–891. doi: 10.1161/CIRCULATIONAHA.114.010757

Antoniak, S., Sparkenbaugh, E., and Pawlinski, R. (2014). Tissue factor, protease activated receptors and pathologic heart remodelling. *Thromb. Haemost.* 112, 893–900. doi: 10.1160/TH14-03-0243

Araz, O. (2020). Current pharmacological approach to ARDS: the place of bosentan. *Eurasian J. Med.* 52, 81–85. doi: 10.5152/eurasianjmed.2020.19218

Araz, O., Demirci, E., Ucar, E. Y., Calik, M., Pulur, D., Karaman, A., et al. (2013). Comparison of reducing effect on lung injury of dexamethasone and bosentan in acute lung injury: an experimental study. *Multidiscip Resp. Med.* 8:74. doi: 10.1186/2049-6958-8-74

Asperen, R. M. W., Lutter, R., Specht, P. A., Moll, G. N., Woensel, J. B., van, Loos, C. M., et al. (2011). Acute respiratory distress syndrome leads to reduced ratio of

ACE/ACE2 activities and is prevented by angiotensin-(1-7) or an angiotensin II receptor antagonist. *J. Pathol.* 225, 618–627. doi: 10.1002/path.2987

Bartsch, P. (1999). High altitude pulmonary edema. *Med. Sci. Sports Exerc.* 31, S23–S27. doi: 10.1097/00005768-199901001-00004

Beiderlinden, M., Kuehl, H., Boes, T., and Peters, J. (2006). Prevalence of pulmonary hypertension associated with severe acute respiratory distress syndrome: predictive value of computed tomography. *Intensive Care Med.* 32, 852–857. doi: 10.1007/s00134-006-0122-9

Bell, T. J., Brand, O. J., Morgan, D. J., Salek-Ardakani, S., Jagger, C., Fujimori, T., et al. (2019). Defective lung function following influenza virus is due to prolonged, reversible hyaluronan synthesis. *Matrix Biol.* 80, 14–28. doi: 10.1016/j.matbio.2018.06.006

Bellani, G., Laffey, J. G., Pham, T., Fan, E., Brochard, L., Esteban, A., et al. (2016). Epidemiology, patterns of care, and mortality for patients with acute respiratory distress syndrome in intensive care units in 50 countries. *JAMA* 315, 788–800. doi: 10.1001/jama.2016.0291

Berhane, K., Margana, R. K., and Boggaram, V. (2000). Characterization of rabbit SP-B promoter region responsive to downregulation by tumor necrosis factor-α. *Am. J. Physiol. Lung Cell Mol. Physiol.* 279, L806–L814. doi: 10.1152/ajplung.2000.279.5.l806

Boissier, F., Katsahian, S., Razazi, K., Thille, A. W., Roche-Campo, F., Leon, R., et al. (2013). Prevalence and prognosis of cor pulmonale during protective ventilation for acute respiratory distress syndrome. *Intensive Care Med.* 39, 1725–1733. doi: 10.1007/s00134-013-2941-9

Brock, M., Trenkmann, M., Gay, R. E., Michel, B. A., Gay, S., Fischler, M., et al. (2009). Interleukin-6 modulates the expression of the bone morphogenic protein receptor type ii through a novel STAT3-microRNA cluster 17/92 pathway. *Circ. Res.* 104, 1184–1191. doi: 10.1161/CIRCRESAHA.109.197491

Brower, R. G., Matthay, M. A., Morris, A., Schoenfeld, D., Thompson, B. T., and Wheeler, A. (2000). Ventilation with lower tidal volumes as compared with traditional tidal volumes for acute lung injury and the acute respiratory distress syndrome. *NEJM* 342, 1301–1308. doi: 10.1056/NEJM200005043421801

Bull, T. M., Clark, B., McFann, K., and Moss, M. (2010). Pulmonary vascular dysfunction is associated with poor outcomes in patients with acute lung injury. *Am. J. Respir. Crit. Care Med.* 182, 1123–1128. doi: 10.1164/rccm.201002-0250OC

Calcaianu, G., Calcaianu, M., Gschwend, A., Canuet, M., Meziani, F., and Kessler, R. (2017). Hemodynamic profile of pulmonary hypertension (PH) in ARDS. *Pulm Circ.* 8, 1–8. doi: 10.1177/2045893217753415

Cheng, H., Wang, Y., and Wang, G.-Q. (2020). Organ-protective effect of angiotensin-converting enzyme 2 and its effect on the prognosis of COVID-19. *J. Med. Virol.* 92, 726–730. doi: 10.1002/jmv.25785

Clozel, M., Maresta, A., and Humbert, M. (2013). Endothelin receptor antagonists. *Handb. Exp. Pharmacol.* 218, 199—227. doi: 10.1007/978-3-642-38664-0_9

Collum, S. D., Chen, N. Y., Hernandez, A. M. M., Hanmandlu, A., Sweeney, H., Mertens, T. C. J. C. J., et al. (2017). Inhibition of hyaluronan synthesis attenuates pulmonary hypertension associated with lung fibrosis. *Br. J. Pharm.* 174, 3284–3301. doi: 10.1111/bph.13947

Collum, S. D., Molina, J. G., Hanmandlu, A., Bi, W., Pedroza, M., Mertens, T. C. J., et al. (2019). Adenosine and hyaluronan promote lung fibrosis and pulmonary hypertension in combined pulmonary fibrosis and emphysema. *Dis. Models Mech.* 12:dmm.038711. doi: 10.1242/dmm.038711

Davenport, A., and Maguire, J. (1994). Is endothelin-induced vasoconstriction mediated only by ETA receptors in humans? *Trends Pharmacol. Sci.* 15:9–11. doi: 10.1016/0165-6147(94)90120-1

Delbrel, E., Soumare, A., Naguez, A., Label, R., Bernard, O., Bruhat, A., et al. (2018). HIF-1α triggers ER stress and CHOP-mediated apoptosis in alveolar epithelial cells, a key event in pulmonary fibrosis. *Sci. Rep.* 8:17939. doi: 10.1038/s41598-018-36063-2

Dessap, A. M., Boissier, F., Charron, C., Bégot, E., Repessé, X., Legras, A., et al. (2016). Acute cor pulmonale during protective ventilation for acute respiratory distress syndrome: prevalence, predictors, and clinical impact. *Intensive Care Med.* 42, 862–870. doi: 10.1007/s00134-015-4141-2

Donoghue, M., Hsieh, F., Baronas, E., Godbout, K., Gosselin, M., Stagliano, N., et al. (2000). A novel angiotensin-converting enzyme–related carboxypeptidase (ACE2) converts angiotensin I to angiotensin 1-9. *Circ. Res.* 87, e1–e9. doi: 10.1161/01.RES.87.5.e1

Dötsch, A., Eisele, L., Rabeling, M., Rump, K., Walstein, K., Bick, A., et al. (2017). Hypoxia inducible factor-2 alpha and prolinhydroxylase 2 polymorphisms in patients with acute respiratory distress syndrome (ARDS). *Int. J. Mol. Sci.* 18:1266. doi: 10.3390/ijms18061266

Druml, W., Steltzer, H., Waldhäusl, W., Lenz, K., Hammerle, A., Vierhapper, H., et al. (1993). Endothelin-1 in adult respiratory distress syndrome. *Am. Rev. Respir. Dis.* 148, 1169–1173. doi: 10.1164/ajrccm/148.5.1169

Eltzschig, H. K., and Carmeliet, P. (2011). Hypoxia and inflammation. *N. Engl. J. Med.* 364, 656–665. doi: 10.1056/NEJMra0910283

Ferreira, A. J., and Santos, R., A. S. (2005). Cardiovascular actions of angiotensin-(1-7). *Braz. J. Med. Biol. Res.* 38, 499–507. doi: 10.1590/s0100-879x2005000400003

Fischer, L., Freise, H., Hilpert, J.-H., Wendholt, D., Lauer, S., Aken, H., et al. (2004). Modulation of hypoxic pulmonary vasoconstriction is time and nitric oxide dependent in a peritonitis model of sepsis. *Intensive Care Med.* 30, 1821–1828. doi: 10.1007/s00134-004-2351-0

Florentin, J., Coppin, E., Vasamsetti, S. B., Zhao, J., Tai, Y.-Y., Tang, Y., et al. (2018). Inflammatory macrophage expansion in pulmonary hypertension depends upon mobilization of blood-borne monocytes. *J. Immunol.* 200, 3612–3625. doi: 10.4049/jimmunol.1701287

Frantzeskaki, F., Armaganidis, A., and Orfanos, S. E. (2017). Immunothrombosis in acute respiratory distress syndrome: cross talks between inflammation and coagulation. *Respiration* 93, 212–225. doi: 10.1159/000453002

Frutos-Vivar, F., Nin, N., and Esteban, A. (2004). Epidemiology of acute lung injury and acute respiratory distress syndrome. *Curr. Opin. Crit. Care* 10, 1–6. doi: 10.1055/s-2006-948287

Fujita, M., Shannon, J. M., Irvin, C. G., Fagan, K. A., Cool, C., Augustin, A., et al. (2001). Overexpression of tumor necrosis factor-α produces an increase in lung volumes and pulmonary hypertension. *Am. J. Physiol. Lung Cell Mol. Physiol.* 280, L39–L49. doi: 10.1152/ajplung.2001.28 0.1.l39

Garcia-Morales, L. J., Chen, N.-Y., Weng, T., Luo, F., Davies, J., Philip, K., et al. (2015). Altered hypoxic–adenosine axis and metabolism in group iii pulmonary hypertension. *Am. J. Respir. Cell Mol. Biol.* 54, 574–583. doi: 10.1165/rcmb.2015-0145OC

Gerasimovskaya, E., Kratzer, A., Sidiakova, A., Salys, J., Zamora, M., and Taraseviciene-Stewart, L. (2012). Interplay of macrophages and T cells in the lung vasculature. *Am. J. Physiol. Lung Cell Mol. Physiol.* 302, L1014–L1022. doi: 10.1152/ajplung.00357.2011

Gong, H., Rehman, J., Tang, H., Wary, K., Mittal, M., Chaturvedi, P., et al. (2015). HIF2α signaling inhibits adherens junctional disruption in acute lung injury. *J. Clin. Invest.* 125, 652–664. doi: 10.1172/JCI77701

Gong, M. N., Thompson, B. T., Williams, P. L., Zhou, W., Wang, M. Z., Pothier, L., et al. (2006). Interleukin-10 polymorphism in position-1082 and acute respiratory distress syndrome. *Eur. Respir. J.* 27, 674–681. doi: 10.1183/09031936.06.00046405

Gong, M. N., Wei, Z., Xu, L. L., Miller, D. P., Thompson, B. T., and Christiani, D. C. (2004). Polymorphism in the surfactant protein-B gene, gender, and the risk of direct pulmonary injury and ARDS. *Chest* 125, 203–211. doi: 10.1378/chest.125.1.203

Gralinski, L., Bankhead, A. III, Jeng, S., Menachery, V., Proll, S., Belisle, S., et al. (2013). Mechanisms of severe acute respiratory syndrome coronavirus-induced acute lung injury. *mBio* 4, e00271-13. doi: 10.1128/mBio.00271-13

Groth, A., Vrugt, B., Brock, M., Speich, R., Ulrich, S., and Huber, L. C. (2014). Inflammatory cytokines in pulmonary hypertension. *Respir. Res.* 15:47. doi: 10.1186/1465-9921-15-47

Guimarães, C., Da-Silva, S., Couture, R., and Rae, G. (2000). Mixed endothelin ET(A) and ET(B) antagonist bosentan inhibits oleic acid-induced lung plasma extravasation in mouse. *J. Cardiovasc. Pharmacol.* 36, S371–S373. doi: 10.1097/00005344-200036051-00107

Hamming, I., Timens, W., Bulthuis, M. L. C., Lely, A. T., Navis, G. J., and van Goor, H. (2004). Tissue distribution of ACE2 protein, the functional receptor for SARS coronavirus. A first step in understanding SARS pathogenesis. *J. Pathol.* 203, 631–637. doi: 10.1002/path.1570

Heinrich, P. C., Castell, J. V., and Andus, T. (1990). Interleukin-6 and the acute phase response. *Biochem. J.* 265, 621–636. doi: 10.1042/bj26 50621

Hellman, U., Karlsson, M. G., Engström-Laurent, A., Cajander, S., Dorofte, L., Ahlm, C., et al. (2020). Presence of hyaluronan in lung alveoli in severe Covid-19: An opening for new treatment options? *J. Biol. Chem.* 295, 15418–15422. doi: 10.1074/jbc.AC120.015967

Helms, J., Tacquard, C., Severac, F., Leonard-Lorant, I., Ohana, M., and Delabranche, X. (2020). High risk of thrombosis in patients in severe SARS-CoV-2 infection: a multicenter prospective cohort study. *Intensive Care Med.* 46, 1089–1098. doi: 10.1007/s00134-020-06062-x

Hemnes, A. R., Rathinasabapathy, A., Austin, E. A., Brittain, E. L., Carrier, E. J., Chen, X., et al. (2018). A potential therapeutic role for angiotensin-converting enzyme 2 in human pulmonary arterial hypertension. *Eur. Respir. J.* 51:1702638. doi: 10.1183/13993003.02638-2017

Hoffmann, M., Kleine-Weber, H., Schroeder, S., Krüger, N., Herrler, T., Erichsen, S., et al. (2020). SARS-CoV-2 cell entry depends on ACE2 and TMPRSS2 and is blocked by a clinically proven protease inhibitor. *Cell* 181, 271–280.e8. doi: 10.1016/j.cell.2020.02.052

Huang, X., Zhang, X., Zhao, D. X., Yin, J., Hu, G., Evans, C. E., et al. (2019). Endothelial hypoxia-inducible factor-1α is required for vascular repair and resolution of inflammatory lung injury through forkhead box protein M1. *Am. J. Pathol.* 189, 1664–1679. doi: 10.1016/j.ajpath.2019.04.014

Imai, Y., Kuba, K., Ohto-Nakanishi, T., and Penninger, J. M. (2010). Angiotensin-converting enzyme 2 (ACE2) in disease pathogenesis. *Circ, J.* 74, 405–410. doi: 10.1253/circj.cj-10-0045

Imai, Y., Kuba, K., Rao, S., Huan, Y., Guo, F., Guan, B., et al. (2005). Angiotensin-converting enzyme 2 protects from severe acute lung failure. *Nature* 436, 112–116. doi: 10.1038/nature03712

Ito, T., Okada, T., Miyashita, H., Nomoto, T., Nonaka-Sarukawa, M., Uchibori, R., et al. (2007). Interleukin-10 expression mediated by an adeno-associated virus vector prevents monocrotaline-induced pulmonary arterial hypertension in rats. *Circ. Res.* 101, 734–741. doi: 10.1161/CIRCRESAHA.107.153023

Itoh, A., Nishihira, J., Makita, H., Miyamoto, K., Yamaguchi, E., and Nishimura, M. (2003). Effects of IL-1β, TNF-α and macrophage migration inhibitory factor on prostacyclin synthesis in rat pulmonary artery smooth muscle cells. *Respirology* 8, 467–472. doi: 10.1046/j.1440-1843.2003.00491.x

Iwai, M., and Horiuchi, M. (2009). Devil and angel in the renin-angiotensin system: ACE-angiotensin II-AT1 receptor axis vs. ACE2-angiotensin-(1-7)-Mas receptor axis. *Hypertension Res.* 32, 533–536. doi: 10.1038/hr.2009.74

Jerng, J.-S., Yu, C.-J., Wang, H.-C., Chen, K.-Y., Cheng, S.-L., and Yang, P.-C. (2006). Polymorphism of the angiotensin-converting enzyme gene affects the outcome of acute respiratory distress syndrome. *Crit. Care Med.* 34, 1001–1006. doi: 10.1097/01.CCM.0000206107.92476.39

Jia, H. (2016). Pulmonary angiotensin-converting enzyme 2 (ACE2) and inflammatory lung disease. *Shock* 46, 239–248. doi: 10.1097/SHK.0000000000000633

José, R. J., Williams, A. E., and Chambers, R. C. (2014). Proteinase-activated receptors in fibroproliferative lung disease. *Thorax* 69, 190–192. doi: 10.1136/thoraxjnl-2013-204367

Kaber, G., Kratochvil, M. J., Burgener, E. B., Peltan, E. L., Barlow, G., Yang, S., et al. (2020). Hyaluronan is abundant in COVID-19 respiratory secretions. *medRxiv*, 2020.09.11.20191692. doi: 10.1101/2020.09.11.20191692

Karmouty-Quintana, H., Thandavarayan, R. A., Keller, S. P., Sahay, S., Pandit, L. M., and Akkanti, B. (2020). Emerging mechanisms of pulmonary vasoconstriction in SARS-CoV-2-induced acute respiratory distress syndrome (ards) and potential therapeutic targets. *Int. J. Mol. Sci.* 21:8081. doi: 10.3390/ijms21218081

Karmouty-Quintana, H., Weng, T., Garcia-Morales, L. J., Chen, N.-Y., Pedroza, M., Zhong, H., et al. (2013a). Adenosine A2B receptor and hyaluronan modulate pulmonary hypertension associated with chronic obstructive pulmonary disease. *Am. J. Respir. Cell Mol. Biol.* 49, 1038–1047. doi: 10.1165/rcmb.2013-0089OC

Karmouty-Quintana, H., Xia, Y., and Blackburn, M. R. (2013b). Adenosine signaling during acute and chronic disease states. *J. Mol. Med. (Berl)* 91, 173–181. doi: 10.1007/s00109-013-0997-1

Karmouty-Quintana, H., Zhong, H., Acero, L., Weng, T., Melicoff, E., West, J. D., et al. (2012). The A2B adenosine receptor modulates pulmonary hypertension associated with interstitial lung disease. *FASEB J.* 26, 2546–2557. doi: 10.1096/fj.11-200907

Khan, A., Benthin, C., Zeno, B., Albertson, T. E., Boyd, J., Christie, J. D., et al. (2017). A pilot clinical trial of recombinant human angiotensin-converting enzyme 2 in acute respiratory distress syndrome. *Crit. Care* 21:234. doi: 10.1186/s13054-017-1823-x

Krege, J. H., John, S. W. M., Langenbach, L. L., Hodgin, J. B., Hagaman, J. R., Bachman, E. S., et al. (1995). Male–female differences in fertility and blood pressure in ACE-deficient mice. *Nature* 375, 146–148. doi: 10.1038/375146a0

Kreutz, R., Algharably, E. A. E.-H., Azizi, M., Dobrowolski, P., Guzik, T., Januszewicz, A., et al. (2020). Hypertension, the renin-angiotensin system, and the risk of lower respiratory tract infections and lung injury: implications for COVID-19. *Cardiovasc. Res.* 116, 1688–1699. doi: 10.1093/cvr/cvaa097

Kuba, K., Imai, Y., and Penninger, J. M. (2006). Angiotensin-converting enzyme 2 in lung diseases. *Curr. Opin. Pharmacol.* 6, 271–276. doi: 10.1016/j.coph.2006.03.001

Kuba, K., Imai, Y., Rao, S., Gao, H., Guo, F., Guan, B., et al. (2005). A crucial role of angiotensin converting enzyme 2 (ACE2) in SARS coronavirus–induced lung injury. *Nat. Med.* 11, 875–879. doi: 10.1038/nm1267

Levi, M., and Van Der Poll, T. (2010). Inflammation and coagulation. *Crit. Care Med.* 38, S26–S34. doi: 10.1097/CCM.0b013e3181c98d21

Li, Y., Jiang, D., Liang, J., Meltzer, E. B., Gray, A., Miura, R., et al. (2011). Severe lung fibrosis requires an invasive fibroblast phenotype regulated by hyaluronan and CD44. *J. Exp. Med.* 208, 1459–1471. doi: 10.1084/jem.20102510

Lumb, A. B., and Slinger, P. (2015). Hypoxic pulmonary vasoconstriction: physiology and anesthetic Implications. *Anesthesiology* 122, 932–946. doi: 10.1042/BSE0430061

Luster, A. D. (1998). Mechanisms of disease: chemokines - chemotactic cytokines that mediate inflammation. *N. Engl. J. Med* 338:436–445. doi: 10.1056/NEJM199802123380706

Machhi, J., Herskovitz, J., Senan, A. M., Dutta, D., Nath, B., Oleynikov, M. D., et al. (2020). The natural history, pathobiology, and clinical manifestations of SARS-CoV-2 infections. *J. Neuroimmune Pharmacol.* 15:359–386. doi: 10.1007/s11481-020-09944-5

MacKman, N. (2009). The role of tissue factor and factor VIIa in hemostasis. *Anesth. Analg.* 108, 1447–1452. doi: 10.1213/ane.0b013e31819bceb1

Mamazhakypov, A., Viswanathan, G., Lawrie, A., Schermuly, R. T., and Rajagopal, S. (2021). The role of chemokines and chemokine receptors in pulmonary arterial hypertension. *Br. J. Pharmacol.* 178:72–89. doi: 10.1111/bph.14826

Maniatis, N. A., Kotanidou, A., Catravas, J. D., and Orfanos, S. E. (2008). Endothelial pathomechanisms in acute lung injury. *Vascul. Pharmacol.* 49, 119–133. doi: 10.1016/j.vph.2008.06.009

Marshall, B. E., Hanson, C. W., Frasch, F., and Marshall, C. (1994). Role of hypoxic pulmonary vasoconstriction in pulmonary gas exchange and blood flow distribution. *Intensive Care Med.* 20, 379–389. doi: 10.1007/BF01720916

Marshall, R. P., Webb, S., Bellingan, G. J., Montgomery, H. E., Chaudhari, B., McAnulty, R. J., et al. (2002). Angiotensin converting enzyme insertion/deletion polymorphism is associated with susceptibility and outcome in acute respiratory distress syndrome. *Am. J. Respir. Crit. Care Med.* 166, 646–650. doi: 10.1164/rccm.2108086

Matthay, M. A., and Zemans, R. L. (2011). The acute respiratory distress syndrome: pathogenesis and treatment. *Annu. Rev. Pathol.* 6, 147–163. doi: 10.1146/annurev-pathol-011110-130158

McKallip, R., Ban, H., and Uchakina, O. (2015). Treatment with the hyaluronic acid synthesis inhibitor 4-methylumbelliferone suppresses LPS-induced lung inflammation. *Inflammation* 38, 1250–1259. doi: 10.1007/s10753-014-0092-y

McKallip, R. J., Hagele, H. F., and Uchakina, O. N. (2013). Treatment with the hyaluronic acid synthesis inhibitor 4-methylumbelliferone suppresses SEB-induced lung inflammation. *Toxins* 5, 1814—1826. doi: 10.3390/toxins5101814

McLoughlin, P. (2018). Hypoxic pulmonary vasoconstriction: Building a solid base [View Point]. *Exp. Physiol.* 103, 1181–1182. doi: 10.1113/EP087179

Meduri, G. U., Annane, D., Chrousos, G. P., Marik, P. E., and Sinclair, S. E. (2009). Activation and regulation of systemic inflammation in ARDS: rationale for prolonged glucocorticoid therapy. *Chest* 136, 1631–1643. doi: 10.1378/chest.08-2408

Mertens, T. C. J., Hanmandlu, A., Tu, L., Phan, C., Collum, S. D., Chen, N.-Y., et al. (2018). Switching-off Adora2b in vascular smooth muscle cells halts the development of pulmonary hypertension. *Front. Physiol.* 9:555. doi: 10.3389/fphys.2018.00555

Miakotina, O. L., and Snyder, J. M. (2002). TNF-α inhibits SP-A gene expression in lung epithelial cells via p38 MAPK. *Am. J. Physiol. Lung Cell Mol. Physiol.* 283, L418–L427. doi: 10.1152/ajplung.00470.2001

Molet, S., Furukawa, K., Maghazechi, A., Hamid, Q., and Giaid, A. (2000). Chemokine- and cytokine-induced expression of endothelin 1 and endothelin-converting enzyme 1 in endothelial cells. *J. Allergy Clin. Immunol.* 105, 333–338. doi: 10.1016/s0091-6749(00)90084-8

Moloney, E. D., and Evans, T. W. (2003). Pathophysiology and pharmacological treatment of pulmonary hypertension in acute respiratory distress syndrome. *Eur. Respir. J.* 21, 720–727. doi: 10.1183/09031936.03.00120102

Monchi, M., Bellenfant, F., Cariou, A., Joly, L.-M., Thebert, D., Laurent, I., et al. (1998). Early predictive factors of survival in the acute respiratory distress syndrome. A multivariate analysis. *Am. J. Respir. Crit. Care Med.* 158, 1076–1081. doi: 10.1164/ajrccm.158.4.9802009

Morrell, N. W., Morris, K. G., and Stenmark, K. R. (1995). Role of angiotensin-converting enzyme and angiotensin II in development of hypoxic pulmonary hypertension. *Am. J. Physiol. Heart Circ. Physiol.* 269, H1186–H1194. doi: 10.1152/ajpheart.1995.269.4.H1186

Morrell, N. W., Upton, P. D., Kotecha, S., Huntley, A., Yacoub, M. H., Polak, J. M., et al. (1999). Angiotensin II activates MAPK and stimulates growth of human pulmonary artery smooth muscle via AT1 receptors. *Am. J. Physiol. Lung Cell Mol. Physiol.* 277, L440–L448. doi: 10.1152/ajplung.1999.277.3.L440

Nakano, Y., Tasaka, S., Saito, F., Yamada, W., Shiraishi, Y., Owaga, Y., et al. (2007). Endothelin-1 level in epithelial lining fluid of patients with acute respiratory distress syndrome. *Respirology* 12, 740–743. doi: 10.1111/j.1440-1843.2007.01115.x

Ñamendys-Silva, S. A., Santos-Martínez, L. E., Pulido, T., Rivero-Sigarroa, E., Baltazar-Torres, J. A., Domínguez-Cherit, G., et al. (2014). Pulmonary hypertension due to acute respiratory distress syndrome. *Braz. J. Med. Biol. Res.* 47, 904–910. doi: 10.1590/1414-431X20143316

Ni, K., Gill, A., Tseng, V., Mikosz, A. M., Koike, K., Beatman, E. L., et al. (2018). Rapid clearance of heavy chain-modified hyaluronan during resolving acute lung injury. *Respir. Res.* 19:107. doi: 10.1186/s12931-018-0812-1

Nieuwenhuizen, L., De Groot, P. G., Grutters, J. C., and Biesma, D. H. (2009). A review of pulmonary coagulopathy in acute lung injury, acute respiratory distress syndrome and pneumonia. *Eur. J. Haematol.* 82, 413–425. doi: 10.1111/j.1600-0609.2009.01238.x

Nong, Z., Stassen, J.-M., Moons, L., Collen, D., and Janssens, S. (1996). Inhibition of tissue angiotensin-converting enzyme with quinapril reduces hypoxic pulmonary hypertension and pulmonary vascular remodeling. *Circulation* 94, 1941–1947. doi: 10.1161/01.CIR.94.8.1941

Orte, C., Polak, J. M., Haworth, S. G., Yacoub, M. H., and Morrell, N. W. (2000). Expression of pulmonary vascular angiotensin-converting enzyme in primary and secondary plexiform pulmonary hypertension. *J. Pathol.* 192, 379–384. doi: 10.1002/1096-9896(2000)9999:9999<::AID-PATH715>3.0.CO;2-Q

Osman, D., Monnet, X., Castelain, V., Anguel, N., Warszawski, J., Teboul, J.-L., et al. (2009). Incidence and prognostic value of right ventricular failure in acute respiratory distress syndrome. *Intensive Care Med.* 35, 69–76. doi: 10.1007/s00134-008-1307-1

Pandolfi, R., Barreira, B., Moreno, E., Lara-Acedo, V., Morales-Cano, D., Martínez-Ramas, A., et al. (2017). Role of acid sphingomyelinase and IL-6 as mediators of endotoxin-induced pulmonary vascular dysfunction. *Thorax* 72, 460–471. doi: 10.1136/thoraxjnl-2015-208067

Parameswaran, N., and Patial, S. (2010). Tumor necrosis factor-a signaling in macrophages. *Crit. Rev. Eukaryot. Gene Expr.* 20, 87–103. doi: 10.1615/CritRevEukarGeneExpr.v20.i2.10

Peek, G. J., Mugford, P. M., Tiruvoipati, R., Wilson, A., Allen, E., Thalanany, M. M., et al. (2009). Efficacy and economic assessment of conventional ventilatory support versus extracorporeal membrane oxygenation for severe adult respiratory failure (CESAR): a multicentre randomised controlled trial. *Lancet* 374, P1351–1363. doi: 10.1016/S0140-6736(09)61069-2

Poor, H., Girgis, R., and Studer, S. (2012). World Health Organization group III pulmonary hypertension. *Prog. Cardiovasc. Dis.* 55, 119–127. doi: 10.1016/j.pcad.2012.08.003

Potus, F. F., Mai, V., Lebret, M., Malenfant, S., Breton-Gagnon, E., Lejoie, A. C., et al. (2020). Novel insights on the pulmonary vascular consequences of COVID-19. *Am. J. Physiol. Lung Cell Mol. Physiol.* 319, L277–L288. doi: 10.1152/ajplung.00195.2020

Price, L. C., McAuley, D. F., Marino, P. S., Finney, S. J., Griffiths, M. J., and Wort, S. J. (2012). Pathophysiology of pulmonary hypertension in acute lung injury. *Am. J. Physiol. Lung Cell Mol. Physiol.* 302, L803–L815. doi: 10.1152/ajplung.00355.2011

Price, L. C., and Wort, J. S. (2017). Pulmonary hypertension in ARDS: inflammation matters! *Thorax* 72, 396–397. doi: 10.1136/thoraxjnl-2016-209199

Puneet, P., Moochhala, S., and Bhatia, M. (2005). Chemokines in acute respiratory distress syndrome. *Am. J. Physiol. Lung Cell Mol. Physiol.* 288, L3–L15. doi: 10.1152/ajplung.00405.2003

Rajagopal, K., Bryant, A. J., Sahay, S., Wareing, N., Zhou, Y., Pandit, L. M., et al. (2021). Idiopathic pulmonary fibrosis and pulmonary hypertension: Heracles meets the Hydra. *Br. J. Pharmacol.* 178, 172–186. doi: 10.1111/bph.15036

Ranieri, V. M., Suter, P. M., Tortorella, C., De Tullio, R., Dayer, J. M., Brienza, A., et al. (1999). Effect of mechanical ventilation on inflammatory mediators in patients with acute respiratory distress syndrome: a randomized controlled trial. *JAMA* 282, 54–61. doi: 10.1001/jama.282.1.54

Rezoagli, E., Fumagalli, R., and Bellani, G. (2017). Definition and epidemiology of acute respiratory distress syndrome. *Ann. Transl. Med.* 5, 1–12. doi: 10.21037/atm.2017.06.62

Rigat, B., Hubert, C., Alhenc-Gelas, F., Cambien, F., Corvol, P., and Soubrier, F. (1990). An insertion/deletion polymorphism in the angiotensin I-converting enzyme gene accounting for half the variance of serum enzyme levels. *JCI* 86, 1343–1346. doi: 10.1172/JCI114844

Ryan, D., Frohlich, S., and McLoughlin, P. (2014). Pulmonary vascular dysfunction in ARDS. *Ann Intensive Care* 4, 1–11. doi: 10.1186/s13613-014-0028-6

Sabat, R., Grütz, G., Warszawska, K., Kirsch, S., Witte, E., Wolk, K., et al. (2010). Biology of interleukin-10. *Cytokine Growth Factor Rev.* 21, 331–344. doi: 10.1016/j.cytogfr.2010.09.002

Samary, C. S., Santos, R. S., Santos, C. L., Felix, N. S., Bentes, M., Barboza, T., et al. (2015). Biological impact of transpulmonary driving pressure in experimental acute respiratory distress syndrome. *Anesthesiology* 123, 423–433. doi: 10.1097/ALN.0000000000000716

Sanai, L., Haynes, W., MacKenzie, A., Grant, I., and Webb, D. (1996). Endothelin production in sepsis and the adult respiratory distress syndrome. *Intensive Care Med.* 22, 52–56. doi: 10.1007/BF01728331

Savale, L., Tu, L., Rideau, D., Izziki, M., Maitre, B., Adnot, S., et al. (2009). Impact of interleukin-6 on hypoxia-induced pulmonary hypertension and lung inflammation in mice. *Respir. Res.* 10:6. doi: 10.1186/1465-9921-10-6

Schuster, D. P., Crouch, E. C., Parks, W. C., Johnson, T., and Botney, M. D. (2012). Angiotensin converting enzyme expression in primary pulmonary hypertension. *Am. J. Respir. Crit. Care Med.* 154, 1087–1091. doi: 10.1164/ajrccm.154.4.8887612

Selimovic, N., Bergh, C. H., Andersson, B., Sakiniene, E., Carlsten, H., and Rundqvist, B. (2009). Growth factors and interleukin-6 across the lung circulation in pulmonary hypertension. *Eur. Respir. J.* 34, 662–668. doi: 10.1183/09031936.00174908

Shi, Y., Wang, Y., Shao, C., Huang, J., Gan, J., Huang, X., et al. (2020). COVID-19 infection: the perspectives on immune responses. *Cell Death Differ* 27, 1451–1454. doi: 10.1038/s41418-020-0530-3

Simonneau, G., Montani, D., Celermajer, D. S., Denton, C. P., Gatzoulis, M. A., Krowka, M., et al. (2019). Haemodynamic definitions and updated clinical classification of pulmonary hypertension. *Eur. Respir. J.* 53, 1–13. doi: 10.1183/13993003.01913-2018

Soon, E., Holmes, A. M., Treacy, C. M., Doughty, N. J., Southgate, L., MacHado, R. D., et al. (2010). Elevated levels of inflammatory cytokines predict survival in idiopathic and familial pulmonary arterial hypertension. *Circulation* 122, 920–927. doi: 10.1161/CIRCULATIONAHA.109.933762

South, A. M., Diz, D. I., and Chappell, M. C. (2020). COVID-19, ACE2, and the cardiovascular consequences. *Am. J. Physiol. Heart Circ. Physiol.* 318, H1084–H1090. doi: 10.1152/ajpheart.00217.2020

Spöhr, F., Busch, C. J., Reich, C., Motsch, J., Gebhard, M. M., Kuebler, W. M., et al. (2007). 4-Aminopyridine restores impaired hypoxic pulmonary vasoconstriction in endotoxemic mice. *Anesthesiology* 107, 597–604. doi: 10.1097/01.anes.0000281897.13703.fd

Squara, P., Dhainaut, J.-F. A., Artigas, A., Carlet, J., and Group ECAW. (1998). Hemodynamic profile in severe ARDS: results of the European Collaborative ARDS Study. *Intensive Care Med.* 24, 1018–1028. doi: 10.1007/s001340050710

Steiner, M. K., Syrkina, O. L., Kolliputi, N., Mark, E. J., Hales, C. A., and Waxman, A. B. (2009). Interleukin-6 overexpression induces pulmonary hypertension. *Circ. Res.* 104, 236–244. doi: 10.1161/CIRCRESAHA.108.182014

Stevens, T., Janssen, P. L., and Tucker, A. (1992). Acute and long-term TNF-α administration increases pulmonary vascular reactivity in isolated rat lungs. *J. Appl. Physiol.* 73, 708–712. doi: 10.1152/jappl.1992.73.2.708

Stow, J. L., Ching Low, P., Offenhäuser, C., and Sangermani, D. (2009). Cytokine secretion in macrophages and other cells: pathways and mediators. *Immunobiology* 214, 601–612. doi: 10.1016/j.imbio.2008.11.005

Sun, X., Wang, T., Cai, D., Hu, Z., Chen, J., Liao, H., et al. (2020). Cytokine storm intervention in the early stages of COVID-19 pneumonia. *Cytokine Growth Factor Rev.* 53, 38–42. doi: 10.1016/j.cytogfr.2020.04.002

Suylen, R. J., Van, A. W. M., Smits, J. F., and Daemen, M. J. (2001). Dissociation of pulmonary vascular remodeling and right ventricular pressure in tissue angiotensin-converting enzyme-deficient mice under conditions of chronic alveolar hypoxia. *Am. J. Respir. Crit. Care Med.* 163, 1241–1245. doi: 10.1164/ajrccm.163.5.2003144

Sylvester, J., Shimoda, L. A., Aaronson, P. I., and Ward, J. P. (2012). Hypoxic pulmonary vasoconstriction. *Physiol. Rev.* 92, 367–520. doi: 10.1152/physrev.00041.2010

Tamosiuniene, R., Tian, W., Dhillon, G., Wang, L., Sung, Y. K., Gera, L., et al. (2011). Regulatory T cells limit vascular endothelial injury and prevent pulmonary hypertension. *Circ. Res.* 109, 867–879. doi: 10.1161/CIRCRESAHA.110.236927

Tang, N., Bai, H., Chen, X., Gong, J., Li, D., and Sun, Z. (2020a). Anticoagulant treatment is associated with decreased mortality in severe coronavirus disease 2019 patients with coagulopathy. *J. Thromb. Haemost.* 18, 1094–1099. doi: 10.1111/jth.14817

Tang, N., Li, D., Wang, X., and Sun, Z. (2020b). Abnormal coagulation parameters are associated with poor prognosis in patients with novel coronavirus pneumonia. *J. Thromb. Haemost.* 18, 1233–1234. doi: 10.1111/jth.14768

The ARDS and Definition Task Force (2012). Acute respiratory distress syndrome: the Berlin definition. *JAMA* 307, 2526–2533. doi: 10.1001/jama.2012.5669

Tipnis, S. R., Hooper, N. M., Hyde, R., Karran, E., Christie, G., and Turner, A. J. (2000). A human homolog of angiotensin-converting enzyme cloning and functional expression as a captopril-insensitive carboxypeptidase. *J. Biol. Chem.* 275, 33238–33243. doi: 10.1074/jbc.M002615200

Tisoncik, J. R., Korth, M. J., Simmons, C. P., Farrar, J., Martin, T. R., and Katze, M. G. (2012). Into the eye of the cytokine storm. *Microbiol. Mol. Biol. Rev.* 76, 16–32. doi: 10.1128/mmbr.05015-11

Tomashefski, J. F., Davies, P., Boggis, C., Greene, R., Zapol, W. M., and Reid, L. M. (1983). The pulmonary vascular lesions of the adult respiratory distress syndrome. *Am. J. Pathol.* 112, 112–126.

Turzo, M., Vaith, J., Lasitschka, F., Weigand, M. A., and Busch, C. J. (2018). Role of ATP-sensitive potassium channels on hypoxic pulmonary vasoconstriction in endotoxemia. *Respir. Res.* 19:29. doi: 10.1186/s12931-018-0735-x

Vieillard-Baron, A., Schmitt, J. M., Augarde, R., Fellahi, J. L., Prin, S., Page, B., et al. (2001). Acute cor pulmonale in acute respiratory distress syndrome submitted to protective ventilation: incidence, clinical implications, and prognosis. *Crit. Care Med.* 29, 1551–1555. doi: 10.1097/00003246-200108000-00009

Villar, J., Blazquez, M. A., Lubillo, S., Quintana, J., and Manzano, J. L. (1989). Pulmonary hypertension in acute respiratory failure. *Crit. Care Med.* 17, 523–526.

Ware, L. B., Fang, X., and Matthay, M. A. (2003). Protein C and thrombomodulin in human acute lung injury. *Am. J. Physiol. Lung Cell Mol. Physiol.* 285, L514–L521. doi: 10.1152/ajplung.00442.2002

Ware, L. B., Matthay, M. A., Parsons, P. E., Thompson, B. T., Januzzi, J. L., Eisner, M. D., et al. (2007). Pathogenetic and prognostic significance of altered coagulation and fibrinolysis in acute lung injury/acute respiratory distress syndrome. *Crit. Care Med.* 35, 1821–1828. doi: 10.1016/s0734-3299(08)70449-0

Welty-Wolf, K. E., Carraway, M. S., Miller, D. L., Ortel, T. L., Ezban, M., Ghio, A. J., et al. (2001). Coagulation blockade prevents sepsis-induced respiratory and renal failure in baboons. *Am. J. Respir. Crit. Care Med.* 164, 1988–1996. doi: 10.1164/ajrccm.164.10.2105027

World Health Organization. (2020). *WHO Coronavirus Disease (COVID-19) Dashboard.* WHO. Available online at: https://covid19.who.int/

Wrapp, D., Wang, N., Corbett, K. S., Goldsmith, J. A., Hsieh, C.-L., Abiona, O., et al. (2020). Cryo-EM structure of the 2019-nCoV spike in the prefusion conformation. *Science* 367, 1260–1263. doi: 10.1126/science.abb2507

Xianwei, W., Magomed, K., Ding, Z., Sona, M., Jingjun, L., Shijie, L., et al. (2012). Cross-talk between inflammation and angiotensin II: studies based on direct transfection of cardiomyocytes with AT1R and AT2R cDNA. *Exp. Biol. Med.* 237, 1394–1401. doi: 10.1258/ebm.2012.012212

Xiaofang, Z., Wang, K., Zuo, P., Liu, Y., Zhang, M., Xie, S., et al. (2020). Early decrease in blood platelet count is associated with poor prognosis in COVID-19 patients—indications for predictive, preventive, and personalized medical approach. *EPMA J.* 11, 1–7. doi: 10.1007/s13167-020-00208-z

Xu, X., Han, M., Li, T., Sun, W., Wang, D., Fu, B., et al. (2020). Effective treatment of severe COVID-19 patients with tocilizumab. *Proc. Natl. Acad. Sci. U.S.A.* 117, 10970–10975. doi: 10.1073/pnas.2005615117

Yamazato, Y., Ferreira, A. J., Hong, K.-H., Sriramula, S., Francis, J., Yamazato, M., et al. (2009). Prevention of pulmonary hypertension by Angiotensin-converting enzyme 2 gene transfer. *Hypertension* 54, 365–371. doi: 10.1161/HYPERTENSIONAHA.108.125468

Zabini, D., Nagaraj, C., Stacher, E., Lang, I. M., Nierlich, P., Klepetko, W., et al. (2012). Angiostatic factors in the pulmonary endarterectomy material from chronic thromboembolic pulmonary hypertension patients cause endothelial dysfunction. *PLoS ONE* 7:e43793. doi: 10.1371/journal.pone.0043793

Zambelli, V., Bellani, G., Borsa, R., Pozzi, F., Grassi, A., Scanziani, M., et al. (2015). Angiotensin-(1-7) improves oxygenation, while reducing cellular infiltrate and fibrosis in experimental acute respiratory distress syndrome. *Intensive Care Med. Exp.* 3:44. doi: 10.1186/s40635-015-0044-3

Zhang, R., Wu, Y., Zhao, M., Liu, C., Zhou, L., Shen, S., et al. (2009). Role of HIF-1α in the regulation ACE and ACE2 expression in hypoxic human pulmonary artery smooth muscle cells. *Am. J. Physiol. Lung Cell Mol. Physiol.* 297, L631–L640. doi: 10.1152/ajplung.90415.2008

Zhiyu, D., Ming, L., John, W., Maggie, M. Z., and You-Yang, Z. (2016). Prolyl-4 Hydroxylase 2 (PHD2) deficiency in endothelial cells and hematopoietic cells induces obliterative vascular remodeling and severe pulmonary arterial hypertension in mice and humans through hypoxia-inducible factor-2α. *Circulation* 133, 2447–2458. doi: 10.1161/CIRCULATIONAHA.116.021494

15

Administration Timing and Efficacy of Tocilizumab in Patients with COVID-19 and Elevated IL-6

Pan Li[1,2†], Zhengmao Lu[2,3†], Qiang Li[2,4†], Zhenmeng Wang[2,5], Yan Guo[2,6], Chen Cai[2,7], Shengyun Wang[2,8], Peng Liu[2,9], Xiaoping Su[10], Yi Huang[11], Yuchao Dong[11], Wenjuan Qiu[2,12], Yueming Ling[2,13], Lonny Yarmus[14], Fengming Luo[15], Li Zeng[2,16], Chong Bai[11,*] and Wei Zhang[2,11*]*

[1] Department of Cardiology, Changhai Hospital, Second Military Medical University, Shanghai, China, [2] Department of Infection Diseases No. 1, The Maternal and Child Health Hospital of Hubei Province, Wuhan, China, [3] Department of Gastrointestinal Surgery, Changhai Hospital, Second Military Medical University, Shanghai, China, [4] Department of Neurosurgery, Changhai Hospital, Second Military Medical University, Shanghai, China, [5] Department of Anesthesia, Third Affiliated Hospital, Second Military Medical University, Shanghai, China, [6] Department of Endocrinology, Changhai Hospital, Second Military Medical University, Shanghai, China, [7] Department of Special Clinic, Changhai Hospital, Second Military Medical University, Shanghai, China, [8] Department of Emergency and Critical Care Medicine, Changzheng Hospital, Second Military Medical University, Shanghai, China, [9] Department of Colorectal Surgery, Changhai Hospital, Second Military Medical University, Shanghai, China, [10] School of Basic Medicine, Wenzhou Medical University, Wenzhou, China, [11] Department of Respiratory and Critical Care Medicine, Changhai Hospital, Second Military Medical University, Shanghai, China, [12] Department of Cardiovascular ICU, Changhai Hospital, Second Military Medical University, Shanghai, China, [13] Department of Clinical Laboratory Science of No. 910 Hospital of PLA Joint Support Force, Quanzhou, China, [14] Division of Pulmonary and Critical Care, Johns Hopkins University School of Medicine, Baltimore, MD, United States, [15] Department of Pulmonary and Critical Care Medicine, West China Hospital, Sichuan University, Chengdu, China, [16] Department of Organ Transplantation, Changhai Hospital, Second Military Medical University, Shanghai, China

***Correspondence:**
Wei Zhang
zhangweismmu@126.com
Chong Bai
bc7878@sohu.com
Li Zeng
Zengli111109@163.com

† These authors have contributed equally to this work and share first authorship

Background: Tocilizumab (TCZ), an interleukin-6 receptor antibody, has previously been used for treating patients with the coronavirus disease 2019 (COVID-19), but there is a lack of data regarding the administration timing of TCZ.

Objectives: This study aimed to evaluate the timing and efficacy of TCZ in the treatment of patients with COVID-19.

Methods: Laboratory-confirmed patients with COVID-19 with an elevated interleukin-6 (IL-6) level (> 10 pg/ml) were offered TCZ intravenously for compassionate use. Clinical characteristics, laboratory tests, and chest imaging before and after the administration of TCZ were retrospectively analyzed.

Results: A total of 58 consecutive patients who met the inclusion criteria and with no compliance to the exclusion criteria were included. Of these 58 patients, 39 patients received TCZ treatment, and 19 patients who declined TCZ treatment were used as the control cohort. In the TCZ-treatment group, 6 patients (15.4%) were in mild condition, 16 (41.0%) were in severe condition, and 17 (43.6%) were in critical condition. After TCZ treatment, the condition of 27 patients (69.2%) improved and 12 (30.8%) died. Compared with the improvement group, patients in the death group had higher baseline levels of IL-6 (*P* = 0.0191) and procalcitonin (PCT) (*P* = 0.0003) and lower lymphocyte percentage (LYM) (*P* = 0.0059). Patients receiving TCZ treatment had better prognoses than those without TCZ treatment (P = 0.0273). Furthermore, patients with a baseline IL-6 level of ≥100 pg/ml in the TCZ-treatment group had poorer clinical outcomes than those with an IL-6 level of <100 pg/ml (P = 0.0051).

Conclusion: The administration of TCZ in an early stage of cytokine storm (IL-6 level < 100 pg/ml) may effectively improve the clinical prognosis of patients with COVID-19 by blocking the IL-6 signal pathway.

Keywords: cytokine storm, interleukin-6, SARS-CoV-2, tocilizumab (TCZ), coronavirus - COVID-19

INTRODUCTION

Ever since the coronavirus disease 2019 (COVID-19) outbreak in December 2019, the disease rapidly continues to spread and has been declared a global pandemic (Wang et al., 2020). According to the real-time statistics released by Johns Hopkins University, the COVID-19 pandemic has led to 77,107,760 confirmed cases with a death toll of 1,696,995 worldwide, as of December 21, 2020. Although the reported incidence rate of COVID-19 is currently lower than that of SARS-CoV and MERS-CoV, the mortality rate among patients with severe COVID-19 is up to 60% (Arabi et al., 2020). More worrisome is the fact that the mechanisms of the underlying pathogenicity of COVID-19 are thus far not fully illustrated. This, in part, has resulted in limited specific antiviral treatments available for COVID-19.

During the SARS-CoV-2 epidemic, it was discovered that the immuno-pathological processes were involved in lung injury (Kuiken et al., 2003). In the biopsy samples of patients with SARS-CoV-2, extensive lung damage revealed the accumulation of monocytes, macrophages, and neutrophils in the lungs, resulting in elevated lung cytokine/chemokine levels (Moore and June, 2020). The levels of serum proinflammatory cytokines and chemokines were also found to increase in patients with COVID-19, including tumor necrosis factor α (TNF-α), interferon-γ (IFN-γ)-induced protein 10 (IP-10), interleukin-6 (IL-6), IL-8, and IL-10 (Chen N. et al., 2020; Huang et al., 2020). Therefore, the clinical deterioration of COVID-19 may partly result from the immunopathology induced by a hypercytokinemia or cytokine storm. Of note is that a large number of studies have shown that the levels of IL-6 were significantly higher in patients with severe COVID-19 as compared to those in uncomplicated individuals (Chen G. et al., 2020; Ye et al., 2020). These findings suggest that IL-6 might play a vital role in the severe deterioration of some patients.

Tocilizumab [TCZ, (Roche Pharma (Schweiz) Ltd., S20171024)], a human monoclonal antibody directed against IL-6, has been commonly used in the therapy of rheumatoid arthritis (RA) (Biggioggero et al., 2018). Recent studies have reported the benefit of TCZ in severely ill patients with COVID-19 (Luo et al., 2020; Stone et al., 2020; Xu et al., 2020). However, to our knowledge, the appropriate timing of the administration of TCZ in patients with COVID-19 is unknown. Herein, this study evaluated the efficacy and timing of the intravenous administration of TCZ for compassionate use in the treatment of patients with COVID-19.

MATERIALS AND METHODS

Study Design and Participants

This single-center retrospective cohort study was performed at the Guanggu district, the Maternal and Child Health Hospital of Hubei Province, China, which is a designated hospital for the treatment of patients with COVID-19. The study protocol was approved by the Medical Ethics Committee of the Maternal and Child Health Hospital of Hubei Province [FYGG (L)-2020-018].

From February 19, 2020 to April 7, 2020, consecutive patients with confirmed COVID-19 were evaluated for inclusion in this study. The inclusion criteria were as follows: (1) age ≥ 18 years; (2) nasal swab samples that were confirmed to be positive for SARS-CoV-2 nucleic acid by real-time reverse-transcriptase-PCR (RT-PCR) or for serum novel coronavirus-specific IgM and IgG antibodies; and (3) IL-6 level exceeding the upper limit of the normal value (>10 pg/ml). The exclusion criteria were as follows: (1) allergic reactions to TCZ or any adjuvant and (2) active inflammatory disease, such as hepatitis, tuberculosis, terminal tumor, or rheumatism immunity.

The diagnosis and severity stratification of COVID-19 were made based on the guidelines released by the National Health Commission of China (trial version 7) (National Health Commission, 2020). Patients with moderate or common type of COVID-19 having fever, dyspnea, and other symptoms with the manifestation of pneumonia seen in imaging data were diagnosed as mild cases; patients with respiratory frequency ≥ 30/min, blood oxygen saturation ≤ 93% at room air, or PaO_2/FiO_2 ratio ≤ 300 mmHg were defined as severe cases; and patients with respiratory failure requiring mechanical ventilation, shock, or other organ dysfunction/failure in addition to COVID-19 needing a stay in the intensive care unit (ICU) for treatment were diagnosed as critical cases. Comparison of the clinical characteristics among patients with COVID-19 treated with or without TCZ (**Table 1**) is a cohort study, while comparison between clinical characteristics of patients in the improvement group and in the death group after receiving TCZ (**Table 2**) is a case-control study.

TCZ Treatment and Observation

Tocilizumab of 4–8 mg/kg, to a maximum dose of 800 mg, was intravenously administered once within 60 min of patients meeting the inclusion criteria. For patients who still had fever 24 h after the administration of the first dose, TCZ was

TABLE 1 | Clinical characteristics of the enrolled patients with coronavirus disease 2019 (COVID-19) treated with or without tocilizumab (TCZ).

	Total (*N* = 58)	TCZ-treatment group (*N* = 39)	Non-TCZ treatment group (*N* = 19)	*p*-value
Age, y	73.9 ± 12.7	74.7 ± 13.4	72.3 ± 11.3	0.2812
Gender, n (%)				0.5685
Male	37 (63.8)	26 (66.7)	11(57.9)	
Female	21 (36.2)	13 (33.3)	8 (42.1)	
BMI	24.1 ± 2.1	24.3 ± 2.1	23.6 ± 2.0	0.2027
Type, n (%)				0.2034
Mild	12 (20.7)	6 (15.4)	6 (31.6)	
Severe	20 (34.5)	16 (41.0)	4 (21.0)	
Critical	26 (44.8)	17 (43.6)	9 (47.4)	
Symptoms, n (%)				
Fever history	39 (67.2)	23 (59.0)	16 (84.2)	0.0756
Fever at admission (°C)	9 (15.5)	6 (15.4)	3 (15.8)	1.0000
Dyspnea	18 (31.0)	7 (18.0)	11 (57.9)	**0.0053**
Fatigue	30 (51.7)	18 (46.2)	12 (63.2)	0.2708
Muscle soreness	9 (15.5)	6 (15.4)	3 (15.8)	1.0000
Chills	8 (13.8)	4 (10.3)	4 (21.1)	0.4179
Cough	30 (51.7)	17 (43.6)	13 (68.4)	0.0973
Throat irritation	8 (13.8)	1 (2.6)	7 (36.8)	**0.0011**
Presence of comorbidities, n (%)				
Hypertension	32 (55.2)	18 (46.1)	14 (73.7)	0.0558
Diabetes	22 (37.9)	10 (25.6)	12 (63.2)	**0.0092**
CHD	18 (31.0)	10 (25.6)	8 (42.1)	0.2367
Cerebrovascular events	6 (10.3)	3 (7.7)	3 (15.8)	0.5894
COPD Renal insufficiency	7 (12.1) 5 (8.6)	4 (10.3) 2 (5.1)	3 (15.8) 3 (15.8)	0.6726 0.3179
Oxygen saturation%	92 (86–95)	90 (85.0–93.0)	92 (87–96)	0.6416
Systolic blood pressure (mmHg)	132 (120–155)	130 (120–155)	136 (125–156)	0.1587
Diastolic blood pressure (mmHg) Body temperature (°C) **Treatment**	78.5 (70–88) 36.4 (36.2–36.8)	78 (69–86) 36.4 (36.2–36.9)	86 (74–90) 36.5 (36.2–36.6)	0.0861 0.9934
Antiviral treatment, n (%)	37 (63.8)	30 (76.9)	11 (57.9)	0.2181
Antibiotic treatment, n (%)	42 (72.4)	31 (79.5)	11 (57.9)	0.1190
Oxygen therapy				0.5801
Low-flow oxygen	24 (41.4)	14 (35.9)	10 (52.6)	
High-flow oxygen Non-invasive ventilation Invasive ventilation	10 (17.2) 9 (15.5) 15 (25.9)	7 (18.0) 6 (15.4) 12 (30.8)	3 (15.8) 3 (15.8) 3 (15.8)	
Glucocorticoid, n (%)	22 (37.9)	21 (53.9)	5 (26.3)	0.0558
Laboratory characteristics				
WBC ($\times 10^9$/L)	7.4 (5.3–11.6)	6.4 (4.1–11.0)	10.9 (6.9–12.3)	**0.0170**
PCT (ng/ml)	0.13 (0.07–0.61)	0.09 (0.05–0.28)	0.20 (0.10–0.81)	0.0721
LDH (U/L)	291 (218–343)	285.5 (212–343)	287.5 (234–312)	0.9203
Lymphocyte count ($\times 10^9$/L)	0.77 (0.45–1.02)	0.70 (0.44–0.93)	0.83 (0.53–1.36)	0.0635
Lymphocyte percentage (%)	8.7 (5.3–17.6)	9.7 (5.2–17.6)	7.6 (5.3–18.4)	0.9208
Hs-CRP (mg/L)	58.3 (24.4–116.8)	35.4 (9.1–92.8)	82.1 (25.5–101.9)	0.9406
IL-6 (pg/ml)	77.8 (34.1–302.0)	63.4 (36.4–129.7)	25.8 (29.8–82.6)	**0.0014**
D-dimer (mg/l)	3.7 (1.3–6.5)	2.9 (1.3–5.3)	4.3 (1.4–12.5)	0.3375

Three methods have been used for testing: the Wilcoxon rank-sum test for continuous variables, the Fisher's exact test for dichotomous variables, and the General Linear Model for categorical variables. All continuous variables were expressed as median (interquartile range [IQR]), except for age, which was represented as mean ± SD. CHD, coronary artery heart disease; COPD, chronic obstructive pulmonary disease; hs-CRP, high-sensitivity C-reactive protein; IL-6, interleukin-6; LDH, lactate dehydrogenase; PCT, procalcitonin; WBC, white blood cell. There was statistical difference in bold type.

TABLE 2 | Clinical characteristics of the patients with COVID-19 in the improvement group or the death group after receiving TCZ.

	Total (*N* = 39)	Improvement group (*N* = 27)	Death group (*N* = 12)	*p*-value
Age, y	74.7 ± 13.4	75.0 ± 12.3	73.8 ± 16.1	0.3413
Gender, n (%)				1.0000
Male	26 (66.7)	18 (66.7)	8 (66.7)	
Female	13 (33.3)	9 (33.3)	4 (33.3)	
BMI	24.3 ± 2.1	24.3 ± 2.3	24.3 ± 1.4	0.9747
Type, n (%)				0.0003
Mild	6 (15.4)	6 (22.2)	0	
Severe	16 (41.0)	15 (55.6)	1 (8.3)	
Critical	17 (43.6)	6 (22.2)	11 (91.7)	
Symptoms, n (%)				
Fever History	23 (59.0)	19 (70.4)	4 (33.3)	**0.0407**
Fever at admission (°C)	6 (15.4)	6 (22.2)	0	0.1508
Dyspnea	7 (18.0)	4 (14.8)	3 (25.0)	0.6536
Fatigue	18 (46.2)	12 (44.4)	6 (50.0)	1.0000
Muscle soreness	6 (15.4)	4 (14.8)	2 (16.7)	1.0000
Chills	4 (10.3)	3 (11.1)	1 (8.3)	1.0000
Cough	17 (43.6)	10 (37.0)	7 (58.3)	0.2994
Throat irritation	1 (2.6)	1 (3.7)	0	1.0000
Presence of comorbidities, n (%)				
Hypertension	18 (46.1)	14 (51.9)	4 (33.3)	0.3221
Diabetes	10 (25.6)	7 (25.9)	3 (25.0)	1.0000
CHD	10 (25.6)	7 (25.9)	3 (25.0)	1.0000
Cerebrovascular events	3 (7.7)	3 (11.1)	0	0.5391
COPD Renal insufficiency	4 (10.3) 2 (5.1)	4 (14.8) 1 (3.7)	0 1 (8.3)	0.2916 0.5263
Oxygen saturation%	90 (85.0–93.0)	92 (88.0–95.0)	86.5 (84.5–92.5)	0.0523
Systolic blood pressure (mmHg)	130 (120–155)	130 (120–155)	128 (120–154)	0.9392
Diastolic blood pressure (mmHg) Body temperature (°C)	78 (69–86) 36.4 (36.2–36.9)	78 (69–84) 36.4 (36.2–36.9)	80 (66.5–88.5) 36.25 (36.15–36.85)	0.7839 0.2983
Treatment				
Antiviral treatment, n (%)	30 (76.9)	21 (77.8)	9 (75.0)	1.0000
Antibiotic treatment, n (%)	31 (79.5)	20 (74.1)	11 (91.7)	0.3938
Oxygen therapy				0.0004
Low-flow oxygen	14 (35.9)	14 (51.9)	0	
High-flow oxygen Non-invasive ventilation Invasive ventilation	7 (18.0) 6 (15.4) 12 (30.8)	6 (22.2) 3 (11.1) 4 (14.8)	1 (8.3) 3 (25.0) 8 (66.7)	
Glucocorticoid, n (%)	21 (53.9)	11 (40.7)	10 (83.3)	**0.0180**
Laboratory characteristics				
WBC (× 10^9/L)	6.4 (4.1–11.0)	6.3 (4.1–8.8)	8.55 (4.9–12.3)	0.3377
PCT (ng/ml)	0.09 (0.05–0.28)	0.07 (0.05–0.11)	0.79 (0.16–1.88)	**0.0003**
LDH (U/L)	285.5 (212–343)	264.5 (192–310)	499.5 (412–614.5)	**0.0056**
Lymphocyte count (× 10^9/L)	0.7 (0.44–0.93)	0.71 (0.44–0.93)	0.65 (0.49–0.89)	0.9515
Lymphocyte percentage (%)	9.7 (5.2–17.6)	14.6 (6.8–20.5)	6.2 (3.0–7.1)	**0.0059**
Hs-CRP (mg/L)	35.4 (9.1–92.8)	24.4 (9.1–87.2)	54.7 (23.9–112.7)	0.1709
IL-6 (pg/ml)	63.4 (36.4–129.7)	53.2 (33.8–91.4)	140.4 (69.9–316.5)	**0.0191**
D-dimer (mg/L)	2.9 (1.3–5.3)	2.7 (1.0–5.1)	3.5 (1.6–6.5)	0.3381

*The tests to determine the laboratory characteristics presented in **Table 2** were conducted at baseline. Three methods have been used for testing: the Wilcoxon rank-sum test for continuous variables, the Fisher's exact test for dichotomous variables, and the General Linear Model for categorical variables. All continuous variables were expressed as median (interquartile range [IQR]), except for age, which was represented as mean ± SD. CHD, coronary artery heart disease; COPD, chronic obstructive pulmonary disease; hs-CRP, high-sensitivity C-reactive protein; IL-6, interleukin-6; LDH, lactate dehydrogenase; PCT, procalcitonin; WBC, white blood cell. There was statistical difference in bold type.*

readministered with an interval of ≥12 h between the two administrations. Other routine treatments such as antiviral, antibiotic, corticosteroid treatment, and oxygen therapy were continued as per physician discretion.

The clinical data including medical history, clinical symptoms, comorbidities, imaging data, treatment measures, and clinical outcomes were collected and analyzed. Laboratory examinations, including complete blood count, liver and renal function, IL-6 levels, high-sensitive C-reactive protein (hs-CRP), procalcitonin (PCT), myocardial enzymes, and coagulation analysis, were collected and analyzed. Elevated IL-6 level was defined to be >10 pg/ml (Pylon immunoassay system); elevated hs-CRP was defined to be >10 mg/L; and elevated PCT was defined to be >0.05 ng/ml, as per the specifications of the manufacturer. The nasopharyngeal swab test for SARS-CoV-2 (Shanghai ZJ Bio-Tech Co., Ltd.) was performed when the patients were admitted to the isolation ward, and it was repeated twice with an interval of at least 24 h before discharge using RT-PCR.

Statistical Analysis

All variables were expressed as the mean ± SD or median (interquartile range [IQR]) or number (%). The Wilcoxon rank-sum test was used for continuous variables, the Fisher's exact test was used for dichotomous variables, and the general linear model was used for categorical variables. The Wilcoxon signed-rank test was used for paired data analysis before and after treatment with TCZ for both patients in the improvement group and those in the death group. The difference of median IL-6 and of median hs-CRP categorized by the outcomes and the difference of median lymphocyte (LYM) count categorized by the baseline IL-6 level were tested by using the Wilcoxon rank-sum test. The Kaplan–Meier methodology was used to estimate the probability of survival. The survival rate was compared between the groups treated with and without TCZ (IL-6, LYM%, hs-CRP, and PCT) using the log-rank test at the two-sided significance level. The multivariable Cox proportional-hazards model analysis was used to explore the role of TCZ in clinical outcomes when adjusted

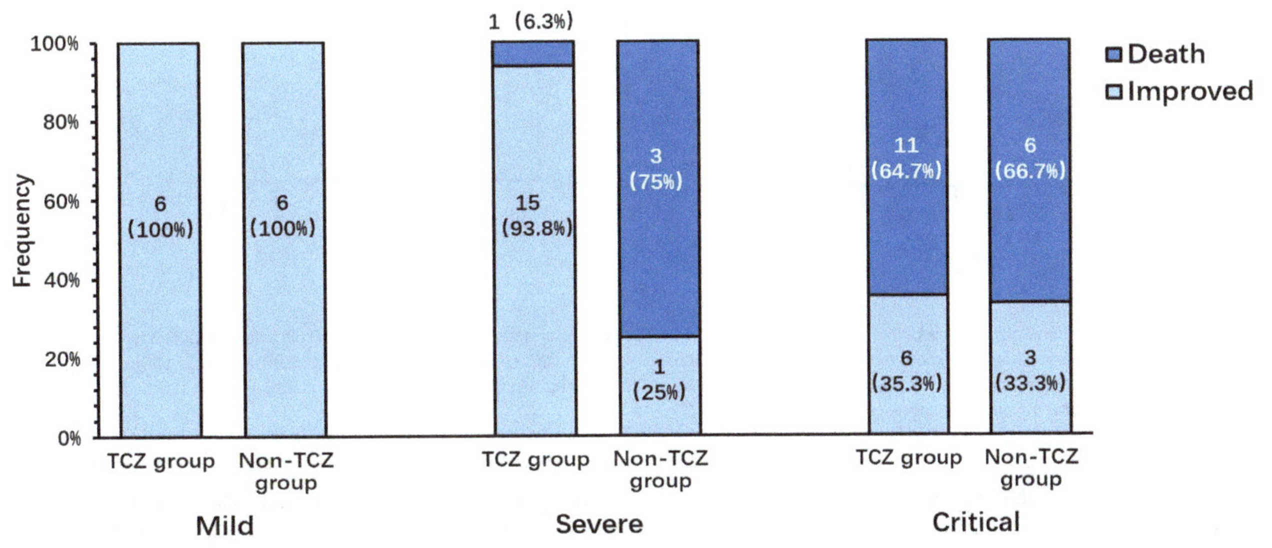

FIGURE 1 | Distribution of disease severity in patients who improved or died after treatment with or without tocilizumab.

TABLE 3 | Laboratory tests before and after the administration of tocilizumab in the improvement group and the death group.

	Improvement group (*N* = 27)		*p*-value	Death group (*N* = 12)		*p*-value
	Before TCZ	After TCZ		Before TCZ	After TCZ	
WBC (× 10^9/L)	6.3 (4.1–8.8)	4.8 (3.9–6.2)	0.0746	8.55 (4.9–12.3)	9.8 (4.6–14.0)	0.8311
PCT (ng/ml)	0.07 (0.05–0.11)	0.05 (0.04–0.06)	0.3088	0.79 (0.16–1.9)	1.75 (0.44–5.5)	0.3750
LDH (U/L)	264.5 (192–310)	219 (193–234)	**0.0096**	499 (412–614.5)	537 (488.5–626.5)	0.8750
Lymphocyte count (× 10^9/L)	0.71 (0.44–0.93)	1.3 (1.1–1.5)	**<0.0001**	0.65 (0.49–0.89)	0.265 (0.12–0.81)	**0.0269**
Lymphocyte percentage (%)	14.6 (6.8–20.5)	24.6 (15.9–29.9)	**<0.0001**	6.15 (3.00–7.05)	7.05 (3.4–11.4)	1.0000
Hs-CRP (mg/L)	24.4 (9.07–87.2)	1.42 (0.56–5.06)	**<0.0001**	54.7 (23.9–112.2)	20.67 (9.5–125.9)	0.7910
IL-6 (pg/ml)	53.2 (33.8–91.4)	110.5 (16.0–3327.1)	**0.0132**	140.4 (69.9–316.5)	1216 (584.9–3504.0)	**0.0059**
D-dimer (mg/L)	2.7 (1.0–5.1)	1.2 (0.73–2.7)	**<0.0001**	3.51 (1.6–6.5)	10.17 (2.8–21.9)	**0.0371**
Oxygen saturation%	92 (88–95)	98 (97–99)	**<0.0001**	86.5 (84.5–92.5)	85 (80–92.5)	0.6240

CHD, coronary artery heart disease; COPD, chronic obstructive pulmonary disease; hs-CRP, high-sensitive C-reactive protein; IL-6, interleukin-6; LDH, lactate dehydrogenase; PCT, procalcitonin; TCZ, tocilizumab; WBC, white blood cell. There was statistical difference in bold type.

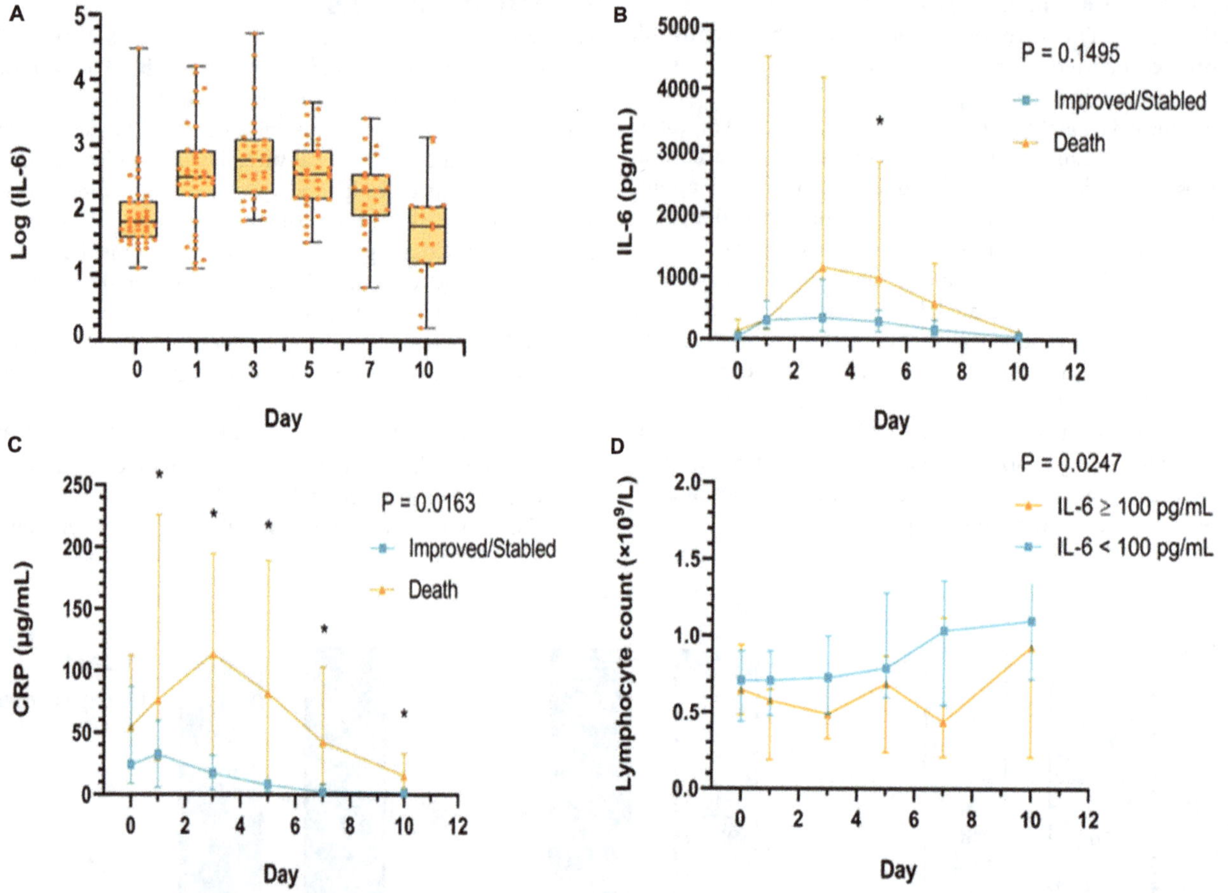

FIGURE 2 | The changing trend of IL-6 levels before and after tocilizumab treatment **(A)**. The change of IL-6 **(B)** and hs-CRP **(C)** levels, respectively, during the tocilizumab treatment categorized by outcomes (improvement and death) at baseline, day 1, day 3, day 5, day 7, and day 10; **(D)** The change of lymphocytes (LYM) during the tocilizumab treatment categorized by baseline IL-6 level (using median value 100 pg/ml as cut-off value) at baseline, day 1, day 3, day 5, day 7, and day 10. $^{*}P < 0.05$ compared with the improvement and death group.

for clinical covariates, including age, body mass index (BMI), diabetes, and glucocorticoid. Statistical analyses were performed using the SAS Studio version 3.7 software. A *P*-value of < 0.05 was considered statistically significant.

RESULTS

Demographic Characteristics

Between February 19, 2020 and April 7, 2020, a total of 58 patients met the inclusion criteria, and no patients who met the exclusion criteria (**Table 1**) were screened. Of these 58 patients, 39 patients signed informed consent and received TCZ treatment and 19 patients, who declined TCZ treatment, were used as the control cohort. The majority of patients (37, 63.8%) were male, with a mean age of 73.9 ± 12.7 years. There were 12 (20.7%) mild cases, 20 (34.5%) severe cases, and 26 (44.8%) critical cases. A total of 39 consecutive patients receiving TCZ treatment were divided into two groups: the improvement group (27 cases, 69.2%) and the death group (12 cases, 30.8%; **Table 2**). Six (22.2%) mild cases, 15 (55.6%) severe cases, and 6 (22.2%) critical cases were observed in the improvement group; meanwhile, 1 (8.3%) severe case and 11 (91.7%) critical cases were present in the death group; no patients with mild cases were present in the death group ($P = 0.0003$). The majority of patients (97.4%) received TCZ once. One patient (2.6%) received a second dose with the same dosage due to the occurrence of fever within 12 h. In contrast, patients in the non-TCZ treatment group had a higher death rate trend (9/19, 47.4%), especially those in the severe case group (3/4, 75%; **Figure 1**).

Clinical Presentations and Safety

A total of 67.2% of the patients presented with fever at the onset, followed by fatigue (51.7%), dry cough (51.7%), dyspnea (31.0%), muscle soreness (15.5%), and chills (13.8%). Among patients treated with TCZ, no significant differences were found between the improvement group and the death group in terms of blood oxygen saturation, blood pressure, and body temperature at baseline. The most common comorbidity was hypertension (55.2%), followed by diabetes (37.0%), coronary heart disease (31.0%), tumor (20.7%), and chronic obstructive pulmonary disease (COPD) (12.1%). There was no difference in the incidence of each comorbidity between the improvement group and the death group (all $P > 0.05$, **Table 1**).

During the hospital stay, 83.3% of patients in the death group and 40.7% of patients in the improvement group received corticosteroids ($P = 0.018$, **Table 2**), but there was no difference in the proportion of corticosteroids administered between the TCZ- and the non-TCZ treatment groups. Patients in the death group received a higher rate of invasive ventilation than those in the improvement group ($P = 0.0004$, **Table 2**). No differences were observed between the death group and the improvement group on receiving other treatments. No adverse effects, such as rash, nausea, thrombocytopenia, neutropenia, and abnormal liver and kidney function, were observed after treatment with TCZ.

Laboratory Examinations

At baseline, patients in the death group had a lower percentage of lymphocytes (6.2 [3.0–7.1]) in comparison to those in the improvement group (14.6 [6.8–20.5], $P = 0.0059$). The values of inflammatory markers including PCT and IL-6 before the use of TCZ were significantly higher in the death group than in the improvement group (PCT: 0.79 [0.16–1.9] vs. 0.07 [0.05-0.11], $P = 0.0003$; IL-6: 140.4 [69.9–316.5] vs. 53.2 [33.8–91.4], $P = 0.0191$). After the treatment with TCZ, the level of lactate dehydrogenase (LDH), hs-CRP, IL-6, and D-dimer decreased significantly (all $P < 0.05$) in the improvement group, while the lymphocyte count and the percentage of lymphocytes increased (all $P < 0.05$, **Table 3**). In contrast, in the death group, there was no significant improvement in the laboratory indexes after the use of TCZ.

The level of IL-6 observed after receiving TCZ treatment is shown in **Figure 2A**. From baseline, the level of IL-6 tended to increase on the first day after the use of TCZ and reached a peak on the third day, and then, it started to decrease on the fifth day and returned to baseline on the tenth day. However, the overall trend of the levels of IL-6 between patients in the improved group and those in the death group after TCZ treatment was not associated with the clinical outcome ($P = 0.1495$). Also, there was no significant difference in the level of IL-6 between the groups at each time point (All $P > 0.05$). After TCZ treatment, there was also a significant difference in hs-CRP levels within 10 days between patients in the improved and patients in the death group ($P = 0.0163$), indicating that the overall trend of the levels of hs-CRP after TCZ treatment was associated with the clinical outcome (**Figure 2C**), whereas the overall trend of the levels of IL-6 was not (**Figure 2B**).

In addition, based on the cut-off value of 100 pg/ml for IL-6 at baseline (10 times the upper limit of normal; e.g., 10 pg/ml), all patients in the study were divided into two groups: patients with an IL-6 level of $\geq$100 pg/ml and patients with an IL-6 level of <100 pg/ml. The elevated trend of the level of lymphocytes was found in both groups after receiving TCZ, and there was a significant difference between the two groups ($P = 0.0247$, **Figure 2D**). The Kaplan-Meier curves showed that the survival rate of patients in the TCZ treatment group was significantly higher than that of patients in the non-TCZ treatment group ($P = 0.0273$, **Figure 3**). The multivariable Cox proportional-hazards model

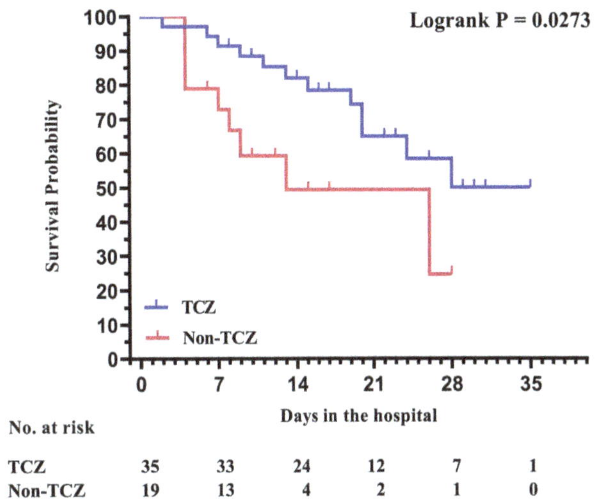

FIGURE 3 | Survival analysis with Kaplan-Meier curves between patients with COVID-19 treated with or without tocilizumab.

showed that TCZ was significantly associated with a lower risk of death (HR 0.383; 95% CI, 0.157 to 0.935; $P = 0.035$; **Supplementary Figure 2**). Furthermore, for patients receiving TCZ, the survival rate of patients with an IL-6 baseline level $\geq$ 100 pg/ml was worse than that of the patients with an IL-6 level < 100 pg/Ml; similar findings were also observed in patients with LYM% < 9.7, hs-CRP > 35.36 mg/L, and PCT $\geq$ 0.09 ng/ml (**Figure 4**).

DISCUSSION

This is the first study assessing the optimal timing of intravenous TCZ in patients with COVID-19. The preliminary data presented in this paper showed that, among the 39 patients with COVID-19 who received TCZ treatment, the majority of patients (27, 69.2%) either improved or stabilized without obvious side effects. TCZ, in this cohort, exhibited a good clinical efficacy and safety profile. Twelve patients (30.8%) in this cohort that died after TCZ therapy during hospitalization showed significantly higher IL-6, PCT, and LDH levels and lower lymphocyte percentages at baseline than those with clinical improvement. Patients receiving TCZ treatment had more survival probability than those that did not receive TCZ treatment. IL-6 levels $\geq$ 100 pg/ml, hs-CRP levels $\geq$ 35.56 mg/L, PCT levels $\geq$ 0.09 ng/ml, and LYM% < 9.7% were closely associated with poor prognoses after TCZ therapy. These findings collectively suggest that TCZ may be considered in the early stages of a cytokine storm (IL-6 level < 100 pg/ml).

Lymphopenia is a common feature in patients with severe COVID-19 and is also a predictor of poor prognosis (Yang et al., 2020). Specifically, the number of T cells, B cells, and natural killer cells decreased dramatically, while the number of neutrophils increased significantly. A cytokine storm in coronavirus disease results in the formation of cytokines storm, indicating an increase

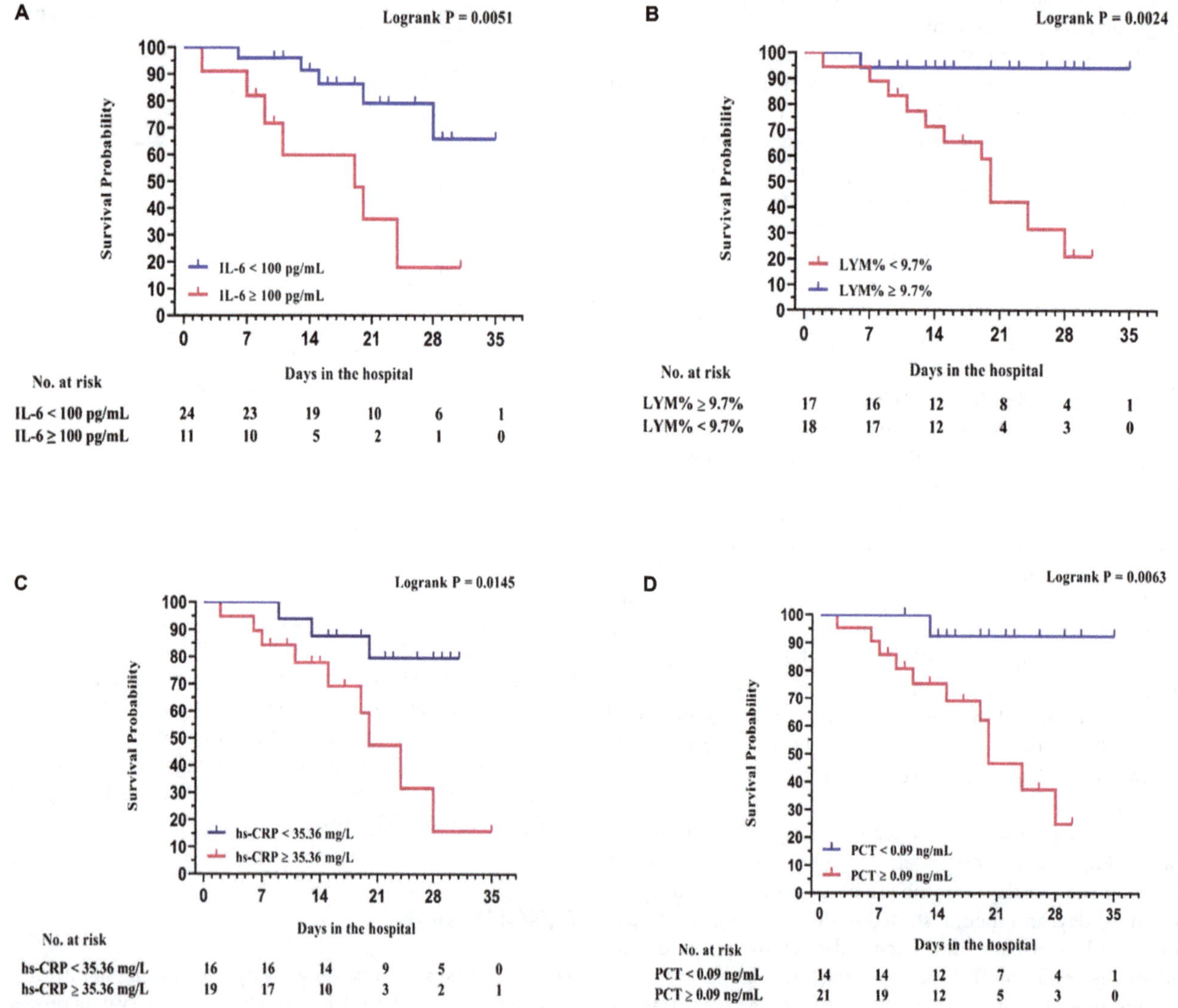

FIGURE 4 | Survival analysis with Kaplan–Meier curves between baseline laboratory examination groups. **(A)** IL-6, using the median value 100 pg/ml as cut-off value; **(B)** LYM%, using the median value of 9.7% as cut-off value; **(C)** hs-CRP, using the median value of 35.36 mg/L as cut-off value; **(D)** PCT, using the median value of 0.09 ng/ml as cut-off value.

in proinflammatory cytokines, such as IL-6, IL-1β, IL-8, and IL-17; granulocyte colony-stimulating factor (G-CSF); granulocyte-macrophage colony-stimulating factor (GM-CSF); monocyte chemoattractant protein 1 (MCP-1); macrophage inflammatory protein-1α (MIP-1α); and TNF-α (Cheung et al., 2005; Law et al., 2005). The abundant release of inflammatory cytokines may mediate acute respiratory distress syndrome (ARDS), leading to inflammatory cell infiltration and diffused alveolar damage within a short time. The cytokine storm can then cause further severe inflammatory damage to multiple organs, including the heart, liver, and kidney. The complex immune process induced by the SARS-CoV-2 could explain why some patients deteriorate suddenly at a later stage or during the recovery period (Special Expert Group for Control of the Epidemic of Novel Coronavirus Pneumonia of the Chinese Preventive Medicine Association, 2020).

Previous studies had reported that IL-6 positively correlated with the severity of COVID-19, with higher levels of IL-6 present in patients with severe and critical COVID-19 than those present in patients with common illness (Chen L. et al., 2020). IL-6 has a prominent proinflammatory effect through binding to the membrane-bound IL-6 receptor (mIL-6R) in a complex with gp130; on the other hand, IL-6-related downstream signal path is mediated by JAKs and STAT3 (Kang et al., 2019). An IL-6 antagonist may effectively reduce mortality in autoimmune diseases by inhibiting cytokine storms (Jones et al., 2011; Wolf et al., 2014). There is pre-existing evidence which suggests that TCZ can improve the clinical outcome in patients with severe and critical COVID-19 (Luo et al., 2020; Price et al., 2020; Toniati et al., 2020; Xu et al., 2020). In the current study, 27 patients (69.2%) who received TCZ had an obvious improvement of clinical symptoms, and the release of an *in vivo* inflammatory response without toxicity or adverse reactions, such as peripheral blood leukocyte decrease or hepatic and renal function abnormity, was observed. The outcomes in the patient cohort in this study suggest that TCZ may be an effective and safe treatment option in patients with COVID-19 with cytokine storms.

Cytokine storm is a highly complex condition, showing an excessive immune response to external stimuli (Davidson et al., 2015). Once a cytokine storm forms during COVID-19 infection and reaches its peak, it may be refractory to treatment. Therefore, the timing of the administration of TCZ is an important factor that affected the prognosis of patients with severe and critical illnesses. In the current study, the rate of death (30.8%) after TCZ treatment is higher than previously reported data. The possible reasons are as follows: (1) the rate of critically ill patients with COVID-19 in the present study is almost 50%, which is higher than that in previously published reports (Xu et al., 2020: 19.0%; Luo et al., 2020: 26.7%; Toniati et al., 2020: 20%; Price et al., 2020: 25%); (2) patients in this study seemed to have a lower baseline oxygen saturation (median SpO_2 90%) than those in the previous studies (SpO_2 range 91–99%) (Xu et al., 2020), suggesting that patients included in this study may be more seriously ill; (3) about 64.7% of critically ill patients in this study died after TCZ treatment, which suggests that later administration of TCZ in critically ill patients with evidence of an existing cytokine storm may be ineffective. Remarkably, of the 12 patients who died during the TCZ treatment, 58.3% patients had higher baseline levels of IL-6 than the cutoff value of 100 pg/ml; whereas, in the improvement group, only 18.5% patients had IL-6 levels above this cutoff value.

Compared to the TCZ treatment group, patients in the non-TCZ treatment group had a numerically higher death rate (47.4% vs. 30.8%) and were closely associated with a lower survival rate ($P = 0.0273$), indicating the improvement effect of TCZ on the prognoses of patients with COVID-19. In particular, a significant improvement was observed in the majority of severe cases (55.6%) receiving TCZ treatment, whereas the improvement rate of severe cases was only 10% in the non-TCZ group. More importantly, the Kaplan–Meier survival curves showed that the baseline IL-6 level of $\geq$100 pg/ml was closely associated with poor prognosis after TCZ treatment whereas at different cutoff values for the IL-6 baseline level, including IL-6 baseline level $\geq$ 30 pg/ml vs. < 30 pg/ml ($P = 0.454$) and IL-6 baseline level $\geq$ 50 pg/ml vs. < 50 pg/ml ($P = 0.076$), both of them have no significant correlation with clinical prognosis (**Supplementary Figure 1**). Accordingly, we recommend that the suitable timing to administer TCZ in patients with COVID-19 is in the early stage of the cytokine storm and, in particular, when the baseline level of IL-6 is less than 100 pg/ml. The early use of TCZ may effectively prevent excessive inflammatory injury and improve the outcome of severely ill patients with COVID-19.

At present, there is no clear conclusion about the time of and dose of administration of TCZ. In this study, based on the guidelines released by the National Health Commission of China, the majority of patients with COVID-19 (97.4%) received TCZ (4–8 mg/kg) once and one patient (2.6%) received a second dose due to the occurrence of fever. The results presented in this paper showed that the patients receiving TCZ treatment had better prognoses than those that did not receive TCZ treatment. Similarly, Xu et al. (2020) reported that TCZ (intravenous infusion of 400 mg) is an effective treatment for severely ill patients with COVID-19. Toniati et al. (2020) treated 100 patients with COVID-19 with TCZ at a dosage of 8 mg/kg (two consecutive intravenous infusions 12 h apart) and found that the treatment was associated with a clinical improvement in more than three-quarters of the patients. Moreover, Luo et al. (2020) suggested that repeated dose of the TCZ is recommended for critically ill patients with COVID-19 with elevated IL-6 levels. However, controversy remains as to whether the use of TCZ improves survival, shortens hospital stay, or reduces the need for mechanical ventilators. A randomized controlled study reported by Salama et al. (2021) demonstrated that TCZ reduced the likelihood of progression to mechanical ventilation or death by day 28 efficiently but that it did not improve the incidence of death from any cause. It appears that the timing of administration of TCZ is a critical factor that affects the prognosis.

The present study has several limitations. Previous data (Zhang et al., 2020) showed that D-dimer on admission could effectively predict the in-hospital mortality of patients with COVID-19. Although the improvement group had a numerically higher D-dimer level at baseline than that of the death group, no statistical difference was observed between the two groups, which may be due to the limited sample size in this study. Moreover, the results of a prospective meta-analysis (Sterne et al., 2020) showed that the administration of systemic corticosteroids among critically ill patients with COVID-19, compared with usual care or placebo, was associated with lower 28-day all-cause mortality. However, in the present study, there was no statistical difference in the use of corticosteroids between the improvement group and the death group after receiving TCZ. This study was conducted in the early stages of the COVID-19 epidemic, and there is a lack of clinical experience in the application of corticosteroids. We believe that the possible reason for the inconsistency of the results presented in this study compared with the reported data may be the different timing and dosages of glucocorticoids among the patients, as well as the limited sample size. Because this is a retrospective study, we did not compare the different dosages and the timing of administration of TCZ prospectively in this study. Therefore, the clinical practice value of the cutoff points of IL-6 in predicting the timing of TCZ administration needs further evaluation in future randomized controlled trials with large sample sizes and long-term clinical follow-up.

CONCLUSION

This study suggests that TCZ may help to improve the prognosis of patients with COVID-19 with the baseline IL-6 level below the cutoff value of 100 pg/ml with an acceptable safety profile. Further clinical trials are required to confirm the observed findings and evaluate the efficacy of TCZ and its scope of clinical application and timing.

AUTHOR CONTRIBUTIONS

PaL: data collection and writing. ZL: data collection and analysis. QL: data interpretation and analysis. ZW and WQ: literature search. YG and LY: manuscript preparation. CC: preparation of figures. SW: preparation of tables. PeL and YD: data interpretation. YH: literature search. YL: data collection. LZ: statistical analysis. CB: data analysis. WZ: study design and writing the manuscript. All authors: contributed to the article and approved the submitted version.

SUPPLEMENTARY MATERIAL

Supplementary Figure 1 | Survival analysis with Kaplan–Meier curves between baseline laboratory examination groups. **(A)** Il-6, using the median value of 30 pg/ml as cut-off value; **(B)** Il-6, using the median value of 50 pg/ml as cut-off value.

Supplementary Figure 2 | Multivariable Cox proportional-hazards model analysis used to explore the role of tocilizumab on clinical outcomes when adjusted for clinical covariates, including age, Bmi, diabetes, and administration of glucocorticoids.

REFERENCES

Arabi, Y. M., Murthy, S., and Webb, S. (2020). Covid-19: a novel coronavirus and a novel challenge for critical care. *Intens. Care Med.* 46, 833–836. doi: 10.1007/s00134-020-05955-1

Biggioggero, M., Crotti, C., Becciolini, A., and Favalli, E. G. (2018). Tocilizumab in the treatment of rheumatoid arthritis: an evidence-based review and patient selection. *Drug Des. Dev. Ther.* 13, 57–70. doi10.2147/DDDT.S150580

Chen, G., Wu, D., Guo, W., Cao, Y., Huang, D., Wang, H., et al. (2020). Clinical and immunological features of severe and moderate coronavirus disease 2019. *J. Clin. Invest.* 130, 2620–2629. doi: 10.1172/JCI137244

Chen, L., Liu, H.-G., Liu, W., Liu, J., Liu, K., Shang, J., et al. (2020). Analysis of clinical features of 29 patients with 2019 novel coronavirus pneumonia. *Chin. J. Tuberc. Respir. Dis.* 43, 203–208.

Chen, N., Zhou, M., Dong, X., Qu, J., Gong, F., Han, Y., et al. (2020). Epidemiological and clinical characteristics of 99 cases of 2019 novel coronavirus pneumonia in Wuhan, China: a descriptive study. *Lancet* 395, 507–513. doi: 10.1016/S0140-6736(20)30211-7

Cheung, C. Y., Poon, L. L., Ng, I. H., Luk, W., Sia, S. F., Wu, M. H., et al. (2005). Cytokine responses in severe acute respiratory syndrome coronavirus-infected macrophages in vitro: possible relevance to pathogenesis. *J. Virol.* 79, 7819–7826. doi: 10.1128/JVI.79.12.7819-7826.2005

Davidson, S., Maini, M. K., and Wack, A. (2015). Disease-promoting effects of type I interferons in viral, bacterial, and coinfections. *J. Interf. Cytokine Res.* 35, 252–264. doi: 10.1089/jir.2014.0227

Huang, C., Wang, Y., Li, X., Ren, L., Zhao, J., Hu, Y., et al. (2020). Clinical features of patients infected with 2019 novel coronavirus in Wuhan, China. *Lancet* 395, 497–506. doi: 10.1016/S0140-6736(20)30183-5

Jones, S. A., Scheller, J., and Rose-John, S. (2011). Therapeutic strategies for the clinical blockade of IL-6/gp130 signaling. *J. Clin. Invest.* 121, 3375–3383. doi: 10.1172/JCI57158

Kang, S., Tanaka, T., Narazaki, M., and Kishimoto, T. (2019). Targeting interleukin-6 signaling in clinic. *Immunity* 50, 1007–1023. doi: 10.1016/j.immuni.2019.03.026

Kuiken, T., Fouchier, R. A. M., Schutten, M., Rimmelzwaan, G. F., van Amerongen, G., van Riel, D., et al. (2003). Newly discovered coronavirus as the primary cause of severe acute respiratory syndrome. *Lancet* 362, 263–270. doi: 10.1016/S0140-6736(03)13967-0

Law, H. K., Cheung, C. Y., Ng, H. Y., Sia, S. F., Chan, Y. O., Luk, W., et al. (2005). Chemokine up-regulation in SARS-coronavirus-infected, monocyte-derived human dendritic cells. *Blood* 106, 2366–2374. doi: 10.1182/blood-2004-10-4166

Luo, P., Liu, Y., Qiu, L., Liu, X., Liu, D., and Li, J. (2020). Tocilizumab treatment in COVID-19: a single center experience. *J. Med. Virol.* 92, 814–818. doi: 10.1002/jmv.25801

Moore, J. B., and June, C. H. (2020). Cytokine release syndrome in severe COVID-19. *Science* 368, 473–474. doi: 10.1126/science.abb8925

National Health Commission (2020). *Diagnosis and Treatment Protocol for Novel Coronavirus Pneumonia. China NHCOTPSRO*, 7th Interim Edn, Available online at: http://www.nhc.gov.cn/yzygj/s7653p/202003/46c9294a7dfe4cef80dc7f5912eb1989/files/ce3e6945832a438eaae415350a8ce964.pdf (accessed March 3, 2020).

Price, C. C., Altice, F. L., Shyr, Y., Koff, A., Pischel, L., Goshua, G., et al. (2020). Tocilizumab treatment for cytokine release syndrome in hospitalized COVID-19. *Chest* doi: 10.1016/j.chest.2020.06.006 [Epub ahead for print],

Salama, C., Han, J., Yau, L., Reiss, W. G., Kramer, B., Neidhart, J. D., et al. (2021). Tocilizumab in patients hospitalized with Covid-19 pneumonia. *N. Engl. J. Med.* 384, 20–30. doi: 10.1056/NEJMoa2030340

Special Expert Group for Control of the Epidemic of Novel Coronavirus Pneumonia of the Chinese Preventive Medicine Association (2020). An update on the epidemiological characteristics of novel Coronavirus pneumonia (COVID-19). *Chin. J. Epidemiol.* 41, 139–144.

Sterne, J. A. C., Murthy, S., Diaz, J. V., Slutsky, A. S., Villar, J., Angus, D. C., et al. (2020). Association between administration of systemic corticosteroids and mortality among critically Ill patients with COVID-19: a meta-analysis. *JAMA* 324, 1330–1341. doi: 10.1001/jama.2020.17023

Stone, J. H., Frigault, M. J., Serling-Boyd, N. J., Fernandes, A. D., Harvey, L., Foulkes, A. S., et al. (2020). Efficacy of Tocilizumab in patients hospitalized with Covid-19. *N. Engl. J. Med.* 383, 2333–2344. doi: 10.1056/NEJMoa2028836

Toniati, P., Piva, S., Cattalini, M., Garrafa, E., Regola, F., Castelli, F., et al. (2020). Tocilizumab for the treatment of severe COVID-19 pneumonia with hyperinflammatory syndrome and acute respiratory failure: a single center study of 100 patients in Brescia, Italy. *Autoimmun. Rev.* 19:102568. doi: 10.1016/j.autrev.2020.102568

Wang, C., Horby, P. W., Hayden, F. G., and Gao, G. F. (2020). A novel coronavirus outbreak of global health concern. *Lancet* 395, 470–473. doi: 10.1016/S0140-6736(20)30185-9

Wolf, J., Rose-John, S., and Garbers, C. (2014). Interleukin-6 and its receptors: a highly regulated and dynamic system. *Cytokine* 70, 11–20. doi: 10.1016/j.cyto.2014.05.024

Xu, X., Han, M., Li, T., Sun, W., Wang, D., Fu, B., et al. (2020). Effective treatment of severe COVID-19 patients with tocilizumab. *Proc. Natl. Acad. Sci. U.S.A.* 117, 10970–10975. doi: 10.1073/pnas.2005615117

Yang, X., Yu, Y., Xu, J., Shu, H., Xia, J., Liu, H., et al. (2020). Clinical course and outcomes of critically ill patients with SARS-CoV-2 pneumonia in Wuhan, China: a single-centered, retrospective, observational study. *Lancet Respir. Med.* 8, 475–481. doi: 10.1016/S2213-2600(20)30079-5

Ye, Q., Wang, B., and Mao, J. (2020). The pathogenesis and treatment of the 'Cytokine Storm' in COVID-19. *J. Infect.* 80, 607–613. doi: 10.1016/j.jinf.2020.03.037

Zhang, L., Yan, X., Fan, Q., Liu, H., Liu, X., Liu, Z., et al. (2020). D-dimer levels on admission to predict in-hospital mortality in patients with Covid-19. *J. Thromb. Haemost.* 18, 1324–1329. doi: 10.1111/jth.14859

16

Derangement of Metabolic and Lysosomal Gene Profiles in Response to Dexamethasone Treatment in Sarcoidosis

Jaya Talreja[1], Christian Bauerfeld[2], Edward Sendler[3], Roger Pique-Regi[3,4], Francesca Luca[3,4] and Lobelia Samavati[1,3]*

[1] Division of Pulmonary, Critical Care and Sleep Medicine, Department of Internal Medicine, School of Medicine and Detroit Medical Center, Wayne State University, Detroit, MI, United States, [2] Division of Critical Care, Department of Pediatrics, School of Medicine and Detroit Medical Center, Wayne State University, Detroit, MI, United States, [3] Center for Molecular Medicine and Genetics, School of Medicine, Wayne State University, Detroit, MI, United States, [4] Department of Obstetrics and Gynecology, School of Medicine, Wayne State University, Detroit, MI, United States

***Correspondence:**
Lobelia Samavati
ay6003@wayne.edu

Glucocorticoids (GCs) play a central role in modulation of inflammation in various diseases, including respiratory diseases such as sarcoidosis. Surprisingly, the specific anti-inflammatory effects of GCs on different myeloid cells especially in macrophages remain poorly understood. Sarcoidosis is a systemic granulomatous disease of unknown etiology that occurs worldwide and is characterized by granuloma formation in different organs. Alveolar macrophages play a role in sarcoidosis granuloma formation and progressive lung disease. The goal of the present study is to identify the effect of GCs on transcriptomic profiles and the cellular pathways in sarcoidosis alveolar macrophages and their corresponding blood myeloid cells. We determined and compared the whole transcriptional signatures of alveolar macrophages from sarcoidosis patients and blood $CD14^+$ monocytes of the same subjects in response to *in vitro* treatment with dexamethasone (DEX) via RNA-sequencing. In response to DEX, we identified 2,834 genes that were differentially expressed in AM. Predominant pathways affected were as following: metabolic pathway ($FDR = 4.1 \times 10^{-10}$), lysosome ($FDR = 6.3 \times 10^{-9}$), phagosome ($FDR = 3.9 \times 10^{-5}$). The DEX effect on AMs is associated with metabolic derangements involving glycolysis, oxidative phosphorylation and lipid metabolisms. In contrast, the top impacted pathways in response to DEX treatment in blood $CD14^+$ monocytes were as following; cytokine-cytokine receptor interaction ($FDR = 6 \times 10^{-6}$) and transcriptional misregulation in cancer ($FDR = 1 \times 10^{-4}$). Pathways similarly affected in both cell types were genes involved in lysosomes, cytoskeleton and transcriptional misregulation in cancer. These data suggest that the different effects of DEX on AMs and peripheral blood monocytes are partly dictated by lineage specific transcriptional programs and their physiological functions.

Keywords: dexamethasone, corticosteroids, gene expression, sarcoidosis, alveolar macrophages, monocytes, RNA-seq

INTRODUCTION

Pulmonary sarcoidosis is characterized by granuloma formation in the lungs. Pulmonary involvement is the leading cause of morbidity and mortality in sarcoidosis patients in the US, while other organ involvements including eyes, central nervous system, cardiac, and skin may lead to severe functional impairments (1, 2). Lungs are constantly exposed to toxins and microbial products and lung macrophages play important roles in the maintenance of immunological homeostasis and are the cornerstone of granuloma formation (1, 3, 4).

Due to their immune-modulatory actions, glucocorticoids (GCs) are one of the most widely prescribed drugs for the treatment of inflammatory and immune mediated disorders, including sarcoidosis (5). The long-term use of GCs is limited due to profound derangements of glucose metabolism, mineral homeostasis, amino acid metabolism, cognition and effects on the cardiovascular system (6). Several studies questioned the long-term benefits of GCs treatment in several respiratory diseases, including chronic obstructive lung disease (COPD). In idiopathic pulmonary fibrosis GCs treatment has been associated with worsening prognosis (7–9). Similarly, the long term benefits of GC treatments in sarcoidosis is unclear (7). While GCs suppress inflammation by decreasing lymphocyte activation, proliferation, and survival, there is a knowledge gap in how GCs modulate the immune response of human myeloid cells and tissue macrophages, especially in sarcoidosis. Recent studies highlighted that GCs have little effect in controlling inflammation in macrophage-dominated diseases (8, 10).

Because AMs originated ontologically from yolk sac and adapt to maintain pulmonary hemostasis and clearance, the effect of GCs on AMs may be different as compared to myeloid derived macrophages and monocytes (11). Additionally, in sarcoidosis the response to GCs treatment is partly dictated by organ involvement. This posits to question if tissue macrophages, especially AMs as compared to monocytes, are less susceptible to GCs treatment. Dissecting the effect of GCs treatment on cellular responses of two different macrophage lineages may uncover important molecular pathways to discriminate beneficial from detrimental effects of this therapy.

The goal of this study was to identify the differential transcriptional signatures and signaling pathways affected by corticosteroids in two relevant macrophage lineages (AMs and peripheral monocytes) in sarcoidosis. We performed transcriptomic analysis of isolated AMs and $CD14^{+}$ monocytes from the same sarcoidosis patients in response to *ex-vivo* treatment with DEX. We identified common as well as unique pathways affected by GCs in sarcoidosis AMs and monocytes.

METHODS

Study Subjects

Sarcoidosis diagnosis was based on the ATS/ERS/WASOG statement (12). The enrollment criteria for sarcoidosis patient were as previously described (13–15). A total of 10 patients with sarcoidosis participated in this study.

Isolation of AMs From BAL

AMs were isolated from BAL fluid as previously described (14, 15). Viability of AMs was routinely about 98%. Immunofluorescent staining with CD68 antibody confirmed >99% purity.

Isolation and Purification of $CD14^{+}$ Monocytes

$CD14^{+}$ monocytes were purified from PBMCs by using the MACS monocyte isolation kit (Miltenyl Biotech, San Diego, CA) according to the manufacturer's instructions (13, 14). The purity of enriched monocytes was evaluated by flow cytometry using fluorochrome-conjugated CD14 antibody; the purity of monocytes was >98%.

mRNA Isolation

Sarcoidosis AMs or monocytes were cultured in the presence of DEX (100 ng/mL) or vehicle for 16 h. After 16 h incubation, mRNA was isolated from purified AMs and monocytes using the Dynabeads mRNA Direct Kit (Ambion) as described earlier (13).

RNA-seq Library Preparation and Sequencing

RNA-seq libraries were prepared using the NEBNext ultradirectional library preparation protocol (New England BioLabs, Ipswich, MA) as described earlier (13). RNA-seq library quality was assessed using an Agilent Bioanalyzer. Individually barcoded RNA-seq libraries were pooled in equimolar quantities. A pooled library of 40 samples: untreated sarcoidosis AMs ($n = 10$), DEX-treated sarcoidosis AMs ($n = 10$), untreated sarcoidosis monocytes ($n = 10$), and DEX-treated sarcoidosis monocytes ($n = 10$) was sequenced on the Illumina Next-Seq 500 (75 cycles, PE).

RNA-seq Data Analysis, Differential Gene Expression, and Canonical Pathway Analysis

RNA-seq data were analyzed using the Illumina Basespace RNA express application. The sequencing reads were aligned to the reference human genome hg19 using STAR aligner and differentially expressed (DE) genes (FDR < 5%) were identified with the DEseq2 analysis tool (16, 17). Enrichment of cellular pathway and gene ontology category was calculated using iPathwayGuidetool and Gene Trail 2 Over-Representation Analysis (ORA) and comparing the list of DE genes with background expressed genes. Pathway enrichment was determined at FDR < 5%, using Benjamini and Hochberg procedure to control for multiple testing (18).

RESULTS

Effect of Dexamethasone on the Transcriptional Signature of Sarcoidosis AMs

Using CD68 antibody as macrophage marker, the purity of isolated AMs was >99% (**Figure S1**). The subject demographics are displayed in **Table 1**. All subjects were non-smokers, and none were on corticosteroid or other immune-suppressive medication. Isolated AMs were cultured either in the presence of DEX (100 ng/mL) for 16 h or vehicle. RNA-seq libraries were prepared from DEX treated AMs ($n = 10$) and untreated AMs ($n = 10$) from the same subjects serving as controls. RNA-seq libraries were sequenced on one lane of the Illumina Next-Seq 500 as described previously (13). Using DeSeq2, we identified 2834 DE genes (log_2-fold change (FC) > 0.6 and FDR < 5%) between DEX-treated vs. untreated AMs from same sarcoidosis patients (**Figure 1A**). The Gene ontology (GO) enrichment analysis of DE genes (FDR < 5%) showed that the significant biological processes impacted after DEX treatment were neutrophil degranulation (FDR = 1.7×10^{-7}), regulation of transcription (FDR = 3.3×10^{-4}), and insulin receptor signaling (FDR = 4.1×10^{-4}) (**Figure 1B**). Most genes involved in neutrophil degranulation were downregulated. CD14 is a general marker for myeloid cells (macrophages and monocytes), but it has been shown that activated neutrophil exhibit surface CD14 (19). The analysis of biological function enrichment showed lysosome and lysosomal membrane as significant cellular components affected by DEX treatment (**Figure 1C**). **Table 2** summarizes the most up and down regulated genes in response to DEX treatment in sarcoidosis AMs. Increased expression of several of these genes has been reported in THP-1 cell lines or monocyte-derived dendritic cells in response to DEX treatment (20–22). We identified that DEX-treatment induced the expression of two novel genes; Ring finger protein (RNF) 175 and amine oxidase copper containing 2 (AOC2). Other upregulated genes were formyl peptide receptor 1 (FPR1) (log_2 FC = 2.6, FDR = 1.8×10^{-7}) and Vanin 1 (VNN1) (log_2 FC = 2.0, FDR = 7.1×10^{-7}). FPR1 is a member of the G-protein coupled receptor 1 family encoding protein (21), which mediates the response of phagocytic cells to microorganisms. Vanin 1 belongs to vanin gene family and has pantetheinase activity and participates in hematopoietic cell trafficking (23). Similarly, complement factor properdin (CFP) (log_2 FC = 1.3, FDR = 7.4×10^{-5}) was upregulated. This gene positively regulates the alternative complement pathway. DEX-treatment downregulated several small nucleolar RNA box genes, solute carrier families and integrin genes in sarcoid AMs.

Pathway enrichment analysis identified over 50 significant pathways affected by DEX treatment (**Figure 1D**). The most significant pathways were metabolic pathway (FDR = 4.1×10^{-10}), lysosome (FDR = 6.3×10^{-9}), phagosome (FDR = 3.9×10^{-5}), FoxO signaling pathway (FDR = 7×10^{-6}), transcriptional misregulation in cancer (FDR = 1.6×10^{-6}), and regulation of actin cytoskeleton (FDR = 5.7×10^{-5}).

TABLE 1 | Subject demographics.

Characteristic	Patients
Age (year)	46.11 ± 14.4
BMI	29 ± 10.4
Gender, *N* (%)	
Female	5 (50)
Male	5 (50)
Self-reported Race, N (%)	
African American	10(100)
White	0 (0)
CXR stage, *N* (%)	
0	0 (0)
1	0 (0)
2	6 (60)
3	4 (40)
Organ Involvements, *N* (%)	
Neuro-ophthalmologic	2 (10)
Lung	10 (100)
Skin	4 (10)
Multiorgans	15 (75)
PPD	Negative
AFB/culture	Negative
IGRA	Negative

BMI, body mass index; CXR, chest X-ray; PPD, purified protein derivative; AFB, acid-fast bacilli; IGRA, interferon gamma release assay.

Effect of Dexamethasone on Metabolic Pathway

We found that 237 DE genes are involved in metabolic pathway of which 65 genes were upregulated and 172 genes were downregulated. To determine the metabolic pathways impacted by DEX treatment, we performed a pathway analysis of these 237 genes using Gene Trail 2. The most significant pathways were as following; oxidative phosphorylation (FDR = 1.4×10^{-36}), carbon (FDR = 4.7×10^{-34}), purine metabolism (FDR = 4.2×10^{-22}), pyrimidine metabolism (FDR = 4.8×10^{-18}), non-alcoholic fatty liver disease (NAFLD) (FDR = 2.3×10^{-17}), glycolysis (FDR = 2.4×10^{-16}), and fatty acid metabolism (FDR = 2.1×10^{-12}). **Figure 2** shows the heatmap of genes involved in fatty acid metabolism (A), oxidative phosphorylation (B), and lysosome pathway (C) in response to DEX-treatment. DEX-treatment led to downregulation of genes involved in glycolysis and oxidative phosphorylation. Specifically, DEX-treatment downregulated the expression of peroxisome proliferator-activated receptor γ (PPARγ) co-activator 1 Beta gene (PPARGC1B) (log_2 FC = −1.4, FDR = 3.08×10^{-9}). PPARγ co-activator is known to be the master regulator of mitochondrial biogenesis, oxidative phosphorylation and lipid metabolism (24, 25). In contrast, DEX increased expression of genes involved in amino sugar and nucleotide sugar metabolism. Fucose-1-phosphate guanylyltransferase (FPGT) increased in response to DEX treatment by 2 folds. Protein encoded by this gene participates in phosphorylation of L-fucose to form beta-L-fucose-1-phosphate which is a substrate of fucose-1-phosphate

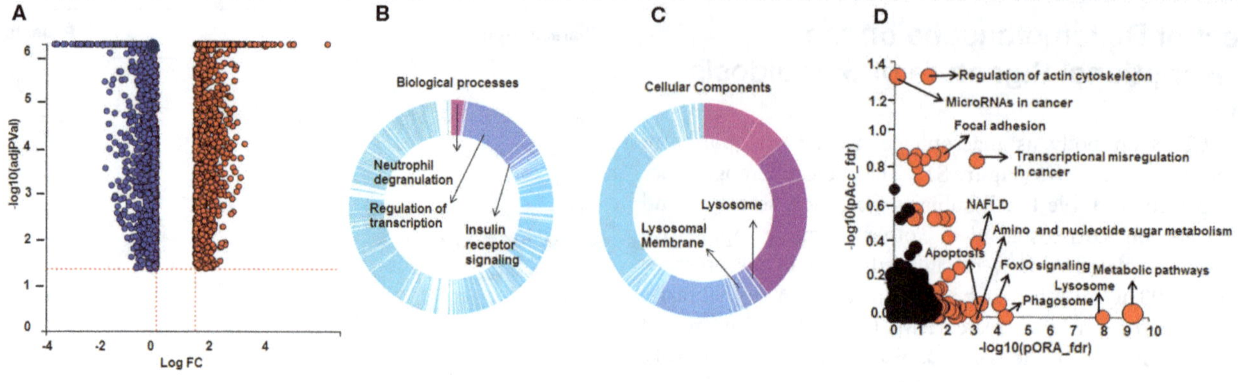

FIGURE 1 | Differential gene expression and Gene Ontology (GO) processes and significant pathways between DEX-treated compared to untreated sarcoid AMs. **(A)** Volcano plot: 2,834 significant DE genes analyzed by DEseq2 analysis tool are represented in terms of their measured expression fold change (log_2FC) on the x-axis and the significance of the change ($-log_{10}$ adj *p*-value) on the y-axis. The dotted lines represent the thresholds used to select the DE genes: log_2-fold change (>0.6) and significance (FDR < 5%). The up-regulated genes (positive log_2FC) are shown in red, while the down-regulated (negative log_2FC) genes are shown in blue. **(B,C)** Gene Ontology (GO) analysis of DE genes. To assess the enrichment of GO terms Elim pruning method was used. GO analysis identified top **(B)** biological processes and **(C)** cellular components. **(D)** Pathway analysis on the DE genes was performed considering a threshold of log_2 FC > 0.6 and FDR < 5% using iPathwayGuide analysis tool that uses two types of evidence: the over-representation on the horizontal axis (pORA) and the perturbation on the vertical axis (pAcc). Significant pathways (FDR < 5%) are shown in red, whereas non-significant are in black. The size of the circle is proportional to the number of genes in that pathway.

guanylyltransferase and GTP to form GDP-beta-L-fucose (26). AOC2 gene (log_2 FC = 3, FDR = 1.1×10^{-13}) catalyzes the oxidative conversion of amines to aldehydes and ammonia in the presence of copper and quinone cofactor and is associated with eye diseases (27). Glutamate-ammonia ligase (GLUL) expression is also increased in response to DEX (log_2 FC = 2, FDR = 3.8×10^{-11}). The protein encoded by this gene catalyzes the synthesis of glutamine from glutamate and ammonia in an ATP-dependent reaction (28). It is a key protein of glutamine synthesis and essential for cellular metabolism including macrophages (29). DEX upregulated the genes involved in insulin receptor signaling. For instance; insulin receptor substrate 2 (IRS2) (log_2 FC = 1.2, FDR = 5.4×10^{-5}), insulin receptor (INSR) (log_2 FC = 1.0, FDR = 2.0×10^{-3}), and phosphoinositide-3-kinase regulatory subunit 1 (PIK3R1) (log_2 FC = 1.0, FDR = 3.4×10^{-6}). AMP-activated protein kinase (AMPK) is an important energy-sensing enzyme that monitors cellular energy status. DEX upregulated the expression of genes that encode AMPK subunits, including catalytic subunit alpha 1 (PRKAA1) (log_2 FC = 0.96, FDR = 1.8×10^{-5}) and non-catalytic subunit beta 2 (PRKAB2) (log_2 FC = 0.95, FDR = 6.2×10^{-11}) (30). The catalytic subunit of AMPK protects cells from ATP depletion by switching off ATP-consuming biosynthetic pathways (30).

Modulation of Phago-Lysosomal Genes by Dexamethasone

The lysosomal pathway was the second most impacted pathway in response to DEX treatment. **Figure 2C** shows the effect of DEX treatment on the gene expression involved in the lysosome pathway in sarcoidosis AMs. Among 44 lysosomal genes only 6 genes were upregulated while the rest were down regulated in response to DEX treatment. Clathrin heavy chain like (CLTCL) 1 expression increased 4 fold (log_2 FC = 2.0, FDR = 8.2×10^{-8}) in response to DEX treatment. Clathrin coated vesicles have been shown to endocytose accumulated protein aggregates and direct them to the lysosome for further degradation (31). Cathepsins represent the major components of the lysosomal proteolytic system. Cathepsin F (CTSF) (log_2 FC = 1.5, FDR = 0.8×10^{-7}) and cathepsin O (CTSO) (log_2 FC = 0.65, FDR= 5.4×10^{-3}) were upregulated. Galactosylceramidase (GALC) hydrolyzes the galactose ester bonds of galactosylceramide and was increased (log_2 FC = 1.0, FDR = 9.1×10^{-5}). Lysosomal related genes involved in V-ATPase dependent organelle acidification such as T Cell Immune Regulator 1 (TCIRG1) (log_2 FC = −1.3, FDR = 1.4×10^{-16}), lysosomal proteases (CTSK) (log_2 FC = −1.1, FDR = 6.3×10^{-4}), sulfatases (ARSB) (log_2 FC = −0.8, FDR = 1.5×10^{-5}), and lysosomal membrane proteins (LAMP) (log_2 FC = −0.7, FDR = 3.5×10^{-3}) were significantly decreased in response to DEX treatment. Cathepsin K (CTSK) expression was downregulated in sarcoid AMs after DEX treatment. CTSK, a lysosomal cysteine protease, is proteolytic for matrix proteins, including gelatin and fibrillar collagens. It has been shown to play a key role in protecting against lung fibrosis (28). The Mucolipin 1 (MCOLN1) gene that encodes a member of the transient receptor potential (TRP) cation channel gene family was downregulated (log_2 FC = −1.1, FDR = 2.6×10^{-10}). MCOLN1 has been suggested to regulate fusion/fission of vesicles in the endocytic pathway (32), and lysosomal ion homeostasis. Mutations in the MCOLN1 gene have been reported with lysosomal storage disease (33). The Transcription factor EB (TFEB) gene was downregulated (log_2 FC = −1.7, FDR = 2.2×10^{-9}). TFEB plays an important role in lysosomal biogenesis, autophagy and cellular metabolism (34). These data show that DEX treatment downregulates genes of the lysosomal pathway and lysosomal biogenesis that are involved in uptake and acidification processes and in the proteolysis of degraded proteins/debris in lysosomes.

TABLE 2 | Top up and down-regulated regulated genes in AMs in response to dexamethasone treatment.

Gene symbol	Gene name	Type	$\log_2$ fold change	FDR *p*-value
pkp2	Plakophilin 2	Cytoskeleton	4.5	7.87E-19
ABLIM3	Actin binding LIM protein family member 3	Cytoskeleton	3.5	1.23E-13
SRPX	Sushi repeat containing protein X-linked	Peroxiredoxin-like domain	3.5	4.03E-10
TSC22D3	TSC22 domain family member 3	Leucine zipper protein	3.4	5.13E-26
METTL7A	Methyltransferase like 7A	Methyltransferase	3.1	6.28E-14
MFGE8	Milk fat globule-EGF factor 8 protein	Membrane glycoprotein	2.9	6.59E-15
RNF175	Ring finger protein 175	E3 ligase	2.9	2.89E-09
AOC2	Amine oxidase copper containing 2	Amine oxidases	2.8	1.1E-13
FMN1	Formin 1	Cytoskeleton	2.7	1.47E-25
MERTK	MER proto-oncogene, tyrosine kinase	Tyrosine kinase	2.7	3.97E-07
FKBP5	FKBP prolyl isomerase 5	Immunophilin protein family	2.7	2.04E-27
RGS2	Regulator of G protein signaling 2	G protein signaling	2.6	3.54E-09
SESN1	Sestrin 1	Sestrin family. P53	2.2	2.20E-19
CD163L1	CD163 molecule like 1	Scavenger receptor	2.7	6.01E-13
FPR1	Formyl peptide receptor 1	G-protein coupled receptor	2.6	1.89E-07
TFPI	Tissue factor pathway inhibitor	Serine protease inhibitor	2.3	3.54E-09
NES	Nestin	Intermediate filament protein family	−3.7	2.74E-12
METTL7B	Methyltransferase like 7B	Methyltransferase	−3.7	1.66E-10
TIE1	Tyrosine kinase with immunoglobulin like and EGF like domains 1	Protein tyrosine kinase	−3.7	1.66E-10
SNORD15B	Small nucleolar RNA, C/D box 15B	Small nucleolar RNAs	−3.7	4.78E-16
SNORA8	Small nucleolar RNA, H/ACA box 8	Small nucleolar RNAs	−3.4	2.04E-11
LGALS2	Galectin 2	Galactoside binding lectin	−3.4	3.58E-13
SNORD97	Small nucleolar RNA, C/D box 97	Small nucleolar RNAs	−2.9	2.04E-12
PRAM1	PML-RARA regulated adaptor molecule 1	Adaptor protein	−2.6	7.21E-25
COL6A1	Collagen type VI alpha 1 chain	Collagen (cytoskeleton)	−2.05	1.52E-06
SLC37A2	Solute carrier family 37 member 2	Solute carrier protein	−2.4	9.65E-07
SLC6A12	Solute carrier family 6 member 12	Solute carrier protein	−2.3	7.21E-15
SLC29A3	Solute carrier family 29 member 3	Solute carrier protein	−1.9	7.68E-13
CASS4	Cas scaffold protein family member 4	Scaffolding protein	−2.4	4.78E-08
UBTD1	Ubiquitin domain containing 1	E3 ligase	−1.7	1.87E-08
ITGB7	Integrin subunit beta 7	Integrin	−2.9	1.92E-11

In response to DEX most genes related to phagosome formation showed decreased expression, only 6 genes were upregulated. Upregulated genes in response to DEX treatment were as following: member RAS oncogene family RAB5A ($\log_2$ FC $= 0.7$, FDR $= 3.39 \times 10^{-11}$) that is required for the fusion of plasma membranes and early endosomes, TLR4 ($\log_2$ FC $=$ 1.5, FDR $= 2.8 \times 10^{-7}$), TLR5 ($\log_2$ FC $= 1.1$, FDR $= 4.1 \times 10^{-2}$), TLR8 ($\log_2$ FC $= 0.8$, FDR $= 4.1 \times 10^{-3}$), dynein cytoplasmic 1 light intermediate chain 2 (DYNC1L) ($\log_2$ FC $= 0.8$, FDR $= 5.7 \times 10^{-15}$) and dynein cytoplasmic 2 heavy chain 1 (DYNC2H1) ($\log_2$ FC $= 1.6$, FDR $=1.3 \times 10^{-6}$). This gene encodes a large cytoplasmic dynein protein involved in retrograde transport in the cilium and intra flagellar transport, a process required for ciliary/flagellar assembly. Cytoplasmic dynein-1 transports cargo into cell interior toward microtubule minus ends (35). Dynein-2, also known as intra flagellar transport dynein, moves cargoes along the axoneme of eukaryotic cilia and flagella (36). They are important for ciliary function, neuron and phagolysosome formation (30, 37). Aberrant function of the protein has been reported in ciliary dysfunction (35). Three genes encoding subunits of NADPH oxidase complex were downregulated. These were CYBA (p22-PHOX) ($\log_2$ FC $= -0.7$, FDR $= 7.2 \times 10^{-9}$), CYBB ($\log_2$ FC $= -0.8$, FDR $= 1.0 \times 10^{-3}$) and NCF2 ($\log_2$ FC $= -0.9$, FDR $= 1.0 \times 10^{-4}$). While NCF-1 gene expression was upregulated ($\log_2$ FC $= 1.72$, FDR $= 3.7 \times 10^{-8}$). NADPH oxidase is a key producer of reactive oxygen species (ROS) participating in killing of bacteria in phagosomes. Mutation in this gene is associated with chronic granulomatous disease (38).

Transcriptional Misregulation in Cancer

DEX treatment of sarcoidosis AMs upregulated the expression of 18 genes and downregulated the expression of 20 genes related to transcriptional misregulation in cancer. The expression of

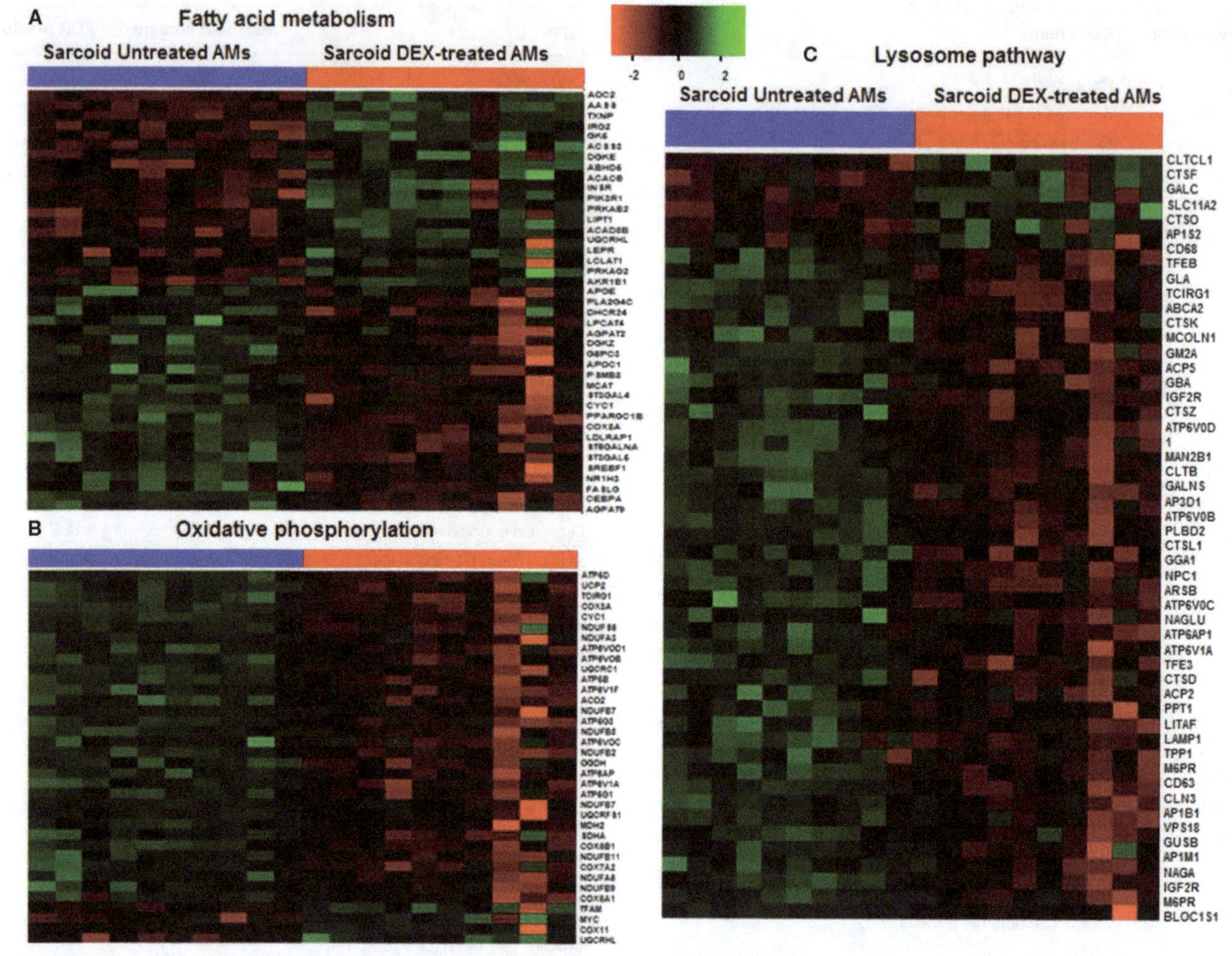

FIGURE 2 | Heat map of DE genes involved in fatty acid metabolism, oxidative phosphorylation and lysosomal pathways. **(A)** Fatty acid metabolism, **(B)** Oxidative phosphorylation, **(C)** Lysosomal pathway. The thresholds used to select the DE genes: $\log_2$ FC > 0.6 and FDR < 5%. Green shade represents high expression and red shade represents low expression.

15-hydroxyprostaglandin dehydrogenase (HPGD) was increased $\log_2$ FC = 1.5, FDR = 9.3×10^{-4}). HPGD is involved in the degradation of prostaglandin E2 (PGE_2) and hence suppresses tumor formation and inhibits inflammation induced by PGE_2 (39, 40). DEX treatment increased the expression of the FLT3 gene ($\log_2$ FC = 1.5, FDR = 1.4×10^{-3}). This gene encodes a receptor tyrosine kinase promoting Ras signaling, which plays a key role in survival, proliferation and differentiation of hematopoietic cells (41–43). Myocyte enhancer factor 2C (MEF2C) expression was upregulated ($\log_2$ FC = 1.0×10^{-6}, FDR = 3.8×10^{-8}). MEF2C, a member of the MADS family of transcription factors, regulates hematopoietic self-renewal and differentiation, supports the proliferation of leukemias, and is associated with increased risk of relapse in leukemia patients as its phosphorylation leads to chemotherapy resistance (44). The NFKB inhibitor zeta (NFKBIZ) gene that encodes for IkappaB-zeta, a transcriptional regulator for NF-kappaB, was upregulated ($\log_2$ FC = 1.5, FDR = 1.0×10^{-5}) with DEX treatment. It has been shown to induce pro-inflammatory responses and lymphoproliferative disorders and in solid tumors (45). The MDM2 proto-oncogene ($\log_2$ FC = 1.5, FDR = 1.0×10^{-6}) encodes a nuclear-localized E3 ubiquitin ligase, promoting tumor formation by targeting tumor suppressor proteins, such as p53, for proteasomal degradation. The upregulated expression of the FLT3, MEF2C, NFKBIZ, and MDM2 genes in sarcoid AMs suggests the potential side effect of DEX and it may lead to increased risk of tumor cell proliferation. DEX treatment modulated expression of several genes related to focal adhesion and cytoskeleton, including integrin families. Cyclin D2 (CCND2) functions as regulators of CDK kinases important for cell cycle G1/S transition was downregulated ($\log_2$ FC = −1.7, FDR = 1.3×10^{-4}) (46).

Regulation of Actin Cytoskeleton

One of the major pathways affected by DEX treatment was regulation of the actin cytoskeleton. Actins are highly conserved proteins that are involved in cell motility, structure, integrity, and intercellular signaling (47). Plakophilin 2 (PKP2) encoding a plakophilin protein, was significantly upregulated ($\log_2 \log_2$ FC = 4.6, FDR = 7.9×10^{-19}). Plakophilin 2 participates in linking cadherins to intermediate filaments in the cytoskeleton and cardiac muscles. It has been shown to be associated with several types of cancers in humans (48). PKP2 regulates calcium signaling in cardiac muscles (49). The slingshot homolog 2 (SSH2) gene was upregulated ($\log_2$ FC = 1.2, FDR = 1.0×10^{-6}). SSH2 encodes a protein tyrosine phosphatase, which regulates actin filaments by dephosphorylating and activating cofilin which promotes actin filament depolymerization (50). The actin regulatory protein, cofilin/actin depolymerization factor (ADF), serves a vital function in cells by severing filaments, thereby increasing the number of filament ends from which polymerization and depolymerization can occur (47). The cofilin pathway is important for actin dynamics, cell movement, cytoskeleton, distribution of receptors and synapse formation and migration of immune cells. It is critical for phagocytosis, motility, and antigen presentation in macrophages, dendritic cells, and neuronal cells (51). Similarly, we found that DEX treatment downregulated the expression of several integrin membrane protein genes. Few of these genes are: Integrin subunit beta and alpha, ITGB7 and ITGA7 ($\log_2$ FC = −1.2, FDR = 4.6×10^{-5}), ITGAM, ITGA6, ITGB2. These genes code for integrins/adhesion receptors involved in leucocyte migration.

Effect of Dexamethasone on Genes Related to Inflammation

The TSC22 domain family member 3 gene (TSC22D3) was found to be highly upregulated in sarcoid AMs after DEX treatment (**Table 2**). TSC22D3 gene encodes GC-induced leucine zipper transcription factor, whose expression is rapidly induced by GC, IL-10 and TGF-β (52, 53). This protein has been shown to play a key role in immunosuppressive effects of GCs. DEX upregulated the expression of genes involved in the negative regulation of inflammation, including Dual specificity phosphatase (DUSP)1, also known as MKP1, which is a phosphatase involved in the dephosphorylation of MAPKs (15), and suppressor of cytokine signaling (SOCS4 and SOCS6). DEX downregulated the expression of various genes that play a key role in inflammation. Gene expression for interleukin 6 receptor complex (IL6R), TNF-receptor superfamily (TNFRSF4) and MyD88, essential signaling molecules in TLR and IL-1 signaling were decreased in response to dexamethasone treatment.

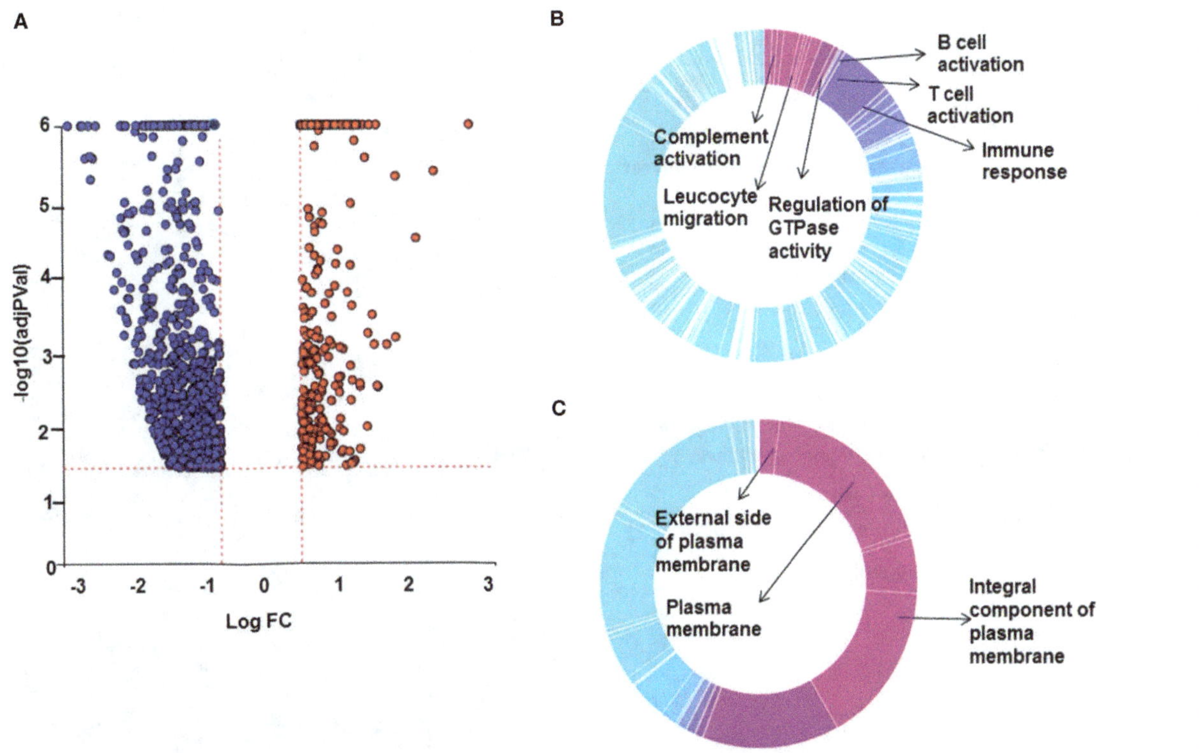

FIGURE 3 | Differential gene expression and Gene Ontology (GO) processes between sarcoid DEX-treated and untreated sarcoid monocytes. **(A)** Volcano plot: All 1,958 significant DE genes analyzed by DEseq2 analysis tool are represented in terms of their measured expression fold change ($\log_2$FC) on x-axis and the significance of the change ($-\log_{10}$ adj *p*-value) on y-axis. The dotted lines represent the thresholds used to select the DE genes: $\log_2$ FC > 0.6 and significance FDR<5%. The up-regulated genes (positive $\log_2$FC) are shown in red, while the down-regulated (negative $\log_2$FC) genes are shown in blue. **(B,C)** Gene Ontology (GO) analysis of DE genes was done using ipathwayGuide analysis tool. To assess the enrichment of GO terms Elim pruning method was used. GO analysis identified top **(B)** biological processes and **(C)** cellular components.

Effect of Dexamethasone on Transcriptional Signature of Sarcoidosis $CD14^+$ Monocytes

To decrease the effect of genetic variation, we used the same cohort of patients used for the AMs study. To identify genes responsive to GC on sarcoidosis monocytes, we isolated $CD14^+$ monocytes from PBMCs and treated in a similar fashion with DEX. In response to DEX treatment 1,958 genes were differentially expressed in monocytes (log_2-fold change of 0.6 and FDR < 5%) (**Figure 3A**). The Gene ontology (GO) enrichment analysis showed that the significant biological processes impacted after DEX treatment were classic complement activation, leukocyte, T and B cell activation as well as phagocytosis (**Figure 3B**) and significant cellular components impacted are shown in **Figure 3C**. Next, we performed pathway enrichment analyses. The top impacted pathways in monocytes were as following: cytokine-cytokine receptor interaction ($FDR = 6 \times 10^{-6}$), transcriptional misregulation in cancer ($FDR = 1 \times 10^{-4}$), Type I DM ($FDR = 2.6 \times 10^{-3}$), cell adhesion (FDR = 0.003), cytoskeleton ($FDR = 2.0 \times 10^{-3}$), RAS signaling ($FDR = 2.0 \times 10^{-3}$), and JAK-STAT pathway ($FDR = 2.0 \times 10^{-3}$) (**Figure 4A**). The top most impacted pathway in $CD14^+$ monocytes in response to DEX treatment was related to cytokine-cytokine receptor interaction. DEX treatment decreased expression of numerous cytokine and chemokine genes in sarcoidosis monocytes, while increasing the expression of CXCL10 and IL-10. In contrast, DEX treatment led to a significant decrease in expression of CCL22 (also known as macrophage-derived chemokine) and CCL24. CCL22 is produced by myeloid cells and regulates migration of leukocytes (54). Many genes related to tumor necrosis factor alpha superfamily members, *TNFRSF8, 9, 11, 14, and 15* were down regulated in response to DEX treatment. **Figure 4B** shows the heatmap of genes involved in cytokine pathways. Similarly, gene expression for several TNF receptor associated factors (TRAFs) that are important for the TLR and TNF signaling activation were decreased. In contrast,

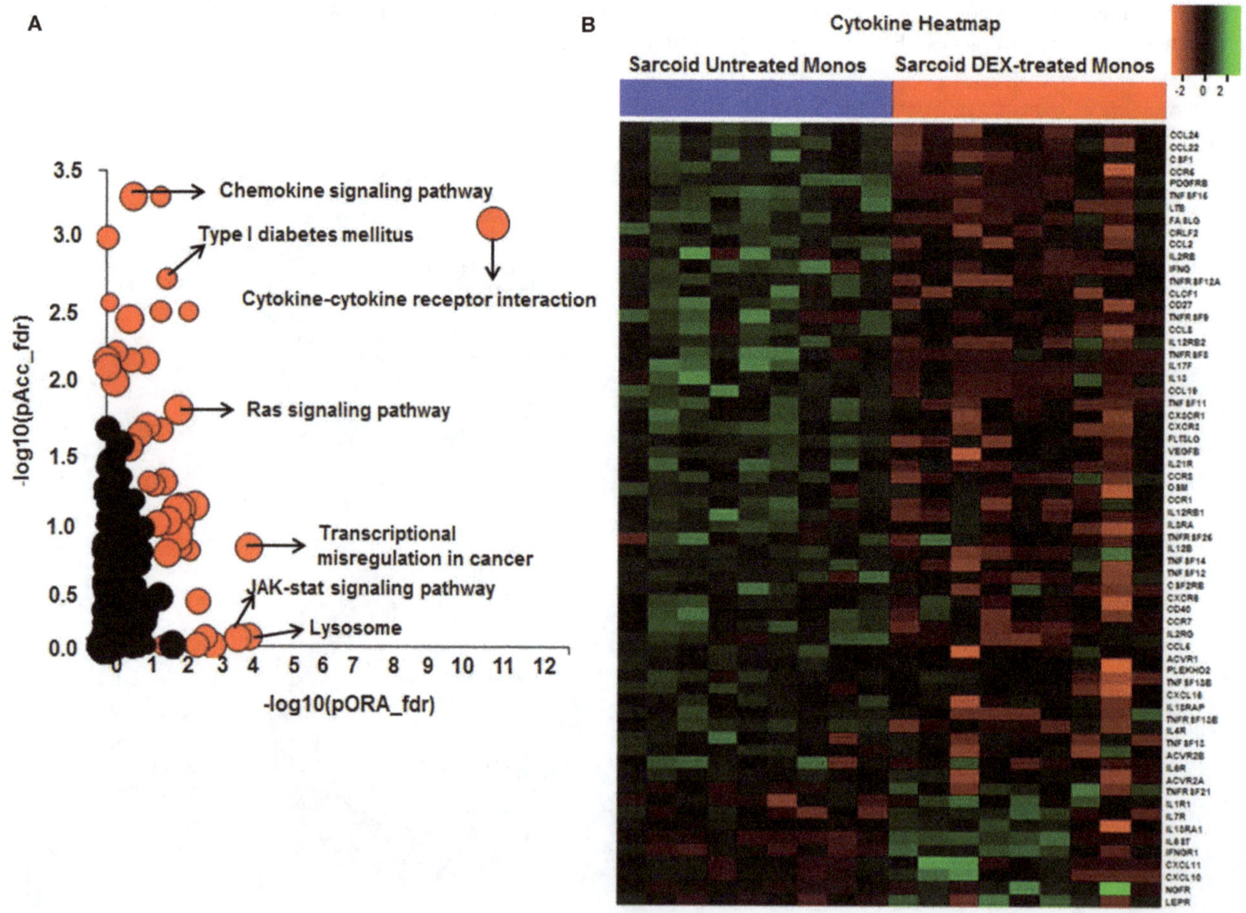

FIGURE 4 | Significant pathways enriched in DEX-treated compared to untreated sarcoid monocytes. **(A)** Pathway analysis was done on the DE genes ($log_2FC > 0.6$ and FDR < 5%) using iPathwayGuide analysis tool that uses two types of evidence: the over-representation on the horizontal axis (pORA) and the perturbation on the vertical axis (pAcc). Significant pathways (FDR < 5%) are shown in red, whereas non-significant are in black. The size of the circle is proportional to the number of genes in that pathway. **(B)** Heat map of DE genes involved in cytokine-cytokine receptor interaction pathway (log_2 FC > 0.6 with FDR < 5%). Green shade represents high expression and red shade represents low expression.

TABLE 3 | 10 top up and down-regulated genes in monocytes in response to dexamethasone treatment.

Gene symbol	Gene name	Type	Log fold change	FDR *p*-value
ABLIM3	Actin binding LIM protein family member 3	Cytoskeleton	3.1	5.89E-09
SERPINE1	Serpin family E member 1	Serine protease	2.4	1.0E-06
MT1G	Metallothionein 1G		2.5	4.37E-06
CD163L1	CD163 molecule like 1		1.9	1.0E-06
FPGT-TNNI3K	FPGT-TNNI3K	Cytoskeleton	2.7	1.0E-06
SLC6A13	Solute carrier family 6 member 13	Solute carrier protein	2.7	1.0E-06
FKBP5	FKBP prolyl isomerase 5	Immunophilin protein family	2.05	5.11E-06
RGS2	Regulator of G protein signaling 2	G protein signaling	2.4	2.82E-06
HSPE1P18	Heat Shock 10kDa Protein 1 Pseudogene 18	Heat shock protein	2.2	1.0E-06
TUBE1	Tubulin epsilon 1	Cytoskeleton	2.3	1.64E-06
RYR2	Ryanodine receptor 2	ER resident	2.7	3.59E-05
CCL24	C-C motif chemokine ligand 24	Cytokine	−3.0	3.70E-08
CCL22	C-C motif chemokine ligand 22	Cytokine	−3.7	3.70E-08
FPR3	Formyl peptide receptor 3	G-protein-coupled receptors	−3.4	3.25E-09
RAPGEF5	Rap guanine nucleotide exchange factor 5	Ras family member	−2.6	2.12E-04
HSD3B7	Hydroxy-delta-5-steroid dehydrogenase	Member of the short-chain dehydrogenase/reductase superfamily	−2.05	2.65E-06
FEZ1	Fasciculation and elongation protein zeta 1	Zygin family	−2.4	9.40E-07
ADAMTS14	ADAM metallopeptidase with thrombospondin type 1 motif 14	Metallopeptidase	−1.9	2.9E-03
KCNN4	Potassium calcium-activated channel subfamily N member 4	Voltage-independent potassium channel	−2.4	1.20E-06
ATP8B4	ATPase phospholipid transporting 8B4	Phospholipid transport	−1.7	1.43E-06
IL32	Interleukin 32	Cytokine	−1.8	1.43E-06

DEX treatment led to increased expression of negative regulators of TLR signaling, TNF alpha induced protein 3 (TNFAIP3-A20). Similar to AMs, the pathway related to transcription misregulation in cancer was significantly impacted in response to DEX treatment of sarcoidosis monocytes.

The top most upregulated gene in response to DEX treatment in sarcoidosis monocytes was actin binding LIM protein family member 3 (ABLIM3) ($\log_2$ FC $= 3.1$, FDR $= 1.0 \times 10^{-6}$) (**Table 3**). The encoded protein interacts with F actin filaments and is a component of adherents junctions in several cell types, including cardiac myocytes (55). Several genes related to retinoid X receptors (RXRs) and retinoic acid receptors (RARs) were downregulated in response to DEX treatment. These are important members of the steroid/thyroid hormone receptors acting predominantly as transcription factors (56).

Concordance Between DEX-Treated Sarcoidosis AMs and Monocytes

In response to DEX 2169 genes were exclusively differentially expressed in sarcoid AMs, while 1293 DE genes were found in sarcoid monocytes as shown in Venn diagram (**Figure 5A**). These results show that the impact of DEX treatment is more profound on sarcoid AMs as compared to monocytes. **Figure 6** shows 665 DE genes overlapping in DEX-treated sarcoidosis AMs and monocytes. We found that the effect of DEX on overlap DE genes was similar except for a few genes. DEX treatment upregulated the expression of activin A receptor type 2B (ACVR2B), MYC proto-oncogene, bHLH transcription factor (MYC), zinc finger and BTB domain containing 18 (ZBTB18) genes in AMs whereas it downregulated their expression in monocytes. ZBTB18 encodes a C2H2-type zinc finger protein and acts a transcriptional repressor of genes involved in neuronal development. Further, we performed the pathway enrichment analysis on the common DE genes in both cell types. The common pathways that were enriched in both DEX-treated AMs and monocytes were Rap1 signaling pathway, lysosomal pathway, PI3kinase signaling pathway, transcriptional misregulation in cancer, Type I diabetes mellitus (**Figure 5B**).

DISCUSSION

Macrophages have a central role in the maintenance of immunological homeostasis and host-defense. They play a crucial role in granuloma formation and provide metabolic cues for T cell responses in sarcoidosis. Alveolar macrophages, similar to other tissue associated macrophages have evolved to perform phagocytic clearance of pathogens and dying cells in the lungs immune-surveillance of the lung for inhaled pathogens as well as homeostatic regulation of lung tissues (11, 57). Circulating monocytes have the potential to differentiate into monocyte derived tissue macrophages and to migrate and interact with antigen-specific T and B lymphocytes to initiate adaptive immune responses.

Glucocorticoids modulate host immune responses to pathogens. In inflammatory diseases, including sarcoidosis, GCs have been used as an immunosuppressive drug to reduce inflammation (58). It has been shown that GCs suppress the expression of inflammatory genes, including TNF-α and

A

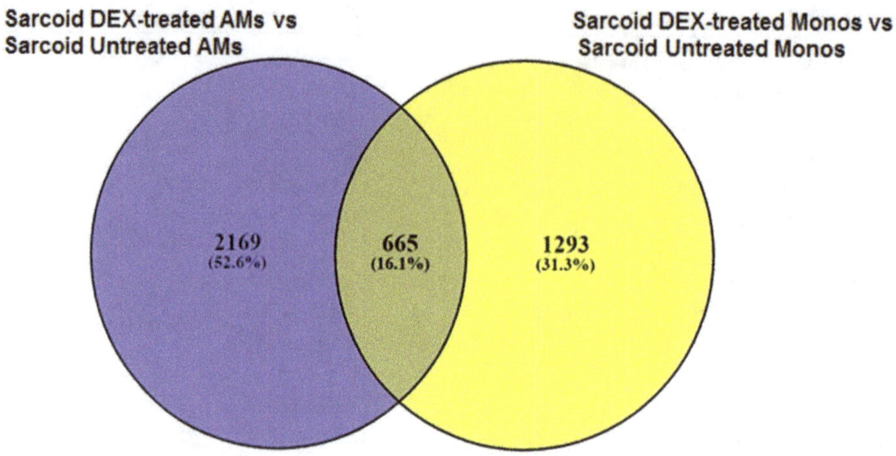

B

Type	Name	Number of hits	Expected score	Adjusted p-value
enriched	Rap1 signaling pathway	17	2.30197	1.21E-006
enriched	Lysosome	13	1.3056	2.28E-006
enriched	Jak-STAT signaling pathway	14	1.67208	2.92E-006
enriched	Insulin signaling pathway	13	1.50029	5.29E-006
enriched	PI3K-Akt signaling pathway	19	3.73354	7.69E-006
enriched	Cytokine-cytokine receptor interaction	16	2.89751	2.52E-005
enriched	Transcriptional misregulation in cancer	13	1.93549	3.76E-005
enriched	MAPK signaling pathway	15	2.72572	4.10E-005
enriched	Ras signaling pathway	14	2.37069	4.22E-005
enriched	Non-alcoholic fatty liver disease (NAFLD)	11	1.61482	1.72E-004
enriched	Regulation of actin cytoskeleton	12	2.24471	5.16E-004
enriched	Glycerophospholipid metabolism	8	0.97347	1.04E-003

FIGURE 5 | Metanalysis of DE genes between two groups: DEX-treated vs. untreated sarcoid AMs and DEX-treated vs. untreated sarcoid monocytes. **(A)** Venn diagram of DE genes showing 2,169 DE genes exclusively expressed in DEX-treated sarcoid AMs whereas 1293 DE genes were exclusively expressed in DEX-treated sarcoid monocytes. 665 DE genes overlap between the two groups **(B)** GeneTrail pathway analysis of common 665 DE genes between DEX treated sarcoid AMs and DEX treated sarcoid monocytes shows top 12 enriched significant pathways.

IFN-γ, and chemokines that are important for the granuloma formation and cell mediated Th1 responses. GCs are the only FDA approved drug to treat pulmonary and extrapulmonary sarcoidosis (59). However, despite their widespread use, there is a lack of evidence for their long term survival benefit in sarcoidosis or prevention of end organ damage such as lung fibrosis (58). In contrast, long term use of GCs has been shown to have significant side effects affecting all systems in the body (60). The most common side effects are excessive weight gain, insomnia, diabetes, osteoporosis, arterial hypertension and depression (60).

To determine the effect of GCs on transcriptome profiling of sarcoid AMs and $CD14^+$ monocytes, we compared the RNA-seq data of sarcoidosis AMs and $CD14^+$ cells treated with dexamethasone *in vitro* vs. untreated sarcoidosis AMs and $CD14^+$ monocytes, respectively. To decrease the confounding factors related to human genetic variation, we isolated the $CD14^+$ peripheral blood monocytes and AMs from the BALs of the same sarcoidosis subjects and compared pairwise RNA seq results. We identified two major pathways impacted after DEX treatment: metabolic and phagolysosomal pathways. Metabolic reprogramming in macrophages is critically important for their effector function (61, 62). **Figure 7** summarizes perturbation of genes related to metabolic pathways. We found that DEX treatment leads to suppression of gene expression related to glycolysis, fatty acid oxidation, TCA cycle and oxidative phosphorylation (**Figure 6**). In contrast, GCs enhance the expression of genes related to amino acid degradation pathways and generation of glutamine from glutamate (GLUL). Dexamethasone effected genes involved in metabolism of glucogenic amino acids (AAs) and ketogenic AAs, suggesting increased glucogenesis and fatty acid precursors (**Figure 6**). These alterations in response to dexamethasone explains some of the adverse effects seen in these patients after treatment with GCs, including loss of muscle mass, and lipodystrophy (63).

Other important dexamethasone effects were its effects on genes involved in lysosome and phagosome functions. Lysosomes are the common platform for endocytosis, phagocytosis, autophagy and biosynthetic routes. They receive both extracellular and intracellular-derived molecular cargo,

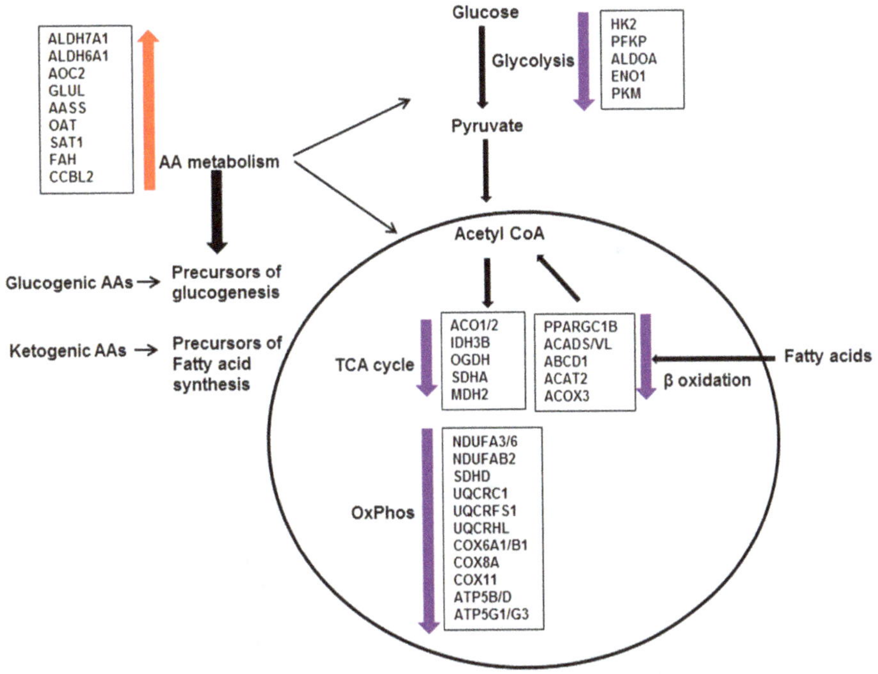

FIGURE 6 | Effect of DEX on metabolic pathways in sarcoid AMs. The pathway analysis of metabolic DE genes showed that the major pathways affected in DEX-treated sarcoid AMs as compared to untreated sarcoid AMS were: Glycolysis, Citric acid cycle (TCA), Oxidative phosphorylation (OxPhos), β-oxidation of fatty acids and Amino acid (AA) metabolism. DEX-treatment resulted in the downregulation of genes involved in glycolysis, TCA cycle, Oxphos and β-oxidation of fatty acids. Alteration in these pathways suggests that glucose metabolism is decreased; glucose is not being utilized completely to generate energy producing molecules ATP and NADH. Reduced β-oxidation of fatty acids suggests that fatty acids are not being transported and degraded optimally in mitochondria to generate energy. Suboptimal fatty acid oxidation may result in the accumulation of long chain fatty acids and metabolites. The upregulation of genes involved in AA metabolism shows that DEX-treated sarcoid AMs may switch to AA catabolism as a source of energy. AAs catabolism results in the conversion of AAs either to pyruvate or intermediates of TCA cycle for energy production or generation of precursors of glucogenesis and fatty acid synthesis.

damaged organelles, engulfed dead cells, and foreign particulates like bacteria for digestion. Tissue macrophages, including AMs, are sentinel cells that are equipped with a series of mechanisms of vesicular trafficking to orchestrate the elimination of bacteria as well as dead cells and debris (60). Clearance of bacteria by macrophages involves internalization of the microorganisms into phagosomes, which are then delivered to endo-lysosomes for enzymatic degradation. Lysosomes are a central organelle in the processing of exogenous and intracellular biomolecules. Thus, the final clearance of pathogens depend on lysosomal function (64). Lysosomes integrate and facilitate cross-talk between nutritional signals such as AA and energy levels, membrane damage and infection, and ultimately enable responses such as autophagy, cell growth, membrane repair and microbe clearance (65, 66). Lysosomes are hubs for cellular signaling and nutritional sensing through interplay with mTOR, AMPK, and GSK signaling (65). DEX-treated AMs show significantly decreased gene expression for the phagosome and lysosome machinery. For instance, transcription factor EB (TFEB), a master regulator of lysosomal biogenesis and fusion (65) was significantly downregulated in sarcoidosis AMs in response to DEX. **Figure 7** shows the downregulation of lysosome pathway genes encoding lysosomal acid hydrolases, membrane proteins, acidification and biogenesis proteins. Our results show that DEX-treatment led to the downregulation of two important genes, TFEB and PPARGC1 (PGC1) that play an important role in lysosomal and mitochondrial biogenesis and cellular metabolism. TFEB has been shown to control lipid catabolism and control the expression of PGC1α (34, 67). The DEX induced downregulation of TFEB, PGC1α, mitochondrial Acyl-CoA Dehydrogenase short chain fatty acid (ACADS) and very long-chain acyl-CoA dehydrogenase (VLCAD), as well as lysosomal genes in sarcoid AMs. This suggests that DEX-treatment decreases fatty acid oxidation and thus may lead to increased lipid deposition. Furthermore, DEX-treatment upregulated the expression of the CLTC1 gene (lysosomal pathway) that may contribute to accumulation of clathrin coated vesicles containing aggregated proteins. In contrast, the downregulation of lysosomal genes involved in proteolysis and acidification suggests that DEX-treatment inhibits the proteolytic degradation. This may result in lysosomal overload with protein aggregates and fatty acid deposits. Decreased lysosomal function may lead to an increase in unfolded protein accumulation and finally to unfolded protein response and ER stress (68). Because pathogens and antigens may play a role in the pathogenesis of sarcoidosis, the downregulation of lysosomes and phagosome by DEX may have negative implications for the disease progression.

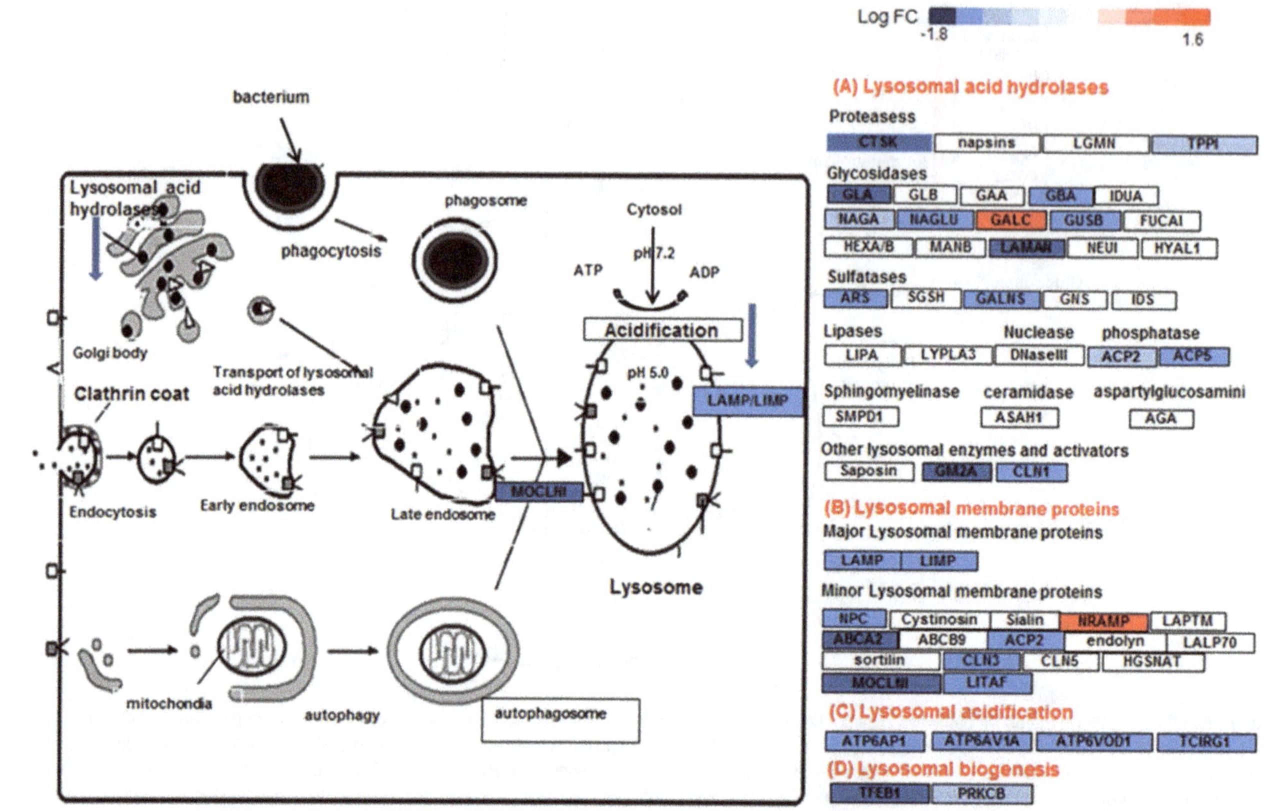

FIGURE 7 | Lysosome pathway in DEX-treated sarcoid AMs. Graphic illustration of pathway analysis of DE ($\log_2$ FC > 0.6 with FDR < 0.05) genes related to lysosome pathway in sarcoid-DEX treated AMs. The pathway diagram is overlaid with the computed perturbation of each gene. The perturbation accounts both for the gene's measured fold changes and for accumulated perturbation propagated from any upstream genes (accumulation). The color intensity corresponds to the level of upregulation (red) or downregulation (blue) of the DE genes in sarcoid-DEX treated AMs vs. sarcoid untreated AMs.

Similar to rheumatoid arthritis, some studies have shown an increased risk of developing cancer in sarcoidosis patients, while others could not confirm such association (69–73). While it is difficult to interpret uncontrolled and retrospective observational studies, the increased risk is partly attributed to uncontrolled inflammation. Our study showed that transcriptional misregulation in cancer was also one of the enriched pathways in response to DEX treatment. We found that DEX treatment upregulated the expression of numerous genes involved in cell proliferation, tumor formation and lymphoproliferative disorders. Interestingly, DEX treatment led to upregulation of this pathway in the monocytes of sarcoidosis subjects, suggesting that this effect is a global effect. These results demonstrate that long-term usage of DEX may lead to uncontrolled proliferation. For example: RAS superfamily gene are proto-oncogene that are involved in the development of various cancers (74, 75). It has been shown that DEX upregulates several members of this family (76). Our data is in line with previous RNA seq data of cultured human pulmonary type II A549 cells showing upregulation of transcriptional misregulation in cancer in response to corticosteroids (77).

In response to DEX treatment, we identified derangement of large numbers of genes regulating the cytoskeleton. Most genes belong to integrin family, but also genes involved in desmosomes such as PKP2 gene encoding a protein which links cadherins to intermediate filaments in the cytoskeleton. Aberrant regulation of these genes, including PKP2, ITGA6, and seven are important for cytoskeleton and cell-cell and cell-matrix interactions and are associated with cardiomyopathy, arrhythmogenic R ventricular cardiomyopathy and hypertrophic cardiomyopathy. Collectively, these data suggest that dexamethasone drives a broad gene expression program promoting matrix stiffening and supporting fibroblast proliferation and selective but coordinated suppression of genes encoding collagen-degrading enzymes.

On the other hand, our results show that DEX treatment altered the expression of genes involved in inflammation and immune responses. DEX treatment led to decreased expression of genes related to inflammation including IL6R, IL-17R, TNFRSF4, and MyD88. Along with this DEX treatment upregulated the expression of several genes that suppress inflammation, including Glucocorticoid-Induced Leucine Zipper Protein (GLIZ, also known as TSC22D3), dual specificity phosphatase 1 (DUSP1, also known as MKP-1), Suppressor of Cytokine Signaling (SOCS) 4 and 6. We have previously shown that DUSP1 expression is decreased in sarcoidosis AMs and monocytes and GCs induced

DUSP1 expression at the protein level (15). Current RNA seq data in an independent cohort of patients is in agreement with our previous results.

CONCLUDING REMARKS

For more than 60 years GCs have been used as anti-inflammatory drugs to treat a variety of inflammatory diseases such as rheumatoid arthritis and pulmonary diseases such as sarcoidosis. Given the fact that macrophages play a critical role in infectious and non-infectious granulomatous diseases (78, 79), it is of surprise that the effects of GCs on macrophages are less well-documented. Here we show that DEX treatment led to profound transcriptomic changes related to cellular metabolisms, lysosomes/phagosomes, and cytoskeleton in lung tissue macrophages. While similar effects were observed after DEX treatment on isolated $CD14^+$ monocytes of the same subjects, the effect on cytokine-cytokine receptor interaction was more prominent in monocytes, suggesting that the effect on lung tissue macrophages are more likely due to lysosomal function metabolic derangement. Further studies need to determine the effects of DEX on proteome profile in different cell types and correlation with RNA seq data.

AUTHOR CONTRIBUTIONS

JT conducted the experiments, analyzed the results, and she contributed in writing the manuscript. CB critically reviewed the manuscript. ES performed the statistical analysis of the RNA-seq data. FL and RP-R reviewed the data analysis and the manuscript. LS conceived and designed the study, participated in all areas of the research such as patients' selection and oversaw patient enrollment, data analysis, and writing of the manuscript.

REFERENCES

Iannuzzi MC, Rybicki BA, Teirstein AS. Sarcoidosis. *N Engl J Med.* (2007) 357:2153–65. doi: 10.1056/NEJMra071714

Kingah P, Alam M, Chugh K, Kamholz J, Samavati L. Role of pulmonary evaluation in diagnosis of neurosarcoidosis. *Sarcoidosis Vasc Diffuse Lung Dis.* (2016) 33:209–15.

Aberdein J, Cole J, Bewley M, Marriott H, Dockrell D. Alveolar macrophages in pulmonary host defence–the unrecognized role of apoptosis as a mechanism of intracellular bacterial killing. *Clin Expe Immunol.* (2013) 174:193–202. doi: 10.1111/cei.12170

Fazel SB, Howie SE, Krajewski AS, Lamb D. B lymphocyte accumulations in human pulmonary sarcoidosis. *Thorax.* (1992) 47:964–7. doi: 10.1136/thx.47.11.964

West SG. Current management of sarcoidosis I: pulmonary, cardiac, and neurologic manifestations. *Curr Opin Rheumatol.* (2018) 30:243–8. doi: 10.1097/BOR.0000000000000489

Ciriaco M, Ventrice P, Russo G, Scicchitano M, Mazzitello G, Scicchitano F, et al. Corticosteroid-related central nervous system side effects. *J Pharmacol Pharmacother.* (2013) 4(Suppl. 1):S94–8. doi: 10.4103/0976-500X.120975

Gottlieb JE, Israel HL, Steiner RM, Triolo J, Patrick H. Outcome in sarcoidosis: the relationship of relapse to corticosteroid therapy. *Chest.* (1997) 111:623- 631. doi: 10.1378/chest.111.3.623

Calverley PM, Anderson JA, Celli B, Ferguson GT, Jenkins C, Jones PW, et al. Salmeterol and fluticasone propionate and survival in chronic obstructive pulmonary disease. *N Engl J Med.* (2007) 356:775–89. doi: 10.1056/NEJMoa063070

Papiris SA, Kagouridis K, Kolilekas L, Papaioannou AI, Roussou A, Triantafillidou C, et al. Survival in idiopathic pulmonary fibrosis acute exacerbations: the non-steroid approach. *BMC Pulm Med.* (2015) 15:162. doi: 10.1186/s12890-015-0146-4

van de Garde MD, Martinez FO, Melgert BN, Hylkema MN, Jonkers RE, Hamann J. Chronic exposure to glucocorticoids shapes gene expression and modulates innate and adaptive activation pathways in macrophages with distinct changes in leukocyte attraction. *J Immunol.* (2014) 192:1196–208. doi: 10.4049/jimmunol.1302138

Epelman S, Lavine KJ, Randolph GJ. Origin and functions of tissue macrophages. *Immunity.* (2014) 41:21–35. doi: 10.1016/j.immuni.2014.06.013

Costabel U, Hunninghake GW. ATS/ERS/WASOG statement on sarcoidosis. Sarcoidosis statement committee. American thoracic society. European respiratory society. World association for sarcoidosis and other granulomatous disorders. *Eur Respir J.* (1999) 14:735–7. doi: 10.1034/j.1399-3003.1999. 14d02.x

Talreja J, Farshi P, Alazizi A, Luca F, Pique-Regi R, Samavati L. RNA- sequencing identifies novel pathways in sarcoidosis monocytes. *Sci Rep.* (2017) 7:2720. doi: 10.1038/s41598-017-02941-4

Talreja J, Talwar H, Ahmad N, Rastogi R, Samavati L. Dual inhibition of rip2 and IRAK1/4 regulates iL-1β and IL-6 in sarcoidosis alveolar macrophages and peripheral blood mononuclear cells. *J Immunol.* (2016) 197:1368–78. doi: 10.4049/jimmunol.1600258

Rastogi R, Du W, Ju D, Pirockinaite G, Liu Y, Nunez G, et al. Dysregulation of p38 and MKP-1 in response to NOD1/TLR4 stimulation in sarcoid bronchoalveolar cells. *Am J Respir Crit Care Med.* (2011) 183:500–10. doi: 10.1164/rccm.201005-0792OC

Dobin A, Davis CA, Schlesinger F, Drenkow J, Zaleski C, Jha S, et al. STAR: ultrafast universal RNA-seq aligner. *Bioinformatics.* (2013) 29:15–21. doi: 10.1093/bioinformatics/bts635

Anders S, Huber W. Differential expression analysis for sequence count data. *Genome Biol.* (2010) 11:R106. doi: 10.1186/gb-2010-11-10-r106

Benjamini Y, Drai D, Elmer G, Kafkafi N, Golani I. Controlling the false discovery rate in behavior genetics research. *Behav Brain Res.* (2001) 125:279– 284. doi: 10.1016/S0166-4328(01)00297-2

Haziot A, B Tsuberi Z, Goyert SM. Neutrophil CD14: biochemical properties and role in the secretion of tumor necrosis factor-alpha in response to lipopolysaccharide. *J Immunol.* (1993) 150:5556–65.

Muzikar KA, Nickols NG, Dervan PB. Repression of DNA-binding dependent glucocorticoid receptor-mediated gene expression. *Proc Natl Acad Sci USA.* (2009) 106:16598–603. doi: 10.1073/pnas.0909192106

García-González PA, Schinnerling K, Sepúlveda-Gutiérrez A, Maggi J, Mehdi AM, Nel HJ, et al. Dexamethasone and monophosphoryl lipid A induce a distinctive profile on monocyte-derived dendritic cells through transcriptional modulation of genes associated with essential processes of the immune response. *Front Immunol.* (2017) 8:1350. doi: 10.3389/fimmu.2017.01350

Zahuczky G, Kristóf E, Majai G, Fésüs L. Differentiation and glucocorticoid regulated apopto-phagocytic gene expression patterns in human macrophages. Role of mertk in enhanced phagocytosis. *PLoS ONE.* (2011) 6:e21349. doi: 10.1371/journal.pone.0021349

Kaskow BJ, Proffit JM, Blangero J, Moses EK, Abraham LJ. Diverse biological activities of the vascular non-inflammatory molecules–the vanin pantetheinases. *Biochem Biophys Res Commun.* (2012) 417:653–658. doi: 10.1016/j.bbrc.2011.11.099

Austin S, St-Pierre, J. PGC1α and mitochondrial metabolism–emerging concepts and relevance in ageing and neurodegenerative disorders. *J Cell Sci.* (2012) 125:4963–71. doi: 10.1242/jcs.113662

Ahmadian M, Suh JM, Hah N, Liddle C, Atkins AR, Downes M, et al. PPARγ signaling and metabolism: the good, the bad and the future. *Nat Med.* (2013) 19:557–66. doi: 10.1038/nm.3159

Kotake T, Hojo S, Tajima N, Matsuoka K, Koyama T, Tsumuraya Y. A bifunctional enzyme with L-fucokinase and GDP-L-fucose pyrophosphorylase activities salvages free L-fucose in arabidopsis. *J Biol Chem.* (2008) 283:8125– 8135. doi: 10.1074/jbc.M710078200

Kaitaniemi S, Elovaara H, Grön K, Kidron H, Liukkonen J, Salminen T, et al. The unique substrate specificity of human AOC2, a semicarbazide- sensitive amine oxidase. *Cell Mol Life Sci.* (2009) 66:2743–57. doi: 10.1007/s00018-009-0076-5

Palmieri EM, Spera I, Menga A, Infantino V, Iacobazzi V, Castegna Glutamine synthetase desensitizes differentiated adipocytes to proinflammatory stimuli by raising intracellular glutamine levels. *FEBS Lett.* (2014) 588:4807–14. doi: 10.1016/j.febslet.2014.11.015

Liu P-S, Wang H, Li X, Chao T, Teav T, Cheng C, et al. α-ketoglutarate orchestrates macrophage activation through metabolic and epigenetic reprogramming. *Nat Immunol.* (2017)18:985–94. doi: 10.1038/ni.3796

Hirokawa N, Niwa S, Tanaka Y. Molecular motors in neurons: transport mechanisms and roles in brain function, development, and disease. *Neuron.* (2010) 68:610–38. doi: 10.1016/j.neuron.2010.09.039

Camus SM, Camus MD, Sadacca LA, Esk C, Gould GW, Kioumourtzoglou D, et al. CHC22 clathrin mediates traffic from early secretory compartments for human GLUT4 pathway biogenesis. *J Cell Biol.* (2020) 219:e201812135. doi: 10.1083/jcb.201812135

Colletti GA, Miedel MT, Quinn J, Andharia N, Weisz OA, Kiselyov K. Loss of lysosomal ion channel transient receptor potential channel mucolipin-1 (TRPML1) leads to cathepsin B-dependent apoptosis. *J Biol Chem.* (2012) 287:8082–91. doi: 10.1074/jbc.M111.285536

LaPlante JM, Falardeau J, Sun M, Kanazirska M, Brown EM, Slaugenhaupt SA, et al. Identification and characterization of the single channel function of human mucolipin-1 implicated in mucolipidosis type IV. A disorder affecting the lysosomal pathway. *FEBS Lett.* (2002) 532:183–7. doi: 10.1016/S0014-5793(02)03670-0

Napolitano G, Ballabio A. TFEB at a glance. *J Cell Sci.* (2016) 129:2475–81. doi: 10.1242/jcs.146365

Roberts AJ. Emerging mechanisms of dynein transport in the cytoplasm versus the cilium. *Biochem Soc Trans.* (2018) 46:967–82. doi: 10.1042/BST20170568

Roberts AJ, Kon T, Knight PJ, Sutoh K, Burgess SA. Functions and mechanics of dynein motor proteins. *Nat Rev Mol Cell Biol.* (2013) 14:713–26. doi: 10.1038/nrm3667

Pu J, Guardia CM, Keren-Kaplan T, Bonifacino JS. Mechanisms and functions of lysosome positioning. *J Cell Sci.* (2016) 129:4329–39. doi: 10.1242/jcs.196287

Porter C, Parkar MH, Verhoeven AJ, Levinsky RJ, Collins M, Kinnon C. p22-phox-deficient chronic granulomatous disease: reconstitution by retrovirus-mediated expression and identification of a biosynthetic intermediate of gp91-phox. *Blood.* (1994) 84:2767–75. doi: 10.1182/blood.V84.8.2767.bloodjournal8482767

Backlund MG, Mann JR, Holla VR, Buchanan FG, H-Tai H, Musiek ES, et al. 15-Hydroxyprostaglandin dehydrogenase is down-regulated in colorectal cancer. *J Biol Chem.* (2005) 280:3217–23. doi: 10.1074/jbc.M411221200

Haworth O, Buckley CD. Resolving the problem of persistence in the switch from acute to chronic inflammation. *Proc Natl Acad Sci.* (2007) 104:20647–8. doi: 10.1073/pnas.0710633105

Grafone T, Palmisano M, Nicci C, Storti S. An overview on the role of FLT3-tyrosine kinase receptor in acute myeloid leukemia: biology and treatment. *Oncol Rev.* (2012) 6:e8. doi: 10.4081/oncol.2012.e8

Ampasavate C, Jutapakdee W, Phongpradist R, Tima S, Tantiworawit A, Charoenkwan P, et al. FLT3, a prognostic biomarker for acute myeloid leukemia (AML): quantitative monitoring with a simple anti-FLT3 interaction and flow cytometric method. *J Clin Lab Anal.* (2019) 33:e22859. doi: 10.1002/jcla.22859

Takahashi S. Downstream molecular pathways of FLT3 in the pathogenesis of acute myeloid leukemia: biology and therapeutic implications. *J Hematol Oncol.* (2011) 4:13. doi: 10.1186/1756-8722-4-13

Brown FC, Still E, Koche RP, Yim CY, Takao S, Cifani P, et al. MEF2C phosphorylation is required for chemotherapy resistance in acute myeloid leukemia. *Cancer Discov.* (2018) 8:478–497. doi: 10.1158/2159-8290.CD-17-1271

Willems M, Dubois N, Musumeci L, Bours V, Robe PA. IκBζ: an emerging player in cancer. *Oncotarget.* (2016) 7:66310–22. doi: 10.18632/oncotarget.11624

Koyama-Nasu R, Nasu-Nishimura Y, Todo T, Ino Y, Saito N, Aburatani H, et al. The critical role of cyclin D2 in cell cycle progression and tumorigenicity of glioblastoma stem cells. *Oncogene.* (2013) 32:3840–5. doi: 10.1038/onc.2012.399

Pfaendtner J, Enrique M, Voth GA. Actin filament remodeling by actin depolymerization factor/cofilin. *Proc Natl Acad Sci USA.* (2010) 107:7299– 304. doi: 10.1073/pnas.0911675107

Hao, XL, Tian Z, Han F, Chen JP, Gao LY, Liu Y. Plakophilin-2 accelerates cell proliferation and migration through activating EGFR signaling in lung adenocarcinoma. *Pathol Res Pract.* (2019) 215:152438. doi: 10.1016/j.prp.2019.152438

Cerrone M, Montnach J, Lin X, Zhao YT, Zhang M, Agullo-Pascual E, et al. Plakophilin-2 is required for transcription of genes that control calcium cycling and cardiac rhythm. *Nat Commun.* (2017) 8:106. doi: 10.1038/s41467-017-00127-0

Endo M, Ohashi K, Mizuno K. LIM kinase and slingshot are critical for neurite extension. *J Biol Chem.* (2007) 282:13692–702. doi: 10.1074/jbc.M610873200

Jönsson F, Gurniak CB, Fleischer B, Kirfel G, Witke W. Immunological responses and actin dynamics in macrophages are controlled by N- cofilin but are independent from ADF. *PLoS ONE.* (2012) 7:e36034. doi: 10.1371/journal.pone.0036034

Godot V, Garcia G, Capel F, Arock M, Durand-Gasselin I, Asselin- Labat M. et al. Dexamethasone and IL-10 stimulate glucocorticoid-induced leucine zipper synthesis by human mast cells. *Allergy.* (2006) 61:886–890. doi: 10.1111/j.1398-9995.2006.01065.x

Nakamura M, Kitaura J, Enomoto Y, Lu Y, Nishimura K, Isobe M, et al. Transforming growth factor-β-stimulated clone-22 is a negative-feedback regulator of Ras/Raf signaling: implications for tumorigenesis. *Cancer Sci.* (2012) 103:26–33. doi: 10.1111/j.1349-7006.2011.02108.x

Yashiro T, Nakano S, Nomura K, Uchida Y, Kasakura K, Nishiyama C. A transcription factor PU. 1 is critical for Ccl22 gene expression in dendritic cells and macrophages. *Sci Rep.* (2019) 9:1161. doi: 10.1038/s41598-018-37894-9

Abraham DM, Marchuk DA. Inhibition of the cardiomyocyte-specific troponin I–interacting kinase limits oxidative stress, injury, and adverse remodeling due to ischemic heart disease. *Circul Res.* (2014) 114:938–40. doi: 10.1161/CIRCRESAHA.113.303238

Dawson MI, Xia Z. The retinoid X receptors and their ligands. *Biochim Biophys Acta.* (2012) 1821:21–56. doi: 10.1016/j.bbalip.2011.09.014

Davies LC, Jenkins SJ, Allen JE, Taylor PR. Tissue-resident macrophages. *Nat Immunol.* (2013) 14:986–95. doi: 10.1038/ni.2705

Grutters J, Van den Bosch J. Corticosteroid treatment in sarcoidosis. *Eur Respir J.* (2006) 28:627–36. doi: 10.1183/09031936.06.00105805

Judson MA. The treatment of pulmonary sarcoidosis. *Respir Med.* (2012) 106:1351–61. doi: 10.1016/j.rmed.2012.01.013

Warrington TP, Bostwick JM. Psychiatric adverse effects of corticosteroids. In: *Mayo Clinic Proceedings.* Elsevier Inc. (2006) 1361–7. doi: 10.4065/81.10.1361

Diskin C, Pålsson-McDermott EM. Metabolic modulation in macrophage effector function. *Front Immunol.* (2018) 9:270. doi: 10.3389/fimmu.2018.00270

Kelly B, O'neill LA. Metabolic reprogramming in macrophages and dendritic cells in innate immunity. *Cell Res.* (2015) 25:771–84. doi: 10.1038/cr.2015.68

Fardet L, Cabane J, Kettaneh A, Lebbe C, Flahault A. Corticosteroid- induced lipodystrophy is associated with features of the metabolic syndrome. *Rheumatology.* (2007) 46:1102–6. doi: 10.1093/rheumatology/kem062

Wong, CO, Gregory S, Hu H, Chao Y, Sepúlveda VE, et al. Lysosomal degradation is required for sustained phagocytosis of bacteria by macrophages. *Cell Host Microbe.* (2017) 21:719–30.e716. doi: 10.1016/j.chom.2017.05.002

Settembre C, Fraldi A, Medina DL, Ballabio A. Signals from the lysosome: a control centre for cellular clearance and energy metabolism. *Nat Rev Mol Cell Biol.* (2013) 14:283–96. doi: 10.1038/nrm3565

Lim CY, Zoncu R. The lysosome as a command-and-control center for cellular metabolism. *J Cell Biol.* (2016) 214:653–664. doi: 10.1083/jcb.201607005

Lin J, Handschin C, Spiegelman BM. Metabolic control through the PGC-1 family of transcription coactivators. *Cell Metab.* (2005) 1:361–70. doi: 10.1016/j.cmet.2005.05.004

Ballabio A, Gieselmann V. Lysosomal disorders: from storage to cellular damage. *Biochim Biophys Acta.* (2009) 1793:684–96. doi: 10.1016/j.bbamcr.2008.12.001

Askling J, Grunewald J, Eklund A, Hillerdal G, Ekbom A. Increased risk for cancer following sarcoidosis. *Am J Respir Crit Care Med.* (1999) 160:1668–72. doi: 10.1164/ajrccm.160.5.9904045

Søgaard KK, Sværke C, Thomsen RW, Nørgaard M. Sarcoidosis and subsequent cancer risk: a danish nationwide cohort study. *Eur Respir J.* (2015) 45:269–72. doi: 10.1183/09031936.00084414

Bologna C, Picot MC, Jorgensen C, Viu P, Verdier R, Sany J. Study of eight cases of cancer in 426 rheumatoid arthritis patients treated with methotrexate. *Ann Rheum Dis.* (1997) 56:97–102. doi: 10.1136/ard.56.2.97

Bonifazi M, Bravi F, Gasparini S, La Vecchia C, Gabrielli A, Wells AU, et al. Sarcoidosis and cancer risk: systematic review and meta-analysis of observational studies. *Chest.* (2015) 147:778–91. doi: 10.1378/chest.14-1475

Romer F, Hommelgaard P, Schou G. Sarcoidosis and cancer revisited: a long- term follow-up study of 555 danish sarcoidosis patients. *Eur Respir J.* (1998) 12:906–12. doi: 10.1183/09031936.98.12040906

Fernández-Medarde A, Santos E. Ras in cancer and developmental diseases. *Genes Cancer.* (2011) 2:344–58. doi: 10.1177/1947601911411084

Simanshu DK, Nissley DV, McCormick F. RAS proteins and their regulators in human disease. *Cell.* (2017) 170:17–33. doi: 10.1016/j.cell.2017.06.009

Kemppainen RJ, Behrend EN. Dexamethasone rapidly induces a novel ras superfamily member-related gene in AtT-20 cells. *J Biol Chem.* (1998) 273:3129–31. doi: 10.1074/jbc.273.6.3129

Mostafa MM, Rider CF, Shah S, Traves SL, Gordon PM, Miller-Larsson A, et al. Glucocorticoid-driven transcriptomes in human airway epithelial cells: commonalities, differences and functional insight from cell lines and primary cells. *BMC Med Genomics.* (2019) 12:29. doi: 10.1186/s12920-018-0467-2

Flynn J, Chan J, Lin P. Macrophages and control of granulomatous inflammation in tuberculosis. *Mucosal Immunol.* (2011) 4:271–8. doi: 10.1038/mi.2011.14

Minton K. Macrophages: granuloma macrophage differentiation. *Nat Rev Immunol.* (2016) 16:718–19. doi: 10.1038/nri.2016.132

17

Efficacy and Safety of Combination Treatment with Apatinib and Osimertinib after Osimertinib Resistance in Epidermal Growth Factor Receptor-Mutant Non-Small Cell Lung Carcinoma

*Xue Yang[1†], Yang Xia[2†], Liyan Xu[3], Li Liang[4], Minglei Zhuo[1], Meina Wu[1], Tongtong An[1], Ziping Wang[1], Yuyan Wang[1], Jianjie Li[1], Jia Zhong[1], Hanxiao Chen[1], Bo Jia[1], Jingjing Wang[1] and Jun Zhao[1]**

[1] Key Laboratory of Carcinogenesis and Translational Research (Ministry of Education), Department of Thoracic Medical Oncology, Peking University Cancer Hospital and Institute, Beijing, China, [2] Key Laboratory of Respiratory Disease of Zhejiang Province, Department of Respiratory and Critical Care Medicine, Second Affiliated Hospital of Zhejiang University School of Medicine, Hangzhou, Zhejiang, China, [3] Department of Medical Oncology, Beijing Chest Hospital, Capital Medical University, Beijing, China, [4] Department of Tumor Chemotherapy and Radiation Sickness, Peking University Third Hospital, Beijing, China

Correspondence:
Jun Zhao
ohjerry@163.com

† These authors have contributed equally to this work

Currently, there are limited treatment options for patients who developed resistance to osimertinib, a third-generation epidermal growth factor receptor (EGFR) inhibitor. Resistance to EGFR inhibitors is frequently associated with enhanced vascular endothelial growth factor (VEGF) levels. This multicenter, retrospective study aimed to evaluate the efficacy of the combination treatment with apatinib and osimertinib in 39 patients with EGFR-mutant non-small cell lung carcinoma (NSCLC) who developed osimertinib resistance. The patients received the combination of oral apatinib 250 mg qd and osimertinib 80 mg qd. The efficacy was evaluated after the first month then every 2 months thereafter. The primary endpoint was progression-free survival (PFS). The overall response rate (ORR) and the disease control rate (DCR) of the combination of apatinib and osimertinib was 12.8% (5/39) and 79.5% (31/39), respectively. The median PFS was 4 months [95% confidence interval (CI): 3.5–4.5 months]. Fourteen patients were administered with at least 6 months of combination therapy, and 11 of them remained on treatment programs. The 6-month PFS rate was 38%. Nine patients underwent biopsies after failing osimertinib treatment, and five of six patients with TP53 mutations had PFS of less than 3 months. The spectrum of resistance to osimertinib mechanisms included c-mesenchymal-epithelial transition factor (c-Met) amplification, phosphatidylinositol-4,5-bisphosphate 3-kinase catalytic subunit alpha (PIK3CA) gain-of-function mutation, phosphatase and tensin homolog (PTEN) loss-of-function mutation, Erb-B2 receptor tyrosine kinase 2 (ERBB2) amplification, and insulin-like growth factor 1 receptor (IGF1R) mutation. The most common adverse events were hypertension (30.7%, 12/39), diarrhea (15.4%, 6/39), and proteinuria (12.8%, 5/39). The combination of apatinib and osimertinib improved the ORR and the DCR of patients with osimertinib-refractory EGFR-positive NSCLC, thus making it a reasonable treatment choice after the development of osimertinib resistance.

Keywords: osimertinib, apatinib, EGFR, NSCLC, resistance

INTRODUCTION

Osimertinib, a third-generation epidermal growth factor receptor-tyrosine kinase inhibitor (EGFR-TKI), can selectively block mutations that are sensitive to EGFR-TKI. It is resistant to EGFR T790M mutation. In patients with non-small cell lung carcinoma (NSCLC) who had EGFR T790M mutations that are resistant to both first- and second-generation EGFR-TKIs, it can help achieve a median progression-free survival (PFS) of approximately 10 months (Mok et al., 2017). However, some patients are becoming resistant to osimertinib, which presents additional challenges. Currently, there are limited treatment options for patients who developed osimertinib resistance (Planchard et al., 2015; Ou et al., 2016; Zhou et al., 2019).

Resistance to EGFR inhibitors is frequently associated with enhanced vascular endothelial growth factor (VEGF) levels. Dual inhibition of the VEGF receptor (VEGFR) and EGFR signaling pathways shows the potential to overcome osimertinib resistance (Naumov et al., 2009; Larsen et al., 2011). Apatinib is an oral tyrosine kinase inhibitor that targets VEGFR-2 (Mi et al., 2010). We previously reported good efficacy and prolonged PFS benefit of using the combination of apatinib and a first-generation EGFR-TKI in cases of EGFR mutation-positive NSCLC (Li et al., 2017) progression. However, there are no data about the efficacy of the combination of a VEGFR inhibitor and osimertinib after third-generation EGFR-TKI failure. Thus, this study aimed to evaluate the efficacy of the combination of apatinib and osimertinib in patients with EGFR-mutant NSCLC who developed osimertinib resistance.

MATERIALS AND METHODS

Study Population

In this analysis, 39 patients were enrolled from four participating institutions, namely, Peking University Cancer Hospital (n = 24), Second Affiliated Hospital of Zhejiang University School of Medicine (n = 9), Beijing Chest Hospital (n = 4), and Peking University Third Hospital (n = 2), between March 1, 2018 and November 1, 2019 (**Figure 1**). Every patient who displayed resistance to osimertinib during treatment for advanced lung adenocarcinoma was identified from the databases of the four institutions. All the patients received the combination of osimertinib and apatinib after progression of osimertinib resistance. None of the enrolled patients received other types of antiangiogenic therapy except for apatinib prior to or during combination therapy. This multicenter, retrospective study was approved by the ethics committee of the four participating institutions. All the patients provided informed consent for treatment in this protocol.

Treatment Regimens

The patients received osimertinib at a dose of 80 mg and apatinib at a dose of 250 mg, taken orally once daily. The treatment would be discontinued in the event of disease progression, unacceptable toxicity, or if the physician or patient opted to end the treatment.

Efficacy and Safety Assessments

Tumor response was radiographically evaluated according to RECIST guidelines version 1.1. Efficacy evaluation was conducted after the first month, then every two months thereafter. The primary endpoint was PFS, which is defined as the time from the first administration of the combination of osimertinib and apatinib to the first documentation of progression of disease according to RECIST guidelines version 1.1. The ORR was calculated as the sum of CR and PR rates, whereas the DCR was calculated as the sum of SD, CR, and PR rates. Toxicities during osimertinib and apatinib combination treatment were assessed

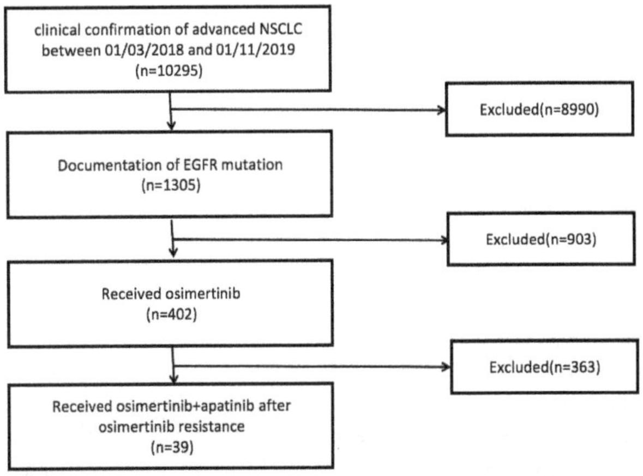

FIGURE 1 | Study cohort selection. EGFR, epidermal growth factor receptor; NSCLC, non-small cell lung carcinoma.

Abbreviations: CR, complete response; CI, confidence interval; DCR, disease control rate; EGFR, epidermal growth factor receptor; EGFR-TKI, epidermal growth factor receptor-tyrosine kinase inhibitor; NGS, next-generation sequencing; NSCLC, non-small cell lung carcinoma; ORR, overall response rate; PR, partial response; PFS, progression-free survival; RECIST, response evaluation criteria in solid tumors; SD, stable disease; VEGF, vascular endothelial growth factor; VEGFR, vascular endothelial growth factor receptor.

according to the Common Terminology Criteria for Adverse Events (CTCAE) 4.0 classification.

Capture-Based Targeted Next-Generation Sequencing

A subgroup of the patients (n = 9) enrolled in the study was subjected to several biopsies (liquid or tumor) once osimertinib resistance progressed and prior to the administration of apatinib. We obtained a biopsy of the tumor of a patient from a lesion, after which we performed targeted next-generation sequencing (NGS) according to previously described methods (Lin et al., 2018; Zhuo et al., 2020). Eight patients underwent liquid biopsy using targeted NGS as previously described (Zhuo et al., 2020). The collected samples of liquid biopsy included peripheral blood (n = 6), pleural effusion (n = 1), and cerebrospinal fluid (n = 1).

TABLE 1 | Baseline clinical features of patients enrolled in the study (n = 39).

Characteristic	Value
Sex	
Male	18 (46%)
Female	21 (54%)
Age (years)	
Median	54
<65	31 (79%)
≥65	8 (21%)
Smoking history	
Yes	9 (24%)
No	30 (76%)
ECOG performance status	
≤1	31 (79%)
2	8 (21%)
Stage	
Iva	14 (36%)
IVb	25 (64%)
Metastasis site	
Brain	18 (46%)
Bone	17 (44%)
Liver	12 (31%)
EGFR mutation status	
EGFR exon 19 del	16 (41%)
EGFR exon 21 L858R	17 (44%)
EGFR exon 18 G719X	6 (15%)
Osimertinib treatment	
First line	4 (10%)
Second line	25 (64%)
Beyond second line	10 (26%)
Previous treatment	
Radiotherapy	5 (13%)
Chemotherapy	10 (26%)
Osimertinib disease progression model	
Intrathoracic progression	24 (62%)
Extrathoracic progression	15 (38%)

ECOG, Eastern Cooperative Oncology Group; EGFR, epidermal growth factor receptor.

Statistical Analysis

The Kaplan–Meier method was used to estimate the median PFS, while we produced 95% CIs with a log–log transformation. Safety analyses were done through descriptive methods as well as percentages. SPSS version 22.0 (IBM, Armonk, NY, United States) was used to calculate and produce the results of all statistical analyses performed in this study. $P < 0.05$ was considered statistically significant.

RESULTS

Patient Characteristics

Of the 39 patients, 18 were male and 21 were female. Thirty patients were never smokers, while nine of them were current or former smokers. Every patient was a carrier of EGFR mutations; and according to their TKI-naïve samples, there were 16 exon 19 deletion, 17 exon 21 L858R mutation, and 6

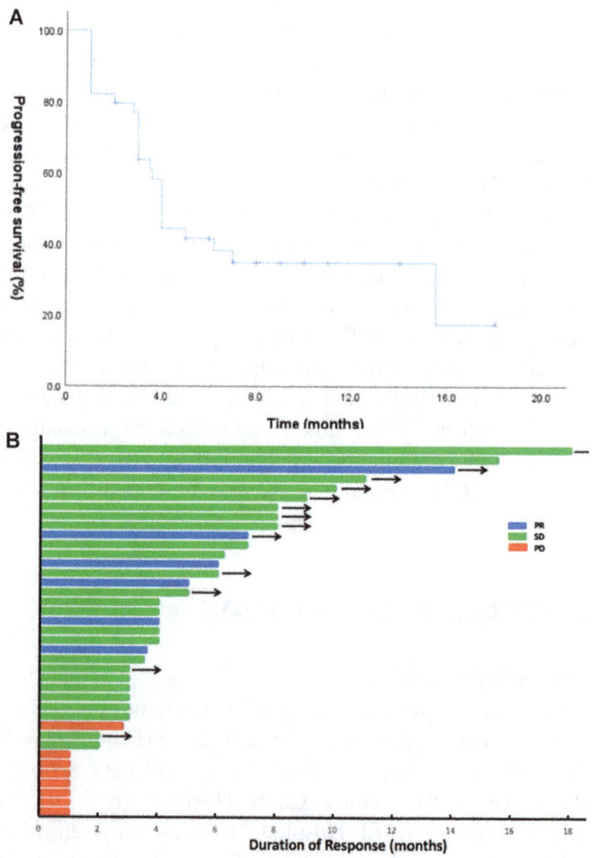

FIGURE 2 | Apatinib and osimertinib activity in osimertinib-resistant EGFR-mutant NSCLC. **(A)** Progression-free survival (PFS) in the 39 patients treated with the combination of apatinib and osimertinib. **(B)** Swimmer plots showing the duration of combination treatment for each patient in the study cohort. Patients who developed a progressive disease are denoted in red, stable disease in green, and partial response in blue. Arrows indicate patients continuing on the combination of apatinib and osimertinib at the time of last follow-up.

exon 18 G719X mutation cases. In total, 4, 25, and 10 patients received osimertinib as first-, second-, and later-line treatment, respectively. The median PFS for osimertinib was 8 months (95% CI: 7.1–8.9). NGS data from 9 patients who developed osimertinib resistance were available for analysis. The clinical characteristics of the patients are listed in **Table 1**.

Molecular Characteristics of Post-osimertinib/Pre-combination Treatment Specimens

Rebiopsy for NGS was performed in nine patients during osimertinib treatment and prior to the combination treatment. We found that of all somatic variations in nine patients, mutations related to EGFR sensitivity were the most common. TP53 mutation was found in seven of nine patients (77.8%), whereas T790M mutation was identified in four of nine patients (44.4%). The spectrum of resistance to osimertinib mechanisms included c-Met amplification (n = 1), PIK3CA gain-of-function mutation (n = 1), PTEN loss-of-function mutation (n = 1), ERBB2 amplification (n = 1), and IGF1R mutation (n = 1).

Outcomes of Combination of Apatinib and Osimertinib Treatment

Until the last follow-up on April 1, 2020, the disease progressed in 25 patients (64.1%), and the remaining 14 patients (35.9%) were still being treated with combination therapy (**Figure 2**). The median follow-up time was 9.8 months (range: 4.8–24.8 months). The ORR and the DCR for the combination of apatinib and osimertinib were 12.8% (5/39) and 79.5% (31/39), respectively. Median PFS was 4 months (95% CI: 3.5–4.5). Fourteen patients had received at least a 6-month combination therapy, and 11 of them were still on treatment. The 6-month PFS rate was 38%. The data are based on treatment length and patient response to the profiling of mutations after the development of osimertinib resistance and are shown in **Figure 3**. Among the 6 patients whose PFS less than 3 months, 5 had pathogenic mutations of TP53 and 3 had maintained T790M (**Table 2**). Examples of three cases with different resistance mechanisms demonstrated various therapeutic effects (**Figure 4**).

The most frequently observed adverse events were hypertension (30.7%, 12/39), diarrhea (15.4%, 6/39), and proteinuria (12.8%, 5/39). Other less common adverse events

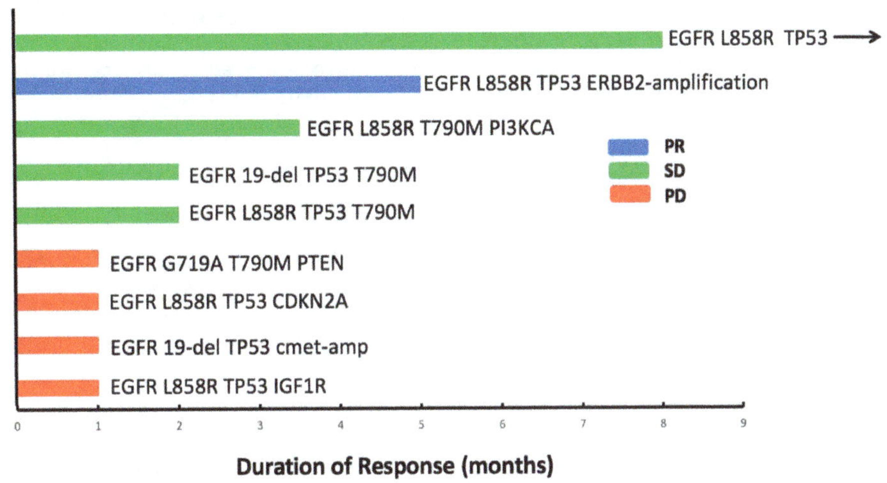

FIGURE 3 | Individual duration of combined treatment in patients with post-osimertinib/pre-combined biopsies. Patients who developed a progressive disease are denoted in red, stable disease in green, and partial response in blue. Arrows indicate patients continuing on the combination of apatinib and osimertinib at the time of last follow-up.

TABLE 2 | Basic characteristics of nine patients with NGS testing.

Patient No.	Gender	Age	Smoking history	ECOG	Stage	EGFR mutation	PFS of Osimertinib (months)	Osimertinib PD model
1	M	61	No	1	IVa	L858R	8	Extrathoracic
2	M	62	No	2	IVb	19-del	8	Extrathoracic
3	F	55	No	1	IVa	L858R	12	Intrathoracic
4	F	44	No	1	IVb	G719A	6	Intrathoracic
5	F	54	No	1	IVa	L858R	2	Intrathoracic
6	F	66	No	2	IVa	19-del	11	Intrathoracic
7	M	35	No	1	IVb	L858R	6	Intrathoracic
8	M	62	No	1	IVb	L858R	12	Extrathoracic
9	F	53	No	1	IVb	L858R	8	Intrathoracic

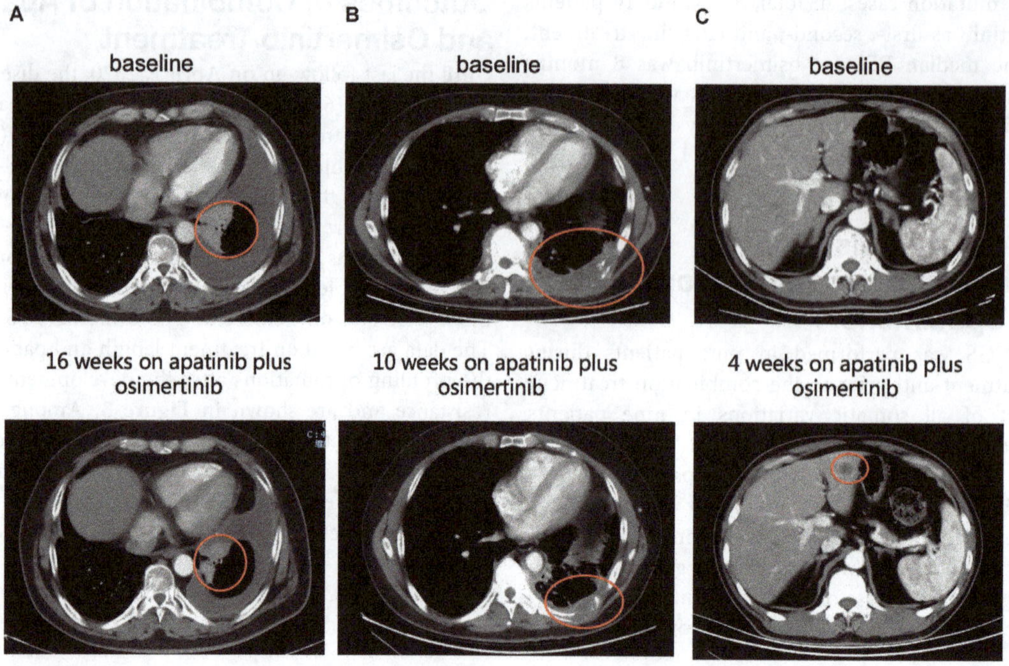

FIGURE 4 | Examples of tumor response to the combination of apatinib and osimertinib in EGFR-positive cases with osimertinib resistance. **(A)** Partial response of a left lung mass to combination therapy in a patient with TP53 mutation detected post-osimertinib/pre-combined treatment biopsy. This patient remained on treatment at the time of last follow-up. **(B)** Partial response of a left chest wall mass to combination therapy in a patient with TP53 mutation and ERBB2-amplification detected post-osimertinib/pre-combined treatment biopsy. **(C)** Progressive disease demonstrated with new hepatic metastases after 1 month of combination treatment in a patient with TP53 and PTEN loss-of-function mutations detected in the post-osimertinib/pre-combined treatment biopsy.

TABLE 3 | Treatment-related adverse events in all patients (*n* = 39).

	Any grade*	Grades 1–2*	Grade 3*
Adverse event	35 (90%)	31 (79%)	4 (11%)
Hypertension	12 (31%)	10 (26%)	2 (5%)
Diarrhea	6 (15%)	6 (15%)	–
Proteinuria	5 (13%)	5 (13%)	–
Rash	3 (8%)	2 (5%)	1 (3%)
Hand–foot syndrome	3 (8%)	3 (8%)	–
Hoarseness	2 (5%)	2 (5%)	–
Thrombocytopenia	2 (5%)	2 (5%)	–
Liver dysfunction	1 (3%)	1 (3%)	–
Decreased left ventricular ejection fraction	1 (3%)	–	1 (3%)

**Grading per the Common Terminology Criteria for Adverse Events, version 4.0.*

included rash (*n* = 3), hand–foot syndrome (*n* = 3), hoarseness (*n* = 2), thrombocytopenia (*n* = 2), and liver dysfunction (*n* = 1). Notably, a patient achieved partial response; however, the combination therapy was terminated because of tachycardia and markedly decreased left ventricular ejection fraction (**Table 3**).

DISCUSSION

Significant research has been conducted on osimertinib resistance, and treatment strategies after osimertinib treatment failure have been evaluated (Le et al., 2018; Leonetti et al., 2019; Zhao et al., 2020). However, there are limited data on the use of apatinib after the development of osimertinib resistance. Given the broad range of resistance mechanisms currently emerging with osimertinib, the potential role of combination therapy in certain osimertinib-refractory settings warrants further investigation. This multicenter retrospective analysis demonstrated that treating patients with the combination of osimertinib and apatinib resulted in a 13% ORR and a median PFS of 4 months, together with a safety profile (Lin et al., 2018). In the scope of our knowledge, this is the first large-scale study to assess the clinical nature of administering combination therapy with osimertinib and apatinib under osimertinib-refractory conditions.

Resistance to osimertinib is related to genomic alterations that are both dependent and independent of EGFR and includes an acquired tertiary mutation related to EGFR resistance (EGFR C797S mutation), MET amplification, aberrations in downstream signaling pathways (mutations in the RAS and RAF genes), and epithelial–mesenchymal transition (Ricordel et al., 2018). For patients with EGFR C797S found alongside T790M, the PFS for the combination treatment of erlotinib and osimertinib was almost 3 months (Wang et al., 2017). Treatment using a combination of cetuximab and brigatinib showed promising results for patients with EGFR-T790M-*cis*-C797S mutations; however, in this study, only few patients were assessed.

To date, For MET-driven acquired resistance, the longest PFS for combination treatment with c-Met inhibitor and osimertinib has been almost 5 months (Sequist et al., 2020). Aside from these types of targeted therapy, the addition of antiangiogenic inhibitors to EGFR-TKI therapy after progression of EGFR-TKI therapy is also an attractive strategy. Preclinical and clinical evidence suggests that EGFR-TKIs may work synergistically with VEGF inhibitors (Naumov et al., 2009; Larsen et al., 2011). We previously showed that apatinib, together with gefitinib, displayed significant antitumor properties in patients with NSCLC because of EGFR-TKI resistance related to T790M, under both *in vitro* and *in vivo* conditions (Li et al., 2017). Moreover, a previous retrospective analysis of patients with advanced NSCLC who failed icotinib treatment showed that the combination of apatinib and icotinib reached a median PFS of 5.33 months (95% CI: 3.63–7.03 months) (Xu et al., 2017). Additionally, patients with EGFR-mutant NSCLC who were first treated with a combination therapy using apatinib and gefitinib demonstrated prolonged PFS inclinations, indicating that the therapy was a reasonable treatment (Zhang et al., 2019). Collectively, these findings support that treatments using the combination of apatinib and a first-generation EGFR-TKI is well tolerated and has good efficacy.

This study produced results similar to those of Liu et al., who assessed three patients afflicted with T790M-positive lung adenocarcinoma. After progression of osimertinib resistance, their patients responded to sustained therapy combining osimertinib and apatinib within a PFS range of 5–7 months (Liu et al., 2019). This suggests that the particular mechanism related to resistance could alter patient response to the apatinib and osimertinib treatment in osimertinib-refractory tumors. EGFR-mutant NSCLC could be affected by changes in TP53, which would result in reduced genomic stability. Previous studies have shown that concomitantTP53 mutations were correlated with lower survival rates in patients with EGFR alterations (Blakely et al., 2017). In our study, we also found that pathogenic TP53 mutation was the most common mutation after the development of osimertinib resistance. In addition to TP53 mutation, maintained T790M mutation was also associated with heterogeneous mechanisms of resistance (PI3KCA mutation and PTEN loss). This finding indicated that subclones with T790M mutants can be found alongside subclones with specific mechanisms related to resistance (Zhao et al., 2020). In this case, targeting T790M alone is unlikely to result in clinical benefit. Among the three of four patients who barely benefited from the combination therapy, with PFS of less than 1 month, T790M loss was related to the progression of other mechanisms related to resistance, such as c-Met amplification and IGF1R and CDKN2A mutations. Our findings underscore the value of conducting multiple biopsies (Lin et al., 2018) in patients who develop progression during osimertinib treatment. In addition, it is essential to explore novel biomarkers predictive of treatment response to the combination of osimertinib and apatinib in patients with osimertinib resistance.

This retrospective study had several limitations and lacked a control group. Moreover, while a multicenter analysis was performed to identify patient eligibility, selection bias was still a potential problem. Thus, further multicenter prospective research is required to validate the experiment results.

In summary, the combination of apatinib and osimertinib in osimertinib-refractory EGFR-positive NSCLC improved the ORR and the DCR. The results promote combination treatment therapy in patients with osimertinib resistance, especially in ones with a non-targetable resistance mechanism. Further studies are warranted to determine biomarkers predictive of treatment response to anti-VEGF therapy for patients with osimertinib-resistant EGFR-mutant NSCLC.

AUTHOR CONTRIBUTIONS

XY and JZa: conception and design. XY, YX, LX, LL, MZ, MW, TA, ZW, YW, and JL: acquisition of data (provided acquired and managed patients, provided facilities, etc.). XY, JZo, HC, BJ, and JW: analysis and interpretation of data (e.g., statistical analysis, biostatistics). XY, YX, LX, LL, and JZa: writing, review, and/or revision of the manuscript. All authors contributed to the article and approved the submitted version.

ACKNOWLEDGMENTS

The authors would like to thank Liting Guo for editing the manuscript. The number of patients and results have been expanded since the data first appeared as conference manuscripts on WCLC 2019.

REFERENCES

Blakely, C. M., Watkins, T. B. K., Wu, W., Gini, B., Chabon, J. J., McCoach, C. E., et al. (2017). Evolution and clinical impact of co-occurring genetic alterations in advanced-stage EGFR-mutant lung cancers. *Nat. Genet.* 49, 1693–1704. doi: 10.1038/ng.3990

Larsen, A. K., Ouaret, D., El Ouadrani, K., and Petitprez, A. (2011). Targeting EGFR and VEGF(R) pathway cross-talk in tumor survival and angiogenesis. *Pharmacol. Ther.* 131, 80–90. doi: 10.1016/j.pharmthera.2011.03.012

Le, X., Puri, S., Negrao, M. V., Nilsson, M. B., Robichaux, J., Boyle, T., et al. (2018). Landscape of EGFR-dependent and -independent resistance mechanisms to osimertinib and continuation therapy beyond progression in EGFR-mutant NSCLC. *Clin. Cancer Res.* 24, 6195–6203. doi: 10.1158/1078-0432.ccr-18-1542

Leonetti, A., Sharma, S., Minari, R., Perego, P., Giovannetti, E., and Tiseo, M. (2019). Resistance mechanisms to osimertinib in EGFR-mutated non-small cell lung cancer. *Br. J. Cancer.* 121, 725–737. doi: 10.1038/s41416-019-0573-8

Li, F., Zhu, T., Cao, B., Wang, J., and Liang, L. (2017). Apatinib enhances antitumour activity of EGFR-TKIs in non-small cell lung cancer with EGFR-TKI resistance. *Eur. J. Cancer.* 84, 184–192. doi: 10.1016/j.ejca.2017.07.037

Lin, J. J., Zhu, V. W., Schoenfeld, A. J., Yeap, B. Y., Saxena, A., Ferris, L. A., et al. (2018). Brigatinib in Patients With Alectinib-Refractory ALK-Positive NSCLC. *J. Thorac. Oncol.* 13, 1530–1538. doi: 10.1016/j.jtho.2018.06.005

Liu, Y., Xiong, Z.-C., Sun, X., Sun, L., Zhang, S.-L., Ma, J.-T., et al. (2019). Impact of apatinib in combination with osimertinib on EGFR T790M-positive lung adenocarcinoma. *Trans Cancer Res.* 8, 2151–2163. doi: 10.21037/tcr.2019.09.35

Mi, Y. J., Liang, Y. J., Huang, H. B., Zhao, H. Y., Wu, C. P., Wang, F., et al. (2010). Apatinib (YN968D1) reverses multidrug resistance by inhibiting the efflux function of multiple ATP-binding cassette transporters. *Cancer Res.* 70, 7981–7991. doi: 10.1158/0008-5472.can-10-0111

Mok, T. S., Wu, Y. L., Ahn, M. J., Garassino, M. C., Kim, H. R., Ramalingam, S. S., et al. (2017). Osimertinib or platinum-pemetrexed in EGFR T790M-positive lung cancer. *N. Engl. J. Med.* 376, 629–640. doi: 10.1056/NEJMoa1612674

Naumov, G. N., Nilsson, M. B., Cascone, T., Briggs, A., Straume, O., Akslen, L. A., et al. (2009). Combined vascular endothelial growth factor receptor and epidermal growth factor receptor (EGFR) blockade inhibits tumor growth in xenograft models of EGFR inhibitor resistance. *Clin. Cancer Res.* 15, 3484–3494. doi: 10.1158/1078-0432.ccr-08-2904

Ou, S. I., Agarwal, N., and Ali, S. M. (2016). High MET amplification level as a resistance mechanism to osimertinib (AZD9291) in a patient that symptomatically responded to crizotinib treatment post-osimertinib progression. *Lung Cancer.* 98, 59–61. doi: 10.1016/j.lungcan.2016.05.015

Planchard, D., Loriot, Y., Andre, F., Gobert, A., Auger, N., Lacroix, L., et al. (2015). EGFR-independent mechanisms of acquired resistance to AZD9291 in EGFR T790M-positive NSCLC patients. *Ann. Oncol.* 26, 2073–2078. doi: 10.1093/annonc/mdv319

Ricordel, C., Friboulet, L., Facchinetti, F., and Soria, J. C. (2018). Molecular mechanisms of acquired resistance to third-generation EGFR-TKIs in EGFR T790M-mutant lung cancer. *Ann. Oncol.* 29, i28–i37. doi: 10.1093/annonc/mdx705

Sequist, L. V., Han, J. Y., Ahn, M. J., Cho, B. C., Yu, H., Kim, S. W., et al. (2020). Osimertinib plus savolitinib in patients with EGFR mutation-positive, MET-amplified, non-small-cell lung cancer after progression on EGFR tyrosine kinase inhibitors: interim results from a multicentre, open-label, phase 1b study. *Lancet Oncol.* 21, 373–386. doi: 10.1016/s1470-2045(19)30785-5

Wang, Z., Yang, J. J., Huang, J., Ye, J. Y., Zhang, X. C., Tu, H. Y., et al. (2017). Lung adenocarcinoma harboring EGFR T790M and in trans C797S responds to combination therapy of first- and third-generation EGFR TKIs and shifts allelic configuration at resistance. *J. Thorac. Oncol.* 12, 1723–1727. doi: 10.1016/j.jtho.2017.06.017

Xu, J., Liu, X., Yang, S., Zhang, X., and Shi, Y. (2017). Apatinib plus icotinib in treating advanced non-small cell lung cancer after icotinib treatment failure: a retrospective study. *Onco. Targets Ther.* 10, 4989–4995. doi: 10.2147/ott.s142686

Zhang, Z., Luo, F., Zhang, Y., Ma, Y., Hong, S., Yang, Y., et al. (2019). The ACTIVE study protocol: apatinib or placebo plus gefitinib as first-line treatment for patients with EGFR-mutant advanced non-small cell lung cancer (CTONG1706). *Cancer Commun.* 39:69. doi: 10.1186/s40880-019-0414-4

Zhao, J., Lin, G., Zhuo, M., Fan, Z., Miao, L., Chen, L., et al. (2020). Next-generation sequencing based mutation profiling reveals heterogeneity of clinical response and resistance to osimertinib. *Lung Cancer* 141, 114–118. doi: 10.1016/j.lungcan.2019.10.021

Zhou, Z., Zhao, Y., Shen, S., Gu, L., Niu, X., Xu, Y., et al. (2019). Durable clinical response of lung adenocarcinoma harboring EGFR 19Del/T790M/in trans-C797S to combination therapy of first- and third-generation EGFR tyrosine kinase inhibitors. *J. Thorac. Oncol.* 14, e157–e159. doi: 10.1016/j.jtho.2019.04.020

Zhuo, M., Guan, Y., Yang, X., Hong, L., Wang, Y., Li, Z., et al. (2020). The prognostic and therapeutic role of genomic subtyping by sequencing tumor or cell-free DNA in pulmonary large-cell neuroendocrine carcinoma. *Clin. Cancer Res.* 26, 892–901. doi: 10.1158/1078-0432.CCR-19-0556

18

T-Bet Expression in Peripheral Th17.0 Cells is Associated with Pulmonary Function Changes in Sarcoidosis

Nicholas K. Arger[1], Siddharth Machiraju[1], Isabel E. Allen[2], Prescott G. Woodruff[1] and Laura L. Koth[1]*

[1] Division of Pulmonary and Critical Care, University of California, San Francisco, San Francisco, CA, United States,
[2] Department of Epidemiology and Biostatistics, University of California, San Francisco, San Francisco, CA, United States

***Correspondence:**
Nicholas K. Arger
nicholas.arger@ucsf.edu

Background: Interferon-gamma (IFN-γ) is a key mediator of sarcoidosis-related granulomatous inflammation. Previous findings of IFN-γ-producing Th17 cells in bronchoalveolar lavage fluid from sarcoidosis patients invokes the transition of Th17.0 cells to Th17.1 cells in the disease's pathogenesis. Since the T-bet transcription factor is crucial for this transition, the goal of this study was to determine if T-bet expression in Th17.0 cells reflects the extent of granulomatous inflammation in sarcoidosis patients as assessed by clinical outcomes.

Methods: Using a case-control study design, we identified two groups of sarcoidosis subjects (total $N = 43$) with pulmonary function tests (PFTs) that either (1) changed (increased or decreased) longitudinally or (2) were stable. We used flow cytometry to measure the transcription factors T-bet and RORγt in Th1, Th17.0, and Th17.1 cell subsets defined by CCR6, CCR4 and CXCR3 in blood samples. We compared the percentages of T-bet$^+$ cells in RORγt$^+$Th17.0 cells (defined as CCR6$^+$CCR4$^+$CXCR3$^-$) based on subjects' PFT group. We also assessed the relationship between the direction of change in PFTs with the changes in %T-bet$^+$ frequencies using mixed effects modeling.

Results: We found that T-bet expression in subjects' RORγt$^+$Th17.0 cells varied based on clinical outcome. The T-bet$^+$ percentage of RORγt$^+$Th17.0 cells was higher in the cases (subject group with PFT changes) as compared to controls (stable group) (27 vs. 16%, $p = 0.0040$). In comparisons before and after subjects' PFT changes, the T-bet$^+$ frequency of RORγt$^+$Th17.0 cells increased or decreased in the opposite direction of the PFT change. The percentage of these T-bet$^+$ cells was also higher in those with greater numbers of involved organs. Serum levels of interferon-γ-induced chemokines, CXCL9, CXCL10, and CXCL11, and whole blood gene expression of IFN-γ-related genes including *GBP1*, *TAP1*, and *JAK2* were independently positively associated with the T-bet$^+$ frequencies of RORγt$^+$Th17.0 cells.

Conclusions: These data suggest that expression of T-bet in Th17.0 cells could reflect the extent of granulomatous inflammation in sarcoidosis patients because they represent a transition state leading to the Th17.1 cell phenotype. These findings indicate that Th17 plasticity may be part of the disease paradigm.

Keywords: sarcoidosis, Th17, Th17.1, Th1, T-bet, RORγt, interferon-gamma, chemokine

INTRODUCTION

Sarcoidosis is a systemic disease in which granulomatous inflammation affects the lungs in the vast majority of patients (1). Its etiology remains unknown and no cure currently exists. Multiple studies have established the importance of IFN-γ-producing CD4$^+$ T helper (Th) cells in sarcoidosis, which have been traditionally designated as "Th1" cells (2–6). In recent years, additional Th cell populations have been recognized in sarcoidosis, including IL-17-producing "Th17" cells (7–10). We previously identified two different CD4$^+$ Th17 subsets in sarcoidosis patients using the expression of chemokine receptors CCR6, CCR4, and CXCR3 (11). In blood, we observed Th17.0 (CCR6$^+$CCR4$^+$CXCR3$^-$) cells with increased frequencies in sarcoidosis compared to health. The majority of these cells produced IL-17 after *ex vivo* stimulation. In contrast, in bronchoalveolar lavage (BAL), we observed "Th17.1" (CCR6$^+$CCR4$^-$CXCR3$^+$) cells, with increased frequencies in sarcoidosis compared to health (11, 12). We found that the majority of Th17.1 cells produced IFN-γ while only a small fraction produced IL-17 upon *ex vivo* stimulation (11). The increased proportion of Th17.0 cells in the circulation accompanied by an increased proportion of Th17.1 cells in the BAL led us to consider whether these findings might be the result of Th17 plasticity, whereby circulating Th17.0 effector cells polarize into Th17.1 cells and accumulate in the lung tissue where the granulomatous inflammation is located.

Prior studies have elucidated how Th17.0 cells can polarize or transition into Th17.1 cells. The initial polarization of Th17.0 effector cells from naïve T cells occurs under the control of the orphan nuclear hormone receptor RORγt (13–17). During this polarization, the chemokine receptors CCR6 and CCR4 are upregulated (18–20). In this context, the transcription factor RORγt is used to define Th17.0 cells (15–17). The mechanism by which Th17.0 cells "polarize" into Th17.1 cells has been elucidated through *in vitro* stimulation with IL-12 and IFN-γ. This stimulation causes upregulation of the transcription factor T-bet (21–24). T-bet is the main transcription factor that controls polarization of naïve T cells to Thl cells (25–29). Once T-bet is activated, several downstream genes are upregulated including those for CXCR3 and IFN-γ (26–28). Based on this collective T cell biology, we speculate that T-bet upregulation in Th17.0 cells in sarcoidosis patients may be initiated by exposure to IL-12 and IFN-γ in lymph nodes or tissues containing granulomatous inflammation (such as the lung). This Th17 plasticity allows them to express both RORγt and T-bet transcription factors and as well as pathogenic cytokines (IFN-γ) and the complement of chemokine receptors including CXCR3 that permit homing from blood to sites of inflammation such as the lung (30). In our study, we hypothesized that the expression of T-bet in circulating Th17.0 cells prior to upregulation of CXCR3 may serve as an indirect measure of the extent of interferon-driven inflammation to which the Th17.0 cells are exposed. To test this, we used flow cytometry to compare the T-bet-expressing frequencies in peripheral blood Th17.0 (RORγt$^+$CCR6$^+$CCR4$^+$CXCR3$^-$) cells between sarcoidosis subjects with different clinical trajectories defined by longitudinal changes in lung function and immunosuppression use.

Abbreviations: ANOVA, analysis of variance; BSA, bovine serum albumin; CI, confidence interval; CS&T, cytometer setup and tracking; DLCO, diffusing capacity of the lungs for carbon monoxide; DMARD, disease modifying antirheumatic drug; DMSO, dimethyl sulfoxide; EDTA, ethylenediaminetetraacetic acid; FBS, fetal bovine serum; FMO, fluorescence minus one; FEV1, forced expiratory volume in 1 s; FVC, forced vital capacity; FEV1/FVC, forced expiratory volume in 1 S to Forced vital capacity ratio; FSC, forward scatter; IFN-γ, interferon-gamma; IFN factor, interferon factor; MFI, median fluorescence intensity; NonTreg, Non-T regulatory; PBMC, peripheral blood mononuclear cell; %pred, percent predicted; RPMI, roswell park memorial institute; SD, standard deviation; SSC, side scatter; Th, T helper; TLC, total lung capacity; TNF-α, tumor necrosis factor alpha.

MATERIALS AND METHODS

Clinical Cohort

We enrolled subjects who met diagnostic criteria for sarcoidosis per guidelines endorsed by the American Thoracic Society (31) as previously described (32). The study design for this cohort did not require individuals to be newly diagnosed to participate. Follow-up visits were performed every 6–12 months for up to 66 months (~5 years). At each visit, we performed blood sampling and collected clinical data. These data included: demographics (age, sex, and self-identified race), chest radiography at initial visit, organ involvement at the initial visit (as assessed by physician review of medical records) (32); and pulmonary function tests (PFTs), which included forced expiratory volume in 1 second (FEV1) percent predicted (%pred), forced vital capacity (FVC %pred), diffusing capacity for carbon monoxide (DLCO %pred), and total lung capacity (TLC %pred). We obtained immunosuppression use history, including dosages of oral corticosteroids or disease-modifying antirheumatic drugs (DMARDs), specifically, methotrexate, azathioprine, mycophenolate, colchicine, hydroxychloroquine, or anti-TNF-α therapy that subjects were actively taking at the time of their study visits. For the current analysis, we also included serum protein (chemokine levels for CXCL9, CXCL10, and CXCL11) and whole blood RNA transcript levels of IFN-γ-related genes that were measured in the same blood samples as previously described (33–35).

Selection of Study Subjects

We used a case-control study design with criteria based on (1) lung function changes and (2) immunosuppressive treatment history to compare cell populations between sarcoidosis subjects with different clinical trajectories. Cases were defined by having a change in absolute FVC or DLCO of 10% or 15% (33, 36, 37), respectively, between any two visits separated by 6 months or greater. Cases could have been on or off treatment at the time of the blood draw (**Figure S1**). For all the cases, we identified the two visits between which the PFT change occurred. We then analyzed blood samples from the first of these two visits (before their lung function change occurred). In a subset of cases, we also analyzed blood samples from the second of these two visits (at the visit in which the change in lung function was measured). This subset of subjects with two measurements included subjects not on immunosuppression with a PFT decline (to avoid the effect of immunosuppression on T cell function) and all subjects with a

PFT increase, some of whom were on immunosuppression (since the sample size was small for this group). We used a change in lung function as a surrogate of on-going granulomatous inflammation or "disease activity" for two main reasons: (1) there is a lack of reliable and accurate non-invasive tests for active granulomatous inflammation and (2) we did not have longitudinal radiographic imaging at each follow up visit, which also can be used to infer disease activity. For controls, we used criteria of (1) no change in FVC and DLCO measurements for at least 24 months following the enrollment blood draw used in this analysis and (2) no use of immunosuppression prior to or during the study period. Of note, we did not include FEV1 in our criteria for PFT changes due to the fact that other processes such airways disease independent of sarcoidosis could affect this value over time; plethysmography was not performed at every visit, therefore TLC was also not used as a criterion.

Flow Cytometry

We employed a 12-parameter flow cytometry panel using an LSRII cytometer (BD Biosciences, San Jose, CA) in the UCSF Flow Cytometry Core (www.flow.ucsf.edu). Samples were blinded and randomized to 8 different batches with cases and controls distributed to each batch. Cases with longitudinal samples were analyzed in the same batch. At time of sample collection, we isolated peripheral blood mononuclear cells (PBMCs) using Leucosep™ tubes then froze them in FBS with 10% DMSO for storage in our liquid nitrogen biorepository. For each batch, samples were thawed in RPMI media, counted, and stained on ice in the dark. Details for antibody staining reagents are listed in **Table S1**. We stained with a Fixed Viability Dye (eBioscience) at 1:500 dilution in PBS per manufacturer's instructions. For surface staining, we incubated cells in flow cytometry buffer (PBS with 2% BSA and 2 mM EDTA) along with 50% Brilliant Stain Buffer (BD Horizon) per manufacturer's instructions. Surface antibodies included CD3 APC-R700, CD4 BUV395, CD25 BV786, CCR6 BV421, CCR4 PE-CF594 (BD Horizon); CD127 BV650, CD45RA APC-Cy7 (BioLegend); and CD45RO PerCP-eFluor710, CXCR3 PE-Cy7 (eBioscience). For intracellular staining, we used T-bet PE and RORγt Alexa Fluor 488 (BD Pharmingen) antibodies along with the Transcription Factor Buffer Set (BD Pharmingen) for both fixation and permeabilization. To set gating parameters for each fluorophore, we used fluorescence minus one (FMO) controls (38–41). We analyzed the same internal reference standard of PBMC for all batches to assess for staining variation with each batch acquisition. To standardize voltages across batches, we used Cytometer Setup and Tracking (CS&T) beads (BD Pharmingen) to measure median fluorescence intensities (MFI) and then matched voltages to these MFI values for each batch (42, 43). We used Ultracomp™ beads (Invitrogen) as compensation controls with each batch. We collected at least 2×10^5 events for each sample.

Gating Strategy

We used FlowJo™ software v10.0.07 (Becton, Dickinson and Company: Ashland, OR) to analyze the flow cytometry data. Compensation was performed using Ultracomp™ beads. We

TABLE 1 | Definitions of Th subsets based on surface chemokine receptor expression.

	CCR6	CXCR3	CCR4
Th17.0	+	−	+
Th17.1	+	+	−
Th1	−	+	−

employed our previous gating strategy to identify Th populations (11). Gating steps were as follows: (**1**) singlets using forward scatter (FSC—height vs. area), (**2**) live cells (negative for the fixed viability dye), (**3**) lymphocytes based on FSC and side scatter (SSC), (**4**) $CD3^+$ cells, (**5**) $CD4^+$ cells, (**6**) Non-T regulatory (NonTreg) cells defined as $CD25^-$ and either $CD127^{Lo}$ or $CD127^{Hi}$, (**7**) T-effectors ($CD45RA^-$ and $CD45RO^+$), and (**8**) the Th17.0, Th17.1, and Th1 subsets were gated based on staining for CCR6, CCR4, and CXCR3 (**Table 1**). We first determined the RORγt and T-bet distributions among the three Th subsets. Because RORγt is the transcription factor that defines the Th17 lineage (13–17), our primary analyses were based on Th17.0 cells that expressed RORγt and we present data for the proportion of these cells that stained positive for T-bet based on FMO control samples.

Data Analysis

Data were analyzed in Stata/SE 15.1 software (StataCorp LLC: College Station, TX) and figures were constructed in GraphPad Prism 6 software (GraphPad Software, Inc.: La Jolla, CA). To compare demographics data, we used *t*-tests for two group comparisons of means from parametric data, analysis of variance analysis (ANOVA) for comparisons of means between three or more groups, and chi-squared testing to compare proportions between groups. We created several linear regression models where the T-bet$^+$ frequency (%) of RORγt$^+$Th17.0 cells was the dependent variable. In these models, we examined case status as a binary predictor with or without adjustment for confounders. In separate models, we compared those with PFT declines and PFT increases along with controls as distinct groups using a categorical predictor with or without adjustment for confounders. Where indicated, we adjusted our regression models for several confounders including age, sex, race, binary designations for immunosuppression use (yes/no), and prior smoking history (yes/no). In a subset of cases with PFT declines (these cases were not on immunosuppression) and PFT increases (these cases were either on or off immunosuppression), we used mixed effects linear regression models to determine if the T-bet$^+$ frequency of RORγt$^+$Th17.0 cells was associated with the direction of PFT change. The fixed effects were the PFT change designations as well as the clinical covariates (age, sex, race, immunosuppression use, and smoking history), and the random effects were the subjects. We specified unstructured covariation matrices in these mixed effects models (44, 45).

We used linear regression models to determine how the T-bet$^+$ frequency of RORγt$^+$Th17.0 cells varied based on the number of total organs involved, where thoracic adenopathy and/or lung parenchymal involvement was considered as one organ. These regression models had either binary (one or greater than one organ) or categorical (each organ number as its own group) designations for total organ number. For the categorical model, five or more organs was considered one group to ensure sufficient numbers of subjects in each category and we also performed a *post-hoc* linear trend test.

We used Pearson correlation analyses to determine the association between T-bet$^+$ frequencies of RORγt$^+$Th17.0 cells and previously measured blood markers related to IFN-γ, including serum levels of the IFN-γ-induced chemokines of CXCL9, CXCL10, and CXCL11 (34, 35) as well whole blood RNA transcript levels for IFN-γ-related genes (33). We also used linear regression models to adjust for potential confounders. We calculated correlation r values for these models by taking the square-root of the adjusted R^2 from the linear regression models. For all regression models, we used robust standard errors (46, 47). We considered an $\alpha < 0.05$ as significant and report two significant digits for all analyses.

TABLE 2 | Sarcoidosis characteristics at enrollment/time of blood draw in cases and controls.

	Cases		Controls	*p*-value*
	PFT Decrease	PFT Increase		
	N = 22	*N* = 11	*N* = 10	
Age (mean years, SD)	56 (12)	50 (13)	46 (9)	0.082
Female (%)	16 (73)	4 (36)	3 (30)	0.089
Race (%)				0.37
African American	1 (5)	2 (18)	0 (0)	
White	19 (86)	7 (64)	8 (80)	
Hispanic	2 (9)	0 (0)	0 (0)	
Other	0 (0)	2 (18)	2 (20)	
Ever Smokers	11 (50)	6 (55)	4 (40)	0.64
Immunosuppression Use (%)	9 (41)	6 (55)	0 (0)	N/A
Extra-thoracic Organ Involvement (%)	75	78	10	0.00056
Initial Visit PFTs: Mean (SD)				
FVC %predicted	97 (16)	80 (18)	99 (13)	0.012†
FEV1 %predicted	89 (18)	75 (24)	89 (17)	0.11
FEV1/FVC	0.72 (0.085)	0.72 (0.14)	0.71 (0.081)	0.95
DLCO %predicted	74 (16)	59 (13)	79 (12)	0.011
TLC %predicted	99 (11)	83 (17)	93 (13)	0.027

**p-values are for comparisons between cases and controls.*
†*p-values for PFTs compare the controls and the cases as two separate groups.*
N/A, not applicable.

RESULTS

Characteristics of Sarcoidosis Subjects

We identified 33 subjects who met the PFT change threshold case definition (22 with declines and 11 with increases) and 10 subjects who met the case definition for control subjects; the clinical characteristics of these subjects are shown in **Table 2** and details regarding their immunosuppression use are shown in **Table S2**. For the cases, the average time between visits where a PFT change occurred was 19 months ($SD = 11$). Cases who had PFT increases had lower values of DLCO and FVC at first measurement than the other groups (cases with declines or controls).

Transcription Factor Expression in Th Cells

Figure 1 shows the gating strategy to identify the Th populations of interest (Th17.0, Th17.1, and Th1) among T-effectors cells based on surface expression of chemokine receptors. Because the polarization of each of these Th cell populations is influenced by the RORγt and T-bet transcription factors (16, 17, 26–28, 48, 49), we also measured the expression of these transcription factors as part of our staining panel (**Figures 2A–C**). We used FMO staining for RORγt and T-bet to set gates for positive and negative expressing cells as shown in **Figures 2D,E** (for FMO controls for each of our staining reagents, please refer to **Figure S2**). **Figures 2A–C,F** shows that using chemokine receptors to identify these Th cell subsets is sensitive but not as specific as also including transcription factors staining. As shown, the majority of Th17.0 cells express RORγt, most of the Th1 cells express T-bet, and the majority of Th17.1 cells express both RORγt and T-bet; further data to illustrate the concordance between these chemokine receptor patterns and transcription factor expression are shown in **Figure S3**. Although Tregs were not the focus of this study, we found that CD25^{Hi}CD127^{Lo}CD4$^+$ T cells were present in the blood and represented 6.7% (95% CI 5.4–8.0) of total CD4$^+$ T cells. Because the Th cell population of interest in this study was the Th17.0 subset, to increase the specificity of this population, we defined these cells by including expression of RORγt as shown by the solid blue box in **Figure 2A** and refer to them as RORγt$^+$Th17.0 cells. We found that some of these RORγt$^+$Th17.0 cells also expressed T-bet as shown in **Figure 2A** by the dashed black box. **Figure 2G** shows the range of T-bet expression in RORγt$^+$Th17.0 cells across subjects. This T-bet$^+$ frequency of RORγt$^+$Th17.0 cells was the focus of our subsequent analyses.

Relationship Between the T-bet$^+$ Frequencies of RORγt$^+$Th17.0 Cells and Clinical Outcomes

We determined how the %T-bet$^+$ frequencies of RORγt$^+$Th17.0 cells varied between cases and controls. Cases had higher T-bet$^+$ frequencies compared to controls (27 vs. 16%, $p = 0.0040$) in unadjusted analysis; this difference was also statistically significant in a model adjusted for age, sex, race, immunosuppression use, and prior smoking status as shown in **Figure 3A**. We also found that as separate groups, those with PFT declines and those with PFT increases had higher T-bet$^+$ frequencies of RORγt$^+$Th17.0 cells compared to controls in both unadjusted and adjusted models (**Figure 3A**). Of note, we did not find any association between the PFT groups and any of the T helper populations as defined by chemokine receptors and also using RORγt and/or T-bet to delineate these populations (Th17.0, Th17.1, Th1, or Th2) (see **Table S3**). We used a mixed effects model adjusted for age, race, sex, immunosuppression use,

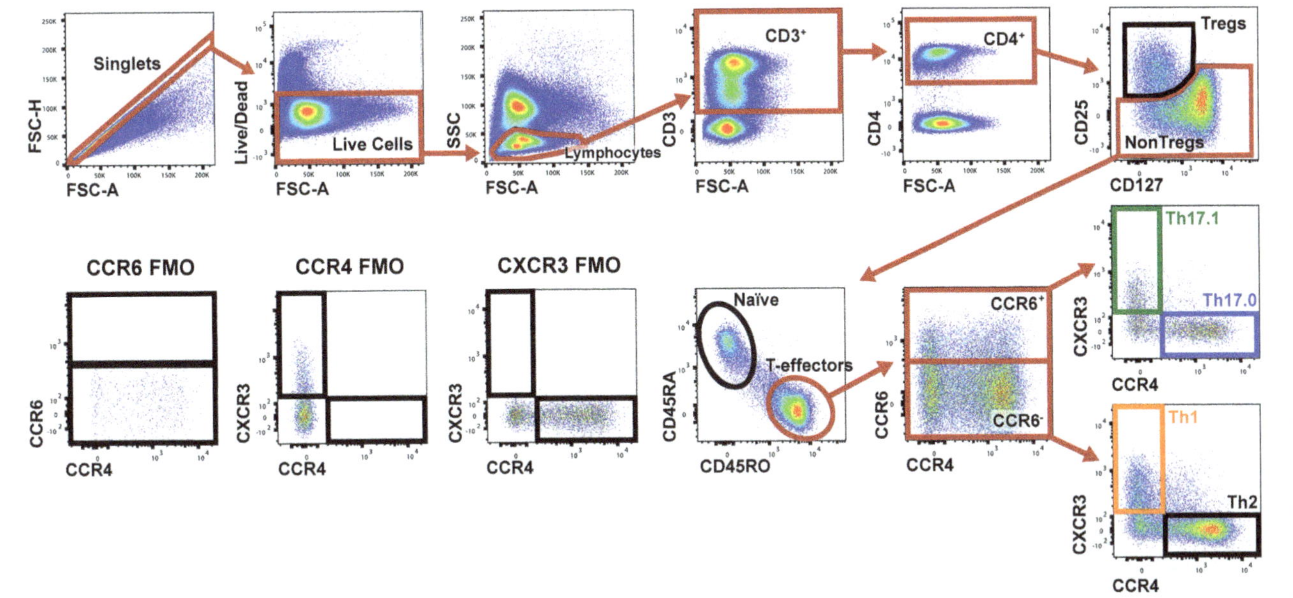

FIGURE 1 | Gating strategy to identify Th populations among T-effector cells. Shown is a representative sarcoidosis subject sample. We gated on singlet cells using FSC-H and FSC-A, then live cells (negative for the fixed viability dye), lymphocytes based on FSC and SSC, then CD3+ and CD4+ cells. We then gated on NonTregs that were CD25− and either CD127^{Lo} or CD127^{Hi} and then T-effectors (CD45RA− and CD45RO+). Among these T-effectors, we enriched for Th subsets using CCR6, CCR4, and CXCR3. Th17.0 cells were CCR6+CCR4+CXCR3−, Th17.1 cells were CCR4−CCR6+CXCR3+ and Th1 cells were CCR6−CCR4−CXCR3+. The gating strategy used for fluorescence minus one (FMO) controls for CCR6, CCR4, and CXCR3 are shown in the lower left corner.

and prior smoking, to examine the T-bet+ frequencies of Th17.0 cells in relation to the direction of PFT change. We found that being in the PFT decline group was associated with an increase in T-bet+ frequency (average change = 8.6%, 95% CI 1.5–16, p = 0.017) (**Figure 3B**). Conversely, being in the PFT increase group was associated with a decrease in T-bet+ frequency (average change = −6.0%, 95% CI −14 to 2.4, p = 0.16) (**Figure 3B**). This model included an interaction term between the PFT change group (decline or increase) and the visit variable to assess if the change in T-bet+ frequency between the two visits differed based on the direction of PFT change. We found that there was a statistically significant interaction between the direction of PFT change and the visit variable. The magnitude of this difference was 15 percentage points (95% CI 3.7–26, p = 0.0089).

Association Between T-bet+ Frequencies of RORγt+Th17.0 Cells and Organ Involvement

We considered the total number of organs involved with sarcoidosis at enrollment into the study as a separate manifestation of granulomatous disease burden. To test if T-bet expression in RORγt+Th17.0 cells varied based on the number of organs involved, we used linear regression models and adjusted for age, sex, race, and immunosuppression use. T-bet+ frequencies of RORγt+Th17.0 cells were 11 percentage points higher on average in those with more than one organ involved relative to those with a single organ involved (**Table 3**). We also constructed a model wherein the number of organs involved was a categorical predictor (from 1 organ to >5 organs) and found that the T-bet+ frequencies increased as the number of organs involved increased, especially with ≥ 5 organs involved (trend test, $p < 0.001$) (**Table 3** and **Figure 4**).

Correlations Between the T-bet+ Frequencies of RORγt+Th17.0 Cells and Other IFN-γ-Related Blood Markers

To assess if T-bet expression in RORγt+Th17.0 cells was associated with other markers of IFN-γ-related inflammation, we determined the correlations between these T-bet+ frequencies and serum levels of IFN-γ-induced chemokines and whole blood gene transcript levels of IFN-γ-related genes, which we had previously measured in the same blood samples (33–35). We found that the T-bet+ frequencies positively correlated with all three serum chemokines (CXCL9, CXCL10, and CXCL11) in models adjusted for age, race, sex, and immunosuppression use (**Table 4**). We previously found that a three gene mean of *GBP1*, *STAT1*, and *STAT2* was higher in a larger number of subjects from this cohort who had either PFT declines or flares requiring immunosuppression use (33). This three gene mean (the "IFN Factor") as well as genes identified to be related to IFN-γ using Ingenuity Pathway Analysis (*TAP1* and *JAK2*) were positively correlated with the T-bet+ frequencies of RORγt+Th17.0 cells (**Table 4**).

DISCUSSION

Sarcoidosis is a systemic disease involving granulomatous inflammation with upregulation of immune pathways related

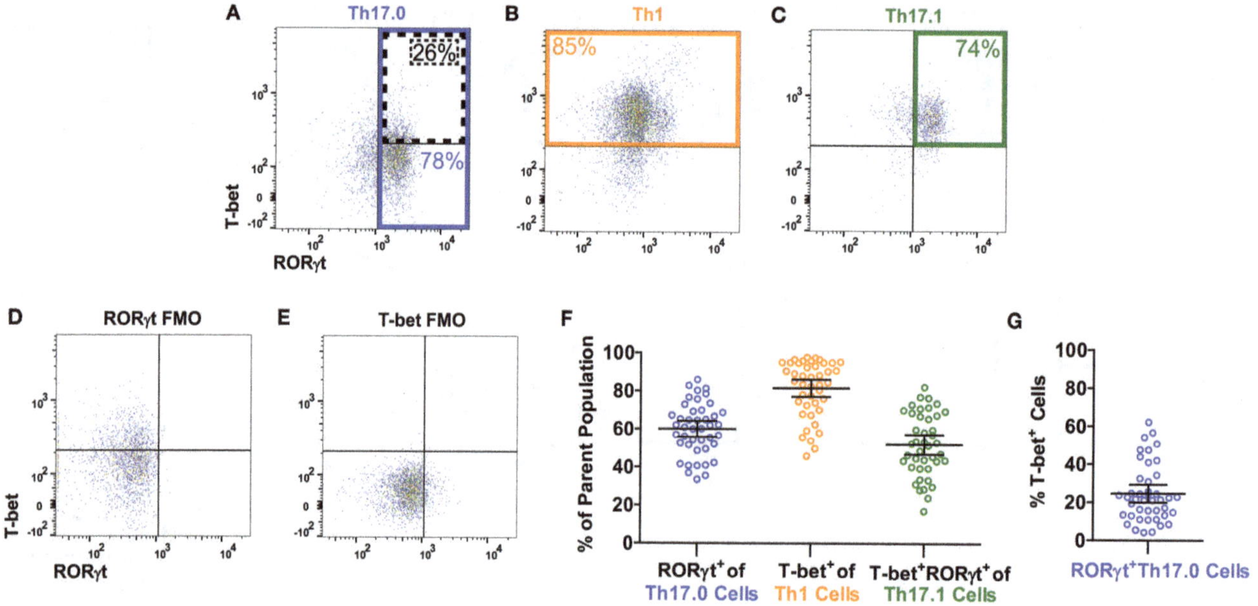

FIGURE 2 | T-bet and RORγt expression in the Th17.0, Th1, and Th17.1 cell populations. For each Th population (as defined in **Figure 1**), we determined the expression of T-bet and RORγt, as shown in a representative sarcoidosis sample. Expression of T-bet and RORγt in **(A)** Th17.0, **(B)** Th1, and **(C)** Th17.1 cells along with fluorescence minus one controls (FMOs) for **(D)** RORγt and **(E)** T-bet are displayed as dot plots. The majority of cells in each Th population had the expected expression pattern of T-bet and RORγt based on its chemokine receptor pattern: **(A)** the majority of Th17.0 cells expressed RORγt (outlined in blue); **(B)** the majority of Th1 cells expressed T-bet (outlined in yellow); and **(C)** the majority of Th17.1 cells expressed both RORγt and T-bet (outlined in green). These frequencies of RORγt$^+$ and/or T-bet$^+$ cells in each of these Th cell populations for this representative subject sample are shown on each plot with corresponding colors. These frequencies are displayed graphically in **(F)** across all subjects where each open circle represents a single subject along with the mean and 95% confidence interval (CI). Our primary population of interest in this study was the Th17.0 subset, so to achieve the highest specificity for the "Th17.0" phenotype, we focused on RORγt$^+$Th17.0 cells as outlined in blue in **(A)**. We found that some of these RORγt$^+$Th17.0 cells also expressed T-bet, as outlined by the dotted black box in **(A)**. There was a range of T-bet$^+$ cells within this RORγt$^+$Th17.0 population across subjects, as shown graphically in **(G)**, where each open circle represents a subject along with the mean and 95% CI. Our subsequent analyses focused on how this T-bet$^+$ frequency among RORγt$^+$Th17.0 cells related to clinical sarcoidosis outcomes.

to IFN-γ (5, 6, 50, 51). In light of recent findings that IFN-γ-producing Th17.1 cells are elevated in the lungs and lymph nodes of sarcoidosis patients with chronic disease (52), the ontogeny and function of these cells may be important in the pathogenesis of sarcoidosis (11, 52). This study was motivated by (1) clinical observations that Th17.0 cells are elevated in blood while Th17.1 cells are elevated in BAL fluid and mediastinal lymph nodes of sarcoidosis patients (11, 52), and (2) scientific evidence from mice and humans demonstrating the plasticity of Th17.0 cells to become Th17.1 cells after exposure to IL-12 and IFN-γ and upregulation of T-bet (21–24). Since granulomas are a source of IL-12 and IFN-γ (53, 54), we hypothesized that T-bet expression in peripheral Th17.0 cells would reflect the extent of granulomatous inflammation in sarcoidosis patients. Therefore, we used transcription factor staining for T-bet and RORγt along with chemokine receptor staining to identify Th17 cell populations, specifically T-bet$^+$ frequencies of RORγt$^+$Th17.0 cells. We found that these T-bet$^+$ frequencies were higher in sarcoidosis subjects with clinical evidence of greater disease burden as manifested by clinically meaningful PFTs changes and organ involvement.

Given the limitations in directly quantifying the degree of inflammation present in our human subjects, our study design utilized clinical features of disease severity as indicators of the extent of granulomatous inflammation. Specifically, we used a case-control study design to compare sarcoidosis subjects with different clinical courses. We assumed that those with any type of PFT change (our cases) had greater amounts of granulomatous inflammation during the study period as compared to those who had stable PFTs and did not require immunosuppression (our controls). The greater T-bet$^+$ frequencies of RORγt$^+$Th17.0 cells in our cases supports our hypothesis that this T-bet$^+$ frequency measure reflects the extent of disease burden. In subgroup analyses of our cases, we found that the T-bet$^+$ frequencies of RORγt$^+$Th17.0 cells were increased following a PFT decline. Conversely, T-bet$^+$ frequencies were decreased following a PFT improvement. We interpret these findings as evidence that these T-bet$^+$ frequencies changed based on disease trajectory and therefore varied based on the extent of granulomatous inflammation over time. We also used the number of organs involved as another indicator of disease burden. Thus, we interpreted the positive association between these T-bet$^+$ frequencies and organ involvement as further evidence that these T-bet$^+$ frequencies were associated with the extent of granulomatous inflammation. As additional support for our findings, we found positive correlations between these T-bet$^+$ frequencies and other measures of IFN-γ-related inflammation, including

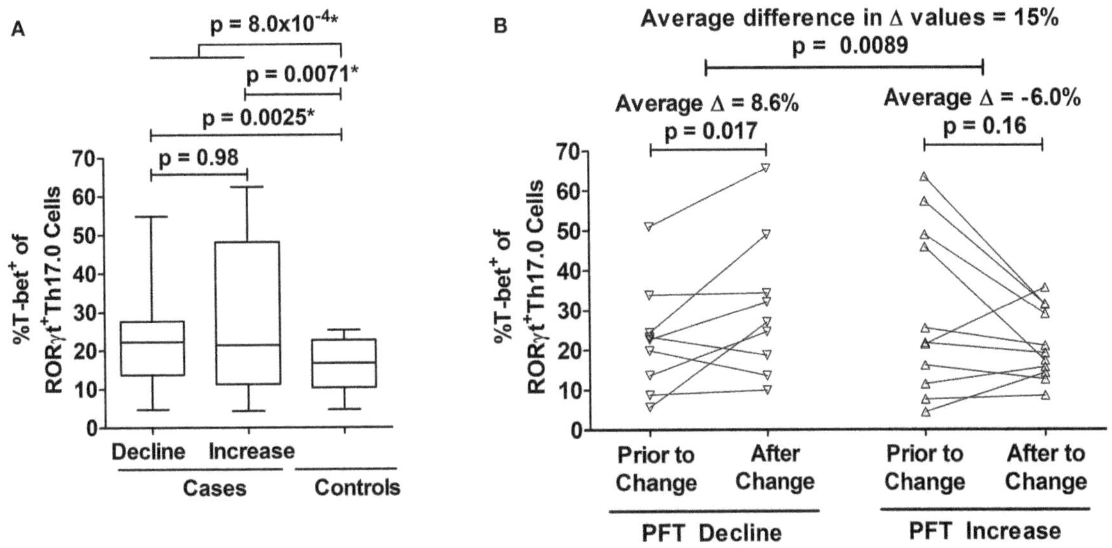

FIGURE 3 | Associations between T-bet$^+$ frequencies of RORγt$^+$Th17.0 cells and pulmonary function changes. **(A)** Cases had higher %T-bet$^+$ frequencies of RORγt$^+$Th17.0 cells compared to controls in either adjusted or unadjusted models (*p-values from model adjusted for age, sex, race, immunosuppression use, and prior smoking). Cases were defined by declines ($n = 22$) or increases ($n = 11$) in either forced vital capacity (FVC) or diffusing capacity (DLCO) of 10 or 15%, respectively during follow up regardless of immunosuppression. Controls ($n = 10$) lacked these same pulmonary function test (PFT) changes and never required immunosuppressive treatment. The upper most *p*-value represents the result from a regression model that compared all cases to controls. The middle two *p*-values represent results from a regression model that distinguished cases as separate groups based on either PFT declines or increases and compared these groups to controls; the lower most *p*-value represents the results from this same regression model where cases with PFT declines were compared to cases with PFT increases. Data are displayed as box-and-whisker plots with median and interquartile ranges. **(B)** As assessed by mixed effects modeling adjusted for age, sex, race, immunosuppression use, and prior smoking, cases had either an increase ($n = 9$) (left panel) or decrease ($n = 11$) (right panel) in T-bet$^+$ frequencies at the visit at which their PFT change occurred. The difference in the magnitude of these changes between those with PFT declines and PFT increases was 15%. In **(B)**, each subject's T-bet$^+$ frequency is represented by an open symbol and are plotted based on when they were sampled relative to the PFT change.

TABLE 3 | Linear regression using two different variables to delineate the number of involved organs[†].

Outcome	Predictor	β-Coefficient	95% CI	*p*-value
%T-bet$^+$ of RORγt$^+$Th17.0 cells	Model (1) Binary: >1 Organ (1 Organ = Ref)	11%	(0.36, 22)	**0.043**
	Model (2) Categorical:		Trend Test:	**1.2×10^{-38}‡**
	1 Organ	(Ref)	(Ref)	(Ref)
	2 Organs	11%	(−2.9, 24)	0.12
	3 Organs	3.5%	(−7, 14)	0.51
	4 Organs	9.4%	(−3.4, 22)	0.15
	≥5 Organs	25%	(16, 34)	**9.8×10^{-8}**

† Adjusted for age, sex, race, and immunosuppression use.
‡ p-value for the test of linear trend for the categorical organ variable.
Ref, Reference.

serum interferon-induced chemokines and whole blood gene transcript levels.

The polarization of Th17.0 cells to Th17.1 cells has been studied both in mice and several human diseases including rheumatoid arthritis, multiple sclerosis, and Crohn's disease (12, 17, 55–62). Mechanisms currently put forth for how Th17.0 can become Th17.1 involve upregulation of T-bet. It has long been established that T-bet expression in naïve T cells leads to the acquisition of a Th1 phenotype after antigenic stimulation in the presence of cytokines such as IL-12 and resulting upregulation of STAT1 (25–29). This process includes T-bet's role in the upregulation of CXCR3 expression, which is essential for trafficking of Th1 cells to sites of inflammation (26, 27, 48). During and post-polarization, T-bet also upregulates IFN-γ through binding to both the promoter and enhancer loci for *IFNG* (29). Mouse models have shown that Th17.0 cells incubated with IFN-γ and IL-12, or TNF-α gain features of Th17.1 cells including CXCR3 expression and the capacity to produce IFN-γ (22–24). This phenomenon of plasticity from IL-17-producing cells to IFN-γ-producing cells has also been observed in mouse models of innate lymphoid cells, where RORγt$^+$ ILC3 cells transition to ILC1 cells through upregulation of T-bet in the presence of specific cytokines such as IL-12 (63–66). A human study of inflammatory bowel disease found that *ex vivo* IL-12 stimulation led to IFN-γ production in Th17 cells that were isolated as CCR6$^+$CXCR3$^-$ cells from mesenteric lymph nodes (17). This observation suggests that upregulation of CXCR3 may occur later in the cellular differentiation of Th17.0 to Th17.1 cell phenotype. Other groups including Cohen et al. (21) showed that polarized Th17.0 cells derived from *ex vivo* human PBMCs could subsequently upregulate the T-bet gene *TBX21* after incubation with IL-12 and IFN-γ. Therefore, T-bet expression in RORγt$^+$Th17.0 cells (CCR6$^+$CXCR3$^-$CCR4$^+$)

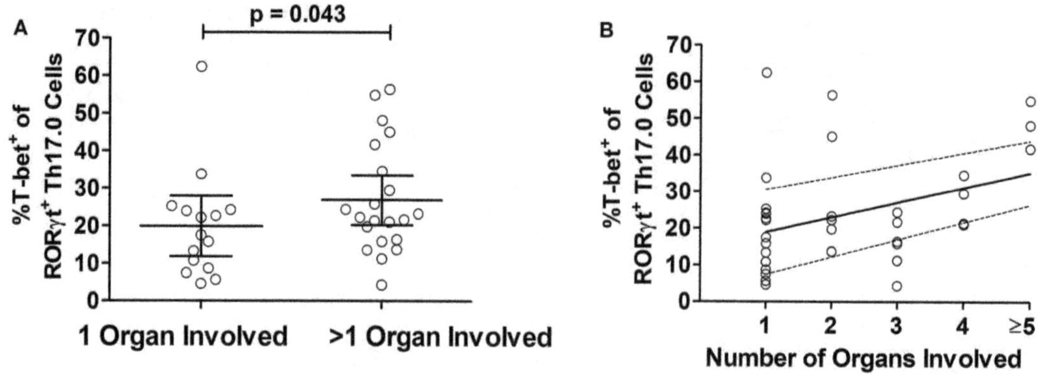

FIGURE 4 | Relationship between T-bet$^+$ frequencies of RORγt$^+$Th17.0 cells and organ involvement. **(A)** The frequencies of %T-bet$^+$ of RORγt$^+$Th17.0 cells were higher in those with greater than one organ involved as compared to only one organ (*p*-value adjusted for age, sex, race, and immunosuppression use). **(B)** The T-bet$^+$ frequencies of RORγt$^+$Th17.0 cells where higher in those with greater number of organs involved. In a linear regression model with total organ involvement as a categorical predicator adjusted for age, sex, race, and immunosuppression use, there was a positive trend toward increasing T-bet$^+$ frequencies of RORγt$^+$Th17.0 cells with greater organ involvement (see **Table 3**). The solid line shows the organ number adjusted for age, sex, race, and immunosuppression use and the dashed lines represent the 95% confidence interval.

TABLE 4 | Results from correlation analyses and regression models for T-bet$^+$ frequencies of RORγt$^+$Th17.0 cells and IFN-γ-related blood markers.

Outcome	Main Predictor	Adj β-coeff†	95% CI	Adj *p*-value	Adj r value	Unadj r value‡
%T-bet$^{\pm}$ of	Log_{10}[CXCL9]§	22	(14, 31)	**1.5×10^{-5}**	0.66	0.65
RORγt$^{\pm}$Th17.0 cells	Log_{10}[CXCL10]	23	(3.6, 42)	**0.022**	0.47	0.41
	Log_{10}[CXCL11]	30	(11, 49)	**0.0028**	0.51	0.50
	IFN Factor††	6.9	(0.81, 13)	**0.028**	0.37	0.58
	JAK2‡‡	4.2	(2.5, 10)	**0.034**	0.29	0.42
	TAP1‡‡	4.8	(0.25, 9.3)	**0.041**	0.26	0.42

†β-coefficient is adjusted for age, race, sex, and immunosuppression use.
‡Unadjusted Pearson r coefficient.
§Serum chemokine values were log_{10}-transformed.
††The "IFN Factor" = a three gene mean of GBP1, STAT1, and STAT2 previously measured from whole blood.
‡‡Whole blood gene expression values in the form of log_2[relative expression].
Adj, Adjusted; CI, Confidence Interval; Coeff, Coefficient; Unadj, Unadjusted.
Bold values indicates p-values for adjusted β-coeffecients.

could potentially represent a transitional state between the Th17 and Th17.1 immune subsets. Our focus on Th17.0 cells (and not Th17.1 cells that also express CXCR3), was motivated by our goal to identify cells prior to upregulation of CXCR3, since expression of this chemokine receptor could lead to trafficking of cells out of the blood.

Where the transition between Th17.0 and Th17.1 occurs *in vivo* has been an on-going question in studies of T cell biology. In the setting of other granulomatous processes such as pulmonary tuberculosis infection, mouse models have shown that dendritic cells present antigen to naïve T cells in mediastinal lymph nodes (67–69). Therefore, the initial polarization of Th1 cells in this disease model does not occur in the alveoli, but instead these polarized cells must traffic to the initial site of infection after their activation in local lymph nodes. For Th17.0 cells, mouse models studying gastrointestinal T cells have shown that Th17.0 cells initially become polarized in the mesenteric lymph nodes then traffic through the blood to the intestine in models of both healthy and inflammatory states (70, 71). The location of Th17.1 polarization potentially includes both lymph nodes and inflamed tissue. In a mouse model of experimental autoimmune encephalitis, single-cell RNA sequencing analysis showed that Th17 cells isolated from lymph nodes and affected central nervous system tissues have several phenotypes with respect to cytokine production (62). These phenotypes ranged from self-renewing IL-17-producing cells and IFN-γ-producing cells in the lymph nodes to IFN-γ-producing cells in inflamed tissues. In a mouse model of colitis, Harbor et al. (59) showed that naïve T cells polarized to Th17.0 cells *ex vivo* and then injected into the peritoneum were later retrieved and found to be competent to produce IFN-γ. These cells were recovered from both mesenteric lymph nodes and inflamed intestinal tissue, suggesting that Th17.0 cells could be subsequently polarized to Th17.1 cells in either compartment. Taken together, these findings suggest that the transition from Th17.0 to Th17.1 cell may occur in both lymph nodes and inflamed tissues.

These mouse and human studies of Th17 plasticity provide a framework for how the transition from Th17.0 to Th17.1 cells might be occurring in sarcoidosis. Although it is unclear *where* the transition is occurring, we speculate that Th17.0 cells exposed to granuloma-related cytokines (i.e., IFN-γ, IL-12 and TNF-α) in the lymph nodes of affected organs, especially mediastinal lymph nodes, could lead to T-bet upregulation. We theorize that we are detecting this early T-bet$^+$ transition state of Th17.0 cells in the blood as these cells exit the lymph nodes and enter the peripheral circulation. Eventually, increased T-bet expression in these Th17.0 cells results in upregulation of CXCR3, which is a key surface marker for the Th17.1 phenotype. Since CXCR3 is a homing receptor, its expression in Th17.1 cells leads to their accumulation in affected tissues. This conceptual framework is supported by several prior and current observations. Previously, we observed elevated frequencies of Th17.0 cells in the blood associated with elevated frequencies of Th17.1 cells in BAL (11). In the current study we observed a positive correlation between T-bet$^+$ frequency in RORγt$^+$Th17.0 cells and several IFN-γ-related blood markers including serum IFN-induced chemokines and gene transcript levels. These observations along with the associations of T-bet$^+$ frequency in RORγt$^+$Th17.0 cells with clinical outcomes lead us to infer that there is a systemic up-regulation of IFN-γ-related pathways and the degree to which these pathways are upregulated may be related to the burden of granulomatous inflammation in the body. Since these responses can be measured in the blood, they could be used to prognosticate patients as well as further our understanding of the underlying immunopathology.

Our findings share commonalities and differences with a prior publication of RORγt and T-bet expression in sarcoidosis subjects. Kaiser *et al.*, showed strong associations between dual expression of CCR6 and CXCR3 in RORγt$^+$T-bet$^+$ T cells (10); we found similar strong associations between CCR6$^+$ and CXCR3$^+$ co-expressing cells we defined as Th17.1 cells that also had dual expression of RORγt and T-bet (see **Figure 2C** and **Figure S3**). However, our study differed in that we did not have BAL specimens and only focused on blood cells. The Kaiser study found that co-expression of RORγt and T-bet in CD4$^+$ cells was higher in the BAL of patients with Löfgren syndrome as compared to non-Löfgren sarcoidosis, suggesting that co-expression predicted a more favorable phenotype. Our study differed in that we did not have patients with Löfgren syndrome, and we used longitudinal PFT changes, immunosuppression use, and total number of organs involved to phenotype subjects. The other difference was that our main focus was on T-bet-expressing RORγt$^+$Th17.0 cells that did not express CXCR3 in order to identify potential transition cells in the blood, which was not addressed in the Kaiser study.

Some of the limitations of our study included our inability to directly assess the potential pathogenicity and IFN-γ-producing capabilities of the RORγt$^+$Th17.0 cells that also expressed T-bet. Staining for transcription factors involves fixation and permeabilization of the cells, which prevents analyses involving stimulation and cytokine measurements after sorting these cells. Nonetheless, the association of the T-bet$^+$ frequencies with clinically meaningful outcomes of sarcoidosis indicates that this cell population may be important to examine in future studies that further define the Th17.0 to Th17.1 transition. Our study was also limited by the lack of serially measured organ involvement and chest radiography, which precluded us from including these clinical findings in our definitions of sarcoidosis outcomes. Another important limitation relates to generalizability since our cohort was heterogeneous, and therefore our study design did not allow us to extrapolate the prognostic value of T-bet$^+$ frequencies of RORγt$^+$Th17.0 cells at initial diagnosis. Similarly, this study also was not designed to address the question of whether T-bet expression in RORγt$^+$Th17.0 cells can predict the likelihood of spontaneous remission. Some of these limitations can be addressed in future studies that enroll subjects at the time of diagnosis. In terms of our study design, we created case and control definitions to maximize the likelihood of identifying those with active and inactive granulomatous inflammation. The limitation of doing this is that we used lack of immunosuppression use to help identify those who were more likely to have inactive disease, therefore use of immunosuppression was not matched between cases and controls. We dealt with this by including immunosuppression as a covariate in all our regression models to control for possible bias in our point estimates. Moreover, we would assume that immunosuppression use would decrease T-bet expression in controls even further, therefore the results we report here are likely more conservative than if we matched based on immunosuppression use.

CONCLUSIONS AND FUTURE DIRECTIONS

In summary, we provide evidence showing that T-bet expression in RORγt$^+$Th17.0 cells was associated with both pulmonary and systemic organ involvement outcomes. These associations were potentially due to the effects of IFN-γ and IL-12 on Th17.0 cells as they circulate through affected lymph nodes where higher levels of these cytokines might be found. Future goals include determining how these frequencies in the blood relate to those in the lung, how they are associated with outcomes when measured at time of diagnosis, and how they change in response to treatment. With this information, we may be able to leverage biological data taken at the time of sarcoidosis diagnosis to inform patient prognosis and guide clinical decision making.

Institutional Review Board. The patients/participants provided their written informed consent to participate in this study.

AUTHOR CONTRIBUTIONS

NA and SM conducted the experiments. NA, IA, PW, and LK analyzed the data. All authors contributed to the writing and editing of the manuscript. All authors read and approved the final manuscript.

ACKNOWLEDGMENTS

The authors thank the following individuals for their specific contributions: Michelle Nguyen, Joris Ramstein, Christine Nguyen, Melissa Ho, Sara Sun, Zoe Lehman, and Victoria Wang for assistance with sample acquisition, analysis, and management of the database; and Owen Solberg, Ph.D., for database programming. We would also like to thank all the participants who volunteered their time for this study.

REFERENCES

Valeyre D, Prasse A, Nunes H, Uzunhan Y, Brillet PY, Muller-Quernheim J. Sarcoidosis. *Lancet.* (2014) 383:1155–67. doi: 10.1016/S0140-6736(13) 60680- 7

Robinson BW, McLemore TL, Crystal RG. Gamma interferon is spontaneously released by alveolar macrophages and lung T lymphocytes in patients with pulmonary sarcoidosis. *J Clin Invest.* (1985) 75:1488–95. doi: 10.1172/JCI111852

Prasse A, Georges CG, Biller H, Hamm H, Matthys H, Luttmann W, et al. Th1 cytokine pattern in sarcoidosis is expressed by bronchoalveolar CD4(+) and CD8(+) T cells. *Clin Exp Immunol.* (2000) 122:241- 8. doi: 10.1046/j.1365-2249.2000.01365.x

Inui N, Chida K, Suda T, Nakamura H. TH1/TH2 and TC1/TC2 profiles in peripheral blood and bronchoalveolar lavage fluid cells in pulmonary sarcoidosis. *J Allergy ClinImmunol.* (2001) 107:337–44. doi: 10.1067/mai.2001.112273

Mollers M, Aries SP, Dromann D, Mascher B, Braun J, Dalhoff K. Intracellular cytokine repertoire in different T cell subsets from patients with sarcoidosis. *Thorax.* (2001) 56:487–93. doi: 10.1136/thorax.56.6.487

Wahlstrom J, Katchar K, Wigzell H, Olerup O, Eklund A, Grunewald J. Analysis of intracellular cytokines in CD4+ and CD8+ lung and blood T cells in sarcoidosis. *Am J RespCrit Care Med.* (2001) 163:115- 21. doi: 10.1164/ajrccm.163.1.9906071

Facco M, Cabrelle A, Teramo A, Olivieri V, Gnoato M, Teolato S, et al. Sarcoidosis is a Th1/Th17 multisystem disorder. *Thorax.* (2011) 66:144- 50. doi: 10.1136/thx.2010.140319

Tondell A, Moen T, Borset M, Salvesen O, Ro AD, Sue-Chu M. Bronchoalveolar lavage fluid IFN-gamma+ Th17 cells and regulatory T cells in pulmonary sarcoidosis. *Mediators Inflamm.* (2014) 2014:438070. doi: 10.1155/2014/438070

Ten Berge B, Paats MS, Bergen IM, van den Blink B, Hoogsteden HC, Lambrecht BN, et al. Increased IL-17A expression in granulomas and in circulating memory T cells in sarcoidosis. *Rheumatology.* (2012) 51:37–46. doi: 10.1093/rheumatology/ker316

Kaiser Y, Lepzien R, Kullberg S, Eklund A, Smed-Sorensen A, Grunewald J. Expanded lung T-bet+RORgammaT+ CD4+ T-cells in sarcoidosis patients with a favourable disease phenotype. *Eur Respir J.* (2016) 48:484- 94. doi: 10.1183/13993003.00092-2016

Ramstein J, Broos CE, Simpson LJ, Ansel KM, Sun SA, Ho ME, et al. Interferon-gamma-producing Th17.1 cells are increased in sarcoidosis and more prevalent than Th1 cells. *Am J Respir Crit Care Med.* (2015) 193:1281- 91. doi: 10.1164/rccm.201507-1499OC

Ramesh R, Kozhaya L, McKevitt K, Djuretic IM, Carlson TJ, Quintero MA, et al. Pro-inflammatory human Th17 cells selectively express P-glycoprotein and are refractory to glucocorticoids. *J Exp Med.* (2014) 211:89–104. doi: 10.1084/jem.20130301

Ivanov, II, McKenzie BS, Zhou L, Tadokoro CE, Lepelley A, et al. The orphan nuclear receptor RORgammat directs the differentiation program of proinflammatory IL-17+ T helper cells. *Cell.* (2006) 126:1121- 33. doi: 10.1016/j.cell.2006.07.035

Sato W, Aranami T, Yamamura T. Cutting edge: human Th17 cells are identified as bearing CCR2+CCR5- phenotype. *J Immunol.* (2007) 178:7525- 9. doi: 10.4049/jimmunol.178.12.7525

Ivanov, II, Zhou L, Littman DR. Transcriptional regulation of Th17 cell differentiation. *Semin Immunology.* (2007) 19:409- 17. doi: 10.1016/j.smim.2007.10.011

Sallusto F, Zielinski CE, Lanzavecchia A. Human Th17 subsets. *Eur J Immunol.* (2012) 42:2215–20. doi: 10.1002/eji.201242741

Bsat M, Chapuy L, Rubio M, Wassef R, Richard C, Schwenter F, et al. Differential pathogenic Th17 profile in mesenteric lymph nodes of crohn's disease and ulcerative colitis patients. *Front Immunol.* (2019) 10:1177. doi: 10.3389/fimmu.2019.01177

Acosta-Rodriguez EV, Rivino L, Geginat J, Jarrossay D, Gattorno M, Lanzavecchia A, et al. Surface phenotype and antigenic specificity of human interleukin 17-producing T helper memory cells. *Nat Immunol.* (2007) 8:639- 46. doi: 10.1038/ni1467

Manel N, Unutmaz D, Littman DR. The differentiation of human T(H)-17 cells requires transforming growth factor-beta and induction of the nuclear receptor RORgammat. *Nat Immunol.* (2008) 9:641–9. doi: 10.1038/ni. 1610

Singh SP, Zhang HH, Foley JF, Hedrick MN, Farber JM. Human T cells that are able to produce IL-17 express the chemokine receptor CCR6. *J Immunol.* (2008) 180:214–21. doi: 10.4049/jimmunol.180.1.214

Cohen CJ, Crome SQ, MacDonald KG, Dai EL, Mager DL, Levings MK. Human Th1 and Th17 cells exhibit epigenetic stability at signature cytokine and transcription factor loci. *J Immunol.* (2011) 187:5615- 26. doi: 10.4049/jimmunol.1101058

Lexberg MH, Taubner A, Albrecht I, Lepenies I, Richter A, Kamradt T, et al. IFN-gamma and IL-12 synergize to convert *in vivo* generated Th17 into Th1/Th17 cells. *Eur J Immunol.* (2010) 40:3017–27. doi: 10.1002/eji.201040539

Wang Y, Godec J, Ben-Aissa K, Cui K, Zhao K, Pucsek AB, et al. The transcription factors T-bet and runx are required for the ontogeny of pathogenic interferon-gamma-producing T helper 17 cells. *Immunity.* (2014) 40:355–66. doi: 10.1016/j.immuni.2014.01.002

Maggi L, Cimaz R, Capone M, Santarlasci V, Querci V, Simonini G, et al. Brief report: etanercept inhibits the tumor necrosis factor alpha-driven shift of Th17 lymphocytes toward a nonclassic Th1 phenotype in juvenile idiopathic arthritis. *Arthr Rheumatol.* (2014) 66:1372–7. doi: 10.1002/art.38355

Murphy KM, Reiner SL. The lineage decisions of helper T cells. *Nat Rev Immunol.* (2002) 2:933–44. doi: 10.1038/nri954

Lametschwandtner G, Biedermann T, Schwarzler C, Gunther C, Kund J, Fassl S, et al. Sustained T-bet expression confers polarized human TH2 cells with TH1-like cytokine production and migratory capacities. *J Allergy Clin Immunol.* (2004) 113:987–94. doi: 10.1016/j.jaci.2004. 02.004

Lord GM, Rao RM, Choe H, Sullivan BM, Lichtman AH, Luscinskas FW, et al. T-bet is required for optimal proinflammatory CD4+ T-cell trafficking. *Blood.* (2005) 106:3432–9. doi: 10.1182/blood-2005-04-1393

Beima KM, Miazgowicz MM, Lewis MD, Yan PS, Huang TH, Weinmann AS. T-bet binding to newly identified target gene promoters is cell type- independent but results in variable context-dependent functional effects. *J Biol Chem.* (2006) 281:11992–2000. doi: 10.1074/jbc.M513613200

Djuretic IM, Levanon D, Negreanu V, Groner Y, Rao A, Ansel KM. Transcription factors T-bet and runx3 cooperate to activate Ifng and silence Il4 in T helper type 1 cells. *Nat Immunol.* (2007) 8:145–53. doi: 10.1038/ni1424

Mikhak Z, Fleming CM, Medoff BD, Thomas SY, Tager AM, Campanella GS, et al. STAT1 in peripheral tissue differentially regulates homing of antigen-specific Th1 and Th2 cells. *J Immunol.* (2006) 176:4959- 67. doi: 10.4049/jimmunol.176.8.4959

Hunninghake GW, Costabel U, Ando M, Baughman R, Cordier JF, du Bois R, et al. ATS/ERS/WASOG statement on sarcoidosis. *Am J Respir Crit Care Med.* (1999) 16:149–73.

Benn BS, Lehman Z, Kidd SA, Ho M, Sun S, Ramstein J, et al. Clinical and biological insights from the university of california san francisco prospective and longitudinal cohort. *Lung.* (2017) 195:553– 61. doi: 10.1007/s00408-017-0037-y

Su R, Li MM, Bhakta NR, Solberg OD, Darnell EP, Ramstein J, et al. Longitudinal analysis of sarcoidosis blood transcriptomic signatures and disease outcomes. *Eur Respir J.* (2014) 44:985– 93. doi: 10.1183/09031936.00039714

Arger NK, Ho M, Woodruff PG, Koth LL. Serum CXCL11 correlates with pulmonary outcomes and disease burden in sarcoidosis. *Respir Med.* (2019) 152:89–96. doi: 10.1016/j.rmed.2019. 04.005

Arger N, Ho M, Allen IE, Benn BS, Woodruff PG, Koth L. CXCL9 and CXCL10 are differentially associated with systemic organ involvement and pulmonary disease severity in sarcoidosis. *Respir Med.* (2020) 161:105822. doi: 10.1016/j. rmed.2019.105822

Judson MA, Baughman RP, Thompson BW, Teirstein AS, Terrin ML, Rossman MD, et al. Two year prognosis of sarcoidosis: the ACCESS experience. *Sarcoidosis Vasc Diffuse Lung Dis.* (2003) 20:204–11.

Khanna D, Mittoo S, Aggarwal R, Proudman SM, Dalbeth N, Matteson EL, et al. Connective tissue disease-associated interstitial lung diseases (CTD-ILD)-report from omeractctd-ild working group. *J Rheumatol.* (2015) 42:2168– 71. doi: 10.3899/jrheum.141182

Roederer M. Spectral compensation for flow cytometry: visualization artifacts, limitations, and caveats. *Cytometry.* (2001) 45:194–205. doi: 10.1002/1097-0320(20011101) 45:3<194::AID-CYTO1163>3.0.CO;2-C

Roederer M. Compensation in flow cytometry. *Curr Protocols Cytometry.* (2002) 22:Unit 1.14. doi: 10.1002/0471142956.cy0114s22

Roederer M. Distributions of autofluorescence after compensation: be panglossian, fret not. *Cytometry A.* (2016) 89:398– 402. doi: 10.1002/cyto.a.22820

Barcelo H, Faul J, Crimmins E, Thyagarajan B.A practical cryopreservation and staining protocol for immunophenotyping in population studies. *Curr Protocols Cytometry.* (2018) 84:e35. doi: 10.1002/cpcy.35

Kalina T, Flores-Montero J, van der Velden VH, Martin-Ayuso M, Bottcher S, Ritgen M, et al. EuroFlow standardization of flow cytometer instrument settings and immunophenotyping protocols. *Leukemia.* (2012) 26:1986– 2010. doi: 10.1038/leu.2012.122

Lanuti P, Simeone P, Rotta G, Almici C, Avvisati G, Azzaro R, et al. A standardized flow cytometry network study for the assessment of circulating endothelial cell physiological ranges. *Sci Rep.* (2018) 8:5823. doi: 10.1038/s41598-018-24234-0

McLean RA, Sanders WL, Stroup WW. A unified approach to mixed linear models. *Am Stat.* (1991) 45:54–64. doi: 10.1080/00031305.1991.10475767

Vittinghoff EV, Glidden DC, Shiboski SE. Exploratory and descriptive methods. In: Dietz K, Gail M, Krickeberg K, Samet J, Tsiatis A, Wong W. Editors. *Regression Methods in Biostatistics. Statistics for Biology and Health.* Boston, MA: Springer (2012) p. 7–26. doi: 10.1007/978-1-4614-1353-0_2

Huber PJ. The behavior of maximum likelihood estimates under nonstandard conditions. In: *Proceedings of the Fifth Berkeley Symposium on Mathematical Statistics and Probability.* Berkeley, CA: University of California Press (1967). p. 221–33.

White H. A heteroskedasticity-consistent covariance matrix estimator and a direct test for heteroskedasticity. *Econometrica.* (1980) 48:817– 38. doi: 10.2307/1912934

Bonecchi R, Bianchi G, Bordignon PP, D'Ambrosio D, Lang R, Borsatti A, et al. Differential expression of chemokine receptors and chemotactic responsiveness of type 1 T helper cells (Th1s) and Th2s. *J Exp Med.* (1998) 187:129–34. doi: 10.1084/jem.187.1.129

Groom JR, Luster AD. CXCR3 in T cell function. *Exp Cell Res.* (2011) 317:620–31. doi: 10.1016/j.yexcr.2010.12.017

Prior C, Haslam PL. Increased levels of serum interferon-gamma in pulmonary sarcoidosis and relationship with response to corticosteroid therapy. *Am Rev Respir Dis.* (1991) 143:53–60. doi: 10.1164/ajrccm/143.1.53

Koth LL, Solberg OD, Peng JC, Bhakta NR, Nguyen CP, Woodruff PG. Sarcoidosis blood transcriptome reflects lung inflammation and overlaps with tuberculosis. *Am J RespCrit Care Med.* (2011) 184:1153– 63. doi: 10.1164/rccm.201106-1143OC

Broos CE, Koth LL, van Nimwegen M, In 't Veen J, Paulissen SMJ, van Hamburg JP, et al. Increased T-helper 17.1 cells in sarcoidosismediastinal lymph nodes. *EurResp J.* (2018) 51:1701124. doi: 10.1183/13993003.01124-2017

Bergeron A, Bonay M, Kambouchner M, Lecossier D, Riquet M, Soler P, et al. Cytokine patterns in tuberculous and sarcoid granulomas: correlations with histopathologic features of the granulomatous response. *J Immunol.* (1997) 159:3034–43.

Sakthivel P, Bruder D. Mechanism of granuloma formation in sarcoidosis. *Curr Opin Hematol.* (2017) 24:59–65. doi: 10.1097/MOH.0000000000000301

Annunziato F, Romagnani S. The transient nature of the Th17 phenotype. *Eur J Immunol.* (2010) 40:3312–6. doi: 10.1002/eji.2010 41145

Domingues HS, Mues M, Lassmann H, Wekerle H, Krishnamoorthy G. Functional and pathogenic differences of Th1 and Th17 cells in experimental autoimmune encephalomyelitis. *PLoS ONE.* (2010) 5:e15531. doi: 10.1371/journal. pone.0015531

Cosmi L, Cimaz R, Maggi L, Santarlasci V, Capone M, Borriello F, et al. Evidence of the transient nature of the Th17 phenotype of CD4+CD161+ T cells in the synovial fluid of patients with juvenile idiopathic arthritis. *Arthr Rheum.* (2011) 63:2504–15. doi: 10.1002/art. 30332

Annunziato F, Cosmi L, Liotta F, Maggi E, Romagnani S. Defining the human T helper 17 cell phenotype. *Trends Immunol.* (2012) 33:505– 12. doi: 10.1016/j. it.2012.05.004

Harbour SN, Maynard CL, Zindl CL, Schoeb TR, Weaver CT. Th17 cells give rise to Th1 cells that are required for the pathogenesis of colitis. *Proc Natl Acad Sci USA.* (2015) 112:7061–6. doi: 10.1073/pnas.1415 675112

Kotake S, Yago T, Kobashigawa T, Nanke Y. The plasticity of Th17 Cells in the pathogenesis of rheumatoid arthritis. *J Clin Med.* (2017) 6:67. doi: 10.3390/ jcm6070067

van Langelaar J, van der Vuurst de Vries RM, Janssen M, Wierenga-Wolf AF, Spilt IM, Siepman TA, et al. T helper 17.1 cells associate with multiple sclerosis disease activity: perspectives for early intervention. *Brain J Neurol.* (2018) 141:1334–49. doi: 10.1093/brain/awy069

Gaublomme JT, Yosef N, Lee Y, Gertner RS, Yang LV, Wu C, et al. Single-cell genomics unveils critical regulators of Th17 cell pathogenicity. *Cell.* (2015) 163:1400–12. doi: 10.1016/j.cell.2015.11.009

Vonarbourg C, Mortha A, Bui VL, Hernandez PP, Kiss EA, Hoyler T, et al. Regulated expression of nuclear receptor RORgammat confers distinct functional fates to NK cell receptor- expressing RORgammat(+) innate lymphocytes. *Immunity.* (2010) 33:736–51. doi: 10.1016/j.immuni.2010.10.017

Sciume G, Hirahara K, Takahashi H, Laurence A, Villarino AV, Singleton KL, et al. Distinct requirements for T-bet in gut innate lymphoid cells. *J Exp Med.* (2012) 209:2331–8. doi: 10.1084/jem.20122097

Klose CS, Kiss EA, Schwierzeck V, Ebert K, Hoyler T, d'Hargues Y, et al. A T-bet gradient controls the fate and function of CCR6-RORgammat+ innate lymphoid cells. *Nature.* (2013) 494:261–5. doi: 10.1038/nature11813

Rankin LC, Groom JR, Chopin M, Herold MJ, Walker JA, Mielke LA, et al. The transcription factor T-bet is essential for the development of NKp46+ innate lymphocytes via the notch pathway. *Nat Immunol.* (2013) 14:389– 95. doi: 10.1038/ni.2545

Wolf AJ, Desvignes L, Linas B, Banaiee N, Tamura T, Takatsu K, et al. Initiation of the adaptive immune response to mycobacterium tuberculosis depends on antigen production in the local lymph node, not the lungs. *J Exp Med.* (2008) 205:105–15. doi: 10.1084/jem.20071367

Olmos S, Stukes S, Ernst JD. Ectopic activation of mycobacterium tuberculosis-specific CD4+ T cells in lungs of CCR7-/- mice. *J Immunol.* (2010) 184:895–901. doi: 10.4049/jimmunol.0901230

Srivastava S, Ernst JD. Cell-to-cell transfer of M. Tuberculosis antigens optimizes CD4 T cell priming. *Cell Host Microbe.* (2014) 15:741–52. doi: 10.1016/j. chom.2014.05.007

Kawabe T, Sun SL, Fujita T, Yamaki S, Asao A, Takahashi T, et al. Homeostatic proliferation of naive CD4+ T cells in mesenteric lymph nodes generates gut-tropic Th17 cells. *J Immunol.* (2013) 190:5788–98. doi: 10.4049/jimmunol.1203111

Kawabe T, Suzuki N, Yamaki S, Sun SL, Asao A, Okuyama Y, et al. Mesenteric lymph nodes contribute to proinflammatory Th17-cell generation during inflammation of the small intestine in mice. *Eur J Immunol.* (2016) 46:1119– 31. doi: 10.1002/eji.201545907

19

Comparison of Immediate and Sequential Withdrawal of a Systemic Glucocorticoid in the Treatment of Acute Exacerbations of Chronic Obstructive Pulmonary Disease

Ling Zhou[1], *Yuanyuan Fang*[1], *Wei Liu*[2], *Jianchu Zhang*[3], *Yingnan Wang*[4], *Sheng Xie*[5], *Minhua Zhong*[6], *Zhengyan Wang*[7], *Guangcai Li*[8], *Hongyan Ai*[9], *Hongrong Guo*[10], *Fanjun Zeng*[11], *Wei Xiao*[12], *Chenghong Li*[13], *Yi Hu*[14], *Yijun Tang*[15] and *Huiguo Liu*[1]*

[1] Department of Respiratory and Critical Care Medicine, Tongji Hospital, Tongji Medical College, Huazhong University of Science and Technology, Wuhan, China, [2] Department of Respiratory and Critical Care Medicine, Renmin Hospital of Wuhan University, Wuhan, China, [3] Department of Respiratory and Critical Care Medicine, Union Hospital, Tongji Medical College, Huazhong University of Science and Technology, Wuhan, China, [4] Department of Respiratory and Critical Care Medicine, The People's Hospital of China Three Gorges University, The First People's Hospital of Yichang, Yichang, China, [5] Department of Respiratory and Critical Care Medicine, Huangshi Central Hospital, Affiliated Hospital of Hubei Polytechnic University, Huangshi, China, [6] Department of Respiratory and Critical Care Medicine, Xiaogan Hospital Affiliated to Wuhan University of Science and Technology, The Central Hospital of Xiaogan, Xiaogan, China, [7] Department of Respiratory Medicine, Suizhou Hospital, Hubei University of Medicine, Suizhou, China, [8] Department of Respiratory and Critical Care Medicine, The Central Hospital of Enshi Tujia and Miao Autonmous Prefecture, Enshi Clinical College of Wuhan University, Enshi Tujia and Miao Autonomous Prefecture, Hubei, China, [9] Department of Respiratory and Critical Care Medicine, Hanyang Hospital Affiliated to Wuhan University of Science and Technology, Wuhan, China, [10] Department of Respiratory and Critical Care Medicine, Wuhan Third Hospital, Tongren Hospital of Wuhan University, Wuhan, China, [11] Department of Respiratory and Critical Care Medicine, The First College of Clinical Medicine Science, China Three Gorges University, Yichang Central People's Hospital, Yichang, China, [12] Department of Respiratory and Critical Care Medicine, The First People's Hospital of Jingzhou, Jingzhou, China, [13] Department of Respiratory and Critical Care Medicine, The Sixth Hospital of Wuhan, Jianghan University, Wuhan, China, [14] Department of Respiratory and Critical Care Medicine, The Central Hospital of Wuhan, Tongji Medical College, Huazhong University of Science and Technology, Wuhan, China, [15] Department of Respiratory and Critical Medical, Taihe Hospital, Affiliated Hospital of Hubei University of Medicine, Shiyan, China

***Correspondence:**
Huiguo Liu
huiguol@163.com

Patients with acute exacerbations of chronic obstructive pulmonary disease (AECOPD) were treated with immediate or sequential withdrawal after 5 days of systemic glucocorticoids. The effects of the two withdrawal methods on the prognosis of patients were compared at 30, 90, 180, and 360 days after discharge. A multicenter, randomized, double-blind, parallel-controlled, open-label study was conducted in the respiratory department of tertiary hospitals in Central China. Patients met inclusion criteria for AECOPD and needed to use systemic glucocorticoids. They were randomly assigned to immediate and sequential withdrawal groups at a 1:1 ratio. The study was completed in August 2020 and is registered at the China Clinical Trials Registry (Chictr.org) (ChiCTR1800018894). According to general data and clinical characteristics, there were no statistically significant differences between the 329 patients in the immediate withdrawal group and the 310 patients in the sequential withdrawal group ($P > 0.05$). At the 30, 90, 180, and 360-days follow-up, the acute exacerbation frequency, rehospitalization rate, mortality, and intensive care unit (ICU) treatment rate were not significantly different between the immediate withdrawal group and sequential withdrawal group ($P > 0.05$). The modified Medical Research Council (mMRC) and COPD assessment test (CAT) scores were also not significantly different between the two groups. At the 180- and 360-day follow-up, forced expiratory volume in 1 s (FEV1%) and peak expiratory flow (PEF) were not significantly different between the two groups ($P > 0.05$). The time from discharge to first acute exacerbation was significantly lower in the immediate withdrawal group (46.12 days) than in sequential withdrawal group (49.02 days) ($P < 0.05$). The time of stay in the hospital for the first time after discharge was not significantly different between the two groups ($P > 0.05$). Adverse events were not significantly different between the immediate withdrawal group and sequential withdrawal group ($P < 0.05$). Subgroup analysis was performed according to age, degree of disease, and relevant indicators. At the 30-day follow-up, the acute exacerbation frequency of patients with advanced age, high global strategy for chronic obstructive lung disease (GOLD), and high fractional exhaled nitric oxide was significantly higher in the immediate withdrawal group than in the sequential withdrawal group ($P < 0.05$). In addition, according to receiver operating characteristic (ROC) curve analysis, the frequency of acute exacerbations at the 30-day follow-up was significantly higher in patients with age > 63.5 years or GOLD > 3 in the immediate withdrawal group than in the sequential withdrawal group, suggesting that the short-term efficacy was poor.

Keywords: glucocorticoids, immediately withdrawal, sequential withdrawal, acute exacerbations of chronic obstructive pulmonary disease, prognosis, methyl predrone, Central China

INTRODUCTION

Chronic obstructive pulmonary disease (COPD) is a chronic, non-specific disease in which inflammation of the airways activates inflammatory epithelial and smooth muscle cells and the release of inflammatory mediators (Doumas et al., 2020). Considering its high rates of morbidity and disability, COPD can pose a serious threat to human health (Rabe et al., 2020). Acute exacerbations of chronic obstructive pulmonary disease (AECOPD) occur when COPD patients show rapid changes within a short period (Vermeersch et al., 2019), with obvious aggravation of clinical symptoms such as cough, sputum production, dyspnea, and shortness of breath. In the absence of timely treatment, the life of the patient may be in jeopardy (Berenyi et al., 2020).

The Global Strategy for Chronic Obstructive Lung Disease (GOLD) guide indicates that glucocorticoids can shorten recovery time and improve lung function and hypoxia during acute exacerbations, in addition to reducing the risk of recurrence and disease progression (Burns et al., 2020). However, the long-term use of glucocorticoids causes a variety of adverse events, such as hyperglycemia, necrosis of the femoral head, reduction in immunity, and increased risk of infection (Lucafo et al., 2020). The GOLD guide recommends methyl prednisone at 40 mg/d for 5 days in cases of AECOPD (Leuppi et al., 2013). The United Kingdom National Institute for Health and Care Excellence (NICE) recommended that COPD be treated with systemic glucocorticoids for 7–14 days (National Collaborating Centre for Chronic, 2004). The Australian and New Zealand guidelines for the diagnosis and treatment of COPD recommend an optimal course of systemic glucocorticoids for 10–14 days (McKenzie et al., 2003). Thus, there is still no consensus on the treatment time and dose of systemic glucocorticoids in the treatment of AECOPD. In this study, a randomized controlled trial was used to compare the short-term efficacy and long-term prognosis of immediate and sequential withdrawal of methyl prednisone treatment of AECOPD.

MATERIALS AND METHODS

Study Design and Subjects

A multicenter, randomized, double-blind, parallel-controlled study was conducted in tertiary hospitals in Central China to compare the effects of systemic glucocorticoid immediate or sequential withdrawal on the prognosis of AECOPD patients at 30, 90, 180, and 360 days after discharge. Patients admitted from July 2017 to August 2019 were randomly assigned to the immediate and sequential withdrawal groups at a 1:1 ratio. Patients in the immediate withdrawal group received intravenous injections of methyl predrone at 40 mg/d for five consecutive days, then withdrawal on day six. Patients in the sequential withdrawal group received the same 5-day treatment, but the dose was reduced to 30 mg/d on days six and seven, to 20 mg/d on days eight and nine, and then stopped completely on day 10. The immediate group received the same amount of saline injection as the sequential withdrawal group from 6 to 10 days. To evaluate the efficacy and prognosis of the two treatment regiments, patient follow-ups were conducted for 1 year from the discharge date. The competent authorities of participating hospitals and the Medical Ethics Committee of Tongji Medical College of Huazhong University of Science and Technology approved the study (2018-S301). The study is registered at the China Clinical Trials Registry (Chictr.org) (ChiCTR1800018894).

All patients agreed to participate in the study and signed the informed consent. The inclusion criteria were as follows: (1) age between 40 years and 70 years; (2) diagnosis of AECOPD: sudden changes in clinical symptoms, including dyspnea, cough, and expectoration of sputum; (3) COPD beyond the range of daily variation; (4) pulmonary function examination indicating that forced expiratory volume in 1 s (FEV1%) < 0.70 after previous use of a bronchodilator. Patients suffering from the following diseases or lesions were excluded: (1) those critically ill patients with assisted respiratory muscle involvement in respiratory movement, thoracic and abdominal contradictory breathing, cyanosis, or need for invasive mechanical ventilation; (2) those with edema, right heart failure, or hemodynamic instability; (3) those with changes in mental state; (4) those with malignant tumors or other serious diseases.

Randomization, Double Blindness, and Follow-ups

The study leader LHG placed the subjects in order of inclusion in either the sequential withdrawal or the immediate withdrawal group. The study leader did not participate in subject recruitment and kept the randomization form confidential. Since the subjects signed the consent form, the researchers and the subjects were informed of the grouping.

Baseline measurements were taken on the day of recruitment, and clinical symptoms were assessed daily during hospitalization (cough assessment score, sputum viscosity, sputum volume, mMRC score). Discharge decisions were made by the attending physician. Clinical symptoms, mMRC score, and CAT score were assessed on days 30, 90, 180, and 360 after discharge, with the frequency of acute exacerbations from the last follow-up recorded. Pulmonary function (FEV1%,PEF) was measured on days 180 and 360 after discharge. There was a focus on adverse events (hypertension, kidney injury, electrolyte disturbance, infection, edema, plasma glucose, and osteoporosis) during and after therapy.

Endpoints

The primary endpoint was the frequency of acute exacerbations at 30, 90, 180, and 360 days after discharge. The key secondary endpoint was mortality. Other secondary endpoints were the mMRC score, CAT score, rehospitalization rate, and ICU treatment rate at 30, 90, 180, and 360 days after discharge and FEV1% and PEF at 180 and 360 days after discharge.

Statistical Analyses

Categorical variables were presented as numbers (percentages) and analyzed using a chi-squared test or Fisher's exact test. Continuous variables with a normal distribution were expressed as the mean ± standard deviation and analyzed using the independent samples *t*-test, whereas those with a skewed distribution were shown as the median (Q_1, Q_3) and analyzed using the Mann–Whitney U test. COX regression analyses were adopted to identify risk factors of prognosis. Receiver operating characteristic (ROC) curves were used to calculate the area under the curve (AUC) of a single continuous variable and the cutoff value. The SPSS software v 25.0 (SPSS Inc., Chicago, IL, United States) was used for statistical analyses. Differences at $P < 0.05$ (two-sided) were considered statistically significant.

RESULTS

General Data and Clinical Characteristics

Trial participant assignment to immediate and sequential withdrawal groups, and inclusion in follow-ups are shown in **Figure 1**. There were 639 COPD patients, including 349 males and 290 females. The average age was 61.02 years, and the average body mass index was 26.03. There were 230 patients that had smoked in the past and 62 patients that were smoking at the time of the study, with 14.93 years being the average time of smoking. Forty-nine cases had COPD exacerbations more than three times in the previous year. Fifteen cases had a history of exposure to biofuels. Among these indicators, there were no statistically significant differences between the immediate and sequential withdrawal group ($P > 0.05$). In addition, the Charlson comorbidity index, admission characteristics, pulmonary function indicators, GOLD grade, mMRC score, CAT score, laboratory indicators, and use of home oxygen therapy were not significantly different between the two groups ($P > 0.05$). We focus on hypertension,kidney injury,electrolyte disturbance, infection, edema, plasma glucose, and osteoporosis in this study, but there were no statistically significant differences between the immediate withdrawal group and sequential withdrawal group ($P > 0.05$, **Table 1**).

Endpoints

The primary endpoint was the frequency of acute exacerbations in the follow-ups at 30, 90, 180, and 360 days after discharge. The frequency of acute exacerbations was not significantly different between immediate and sequential withdrawal groups at 30, 90, 180, and 360 days after discharge ($P > 0.05$, **Figure 2**).

The key secondary endpoint was mortality. Mortality was not significantly different between immediate and sequential withdrawal groups at 30, 90, 180, and 360 days ($P > 0.05$). The other secondary endpoints were mMRC score, CAT score, admission rate, and ICU treatment rate at 30, 90, 180, and 360 days after discharge and FEV1% and PEF at 180 and 360 days

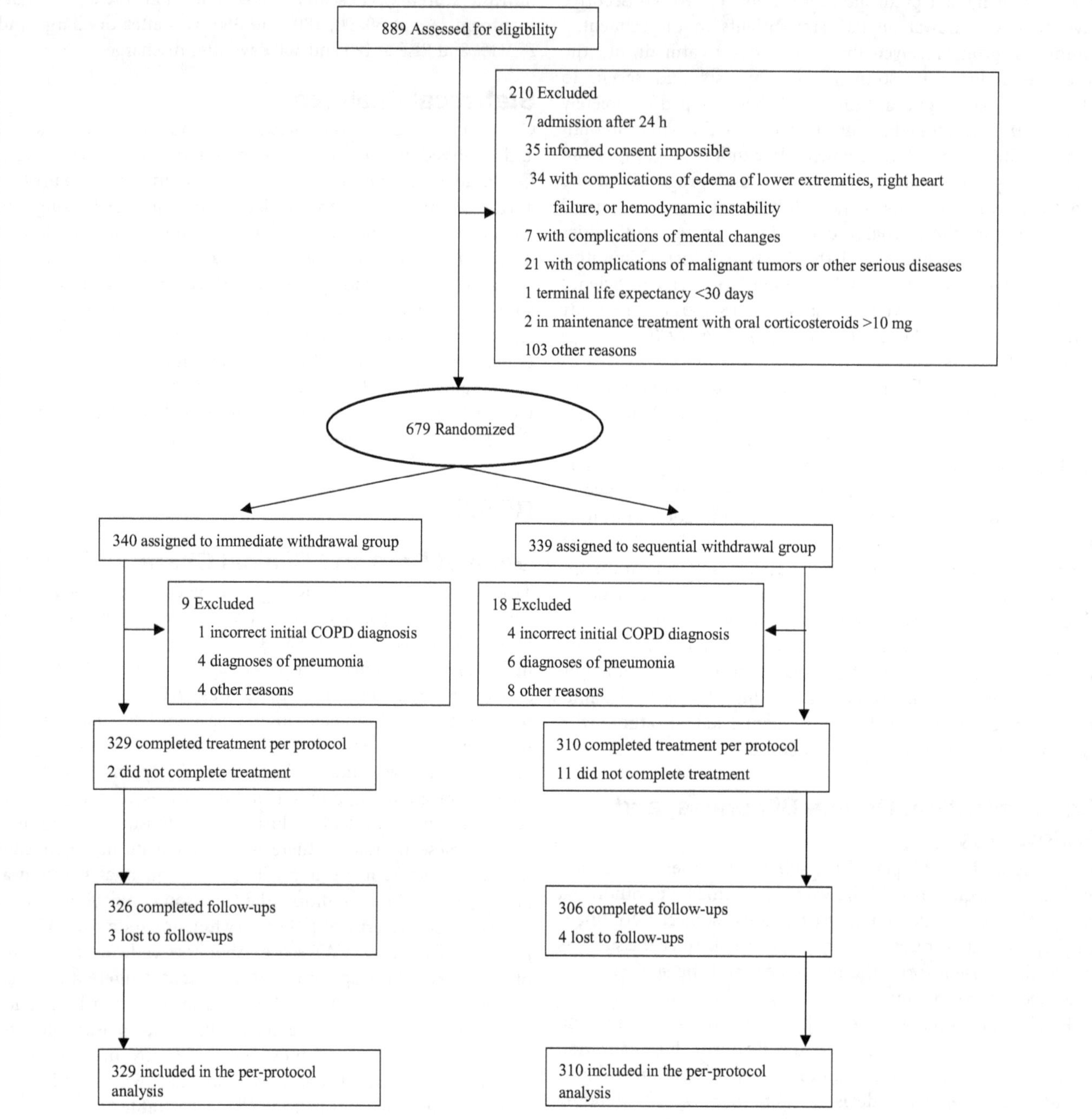

FIGURE 1 | Trial participant enrollment, assignment to immediate and sequential withdrawal groups, and inclusion in follow-ups.

after discharge. There were no statistically significant differences in these indicators between the two groups ($P > 0.05$). The time from discharge to first acute exacerbation was significantly lower in the immediate withdrawal group (46.12 days) than in the sequential withdrawal group (49.02 days) ($P < 0.05$). The time of stay in the hospital for the first time after discharge was longer in the immediate withdrawal group (6.28 days) than in the sequential withdrawal group (6.17 days), but the difference was not statistically significant ($P > 0.05$, **Table 2**).

Subgroup Analysis

Subgroup Analysis at the 30-day Follow-Up

Prognostic evaluation was defined according to acute exacerbation frequency in the follow-up at 30 days after discharge. Subgroup analysis was performed according to the history of frequent acute exacerbations, C-reactive protein (CRP), eosinophils, fractional exhaled nitric oxide (FeNO), GOLD grade, and age (**Figure 3**). In patients with either frequent or infrequent acute exacerbation history, high CRP or low CRP,

TABLE 1 | Baseline characteristics of the intention-to-treat population.

Items	Total ($n = 639$)	Immediate withdrawal ($n = 329$)	Sequential withdrawal ($n = 310$)	Statistic	P
Age (y)	61.02 ± 0.19	61.19 ± 0.28	60.87 ± 0.27	0.802*	0.423
Sex					
Male	349 (54.6)	177 (53.8)	172 (55.5)	0.183†	0.669
Female	290 (45.4)	152 (46.2)	138 (44.5)		
BMI	26.30 ± 0.18	26.00 ± 0.26	26.61 ± 0.27	1.597*	0.111
Smokers					
Never	347 (54.3)	178 (54.1)	169 (54.5)	0.779†	0.677
Past	230 (36.0)	122 (37.1)	108 (34.8)		
Current	62 (9.7)	29 (8.8)	33 (10.7)		
Pack-years smoked (y)	14.93 ± 0.48	14.85 ± 0.70	15.01 ± 0.65	0.167*	0.868
Course of COPD (y)	3.38 ± 0.06	3.38 ± 0.08	3.36 ± 0.09	0.217*	0.829
Number of AECOPD in previous year				2.837†	0.586
0	45 (7.0)	24 (7.3)	21 (6.8)		
1	74 (11.6)	41 (12.5)	33 (10.6)		
2	292 (45.7)	156 (47.4)	136 (43.9)		
3	179 (28.0)	83 (25.2)	96 (31.0)		
> 3	49 (7.7)	25 (7.6)	24 (7.7)		
History of biofuel use	15 (2.3)	6 (1.8)	9 (2.9)	0.811†	0.368
Charlson comorbidity index	2.86 ± 0.03	2.87 ± 0.04	2.86 ± 0.05	0.834*	0.834
Admission presentation					
Cough symptom score	2.05 ± 0.04	2.09 ± 0.05	2.01 ± 0.04	1.207*	0.228
Sputum viscosity	1.98 ± 0.03	2.02 ± 0.06	1.92 ± 0.05	1.393*	0.164
Sputum volume	1.66 ± 0.02	1.62 ± 0.03	1.70 ± 0.04	1.195*	0.232
Pulmonary function					
FEV1%	60.34 ± 0.27	59.99 ± 0.40	60.71 ± 0.35	1.360*	0.174
PEF	7.76 ± 0.08	7.62 ± 0.11	7.91 ± 0.10	1.852*	0.065
GOLD				7.273†	0.064
GOLD1	30 (4.6)	14 (4.3)	16 (5.2)		
GOLD2	229 (35.9)	105 (31.9)	124 (40.0)		
GOLD3	275 (43.0)	158 (48.0)	117 (37.7)		
GOLD4	105 (16.5)	52 (15.8)	53 (17.1)		
mMRC score	1.99 ± 0.03	1.96 ± 0.04	2.03 ± 0.05	0.997*	0.319
CAT score	18.21 ± 0.29	18.11 ± 1.15	17.18 ± 0.46	0.814*	0.416
Laboratory					
Leucocytes (10^9/L)	6.83 ± 0.11	6.66 ± 0.16	7.02 ± 0.14	1.687*	0.092
Eosinophils (10^9/L)	0.55 ± 0.05	0.55 ± 0.03	0.56 ± 0.11	0.129*	0.897
C-reactive protein (mg/L)	2.50 ± 0.16	2.22 ± 0.18	2.69 ± 0.24	1.475*	0.141
FeNO	29.62 ± 0.71	31.05 ± 1.08	28.10 ± 0.91	0.454*	0.224
$PaCO_2$ (kPa)	40.32 ± 0.31	39.91 ± 0.401	40.92 ± 0.50	1.589*	0.114
PaO_2 (kPa)	66.82 ± 1.35	67.11 ± 1.95	66.38 ± 1.73	0.265*	0.791
Home oxygen therapy	76 (11.9)	34 (10.3)	42 (13.5)	1.573*	0.209
Clinical findings					
Diastolic blood pressure (mm Hg)	79 ± 0.36	78 ± 0.56	80 ± 0.44	1.273*	0.204
Systolic blood pressure (mm Hg)	116 ± 0.32	116 ± 0.42	117 ± 0.49	1.168*	0.243
Heart rate (beats/min)	92 ± 0.47	91 ± 0.67	92 ± 0.46	0.659*	0.510
Oxygen saturation (%)	94 ± 0.24	94 ± 0.39	95 ± 0.27	1.931*	0.054
Respiratory rate (breaths/min)	21 ± 0.71	21 ± 0.34	20 ± 0.35	0.863*	0.389
Adverse events					
Hypertension	0	0	0	–	–
Electrolyte disturbance	3 (0.5)	2 (0.6)	1 (0.3)	0.278†	0.598
Kidney injury	0	0	0	–	–

(Continued)

TABLE 1 | Continued

Items	Total ($n = 639$)	Immediate withdrawal ($n = 329$)	Sequential withdrawal ($n = 310$)	Statistic	*P*
Infection	0	0	0	–	–
Edema	4 (0.6)	1 (0.3)	3 (1.0)	1.131†	0.287
Elevated plasma glucose	6 (0.9)	2 (0.6)	4 (1.3)	0.667†	0.414
Osteoporosis	0	0	0	–	–

*Data are shown as the mean ± standard deviation or n (%). *t-test; †χ^2-value. BMI, Body Mass Index; COPD, chronic obstructive pulmonary disease; AECOPD, acute exacerbation of chronic obstructive pulmonary disease; FEV1, forced expiratory volume in 1 s; PEF, peak expiratory flow; GOLD, global initiative for chronic obstructive lung disease;mMRC, Modified Medical Research Council Dyspnea Scale; CAT, COPD Assessment Test; FeNO, Fractional exhaled nitric oxide; PaO_2, partial pressure of oxygen; $PaCO_2$, partial pressure of carbon dioxide. Degree of sputum viscosity: (1), sputum clings to the wall of phlegm cup during rotation; (2), sputum slides slowly along the wall of phlegm cup during rotation; (3), sputum can be poured out quickly but some remains attached to the wall of phlegm cup; (4), sputum can be poured out quickly and completely. Sputum volume: 1, mild, with less than 10 mL/day; 2, moderate, with 10–150 mL/day; 3, severe, with more than 150 mL/day.*

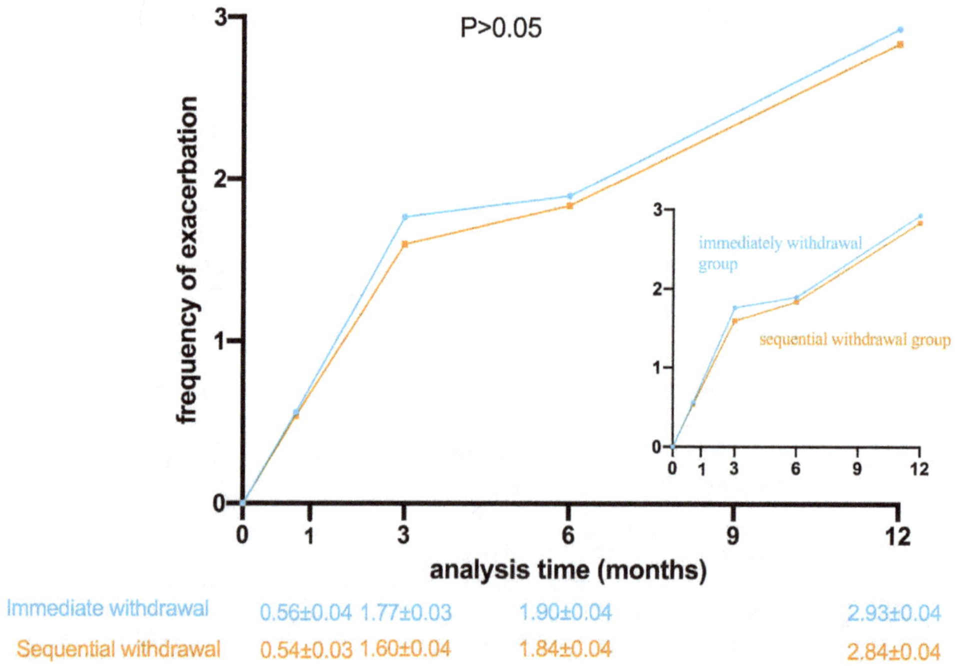

FIGURE 2 | Frequency of acute exacerbations in the immediate withdrawal group and the sequential withdrawal group with time following discharge. ($P > 0.05$).

high eosinophils or low eosinophils, there was no statistically significant difference in acute exacerbation frequency between immediate and sequential withdrawal groups at the 30-day follow-up ($P > 0.05$). Although the acute exacerbation frequency of patients with high FeNO showed no statistically significant difference between the two groups ($P > 0.05$), in patients with low FeNO, the difference was significant between immediate and sequential withdrawal groups ($P < 0.05$). Although the acute exacerbation frequency of patients with a low GOLD grade was not different between the two withdrawal groups, in patients with a high GOLD grade, the difference was significant between immediate and sequential withdrawal groups at the 30-day follow-up ($P < 0.05$). The acute exacerbation frequency in patients with age ≤ 59 years showed no statistically significant difference between the immediate and sequential withdrawal groups ($P > 0.05$). However, in patients with age > 59 years, the difference between withdrawal methods was significant ($P < 0.05$). Thus, the results of the 30-day follow-up show acute exacerbation frequency in patients with advanced age, high GOLD grade, and low FeNO, and was significantly higher in the immediate withdrawal group than in the sequential withdrawal group ($P < 0.05$, **Figure 3**).

Subgroup Analysis at the 360-day Follow-up

Prognostic evaluation was defined according to acute exacerbation frequency in the follow-up at 360 days. Subgroup analysis was performed according to the history of frequent acute exacerbations, CRP, eosinophils, FeNO, GOLD grade, and age (**Figure 4**). In patients with a history of either previous frequent aggravation or infrequent aggravation, there was no statistically significant difference in acute exacerbation frequency between immediate and sequential withdrawal groups at the 360-day follow-up ($P > 0.05$). Similarly, in patients with either high or low CRP, high or low eosinophils, high or low FeNO, high or low GOLD grade, age ≤ 59 years or age > 59 years, there was no statistically significant difference

TABLE 2 | Secondary endpoints.

	Visit time (days)	Immediate withdrawal group	Sequential withdrawal group	Statistic	*P*-value
Key secondary endpoint					
Mortality	30	0	0	–	–
	90	3 (0.9)	3 (1)	0.073*	0.942
	180	5 (1.5)	6 (1.9)	1.163†	0.686
	360	7 (2.1)	8 (2.6)	0.143†	0.705
Other secondary endpoints					
mMRC score	30	1.97 ± 0.05	1.99 ± 0.05	0.380‡	0.704
	90	2.01 ± 0.05	2.06 ± 0.05	0.679‡	0.497
	180	1.95 ± 0.04	2.08 ± 0.05	1.923‡	0.055
	360	1.96 ± 0.05	2.04 ± 0.05	0.997‡	0.319
CAT score	30	18.93 ± 0.38	17.15 ± 0.44	3.045‡	0.770
	90	19.31 ± 0.37	17.61 ± 0.45	2.875‡	0.841
	180	19.04 ± 0.36	17.35 ± 0.47	2.854‡	0.312
	360	19.09 ± 0.36	17.66 ± 0.49	2.354‡	0.162
Rehospitalization rate	30	63 (19.1)	44 (14.2)	2.811†	0.094
	90	107 (32.5)	90 (29.0)	0.912†	0.339
	180	123 (37.4)	132 (42.6)	1.796†	0.180
	360	144 (43.8)	145 (46.8)	0.582†	0.446
ICU treatment rate	30	3 (0.9)	6 (1.9)	1.097*	0.328
	90	12 (3.6)	15 (4.8)	0.559†	0.454
	180	25 (7.6)	26 (8.4)	0.135†	0.713
	360	47 (14.3)	45 (14.5)	0.007†	0.934
FEV1%	180	61.00 ± 0.48	61.80 ± 0.42	1.501‡	0.134
	360	62.92 ± 0.51	61.57 ± 0.47	1.665‡	0.097
PEF	180	7.54 ± 0.11	7.89 ± 0.14	1.263‡	0.207
	360	7.73 ± 0.15	7.89 ± 0.14	1.075‡	0.283
Time from discharge to first acute exacerbation	–	46.12 ± 1.28	49.02 ± 1.33	0.489‡	0.030
Time of stay in hospital for the first time after discharge	–	6.28 ± 0.07	6.17 ± 0.05	1.275‡	0.203

*Data are shown as the mean ± standard deviation or n (%). *Fisher's test; †χ^2-value; ‡t-test. mMRC, Modified Medical Research Council Dyspnea Scale; CAT, COPD Assessment Test; ICU, intensive-care unit; FEV1, forced expiratory volume in 1 s; PEF, peak expiratory flow.*

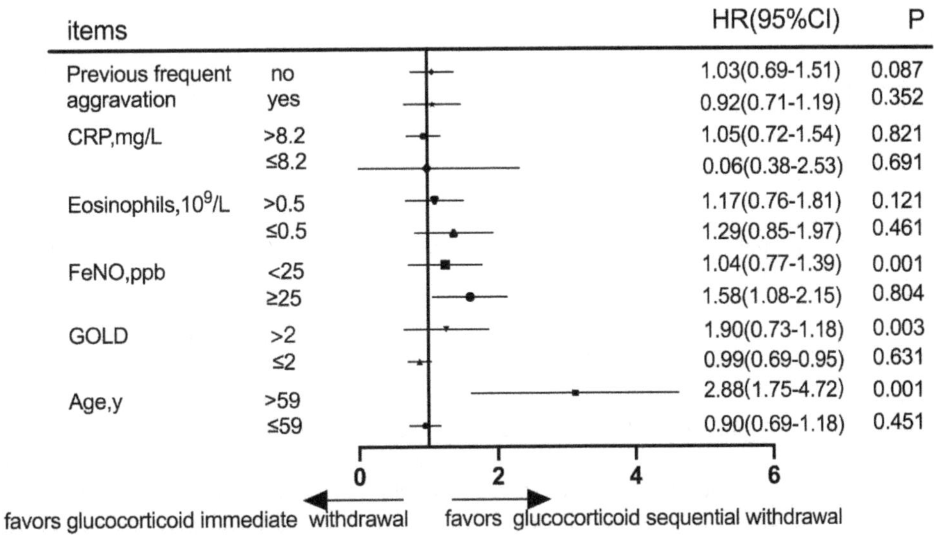

FIGURE 3 | Subgroup analysis according to previous frequent aggravation, CRP, eosinophils, FeNO, GOLD grade, and age at the 30-day follow-up. CRP, C-reactive protein; FeNO, Fractional exhaled nitric oxide; GOLD, global initiative for chronic obstructive lung disease.

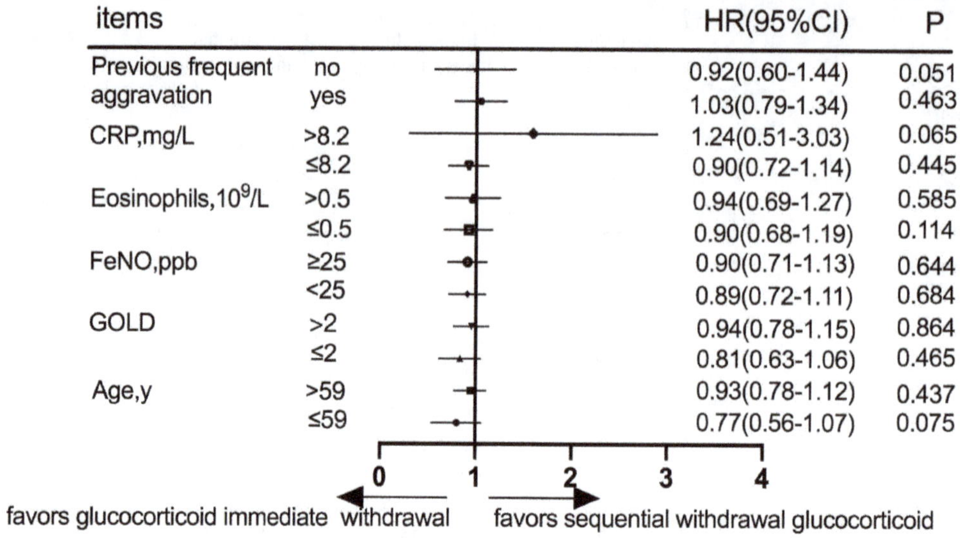

FIGURE 4 | Subgroup analysis according to previous frequent aggravation, CRP, eosinophils, FeNO, GOLD grade, and age at the 360-day follow-up. CRP, C-reactive protein; FeNO, Fractional exhaled nitric oxide; GOLD, global initiative for chronic obstructive lung disease.

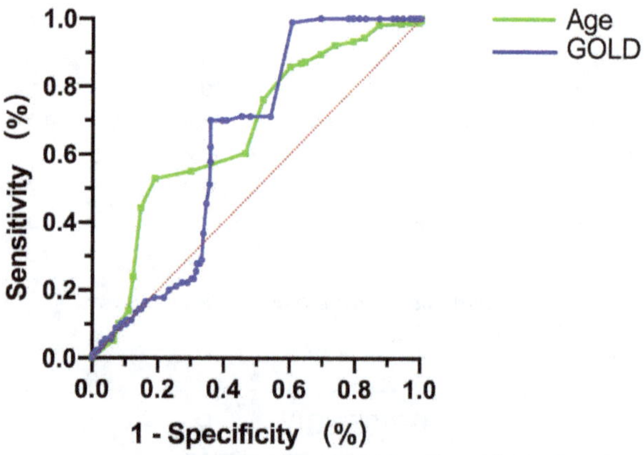

FIGURE 5 | Receiver operating characteristic curves for age and GOLD in the diagnosis of short-term efficacy.

in acute exacerbation frequency between immediate and sequential withdrawal groups at the 360-day follow-up ($P > 0.05$, **Figure 4**).

Efficacy Analysis of Each Indicator at the 30-day Follow-up

Subgroup analysis showed that different ages, GOLD grading, and FeNO values could affect short-term efficacy. ROC curve analysis was performed based on the significant index values (age, GOLD, FeNO) to analyze short-term efficacy. Although FeNO had no diagnostic value for short-term efficacy ($P > 0.05$), age and GOLD grading had diagnostic value in evaluating the short-term efficacy ($P < 0.05$). Thus, age > 63.5 years with an AUC = 0.668 (95%CI: 0.627–0.711) and GOLD > 3 with an AUC = 0.638 (95%CI: 0.586–0.689) were risk factors for short-term efficacy (**Figure 5** and **Table 3**).

DISCUSSION

The treatment goal for AECOPD is to minimize the adverse effects of the current deterioration of the disease as soon as possible and prevent the development of subsequent events (Zhang et al., 2020). Standardized diagnosis and treatment measures play an important role in the prognosis of patients. Current recommendations from the Global Initiative for Chronic Obstructive Lung Disease suggest that patients who continue to have exacerbations should initially step up to glucocorticoid therapy (Terry and Dhand, 2019, 2020). GOLD point out AECOPD treatment strategies: "A dose of 40 mg prednisone per day for 5 days is recommended." and "Intensified combination therapy with ICS/LABA for 10 days at Upper Respiratory Tract Infection onset could be associated with a reduction of exacerbations, particularly in patients with severe disease" (Singh et al., 2019). Immediate withdrawal for 5-days can reduce the treatment dose of glucocorticoid, but rapid withdrawal or dose reduction may result in a rebound effect, causing aggravation and deterioration of the original disease. Prolonged use of glucocorticoid can reverse severe illness and reduce the acute acerbation frequency in specific subgroups. some diseases, such as hypopituitarism, adrenocortical dysfunction, nephrotic syndrome, systemic lupus erythematosus, rheumatoid arthritis and other diseases need long-term use, or even lifelong use. long-term use of glucocorticoids may cause some adverse events, such as obesity, peptic ulcer, or even gastrointestinal bleeding, which can also cause high blood pressure, high plasma glucose, osteoporosis, and aseptic necrosis of the femoral head. In this study, a randomized controlled trial comparing the short-term

TABLE 3 | Efficacy analysis of each indicator at the 30-day follow-up.

Items	AUC (95%CI)	*P*-value	Cut-off	Sensitivity (%)	Specificity (%)	Yoden index
Age	0.668 (0.627–0.711)	0.001	63.5	52.81	81.96	0.347
GOLD	0.638 (0.586–0.689)	0.007	3	40.47	98.89	0.393
FeNO	0.541 (0.497–1.586)	0.067	/	/	/	/

efficacy and long-term prognosis of immediate and sequential withdrawal of methyl prednisone was performed.

The trial included more than 600 patients with COPD, and all patients were randomly assigned to either the immediate withdrawal group or the sequential withdrawal group. The general data were analyzed to ensure there were no statistically significant differences between the immediate and sequential withdrawal groups ($P > 0.05$). Follow-up results show the frequency of acute exacerbations had no statistically significant differences between the immediate and sequential withdrawal groups at 30, 90, 180, and 360 days after discharge ($P > 0.05$). The mMRC dyspnea score is a 5-point (0–4) scale based on the severity of dyspnea (Cheng et al., 2019), and the CAT score is a patient-completed instrument used to assess and quantify health-related quality of life and symptom burden in COPD patients (Jones et al., 2009). As indicators of prognosis, mMRC and CAT scores were not statistically significant difference between the immediate and sequential withdrawal groups during follow-up ($P > 0.05$). The 2011 GOLD consensus report uses symptoms, exacerbation history, and FEV1% to improve the clinical assessment and to guide treatment of COPD patients (Vestbo et al., 2012). In this study, there were no statistically significant differences in FEV1% and PEF between immediate and sequential withdrawal groups at 180 and 360 days ($P > 0.05$). The time from discharge to first acute exacerbation was significantly lower ($P < 0.05$) in the immediate withdrawal group (46.12 days) than in the sequential withdrawal group (49.02 days), indicating that sequential withdrawal of glucocorticoid can hold a longer disease stabilization time.

Different studies recommend different durations of glucocorticoid application, Yii et al. (2019) found that a history of frequent acute exacerbations is a strong and independent predictor of prognosis. In addition, the history of exacerbations is independent of severe exacerbations (Han et al., 2017). Moreover, Motegi et al. (2013) found that no index was significantly better than history of exacerbation alone to predict future exacerbations. In this study, subgroup analysis was performed according to the history of frequent acute exacerbation, but there was no statistically significant difference between the two withdrawal groups ($P > 0.05$).

The CRP is a type of acute protein that increases sharply in the plasma when the body is infected or damaged (Aksu et al., 2013). It can activate, complement, and enhance phagocytosis of phagocytes and play a regulatory role in clearing invading pathogenic microorganisms and injured, necrotic, and apoptotic cells (Sacks, 2019). The value of CRP as a prognostic biomarker in AECOPD patients has been extensively investigated (Sneh et al., 2020). The association of blood eosinophil levels with rehospitalization rates is a question that remains to be answered: some studies show increased rehospitalizations (Vedel-Krogh et al., 2016; Couillard et al., 2017), whereas others find no significant effect (Bafadhel et al., 2016). In this study, subgroup analysis was performed according to CRP and eosinophils, but there was no statistically significant difference between the two methods of withdrawal ($P > 0.05$). This result might be due to CRP having a half-life of 19 h and therefore there is no significant difference in a long-term follow-up. Thus, the study was expanded to identify the relevant indicators. The GOLD was developed to spread awareness of COPD as a major public health problem and facilitate its prevention and treatment (Nowak et al., 2020). To explore the effect of the GOLD on patient prognosis, patients were divided into high or low GOLD grade groups, and the difference was significant ($P < 0.05$). The GOLD attempts to promote spirometry not only as a case-finding and prognostication tool for airflow obstruction but also as a marker for good health (Bhatt et al., 2019). According to this study, patients with an elevated GOLD grade should be treated with sequential withdrawal.

The FeNO measurement was considered to be a biomarker for airway eosinophilic inflammation (Zhou et al., 2020), because its concentration is highly correlated with the number of inflammatory cells (Hogman et al., 2019). In this study, subgroup analysis was performed according to FeNO, and the difference was not statistically significant ($P > 0.05$). FeNO is significantly elevated in asthmatic patients (Heaney et al., 2019), and FeNO values in stable COPD patients were slightly higher than those in healthy individuals (Matsunaga et al., 2020). The relationship between FeNO and AECOPD needs to be explored further. The elderly are the main patients with chronic diseases (Zhou et al., 2019), COPD is one of the major chronic diseases. In this study, subgroup analysis was performed according to age, and the difference was significant ($P < 0.05$). The ROC curve analysis showed sequential withdrawal at age > 59 years could decrease acute exacerbation frequency at the 30-day follow-up. Elderly patients are likely to have many complications that affect treatment (Rydberg et al., 2020). Clinicians should consider increasing age as a key risk factor in the management of COPD and develop correct treatment to improve the therapeutic effect (Stone et al., 2012). Because there was no consensus for the time and dose of systemic glucocorticoids in treating AECOPD, they should be explored in further studies.

The study had some deficiencies: (1) although the study was a randomized, double-blind, controlled trial, the open labeling might have affected clinical decisions and outcome endpoints; (2) the number of patients were insufficient to distinguish causes of death, and mortality assessment was not targeted, therefore, adverse reactions of glucocorticoid therapy might not have been detected.

CONCLUSION

In this study, the glucocorticoid schemes for AECOPD treatment were analyzed. sequential withdrawal of glucocorticoid can hold a longer disease stabilization time. The frequency of acute exacerbations at the 30-day follow-up was significantly higher in patients with age > 63.5 years or GOLD > 3 in the immediate withdrawal group than in the sequential withdrawal group, suggesting that the short-term efficacy was poor. AECOPD patients who are elderly or with a high GOLD grade should be treated with glucocorticoid sequential withdrawal to reduce the acute exacerbation frequency of the 30-day follow-up.

AUTHOR CONTRIBUTIONS

All authors contributed to data analysis, drafting or revising the article, gave final approval of the version to be published, and agreed to be accountable for all aspects of the work.

REFERENCES

Aksu, F., Capan, N., Aksu, K., Ofluoglu, R., Canbakan, S., Yavuz, B., et al. (2013). C-reactive protein levels are raised in stable Chronic obstructive pulmonary disease patients independent of smoking behavior and biomass exposure. *J. Thorac. Dis.* 5, 414–421.

Bafadhel, M., Greening, N. J., Harvey-Dunstan, T. C., Williams, J. E., Morgan, M. D., Brightling, C. E., et al. (2016). Blood eosinophils and outcomes in severe hospitalized exacerbations of COPD. *Chest* 150, 320–328. doi: 10.1016/j.chest.2016.01.026

Berenyi, F., Steinfort, D. P., Abdelhamid, Y. A., Bailey, M. J., Pilcher, D. V., Bellomo, R., et al. (2020). Characteristics and outcomes of critically Ill patients with acute exacerbation of Chronic obstructive pulmonary disease in Australia and New Zealand. *Ann. Am. Thorac. Soc.* 17, 736–745. doi: 10.1513/annalsats.201911-821oc

Bhatt, S. P., Balte, P. P., Schwartz, J. E., Cassano, P. A., Couper, D., Jacobs, D. R., et al. (2019). Discriminative accuracy of FEV1:FVC thresholds for COPD-related hospitalization and mortality. *JAMA* 321, 2438–2447. doi: 10.1001/jama.2019.7233

Burns, R. B., Anandaiah, A., Rice, M. B., and Smetana, G. W. (2020). Should you recommend inhaled corticosteroids for this patient with chronic obstructive pulmonary disease: grand rounds discussion from Beth Israel deaconess medical center. *Ann. Intern. Med.* 172, 735–742. doi: 10.7326/m20-1058

Cheng, S. L., Lin, C. H., Wang, C. C., Chan, M. C., Hsu, J. Y., Hang, L. W., et al. (2019). Comparison between COPD assessment test (CAT) and modified medical research council (mMRC) dyspnea scores for evaluation of clinical symptoms, comorbidities and medical resources utilization in COPD patients. *J. Formos. Med. Assoc.* 118, 429–435. doi: 10.1016/j.jfma.2018.06.018

Couillard, S., Larivee, P., Courteau, J., and Vanasse, A. (2017). Eosinophils in COPD exacerbations are associated with increased readmissions. *Chest* 151, 366–373. doi: 10.1016/j.chest.2016.10.003

Doumas, M., Imprialos, K. P., and Stavropoulos, K. (2020). Metoprolol for the prevention of exacerbations of COPD. *N. Engl. J. Med.* 382, 1374–1375. doi: 10.1056/nejmc2000638

Han, M. K., Quibrera, P. M., Carretta, E. E., Barr, R. G., Bleecker, E. R., Bowler, R. P., et al. (2017). Frequency of exacerbations in patients with chronic obstructive pulmonary disease: an analysis of the SPIROMICS cohort. *Lancet Respir. Med.* 5, 619–626.

Heaney, L. G., Busby, J., Bradding, P., Chaudhuri, R., Mansur, A. H., Niven, R., et al. (2019). Remotely monitored therapy and Nitric Oxide suppression identifies nonadherence in severe asthma. *Am. J. Respir. Crit. Care Med.* 199, 454–464. doi: 10.1164/rccm.201806-1182oc

Hogman, M., Thornadtsson, A., Broms, K., Janson, C., Lisspers, K., Stallberg, B., et al. (2019). Different relationships between FENO and COPD characteristics in smokers and Ex-Smokers. *COPD* 16, 227–233. doi: 10.1080/15412555.2019.1638355

Jones, P. W., Harding, G., Berry, P., Wiklund, I., Chen, W. H., and Kline Leidy, N. (2009). Development and first validation of the COPD assessment test. *Eur. Respir. J.* 34, 648–654. doi: 10.1183/09031936.00102509

Leuppi, J. D., Schuetz, P., Bingisser, R., Bodmer, M., Briel, M., Drescher, T., et al. (2013). Short-term vs conventional glucocorticoid therapy in acute exacerbations of chronic obstructive pulmonary disease: the REDUCE randomized clinical trial. *JAMA* 309, 2223–2231. doi: 10.1001/jama.2013.5023

Lucafo, M., Franzin, M., Decorti, G., and Stocco, G. (2020). A patent review of anticancer glucocorticoid receptor modulators (2014-present). *Expert Opin. Ther. Pat.* 30, 313–324. doi: 10.1080/13543776.2020.1740206

Matsunaga, K., Kuwahira, I., Hanaoka, M., Saito, J., Tsuburai, T., Fukunaga, K., et al. (2020). An official JRS statement: the principles of fractional exhaled nitric oxide (FeNO) measurement and interpretation of the results in clinical practice. *Respir. Investig.* 59, 34–52. doi: 10.1016/j.resinv.2020.05.006

McKenzie, D. K., Frith, P. A., Burdon, J. G., Town, G. I., Australian Lung Foundation, Thoracic Society of Australia and New Zealand, et al. (2003). The COPDX plan: Australian and New Zealand guidelines for the management of Chronic obstructive pulmonary disease 2003. *Med. J. Aust.* 178, S1–S39.

Motegi, T., Jones, R. C., Ishii, T., Hattori, K., Kusunoki, Y., Furutate, R., et al. (2013). A comparison of three multidimensional indices of COPD severity as predictors of future exacerbations. *Int. J. Chron. Obstruct. Pulmon. Dis.* 8, 259–271. doi: 10.2147/COPD.S42769

National Collaborating Centre for Chronic (2004). Chronic obstructive pulmonary disease. national clinical guideline on management of chronic obstructive pulmonary disease in adults in primary and secondary care. *Thorax* 59(Suppl. 1), 1–232.

Nowak, M., Brozek, G. M., Zejda, J. E., Jankowski, M., and Pierzchala, W. (2020). Impact of changing GOLD guidelines (2007-2011-2017) on assignment of a COPD patient to disease severity category. *Postepy Dermatol. Alergol.* 37, 221–228. doi: 10.5114/ada.2018.79143

Rabe, K. F., Martinez, F. J., Ferguson, G. T., Wang, C., Singh, D., Wedzicha, J. A., et al. (2020). Triple inhaled therapy at two glucocorticoid doses in moderate-to-very-severe COPD. *N. Engl. J. Med.* 383, 35–48. doi: 10.1056/nejmoa1916046

Rydberg, D. M., Linder, M., Malmstrom, R. E., and Andersen, M. (2020). Risk factors for severe bleeding events during warfarin treatment: the influence of sex, age, comorbidity and co-medication. *Eur. J. Clin. Pharmacol.* 76, 867–876. doi: 10.1007/s00228-020-02856-6

Sacks, H. S. (2019). In primary care, CRP testing reduced antibiotic use in COPD exacerbations without worsening health. *Ann. Intern. Med.* 171:JC51.

Singh, D., Agusti, A., Anzueto, A., Barnes, P. J., Bourbeau, J., Celli, B. R., et al. (2019). Global strategy for the diagnosis, management, and prevention of Chronic obstructive lung disease: the GOLD science committee report 2019. *Eur. Respir. J.* 53:1900164.

Sneh, A., Pawan, T., Randeep, G., Anant, M., Mani, K., Hadda, V., et al. (2020). Acute phase proteins as predictors of survival in patients with acute exacerbation of Chronic obstructive pulmonary disease requiring mechanical ventilation. *COPD* 17, 22–28. doi: 10.1080/15412555.2019.1698019

Stone, R. A., Lowe, D., Potter, J. M., Buckingham, R. J., Roberts, C. M., and Pursey, N. J. (2012). Managing patients with COPD exacerbation: does age matter? *Age Ageing* 41, 461–468. doi: 10.1093/ageing/afs039

Terry, P. D., and Dhand, R. (2020). Inhalation therapy for stable COPD: 20 Years of GOLD reports. *Adv. Ther.* 37, 1812–1828. doi: 10.1007/s12325-020-01289-y

Vedel-Krogh, S., Nielsen, S. F., Lange, P., Vestbo, J., and Nordestgaard, B. G. (2016). Blood Eosinophils and Exacerbations in Chronic obstructive pulmonary disease. the Copenhagen general population study. *Am. J. Respir. Crit. Care Med.* 193, 965–974. doi: 10.1164/rccm.201509-1869oc

Vermeersch, K., Gabrovska, M., Aumann, J., Demedts, I. K., Corhay, J. L., Marchand, E., et al. (2019). Azithromycin during acute Chronic obstructive pulmonary disease exacerbations requiring hospitalization (BACE). a multicenter, randomized, double-blind, placebo-controlled trial. *Am. J. Respir. Crit. Care Med.* 200, 857–868. doi: 10.1164/rccm.201901-0094oc

Vestbo, J., Hurd, S. S., and Rodriguez-Roisin, R. (2012). The 2011 revision of the global strategy for the diagnosis, management and prevention of COPD (GOLD)-why and what? *Clin. Respir. J.* 6, 208–214. doi: 10.1111/crj.12002

Yii, A. C. A., Loh, C. H., Tiew, P. Y., Xu, H., Taha, A. A. M., Koh, J., et al. (2019). A clinical prediction model for hospitalized COPD exacerbations based on "treatable traits". *Int. J. Chron. Obstruct. Pulmon. Dis.* 14, 719–728. doi: 10.2147/COPD.S194922

Zhang, R., Zhu, J., Liu, Y., Li, Y., Liu, W., Zhang, M., et al. (2020). Optimization of Nebulized Budesonide in the treatment of Acute Exacerbation of Chronic obstructive pulmonary disease. *Int. J. Chron. Obstruct. Pulmon. Dis.* 15, 409–415. doi: 10.2147/copd.s235125

Zhou, A., Zhou, Z., Deng, D., Zhao, Y., Duan, J., Cheng, W., et al. (2020). The value of FENO measurement for predicting treatment response in patients with acute exacerbation of Chronic obstructive pulmonary disease. *Int. J. Chron. Obstruct. Pulmon. Dis.* 15, 2257–2266. doi: 10.2147/copd.s263673

Zhou, M., Wang, H., Zeng, X., Yin, P., Zhu, J., and Chen, W. (2019). Mortality, morbidity, and risk factors in China and its provinces, 1990-2017: a systematic analysis for the global burden of disease study 2017. *Lancet* 394, 1145–1158. doi: 10.1016/s0140-6736(19)30427-1

20

Environmental Risk Factors for Sarcoidosis

*Marc A. Judson**

Albany Medical College, Albany, NY, United States

Correspondence:
Marc A. Judson
judsonm@amc.edu

Sarcoidosis is a multisystem granulomatous disease that may affect any body organ. Sarcoidosis is associated with many environmental and occupational exposures. Because the exact immunopathogenesis of sarcoidosis is unknown, it is not known whether these exposures are truly causing sarcoidosis, rendering the immune system more susceptible to the development of sarcoidosis, exacerbating subclinical cases of sarcoidosis, or causing a granulomatous condition distinct from sarcoidosis. This manuscript outlines what is known about the immunopathogenesis of sarcoidosis and postulates mechanisms whereby these exposures could cause or exacerbate the disease. We also describe the varied environmental and occupational exposures that have been associated with sarcoidosis. This includes potential infectious exposures such as mycobacteria and Propionibacterium acnes, a skin commensal bacterium, as well as non-infectious environmental exposures including inhaled bioaerosols, metal dusts and products of combustion. Further insights concerning the relationship of environmental exposures to the development of sarcoidosis may have a major impact on the prevention and treatment of this enigmatic disease.

Keywords: sarcoidosis, antigen, environment, infection, immunity

INTRODUCTION

Sarcoidosis is a multisystem granulomatous disease of unknown cause. The lung is the most common organ involved with sarcoidosis at a frequency of ~90 percent (1, 2). The skin, eyes, peripheral lymph nodes and liver are also commonly involved (1, 2). Unlike sarcoidosis, the causes of many granulomatous diseases are known. Exposures that may cause granulomatous inflammation include mycobacteria and fungi that may cause granulomatous infection, (3, 4) bioaerosols including bird antigens that cause hypersensitivity pneumonitis (5) and metals including beryllium that causes chronic beryllium disease (CBD) (6). It is plausible that sarcoidosis is caused by one or several antigen exposures that initiates and possibly perpetuates the granulomatous process. Several environmental exposures have been linked to sarcoidosis. Because these exposures are disparate, they may lead to the development of sarcoidosis via different mechanisms; and in fact, it is possible that sarcoidosis represents a conglomeration of several dissimilar diseases ["the sarcoidoses" (7)]. This manuscript will explore environmental risk factors for sarcoidosis. We will briefly describe the potential role of environment antigens in leading to the granulomatous inflammation of sarcoidosis, and then focus on the available evidence supporting an association of specific environmental exposures with the development of sarcoidosis.

OVERVIEW OF IMMUNOPATHOGENESIS OF SARCOIDOSIS RELATIVE TO ENVIRONMENTAL RISK FACTORS

Environmental exposures are postulated to be associated with the development of sarcoidosis in four general ways. The first mechanism involves the detection and processing of antigen by antigen presenting cells such as macrophages and dendritic cells. These processed antigens are subsequently presented via human leukocyte antigen (HLA) Class II molecules to a restricted set of T-cell receptors on naive T lymphocytes that are primarily of the $CD4^+$ class (8). An interplay of antigen, HLA class II molecules, and T-cell receptors occurs at the HLA molecule binding site and is thought to be essential for sarcoidosis to develop (9). These events induce a polarization of the T lymphocytes to a Thl/Th17 phenotype, (10) followed by cellular recruitment, proliferation, and differentiation leading to formation of the sarcoid granuloma. This mechanism is thought to be common across most granulomatous lung diseases known to be caused by a specific antigen, and therefore it is possible that the immune system may not be dysregulated in this instance.

There is a large body of evidence to support this proposed mechanism for the immunopathogenesis of sarcoidosis. Various HLA gene alleles have been associated with development of sarcoidosis, (11, 12) protection from developing sarcoidosis, (11, 12) and specific disease phenotypes (11, 12). Further analyses have suggested that such HLA gene polymorphisms result in conformational changes in the antigen binding pockets of HLA molecules (13). Additional evidence supporting this proposed mechanism for sarcoidosis relates to CBD, a phenotypic mimic of sarcoidosis both radiographically and pathologically, (14, 15) which is associated with specific amino acid substitutions in the HLA molecule (16, 17) Beryllium-specific oligoclonal CD4+ T lymphocytes recognize beryllium within HLA molecules with these amino acid substitutions and this recognition leads to CD4+ lymphocyte proliferation, recruitment of other T cells and monocytes to the lung, (18) and the production of Thl/Th17 cytokines that eventually results in granuloma formation (18, 19). Further indirect support of this mechanism of sarcoidosis granuloma formation is that the lung and the skin are the two most common organs involved with sarcoidosis when the disease is clinically isolated to one organ (20). The skin and the lung are particularly conductive sites for antigen capture (21) and adaptive immune responses (22). It may be that these two organs are the main "portal of entry" for antigens that elicit the sarcoidosis granulomatous response, with further organ involvement requiring dissemination of antigen and/or other inflammatory mechanisms, (20) such as T-cell homing (23).

Although there is abundant evidence supporting the aforementioned mechanism of antigen-induced granulomatous inflammation in sarcoidosis, this mechanism is inconsistent with several available clinical and epidemiologic data. First, the associations between various HLA alleles and sarcoidosis phenotypes are not universal, but rather ethnicity-specific (11, 12, 24). Second, although sarcoidosis patients with specific phenotypic features of sarcoidosis have statistically higher percentages of certain HLA alleles than sarcoidosis patients without those specific phenotypic features or the general population, a significant percentage of individuals in these latter two groups carry the allele of risk (12, 25). In addition, most of these allele-specific phenotypes explain a small minority of cases (12, 13, 25). Another criticism of this mechanism is that it is problematic to account for the systemic features of sarcoidosis. The granulomas of sarcoidosis are often found in multiple and disparate organs. It is unclear how causative sarcoidosis antigens could disseminate throughout the body.

The second mechanism by which environmental antigens may induce a granulomatous response in sarcoidosis involves dysregulation of the immune system leading to autoimmunity. Evidence is accumulating that autoimmunity may be involved in some forms of sarcoidosis (26–30). Autoimmunity in sarcoidosis may occur via molecular mimicry whereby antigens trigger inflammation leading to exposure of self-peptides (31). Immunologic similarities between the "foreign" trigger and the "self" peptide promote autoreactive T or B cells in a susceptible individual. It is possible that the initial granulomatous reaction in sarcoidosis is a direct consequence of an antigen exposure in a target organ, but that subsequent granulomatous reactions in other organs are the result of molecular mimicry. This mechanism might explain how sarcoidosis manifests as a systemic disease without the need for a putative antigen to disseminate throughout the body. The best evidence for autoimmunity has been demonstrated in Lofgren's syndrome, a self-limiting form of the sarcoidosis where independent groups have identified vimentin as a possible autoantigen using proteomic techniques on lung macrophages and homogenized spleen tissue (32–36). Molecular mimicry may also by alteration of the binding pocket of the HLA molecule causing a granulomatous reaction to self-antigens. This mechanism appears to be relevant in the case of chronic beryllium disease, (37) and may explain other associations of metal exposures to the development of sarcoidosis or sarcoidosis-like reactions (vide infra). Antinuclear antibodies have been found in more than one-quarter of sarcoidosis patients in some cohort, suggesting autoimmunity may occur in sarcoidosis and may cause overlap syndromes with connective tissue diseases (38). Another form of "autoimmunity" could occur from autophagy that has been shown to promote MHC-II (major histocompatibility complex-II) presentation of proteins from intracellular sources (39). Perhaps environmental antigens first stimulate HLA molecules that interact with intracellular proteins as the result of autophagy.

A third mechanism by environmental exposures may induce sarcoidosis is by acting as an adjuvant and/or as a non-specific stimulator/dysregulator of the immune system. Such a mechanism would not directly cause sarcoidosis but would render the immune system more susceptible to another antigen or mechanism that could cause sarcoidosis. Such a mechanism may be analogous to a drug-induced sarcoidosis (DISR) like reaction that occurs with immune checkpoint inhibitor (ICI) therapy (40). ICIs are drugs that not only enhance anti-tumor activity, but also stimulate the immune system resulting in numerous immune-related adverse events (irAEs) One of several of these irAEs is a DISR, although $< 10\%$ of irAEs were DISRs in one series (41). It is therefore plausible that ICIs are not stimulating the immune system specifically to cause sarcoidosis but enhancing the risk of sarcoidosis in susceptible individuals.

Finally, environmental exposures that are epidemiologically associated with sarcoidosis may not be involved in any mechanism of disease development, as association does not prove causation. **Figure 1** outlines the possible mechanisms to explain the association of environmental exposures to sarcoidosis.

THE ROLE OF GENETICS

The aforementioned discussion concerning the relationship between sarcoidosis and potential environmental exposures is incomplete without a discussion of the importance of genetics. It is hypothesized that a combination of genetic and environmental factors contribute to the development of sarcoidosis (42). A recent large familial aggregation study showed that heritability of the disease was 39%, (43) suggesting that genetic variation is an important contributing factor to the risk of sarcoidosis. Various HLA polymorphisms have been associated with development of sarcoidosis, protection from sarcoidosis and certain phenotypic expressions of sarcoidosis (11, 13). In addition, genome-wise association studies have reported variations numerous non-HLA genes that are associated with sarcoidosis. These include annexin A11 (44) that is involved in cell division and apoptosis, NOTCH4 (45) that regulates the activity of T cell immune responses, and BTNL2 (45, 46) that is involved in T cell activation. We suspect that many of the aforementioned mechanisms described concerning the association of environmental exposures to sarcoidosis depend on specific genetic factors. We envision that in the future, the etiology of sarcoidosis will be personalized whereby certain genetics traits present in an individual will suggest that certain specific exposures will place the subject at risk of developing sarcoidosis.

POTENTIAL INFECTIOUS CAUSES OF SARCOIDOSIS

Infectious agents have been suspected as being a possible cause of sarcoidosis. However, data supporting this conjecture are inconsistent and unconvincing. There is an abundance of indirect evidence that mycobacteria are involved in the development of sarcoidosis. Two meta-analyses of studies evaluating infectious agents as a cause of sarcoidosis have suggested an etiologic link between mycobacteria and sarcoidosis (47, 48). Molecular techniques have identified mycobacterial components in sarcoidosis tissues in some (49–51) but not all (52, 53) studies. Mycobacterial catalase-peroxidase protein (mKatG) has been identified in sarcoidosis tissues. mKatG has similar physicochemical properties to the Kveim-Siltzbach reagent that induces granulomatous inflammation almost exclusively in

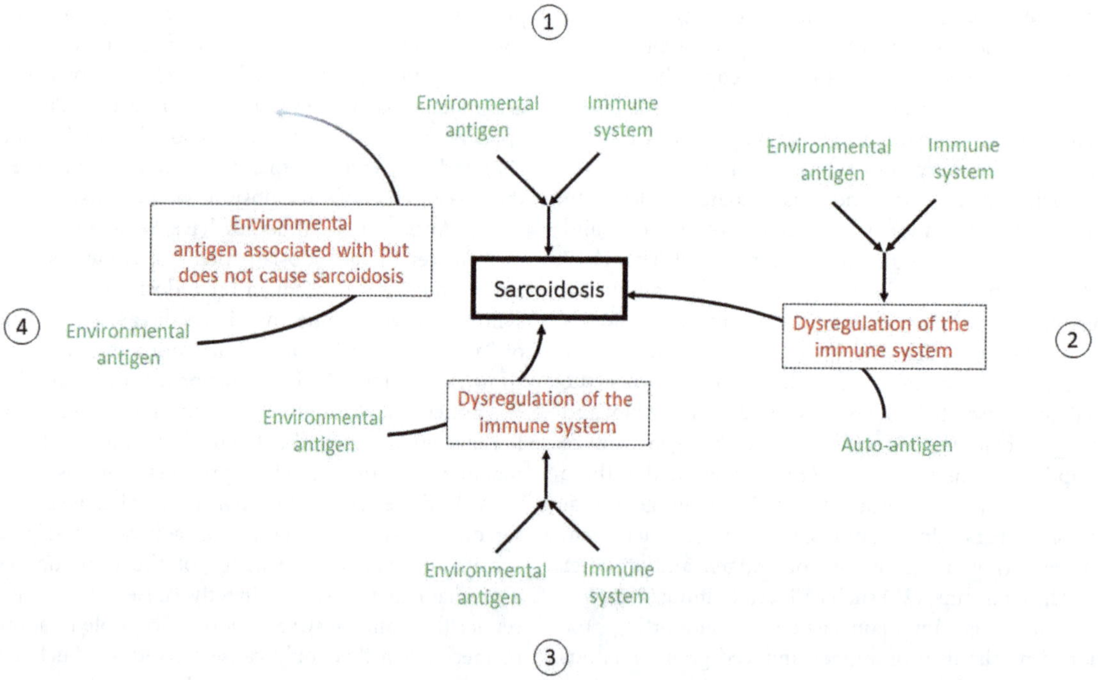

FIGURE 1 | A depiction of the possible mechanisms to explain the association of environmental exposures to sarcoidosis. 1: The environmental exposure may act as an antigen to stimulate the immune system to directly cause sarcoidosis. The immune system is functioning normally with a appropriate response to the antigen. 2: The antigen interacts with the immune system to cause its deregulation. The immune system then acts abnormally to cause sarcoidosis. 3: The antigen acts as an adjuvant that acts as an adjuvant to stimulate or dysregulate the immune system but not directly cause sarcoidosis. However, the immune system is now "primed" such that another antigen or stimulus can now interact with the immune system to cause sarcoidosis. 4: The environmental exposure is a cofounder. Although this exposure is associated with sarcoidosis, it does not cause sarcoidosis.

sarcoidosis patients (54) T-cell responses to mKatG have been demonstrated in peripheral blood monocytes of sarcoidosis patients (55, 56) with even more robust T-cell responses in bronchoalveolar lavage fluid (55, 57) and strongest responses in those with active disease (55, 57) Similar findings have not been demonstrated in other lung diseases (55, 57). It should be noted that the demonstration of mycobacterial antigens in sarcoidosis patients and granulomatous immune responses to mycobacterial antigens does not imply that sarcoidosis is a form of mycobacterial infection. Rather, it may be that some poorly degraded mycobacterial antigens contribute to the immune process of sarcoidosis without the presence of viable invasive mycobacterial organisms (48).

There is abundant evidence that Propionibacterium acnes, a skin commensal bacterium, is associated with sarcoidosis. This microorganism is the only one that has been cultured from sarcoidosis lesions (58, 59). Numerous studies have identified specific immune responses to Propionibacterium acnes in sarcoidosis patients but much less to none in non-sarcoidosis controls (52, 60, 61). Propionibacterium acnes was highly associated with sarcoidosis in a meta-analysis of studies evaluating infectious agents as a cause of the disease (47).

Numerous other infectious agents have been implicated in the immunopathogenesis of sarcoidosis. Several of these infectious agents are listed in **Table 1**. Implicated infectious agents include bacteria, mycobacteria, and fungi.

Several trials of antibiotics for sarcoidosis have targeted suspected infectious pathogens. Therapy with concomitant levofloxacin, ethambutol, erythromycin and rifampin (CLEAR) has been used for the treatment of sarcoidosis by targeting presumed mycobacterial pathogens. An open label trail of CLEAR for pulmonary sarcoidosis showed an improvement in forced vital capacity in 8 of the 15 enrolled patients who were able to tolerate the study drugs for the full 8 weeks of the study (72). A subsequent small ($N = 29$) single-blind placebo-control trial of the CLEAR regimen for cutaneous sarcoidosis showed a statistically significant greater reduction in lesion size with CLEAR than placebo (73). A larger randomized double-blind placebo-controlled trial of CLEAR for pulmonary sarcoidosis is currently underway. Several case series of tetracyclines, including doxycycline and minocycline, have been reported as effective for cutaneous sarcoidosis (74, 75). These reports were unblinded descriptions of treated cases without comparisons with a control group. Furthermore, it is unclear if the mechanism of action of these tetracyclines was antibacterial or anti-inflammatory (76). Case reports and case series have shown a benefit from with clarithromycin for presumed Propionibacterium acnes infection in sarcoidosis patients, (77) as well as a benefit from empiric anti-fungal therapy (78). However, these reports also contained no control patients and/or were poorly designed to rigorously demonstrate a clinically relevant endpoint. In summary, the available evidence does not clearly demonstrate that therapy vs. a specific infectious pathogen is useful for the treatment of sarcoidosis. As previously mentioned, this does not exclude infectious organisms being involved in the immunopathogenesis of sarcoidosis, as an antigen of a microorganism may stimulate the immune system in ways that promote the granulomatous inflammation of sarcoidosis.

Besides examining individual infectious pathogens as causes of sarcoidosis, human microbiotica may have an important role in disease development. Human microbiotica regulate several physiological processes including metabolic functions and immune homeostasis (79). Alterations in the gut and respiratory microbiome have been associated with several inflammatory diseases including autoimmune diseases and cancer (80–83). It is plausible that sarcoidosis may be associated with specific changes in the composition of lung or gut microbiotica. However, a few studies examining changes in the lung microbiome have failed to identify distributions that are specific for sarcoidosis (84, 85). One recent study did suggest that Atopobium and Fusobacterium may be associated with sarcoidosis, (86) and another found that microbiota in bronchoalveolar lavage of sarcoidosis patients was less diverse and abundant compared to healthy controls (87). However, it is unclear whether these changes in the lung microbiome are causing sarcoidosis or are a result of the disease.

TABLE 1 | Selected infectious agents associated with sarcoidosis*.

Infectious agents	Immunologic	Molecular	Culture
Mycobacterium tuberculosis	√(50, 55, 62)	√(49, 56, 63)	
Other Mycobacteria	√(57, 64)	√(49, 51)	
Propionibacterium acnes	√(52, 65, 66)	√(60)	√(58, 59)
Fungi	√(67, 68)		
Borrelia	√(69)	√(70, 71)	

*References are in parentheses.

POTENTIAL NON-INFECTIOUS ENVIRONMENTAL RISK FACTORS FOR SARCOIDOSIS

There are numerous non-infectious environmental risk factors associated with sarcoidosis. These risk factors include working in various occupations, exposure to various substances, and dwelling in particular environments (**Table 2**). Most of these associations are epidemiologic. Numerous epidemiologic studies have demonstrated that sarcoidosis occurs most commonly in the Spring season (88–91). This suggests that some sarcoidosis cases may result from inhalation of an organic bioaerosol that is more abundant in the springtime, possibly analogous to summer-type hypersensitivity which is a form of hypersensitivity pneumonitis in Japan caused by inhalation of certain fungi that reach high concentrations in the summer air (113). Several other epidemiologic analyses have found that the prevalence of sarcoidosis is associated with exposure to other organic bioaerosols such as exposure to musty odors at the workplace (103) and exposure to industrial organic dusts (104, 105).

Sarcoidosis is also associated with inorganic aerosol exposures, particularly with several metal dusts. This association is not surprising, as CBD from beryllium exposure is a clinical mimic of sarcoidosis. Sarcoidosis is not only associated with

TABLE 2 | Non-infectious environmental risk factors associated with sarcoidosis.

General category	Type of study	Study population	Findings	Reference
Space and/or time clustering: Seasonal variation in disease incidence	Space-time analysis	(88)- Rochester, MN; (89)-Turkey; (90)-New Zealand; (91)-Catlonia, Spain	Increased risk in the Spring	(88–91)
	Space-time analysis	USA Veterans	Increased risk in the Summer	(92)
	Space-time analysis	Rochester, MN	Decreased incidence in Autumn	(93)
Space clustering	Space clustering analysis	Ireland	Increased prevalence in certain regions of Ireland	(94)
	Space clustering analysis	Ireland	Higher risks in the North than South	(94)
	Space clustering analysis	Japan	Higher rates of sarcoidosis in Northern than Southern Japan	(95)
	Space clustering analysis	Hospitalized patients US military	Higher frequency in the Southeast US than other US locations	(96)
	Space clustering analysis	South Carolina	Increased prevalence near the coastline of South Carolina	(97)
	Space-time analysis vs. standard incidence and prevalence rates of sarcoidosis	Poland, living in forest of arable land	Increased incidence	(98)
	Co-inertia analysis plus linear model of hospitalized patients	Switzerland, Living near areas with metal industries	Increased prevalence	(99)
	Co-inertia analysis plus linear model of hospitalized patients	Switzerland, living in areas with potato production, artificial meadows, grain production	Increased prevalence	(99)
Occupational exposure	firefighter cohort vs. EMT cohort	NYC, Firefighters	Increased incidence and/or prevalence	(100)
	firefighter cohort vs. police cohort	Prov, RI, Firefighters	Increased incidence and/or prevalence	(101)
	Hospitalizations rates of Blacks in the US Navy	Black US Navy ship servicemen	Increased risk	(102)
	Hospitalizations rates of Blacks in the US Navy	Black US Navy Aviation structural mechanics	Increased risk	(102)
	Hospitalizations rates of Blacks in the US Navy	White US Navy ship culinary specialists	Increased risk	(102)
	Case-control US	Using insecticides	Increased risk	(103)
	Case-control US	Musty odor at work	Increased risk	(103)
	Case-control US	Building materials	Increased risk	(104)
	Case-control US	Hardware	Increased risk	(104)
	Case-control US	Garden supplies	Increased risk	(104)
	Case-control US	Mobile homes	Increased risk	(104)
	Case control US	Industrial organic dusts	Increased risk	(104)
	Case-control*AA Detroit, MI	Education	Increased risk	(105)
	Case-control*AA Detroit, MI	Metal machining	Increased risk	(105)
	Case-control*AA Detroit, MI	Metal working	Increased risk	(105)
	Case-control*AA Detroit, MI	Transportation services	Increased risk	(105)
	Incidence vs. exposure	Sweden: Silica exposure in foundry workers	Increased risk	(106)
	Longitudinal cohort of construction workers, exposed vs. unexposed to silica	Sweden, construction workers	Increased risk	(107)
	Silica in lung and lymph node biopsy, Case series: 2 cases	Silica (metal-halide lamp production)	Increased risk	(108)
	Case-control with sarcoidosis patients and their siblings who did not have sarcoidosis	AAs USA, Photocopier toner exposure	Increased risk	(109)

(Continued)

TABLE 2 | Continued

General category	Type of study	Study population	Findings	Reference
	Tracking sarcoidosis incidence in FDNY workers pre and post WTC disaster	NYC, World Trade Center dust exposure	Increased incidence	(110)
	Case-control*AA Detroit MI	AA Detroit MI, Working in high humidity	Increased risk	(105)
	Case-Control*AA Detroit MI	AA Detroit MI, Working with titanium	Increased risk	(105)
	Case-Control*AA Detroit MI	AA Detroit MI, Working with vegetable dust	Increased risk	(105)
	Elicited history of exposure and analyzed lung biopsy specimens	Man-made mineral fibers	Increased risk	(111)
Environmental exposure	Case-Control with dose response SC	SC, Wood stove use	Increased risk	(112)
	Case-Control with dose response SC	SC, Fireplace use	Increased risk	(112)
	Case-Control*AA Detroit MI	AA Detroit MI, Musty odors	Increased risk	(105)
	Case-control SC	SC, Non-public water use	Increased risk	(112)
	Case-control SC	SC, Living/working on a farm	Increased risk	(112)

**Controls were unaffected siblings of sarcoidosis cases; MN, Minnesota; NYC, New York City; RI, Rhode Island; AA, African American; FDNY, Fire Department of New York City; WTC, World Trade Center; SC, South Carolina.*

several occupations directly involved with manipulations of metals (102, 105) but also more subtle exposures including photocopier toner (109) that contains copper, iron, and silica (114). One report found a significant association of man-made mineral fiber exposure and the development of sarcoidosis, and then went further to perform electron microscopy quantitative analysis on previous lung specimens in the sarcoidosis group and found that half of them silica, aluminum and/or titanium (111).

Exposure to combustible products, especially combustible wood, has been associated with the development of sarcoidosis. A prototypical example of this association is the high incidence and prevalence rates sarcoidosis that is observed in firefighters (100, 101). In one analysis, emergency medical technicians (EMTs) served as a control group to the firefighters because both groups went to fire sites (100). The annual incidence rate of sarcoidosis was extremely high (44/100,000) in the firefighters whereas it was 0 in the EMTs. Wood stove use and fireplace use have also been associated with the development of sarcoidosis (112). The rigor of this association was strengthened by demonstrating a significant dose-response relationship of both wood stove and fireplace use to the frequency of sarcoidosis. Dust from the World Trade Center disaster has been associated with increased rates of developing sarcoidosis within the first 4 years after exposure (110). However, World Trade Center dust was a heterogenous exposure, and it is unclear whether the causative substance(s) was a combustible product, metal or gas.

Higher prevalence rates of sarcoidosis have been observed in Northern latitudes such as Northern Europe and Northern Japan, (95, 115) and it has been postulated that this relates to decreased sunlight exposure causing a deficiency in 1,25-dihydroxy-vitamin D (116). A deficiency in 1,25-dihydroxy-vitamin D is associated with decreased production of the antimicrobial peptide cathelicidin that contributes to the development of infectious granulomatous diseases such as tuberculosis (95, 117). A relative deficiency in 1,25-dihydroxy-vitamin D may also explain the increased frequency of sarcoidosis in Blacks, as the ability to convert 7-dehydrocholesterol to previtamin D is suppressed because of skin pigmentation (118).

Some exposures associated with sarcoidosis are problematic to explain such as working in education (105) or the culinary arts (102). This may relate to the aforementioned concept that sarcoidosis may involve an initial portal of entry where a causative antigen first interacts with the immune system and then requires additional inflammatory modulation to cause disease. In an analysis that focused on mortality from sarcoidosis and not the incidence or prevalence of disease, women with sarcoidosis were more likely to have exposure from person-to-person contact (administration and banking) whereas men who were more likely to have inhalational exposures (119). This may explain why woman are more likely to develop non-pulmonary sarcoidosis than men, (20) and it might also explain how non-respiratory exposures may be mechanistically linked to the development of sarcoidosis.

ANIMAL AND EXPERIMENTAL MODELS OF GRANULOMATOUS DISEASE

Various animal and experimental models of granulomatous have been developed that have involved exposure to environmental substances (120). Carbon nanotube induced granulomatous lung disease has been demonstrated in an animal model and has shown several similarities to sarcoidosis (121, 122). Numerous components of infectious agents, particularly mycobacteria and Propionibacterium acnes have mimicked features of sarcoidosis in animal models (123–126). These models have demonstrated similar immune responses in terms of T-cell function and the production of cytokines seen in sarcoidosis (120).

SUMMARY

In conclusion, sarcoidosis is associated with several environmental exposures including infectious agents, non-infectious organic antigens, metals, combustible products, and other inorganic substances. These disparate exposures may suggest that sarcoidosis represents a collection of different disorders that all result in the development of a multisystem granulomatous disease. Alternatively, these varied exposures may each stimulate the immune system in different ways such that a specific immune pathway that leads to sarcoidosis is promoted. This could include the induction of autoimmunity. Genetics factors are most probably an important aspect of these mechanisms. Further insights concerning the relationship of environmental exposures to the development of sarcoidosis may have a major impact on the prevention and treatment of this enigmatic disease.

AUTHOR CONTRIBUTIONS

The author confirms being the sole contributor of this work and has approved it for publication.

REFERENCES

Baughman RP, Teirstein AS, Judson MA, Rossman MD, Yeager H, Bresnitz EA, et al. Clinical characteristics of patients in a case control study of sarcoidosis. *Am J Respir Crit Care Med.* (2001) 164(10 Pt 1):1885- 9. doi: 10.1164/ajrccm.164.10.2104046

Judson MA, Boan AD, Lackland DT. The clinical course of sarcoidosis: presentation, diagnosis, and treatment in a large white and black cohort in the United States. *Sarcoidosis Vasc Diffuse Lung Dis.* (2012) 29:119–27.

Ehlers S, Schaible UE. The granuloma in tuberculosis: dynamics of a host-pathogen collusion. *Front Immunol.* (2012) 3:411. doi: 10.3389/fimmu.2012.00411

Zumla A, James DG. Granulomatous infections: etiology and classification. *Clin Infect Dis.* (1996) 23:146–58. doi: 10.1093/clinids/23.1.146

Selman M, Pardo A, King TE. Hypersensitivity pneumonitis: insights in diagnosis and pathobiology. *Am J Respir Crit Care Med.* (2012). 186:314- 24. doi: 10.1164/rccm.201203-0513CI

Rossman MD. Chronic beryllium disease: diagnosis and management. *Environ Health Perspect.* (1996) 104(Suppl. 5):945–7. doi: 10.1289/ehp.96104s5945

Newman LS, Rose CS, Maier LA. Sarcoidosis. *N Engl J Med.* (1997) 336:1224- 34. doi: 10.1056/NEJM199704243361706

Baughman RP, Culver DA, Judson MA. A concise review of pulmonary sarcoidosis. *Am J Respir Crit Care Med.* (2011) 183:573–81. doi: 10.1164/rccm.201006-0865CI

Moller DR, Chen ES. Genetic basis of remitting sarcoidosis: triumph of the trimolecular complex? *Am J Respir Crit Care Med.* (2002) 27:391- 5. doi: 10.1165/rcmb.2002-0164PS

Broos CE, Koth LL, van Nimwegen M, Veen JCCM, Paulissen SMJ, Hamburg JP, et al. Increased T-helper 17.1 cells in sarcoidosis mediastinal lymph nodes. *Eur Respir J.* (2018) 51:170112. doi: 10.1183/13993003.011 24-2017

Martinetti M, Luisetti M, Cuccia M. HLA and sarcoidosis: new pathogenetic insights. *Sarcoidosis Vasc Diffuse Lung Dis.* (2002) 19:83–95.

Du Bois R, Beirne PA, Anevlavis SE. Genetics. In: Drent M, Costabel U, editors. *Sarcoidosis: European Respiratory Monograph.* Sheffield: European respiroatry Society Journals Ltd. (2005). p. 64–81. doi: 10.1183/1025448x.00032005

Rossman MD, Thompson B, Frederick M, Maliarik M, Iannuzzi MC, Rybicki BA, et al. HLA-DRB11101: a significant risk factor for sarcoidosis in blacks and whites. *Am J Hum Genet.* (2003) 73:720–35. doi: 10.1086/378097

Mayer AS, Hamzeh N, Maier LA. Sarcoidosis and chronic beryllium disease: similarities and differences. *Semin Respir Crit Care Med.* (2014) 35:316- 29. doi: 10.1055/s-0034-1377059

Müller-Quernheim J, Gaede KI, Fireman E, Zissel G. Diagnoses of chronic beryllium disease within cohorts of sarcoidosis patients. *Eur Respir J.* (2006) 27:1190–5. doi: 10.1183/09031936.06.00112205

Van Dyke MV, Martyny JW, Mroz MM, Silveira LJ, Strand M, Fingerlin TE, et al. Risk of chronic beryllium disease by HLA-DPB1 E69 genotype and beryllium exposure in nuclear workers. *Am J Respir Crit Care Med.* (2011) 183:1680–8. doi: 10.1164/rccm.201002-0254OC

Van Dyke MV, Martyny JW, Mroz MM, Silveira LJ, Strand M, Cragle DL, et al. Exposure and genetics increase risk of beryllium sensitisation and chronic beryllium disease in the nuclear weapons industry. *Occup Environ Med.* (2011) 68:842–8. doi: 10.1136/oem.2010.064220

Fontenot AP, Torres M, Marshall WH, Newman LS, Kotzin BL. Beryllium presentation to CD4+ T cells underlies disease-susceptibility HLA-DP alleles in chronic beryllium disease. *Proc Natl Acad Sci USA.* (2000) 97:12717- 22. doi: 10.1073/pnas.220430797

Tinkle SS, Schwitters PW, Newman LS. Cytokine production by bronchoalveolar lavage cells in chronic beryllium disease. *Environ Health Perspect.* (1996) 104(Suppl. 5):969–71. doi: 10.1289/ehp.96104s5969

James WE, Koutroumpakis E, Saha B, Nathani A, Saavedra L, Yucel RM, et al. Clinical Features of Extrapulmonary Sarcoidosis Without Lung Involvement. *Chest.* (2018) 154:349–56. doi: 10.1016/j.chest.2018.02.003

Kurata A, Terado Y, Izumi M, Fujioka Y, Franke FE. Where does the antigen of cutaneous sarcoidosis come from? *J Cutan Pathol.* (2010) 37:211- 21. doi: 10.1111/j.1600-0560.2009.01309.x

Bordignon M, Rottoli P, Agostini C, Alaibac M. Adaptive immune responses in primary cutaneous sarcoidosis. *Clin Dev Immunol.* (2011) 2011:235142. doi: 10.1155/2011/235142

Brinkman CC, Rouhani SJ, Srinivasan N, Engelhard VH. Peripheral tissue homing receptors enable T cell entry into lymph nodes and affect the anatomical distribution of memory cells. *J Immunol.* (2013) 191:2412- 25. doi: 10.4049/jimmunol.1300651

Judson MA. A sarcoidosis clinician's perspective of MHC functional elements outside the antigen binding site. *Hum Immunol.* (2019) 80:85- 9. doi: 10.1016/j.humimm.2018.05.007

Rossman MD, Thompson B, Frederick M, Iannuzzi MC, Rybicki BA, Pander JP, et al. HLA and environmental interactions in sarcoidosis. *Sarcoidosis Vasc Diffuse Lung Dis.* (2008) 25:125–32.

Zissel G, Muller-Quernheim J. Specific antigen(s) in sarcoidosis: a link to autoimmunity? *Eur Respir J.* (2016) 47:707- 9. doi: 10.1183/13993003.01791-2015

Häggmark A, Hamsten C, Wiklundh E, Lindskog C, Mattsson C, Andersson E, et al. Proteomic profiling reveals autoimmune targets in sarcoidosis. *Am J Respir Crit Care Med.* (2015) 191:574–83. doi: 10.1164/rccm.201407-1341OC

Tchernev G, Lotti T, Cardoso JC, Kanazawa N, Guarneri C, Wollina U. Cancer, infection and disturbances of the integrity of tissue homeostasis: the most significant triggers for molecular mimicry and autoimmunity in dermatology? *Wien Med Wochenschr.* (2014) 164:245–6. doi: 10.1007/s10354-014-0280-2

Tchernev G, Wollina U. Bacterial antigens and molecular mimicry: the bridging common problematic link in the pathogenesis of sarcoidosis and sarcoid-like reactions: isn't it time to wake up? *Wien Med Wochenschr.* (2014). 164:260–2. doi: 10.1007/s10354-014-0283-z

Kinloch AJ, Kaiser Y, Wolfgeher D, Ai J, Eklund A, Clark MR, et al. *In situ* humoral immunity to vimentin in HLA-DRB1 03(+) patients with pulmonary sarcoidosis. *Front Immunol.* (2018) 9:1516. doi: 10.3389/fimmu.2018.01516

Rojas M, Restrepo-Jimenez P, Monsalve DM, Pacheco Y, Acosta-Ampudia Y, Ramírez-Santana C, et al. Molecular mimicry and autoimmunity. *J Autoimmun.* (2018) 95:100–23. doi: 10.1016/j.jaut.2018.10.012

Grunewald J, Kaiser Y, Ostadkarampour M, Rivera NV, Vezzi F, Lötstedt B, et al. T-cell receptor-HLA-DRB1 associations suggest specific antigens in pulmonary sarcoidosis. *Eur Respir J.* (2016) 47:898–909. doi: 10.1183/13993003.01209-2015

Eberhardt C, Thillai M, Parker R, Siddiqui N, Potiphar L, Goldin R, et al. Proteomic analysis of kveim reagent identifies targets of cellular immunity in sarcoidosis. *PLoS ONE.* (2017) 12:e0170285. doi: 10.1371/journal.pone.0170285

Heyder T, Kohler M, Tarasova NK, Haag S, Rutishauser D, Rivera NV, et al. Approach for identifying human leukocyte antigen (HLA)-DR bound peptides from scarce clinical samples. *Mol Cell Proteomics.* (2016) 15:3017– 29. doi: 10.1074/mcp.M116.060764

Wahlström J, Dengjel J, Winqvist O, Targoff I, Persson B, Duyar H, et al. Autoimmune T cell responses to antigenic peptides presented by bronchoalveolar lavage cell HLA-DR molecules in sarcoidosis. *Clin Immunol.* (2009) 133:353–63. doi: 10.1016/j.clim.2009.08.008

Wahlström J, Dengjel J, Persson B, Duyar H, Rammensee HG, Stevanovic´ S, et al. Identification of HLA-DR-bound peptides presented by human bronchoalveolar lavage cells in sarcoidosis. *J Clin Invest.* (2007) 117:3576– 82. doi: 10.1172/JCI32401

Fontenot AP, Falta MT, Kappler JW, Dai S, McKee AS. Beryllium- induced hypersensitivity: genetic susceptibility and neoantigen generation. *J Immunol.* (2016) 196:22–7. doi: 10.4049/jimmunol.1502011

Kobak S, Yilmaz H, Sever F, Duran A, Sen N, Karaarslan A. The prevalence of antinuclear antibodies in patients with sarcoidosis. *Autoimmune Dis.* (2014) 2014:351852. doi: 10.1155/2014/351852

Dengjel J, Schoor O, Fischer R, Reich M, Kraus M, Müller M, et al. Autophagy promotes MHC class II presentation of peptides from intracellular source proteins. *Proc Natl Acad Sci USA.* (2005) 102:7922– 7. doi: 10.1073/pnas.0501190102

Gkiozos I, Kopitopoulou A, Kalkanis A, Vamvakaris IN, Judson MA, Syrigos KN. Sarcoidosis-like reactions induced by checkpoint inhibitors. *J Thorac Oncol.* (2018) 13:1076–82. doi: 10.1016/j.jtho.2018.04.031

Le Burel S, Champiat S, Mateus C, Marabelle A, Michot JM, Robert C, et al. Prevalence of immune-related systemic adverse events in patients treated with anti-Programmed cell Death 1/anti-Programmed cell Death-Ligand 1 agents: a single-centre pharmacovigilance database analysis. *Eur J Cancer.* (2017) 82:34–44. doi: 10.1016/j.ejca.2017.05.032

Arkema EV, Cozier YC. Epidemiology of sarcoidosis: current findings and future directions. *Ther Adv Chronic Dis.* (2018) 9:227–40. doi: 10.1177/2040622318790197

Rossides M, Grunewald J, Eklund A, Kullberg S, Di Giuseppe D, Askling J, et al. Familial aggregation and heritability of sarcoidosis: a Swedish nested case-control study. *Eur Respir J.* (2018) 52:1800385. doi: 10.1183/13993003.00385-2018

Levin AM, Iannuzzi MC, Montgomery CG, Trudeau S, Datta I, McKeigue P, et al. Association of ANXA11 genetic variation with sarcoidosis in African Americans and European Americans. *Genes Immun.* (2013) 14:13– 8. doi: 10.1038/gene.2012.48

Adrianto I, Lin CP, Hale JJ, Levin AM, Datta I, Parker R, et al. Genome-wide association study of African and European Americans implicates multiple shared and ethnic specific loci in sarcoidosis susceptibility. *PLoS ONE.* (2012) 7:e43907. doi: 10.1371/journal.pone.0043907

Morais A, Lima B, Peixoto MJ, Alves H, Marques A, Delgado L. BTNL2 gene polymorphism associations with susceptibility and phenotype expression in sarcoidosis. *Respir Med.* (2012) 106:1771–7. doi: 10.1016/j.rmed.2012.08.009

Esteves T, Aparicio G, Garcia-Patos V. Is there any association between Sarcoidosis and infectious agents?: a systematic review and meta-analysis. *BMC Pulm Med.* (2016) 16:165. doi: 10.1186/s12890-016-0332-z

Fang C, Huang H, Xu Z. Immunological evidence for the role of mycobacteria in sarcoidosis: a meta-analysis. *PLoS ONE.* (2016) 11:e0154716. doi: 10.1371/journal.pone.0154716

Lee H, Eom M, Kim SH, Wang HY, Lee H, Choi EH. Identification of Mycobacterium tuberculosis and non-tuberculous mycobacteria from cutaneous sarcoidosis lesions by reverse blot hybridization assay. *J Dermatol.* (2019) 46:917–21. doi: 10.1111/1346-8138.15042

Goyal B, Sheikh JA, Agarwal R, Verma I. Levels of circulating immune complexes containing Mycobacterium Tuberculosis-specific antigens in pulmonary tuberculosis and sarcoidosis patients. *Indian J Med Microbiol.* (2017) 35:290–2. doi: 10.4103/0255-0857.209569

Rotsinger JE, Celada LJ, Polosukhin VV, Atkinson JB, Drake WP. Molecular analysis of sarcoidosis granulomas reveals antimicrobial targets. *Am J Respir Cell Mol Biol.* (2016) 55:128–34. doi: 10.1165/rcmb.2015-0212OC

Eishi Y, Suga M, Ishige I, Kobayashi D, Yamada T, Takemura T, et al. Quantitative analysis of mycobacterial and propionibacterial DNA in lymph nodes of Japanese and European patients with sarcoidosis. *J Clin Microbiol.* (2002) 40:198–204. doi: 10.1128/JCM.40.1.198-204.2002

Milman N, Lisby G, Friis S, Kemp L. Prolonged culture for mycobacteria in mediastinal lymph nodes from patients with pulmonary sarcoidosis. A negative study. *Sarcoidosis Vasc Diffuse Lung Dis.* (2004) 21:25–8.

Song Z, Marzilli L, Greenlee BM, Chen ES, Silver RF, Askin FB, et al. Mycobacterial catalase-peroxidase is a tissue antigen and target of the adaptive immune response in systemic sarcoidosis. *J Exp Med.* (2005) 201:755–67. doi: 10.1084/jem.20040429

Chen ES, Wahlström J, Song Z, Willett MH, Wikén M, Yung RC, et al. T cell responses to mycobacterial catalase-peroxidase profile a pathogenic antigen in systemic sarcoidosis. *J Immunol.* (2008) 181:8784– 96. doi: 10.4049/jimmunol.181.12.8784

Drake WP, Dhason MS, Nadaf M, Shepherd BE, Vadivelu S, Hajizadeh R, et al. Cellular recognition of Mycobacterium tuberculosis ESAT-6 and KatG peptides in systemic sarcoidosis. *Infect Immun.* (2007) 75:527– 30. doi: 10.1128/IAI.00732-06

Oswald-Richter KA, Culver DA, Hawkins C, Hajizadeh R, Abraham S, Shepherd BE, et al. Cellular responses to mycobacterial antigens are present in bronchoalveolar lavage fluid used in the diagnosis of sarcoidosis. *Infect Immun.* (2009) 77:3740–8. doi: 10.1128/IAI.00142-09

Homma JY, Abe C, Chosa H, Ueda K, Saegusa J, Nakayama M, et al. Bacteriological investigation on biopsy specimens from patients with sarcoidosis. *Jpn J Exp Med.* (1978) 48:251–5.

Abe C, Iwai K, Mikami R, Hosoda Y. Frequent isolation of Propionibacterium acnes from sarcoidosis lymph nodes. *Zentralbl Bakteriol Mikrobiol Hyg A.* (1984) 256:541–7. doi: 10.1016/S0174-3031(84)80032-3

Nagata K, Eishi Y, Uchida K, Yoneda K, Hatanaka H, Yasuhara T, et al. Immunohistochemical detection of propionibacterium acnes in the retinal granulomas in patients with ocular sarcoidosis. *Sci Rep.* (2017) 7:15226. doi: 10.1038/s41598-017-15710-0

Suzuki Y, Uchida K, Takemura T, Sekine M, Tamura T, Furukawa A, et al. Propionibacterium acnes-derived insoluble immune complexes in sinus macrophages of lymph nodes affected by sarcoidosis. *PLoS ONE.* (2018) 13:e0192408. doi: 10.1371/journal.pone.0192408

Hajizadeh R, Sato H, Carlisle J, Nadaf MT, Evans W, Shepherd BE, et al. Mycobacterium tuberculosis Antigen 85A induces Th-1 immune responses in systemic sarcoidosis. *J Clin Immunol.* (2007) 27:445– 54. doi: 10.1007/s10875-007-9080-4

Dubaniewicz A, Dubaniewicz-Wybieralska M, Sternau A, Zwolska Z, Izycka-Swieszewska E, Augustynowicz-Kopec E, et al. Mycobacterium tuberculosis complex and mycobacterial heat shock proteins in lymph node tissue from patients with pulmonary sarcoidosis. *J Clin Microbiol.* (2006) 44:3448– 51. doi: 10.1128/JCM.01433-06

Carlisle J, Evans W, Hajizadeh R, Nadaf M, Shepherd B, Ott RD, et al. Multiple Mycobacterium antigens induce interferon-gamma production from sarcoidosis peripheral blood mononuclear cells. *Clin Exp Immunol.* (2007) 150:460–8. doi: 10.1111/j.1365-2249.2007.03510.x

Nakata Y, Ejiri T, Kishi T, Mori Y, Hioka T, Kataoka M, et al. Alveolar lymphocyte proliferation induced by Propionibacterium acnes in sarcoidosis patients. *Acta Med Okayama.* (1986) 40:257–64.

Furusawa H, Suzuki Y, Miyazaki Y, Inase N, Eishi Y. Th1 and Th17 immune responses to viable Propionibacterium acnes in patients with sarcoidosis. *Respir Investig.* (2012) 50:104–9. doi: 10.1016/j.resinv.2012.07.001

Terc˘elj M, Stopinšek S, Ihan A, Salobir B, Simc˘ic˘ S, Wraber B, et al. *In vitro* and *in vivo* reactivity to fungal cell wall agents in sarcoidosis. *Clin Exp Immunol.* (2011) 166:87–93. doi: 10.1111/j.1365-2249.2011.04456.x

Suchankova M, Paulovicova E, Paulovicova L, Majer I, Tedlova E, Novosadova H, et al. Increased antifungal antibodies in bronchoalveolar lavage fluid and serum in pulmonary sarcoidosis. *Scand J Immunol.* (2015) 81:259–64. doi: 10.1111/sji.12273

Ishihara M, Ohno S, Ono H, Isogai E, Kimura K, Isogai H, et al. Seroprevalence of anti-Borrelia antibodies among patients with confirmed sarcoidosis in a region of Japan where Lyme borreliosis is endemic. *Graefes Arch Clin Exp Ophthalmol.* (1998) 236:280–4. doi: 10.1007/s004170050078

Xu Z, Ma D, Luo W, Zhu Y. Detection of Borrelia burgdorferi DNA in granulomatous tissues from patients with sarcoidosis using polymerase chain reaction *in situ* technique. *Chin Med Sci J.* (1996) 11:220–3.

Lian W, Luo W. Borrelia burgdorferi DNA in biological samples from patients with sarcoidosis using the polymerase chain reaction technique. *Chin Med Sci J.* (1995) 10:93–5.

Drake WP, Richmond BW, Oswald-Richter K, Yu C, Isom JM, Worrell JA, et al. Effects of broad-spectrum antimycobacterial therapy on chronic pulmonary sarcoidosis. *Sarcoidosis Vasc Diffuse Lung Dis.* (2013) 30:201–11.

Drake WP, Oswald-Richter K, Richmond BW, Isom J, Burke VE, Algood H, et al. Oral antimycobacterial therapy in chronic cutaneous sarcoidosis: a randomized, single-masked, placebo-controlled study. *JAMA Dermatol.* (2013) 149:1040–9. doi: 10.1001/jamadermatol.2013.4646

Steen T, English JC. Oral minocycline in treatment of cutaneous sarcoidosis. *JAMA Dermatol.* (2013) 149:758–60. doi: 10.1001/jamadermatol.2013.2977

Bachelez H, Senet P, Cadranel J, Kaoukhov A, Dubertret L. The use of tetracyclines for the treatment of sarcoidosis. *Arch Dermatol.* (2001) 137:69– 73. doi: 10.1001/archderm.137.1.69

Miyazaki E, Ando M, Fukami T, Nureki S, Eishi Y, Kumamoto T. Minocycline for the treatment of sarcoidosis: is the mechanism of action immunomodulating or antimicrobial effect? *Clin Rheumatol.* (2008) 27:1195–7. doi: 10.1007/s10067-008-0903-3

Takemori N, Nakamura M, Kojima M, Eishi Y. Successful treatment in a case of Propionibacterium acnes-associated sarcoidosis with clarithromycin administration: a case report. *J Med Case Rep.* (2014) 8:15. doi: 10.1186/1752-1947-8-15

Tercelj M, Salobir B, Zupancic M, Rylander R. Antifungal medication is efficient in the treatment of sarcoidosis. *Ther Adv Respir Dis.* (2011) 5:157– 62. doi: 10.1177/1753465811401648

Inaoka PT, Shono M, Kamada M, Espinoza JL. Host-microbe interactions in the pathogenesis and clinical course of sarcoidosis. *J Biomed Sci.* (2019) 26:45. doi: 10.1186/s12929-019-0537-6

Espinoza JL, Minami M. Sensing bacterial-induced DNA damaging effects via natural killer group 2 member D immune receptor: from dysbiosis to autoimmunity and carcinogenesis. *Front Immunol.* (2018) 9:52. doi: 10.3389/fimmu.2018.00052

Kriss M, Hazleton KZ, Nusbacher NM, Martin CG, Lozupone CA. Low diversity gut microbiota dysbiosis: drivers, functional implications and recovery. *Curr Opin Microbiol.* (2018) 44:34– 40. doi: 10.1016/j.mib.2018.07.003

Costa AN, Costa FMD, Campos SV, Salles RK, Athanazio RA. The pulmonary microbiome: challenges of a new paradigm. *J Bras Pneumol.* (2018) 44:424–32. doi: 10.1590/s1806-37562017000000209

Sulaiman I, Wu BG, Li Y, Scott AS, Malecha P, Scaglione B, et al. Evaluation of the airway microbiome in nontuberculous mycobacteria disease. *Eur Respir J.* (2018) 52:1800810. doi: 10.1183/13993003.00810-2018

Garzoni C, Brugger SD, Qi W, Wasmer S, Cusini A, Dumont P, et al. Microbial communities in the respiratory tract of patients with interstitial lung disease. *Thorax.* (2013) 68:1150–6. doi: 10.1136/thoraxjnl-2012-202917

Clarke EL, Lauder AP, Hofstaedter CE, Hwang Y, Fitzgerald AS, Imai I, et al. Microbial Lineages in Sarcoidosis. A Metagenomic Analysis Tailored for Low-Microbial Content Samples. *Am J Respir Crit Care Med.* (2018) 197:225–34. doi: 10.1164/rccm.201705-0891OC

Zimmermann A, Knecht H, Häsler R, Zissel G, Gaede KI, Hofmann S, et al. Atopobium and Fusobacterium as novel candidates for sarcoidosis-associated microbiota. *Eur Respir J.* (2017) 50:1600746. doi: 10.1183/13993003.00746-2016

Scher JU, Joshua V, Artacho A, Abdollahi-Roodsaz S, Öckinger J, Kullberg S, et al. The lung microbiota in early rheumatoid arthritis and autoimmunity. *Microbiome.* (2016) 4:60. doi: 10.1186/s40168-016-0206-x

Henke CE, Henke G, Elveback LR, Beard CM, Ballard DJ, Kurland LT. The epidemiology of sarcoidosis in Rochester, Minnesota: a population- based study of incidence and survival. *Am J Epidemiol.* (1986) 123:840–5. doi: 10.1093/oxfordjournals.aje.a114313

Demirkok SS, Basaranoglu M, Coker E, Karayel T. Seasonality of the onset of symptoms, tuberculin test anergy and Kveim positive reaction in a large cohort of patients with sarcoidosis. *Respirology.* (2007) 12:591– 3. doi: 10.1111/j.1440-1843.2007.01062.x

Wilsher ML. Seasonal clustering of sarcoidosis presenting with erythema nodosum. *Eur Respir J.* (1998) 12:1197– 9. doi: 10.1183/09031936.98.12051197

Fité E, Alsina JM, Mañá J, Pujol R, Ruiz J, Morera J. Epidemiology of sarcoidosis in Catalonia: 1979-1989. *Sarcoidosis Vasc Diffuse Lung Dis.* (1996) 13:153–8.

Gupta D, Agarwal R, Aggarwal AN. Seasonality of sarcoidosis: the 'heat' is on. *Sarcoidosis Vasc Diffuse Lung Dis.* (2013) 30:241–3.

Ungprasert P, Crowson CS, Matteson EL. Seasonal variation in incidence of sarcoidosis: a population-based study, 1976-2013. *Thorax.* (2016) 71:1164– 6. doi: 10.1136/thoraxjnl-2016-209032

Nicholson TT, Plant BJ, Henry MT, Bredin CP. Sarcoidosis in Ireland: regional differences in prevalence and mortality from 1996-2005. *Sarcoidosis Vasc Diffuse Lung Dis.* (2010) 27:111–20.

Hosoda Y, Sasagawa S, Yamaguchi T. Sarcoidosis and tuberculosis: epidemiological similarities and dissimilarities. A review of a series of studies in a Japanese work population. (1941-1996) and the general population (1959-1984). *Sarcoidosis Vasc Diffuse Lung Dis.* (2004). 21:85–93.

McDonough C, Gray GC. Risk factors for sarcoidosis hospitalization among U.S. Navy and Marine Corps personnel, 1981 to 1995. *Mil Med.* (2000). 165:630–2. doi: 10.1093/milmed/165.8.630

Kajdasz DK, Judson MA, Mohr LC, Lackland DT. Geographic variation in sarcoidosis in South Carolina: its relation to socioeconomic status and health care indicators. *Am J Epidemiol.* (1999) 150:271–8. doi: 10.1093/oxfordjournals.aje.a009998

Kowalska M, Niewiadomska E, Zejda JE. Epidemiology of sarcoidosis recorded in 2006-2010 in the Silesian voivodeship on the basis of routine medical reporting. *Ann Agric Environ Med.* (2014) 21:55–8.

Deubelbeiss U, Gemperli A, Schindler C, Baty F, Brutsche MH. Prevalence of sarcoidosis in Switzerland is associated with environmental factors. *Eur Respir J.* (2010) 35:1088–97. doi: 10.1183/09031936.00197808

Prezant DJ, Dhala A, Goldstein A, Janus D, Ortiz F, Aldrich TK, et al. The incidence, prevalence, and severity of sarcoidosis in New York City firefighters. *Chest.* (1999) 116:1183–93. doi: 10.1378/chest.116.5.1183

Kern DG, Neill MA, Wrenn DS, Varone JC. Investigation of a unique time- space cluster of sarcoidosis in firefighters. *Am Rev Respir Dis.* (1993) 148(4 Pt 1):974–80. doi: 10.1164/ajrccm/148.4_Pt_1.974

Gorham ED, Garland CF, Garland FC, Kaiser K, Travis WD, Centeno JA. Trends and occupational associations in incidence of hospitalized pulmonary sarcoidosis and other lung diseases in Navy personnel: a 27-year historical prospective study, 1975-2001. *Chest.* (2004) 126:1431– 8. doi: 10.1378/chest.126.5.1431

Newman LS, Rose CS, Bresnitz EA, Rossman MD, Barnard J, Frederick M, et al. A case control etiologic study of sarcoidosis: environmental and occupational risk factors. *Am J Respir Crit Care Med.* (2004) 170:1324– 30. doi: 10.1164/rccm.200402-249OC

Barnard J, Rose C, Newman L, Canner M, Martyny J, McCammon C, et al. Job and industry classifications associated with sarcoidosis in A Case- Control Etiologic Study of Sarcoidosis (ACCESS). *J Occup Environ Med.* (2005) 47:226–34. doi: 10.1097/01.jom.0000155711.88781.91

Kucera GP, Rybicki BA, Kirkey KL, Coon SW, Major ML, Maliarik MJ, et al. Occupational risk factors for sarcoidosis in African-American siblings. *Chest.* (2003) 123:1527–35. doi: 10.1378/chest.123.5.1527

Vihlborg P, Bryngelsson IL, Andersson L, Graff P. Risk of sarcoidosis and seropositive rheumatoid arthritis from occupational silica exposure in Swedish iron foundries: a retrospective cohort study. *BMJ Open.* (2017) 7:e016839. doi: 10.1136/bmjopen-2017-016839

Jonsson E, Järvholm B, Andersson M. Silica dust and sarcoidosis in Swedish construction workers. *Occup Med.* (2019) 69:482– 6. doi: 10.1093/occmed/kqz118

Ronsmans S, Verbeken EK, Adams E, Keirsbilck S, Yserbyt J, Wuyts WA, et al. Granulomatous lung disease in two workers making light bulbs. *Am J Ind Med.* (2019) 62:908–3. doi: 10.1002/ajim.23030

Rybicki BA, Amend KL, Maliarik MJ, Iannuzzi MC. Photocopier exposure and risk of sarcoidosis in African-American sibs. *Sarcoidosis Vasc Diffuse Lung Dis.* (2004) 21:49–55. doi: 10.1007/s11083-004-2862-x

Izbicki G, Chavko R, Banauch GI, Weiden MD, Berger KI, Aldrich TK, et al. World Trade Center "sarcoid-like" granulomatous pulmonary disease in New York City Fire Department rescue workers. *Chest.* (2007) 131:1414– 23. doi: 10.1378/chest.06-2114

Drent M, Bomans PH, Van Suylen RJ, Lamers RJ, Bast A, Wouters EF. Association of man-made mineral fibre exposure and sarcoidlike granulomas. *Respir Med.* (2000) 94:815–20. doi: 10.1053/rmed.2000.0827

Kajdasz DK, Lackland DT, Mohr LC, Judson MA. A current assessment of rurally linked exposures as potential risk factors for sarcoidosis. *Ann Epidemiol.* (2001) 11:111–7. doi: 10.1016/S1047-2797(00) 00179-4

Nakajima A, Saraya T, Mori T, Ikeda R, Sugita T, Watanabe T, et al. Familial summer-type hypersensitivity pneumonitis in Japan: two case reports and review of the literature. *BMC Res Notes.* (2013) 6:371. doi: 10.1186/1756-0500-6-371

Armbruster C, Dekan G, Hovorka A. Granulomatous pneumonitis and mediastinal lymphadenopathy due to photocopier toner dust. *Lancet.* (1996) 348:690. doi: 10.1016/S0140-6736(05)65119-7

Arkema EV, Grunewald J, Kullberg S, Eklund A, Askling J. Sarcoidosis incidence and prevalence: a nationwide register-based assessment in Sweden. *Eur Respir J.* (2016) 48:1690–9. doi: 10.1183/13993003.004 77-2016

Sawahata M, Sugiyama Y. An epidemiological perspective of the pathology and etiology of sarcoidosis. *Sarcoidosis Vasc Diffuse Lung Dis.* (2016) 33:112–6.

Hill AB. The environment and disease: association or causation? (1965). *J R Soc Med.* (2015). 108:32–7. doi: 10.1177/0141076814562718

Harris SS. Vitamin D and African Americans. *J Nutr.* (2006) 136:1126– 9. doi: 10.1093/jn/136.4.1126

Yanardag H, Pamuk ON, Karayel T. Cutaneous involvement in sarcoidosis: analysis of the features in 170 patients. *Respir Med.* (2003) 97:978– 82. doi: 10.1016/S0954-6111(03)00127-6

Hu Y, Yibrehu B, Zabini D, Kuebler WM. Animal models of sarcoidosis. *Cell Tissue Res.* (2017) 367:651–61. doi: 10.1007/s00441-016-2526-3

Barna BP, Judson MA, Thomassen MJ. Carbon Nanotubes and Chronic Granulomatous Disease. *Nanomaterials.* (2014) 4:508–21. doi: 10.3390/nano4020508

Barna BP, Huizar I, Malur A, McPeek M, Marshall I, Jacob M, et al. Carbon nanotube-induced pulmonary granulomatous disease: Twist1 and alveolar macrophage M1 activation. *Int J Mol Sci.* (2013) 14:23858– 71. doi: 10.3390/ijms141223858

Chen ES, Song Z, Willett MH, Heine S, Yung RC, Liu MC, et al. Serum amyloid A regulates granulomatous inflammation in sarcoidosis through Toll-like receptor-2. *Am J Respir Crit Care Med.* (2010) 181:360– 73. doi: 10.1164/rccm.200905-0696OC

Herndon B, Quinn T, Wasson N, Nzabi M, Molteni A. Urease and *Helicobacter* spp. antigens in pulmonary granuloma. *J Comp Pathol.* (2013) 148:266–77. doi: 10.1016/j.jcpa.2012.06.011

Swaisgood CM, Oswald-Richter K, Moeller SD, Klemenc JM, Ruple LM, Farver CF, et al. Development of a sarcoidosis murine lung granuloma model using Mycobacterium superoxide dismutase A peptide. *Am J Respir Cell Mol Biol.* (2011) 44:166–74. doi: 10.1165/rcmb.2009-0350OC

Werner JL, Escolero SG, Hewlett JT, Mak TN, Williams BP, Eishi Y, et al. Induction of pulmonary granuloma formation by propionibacterium acnes is regulated by MyD88 and Nox2. *Am J Respir Cell Mol Biol.* (2017) 56:121– 30. doi: 10.1165/rcmb.2016-0035OC

21

Exhaled Volatile Organic Compounds for Identifying Patients with Chronic Pulmonary Aspergillosis

Zheng-Tu Li[1†], Pei-Ying Zeng[1†], Zhao-Ming Chen[1†], Wei-Jie Guan[1,2†], Tong Wang[3,4], Ye Lin[1], Shao-Qiang Li[1], Zhi-Juan Zhang[3,4,5], Yang-Qing Zhan[1], Ming-Die Wang[1], Guo-Bin Tan[3,4,6], Xue Li[3,4] and Feng Ye[1*]*

[1] State Key Laboratory of Respiratory Disease, National Clinical Research Center for Respiratory Disease, National Center for Respiratory Medicine, Guangzhou Institute of Respiratory Health, The First Affiliated Hospital of Guangzhou Medical University, Guangzhou, China, [2] Department of Thoracic Surgery, Guangzhou Institute for Respiratory Health, The First Affiliated Hospital of Guangzhou Medical University, Guangzhou, Guangdong, China, [3] Institute of Mass Spectrometry and Atmospheric Environment, Jinan University, Guangzhou, China, [4] Guangdong Provincial Engineering Research Center for On-Line Source Apportionment System of Air Pollution, Guangzhou, China, [5] College of Pharmacy, Hena University of Chinese Medicine, Zhengzhou, China, [6] Guangzhou Hexin Instrument Co., Ltd., Guangzhou, China

Correspondence:
Xue Li
tamylee@jnu.edu.cn
Feng Ye
tu276025@gird.cn; yefeng@gird.cn

† These authors have contributed equally to this work and share first authorship

Background: Diagnosing chronic pulmonary aspergillosis is a major challenge in clinical practice. The development and validation of a novel, sensitive and specific assay for diagnosing chronic pulmonary aspergillosis is urgently needed.

Methods: From April 2018 to June 2019, 53 patients with chronic pulmonary aspergillosis (CPA), 32 patients with community-acquired pneumonia (CAP) and 48 healthy controls were recruited from the First Affiliated Hospital of Guangzhou Medical University. Clinical characteristics and samples were collected at enrollment. All exhaled breath samples were analyzed offline using thermal desorption single-photon ionization time-of-flight mass spectrometry; to analyze the metabolic pathways of the characteristic volatile organic compounds, serum samples were subjected to ultrahigh-performance liquid chromatography.

Results: We identified characteristic volatile organic compounds in patients with chronic pulmonary aspergillosis, which mainly consisted of phenol, neopentyl alcohol, toluene, limonene and ethylbenzene. These compounds were assessed using a logistic regression model. The sensitivity and specificity were 95.8 and 96.9% for discriminating patients in the CPA group from those in the CAP group and 95.8 and 97.9% for discriminating patients in the CPA group from healthy controls, respectively. The concentration of limonene (*m/z* 136) correlated significantly positively with anti-*Aspergillus fumigatus* IgG antibody titers ($r = 0.420$, $P < 0.01$). After antifungal treatment, serum IgG and the concentration of limonene (*m/z* 136) decreased in the subgroup of patients with chronic pulmonary aspergillosis.

Conclusions: We identified VOCs that can be used as biomarkers for differential diagnosis and therapeutic response prediction in patients with chronic pulmonary aspergillosis.

Keywords: chronic pulmonary aspergillosis, volatile organic compounds, metabolomics, exhalation, single-photon ionization-mass spectrometry

IMPORTANCE

In this study, it is promising to apply TD-SPI-TOF-MS to quickly evaluate the possibility of using breath VOCs to fast screen chronic pulmonary aspergillosis (CPA) patients. And several characteristic volatile organic compounds were identified as potential biomarkers for differential diagnosis and therapeutic response prediction in patients with CPA. Furthermore, the serum metabolism also used to preliminarily explore the source of exhaled VOCs. The findings of our study will provide a new, relatively non-invasive and easy to operate diagnostic method for the future clinical diagnosis of CPA.

INTRODUCTION

Pulmonary aspergillosis is common in immunosuppressed patients and a major global health burden, affecting more than 3 million people worldwide (1, 2). Patients with chronic pulmonary aspergillosis (CPA) frequently have comorbidities and atypical clinical symptoms, making early diagnosis and treatment difficult. To date, the diagnosis of CPA mainly relies on pathology, serology and imaging. However, these diagnostic methods are time consuming and may be invasive, and personnel performing microscopy analyses need to be professional and experienced; therefore, missed or delayed diagnosis occurs in a considerable proportion of patients, which might increase the mortality rate (3, 4).

Recent scientific advances have allowed for the rapid, non-invasive, and convenient diagnosis of respiratory disease with cutting-edge technologies (5). Measuring the patterns of volatile organic compounds (VOCs) in exhaled breath is a novel non-invasive metabolomic approach for studying the molecular signatures of respiratory disease (6–10), and gas chromatography-mass spectrometry (GC-MS) has identified several characteristic VOCs in patients with pulmonary aspergillosis (11–13). Nonetheless, breath analysis of pulmonary aspergillosis is mostly based on *Aspergillus* strains *in vitro*, and there are a limited number of volatile substances that can be detected by GC-MS. Thermal desorption—single-photon ionization—mass spectrometry (TD-SPI-MS) has a high sensitivity, is user-friendly, and can be applied to detect VOCs with a low concentration or a wide range of substances (9, 14). In general, metabolomic analysis can quantitatively analyze all metabolites, which helps in evaluating associations between metabolites and pathophysiological changes (15). Indeed, a number of studies have reported that serum metabolites can be used as biomarkers of infectious diseases for diagnosing and evaluating clinical severity (16–19).

In this study, we aimed to perform broad-spectrum screening of exhaled VOCs and metabolomic analysis by applying TD-SPI-MS for patients with CPA. The metabolic pathways of such metabolites may further reveal the components and biological roles of the characteristic VOCs in exhaled breath associated with pulmonary aspergillosis. Our findings provide a novel tool for the non-invasive, simple and reliable clinical diagnosis of CPA.

METHODS

Patients

Between April 2018 and June 2019, patients with CPA, patients with community-acquired pneumonia (CAP) and healthy controls were recruited from the First Affiliated Hospital of Guangzhou Medical University. Patients with CPA according to the guidelines of diagnosis and management of *Aspergillus* diseases were enrolled (group CPA) (20). The diagnosis of CAP was made according to the guidelines of diagnosis and treatment of CAP (group CAP) (21). The healthy controls did not have any documented pulmonary infectious, interstitial or malignant lung diseases (group N). We excluded patients who were younger than 18 years old, declined exhaled breath analysis, had ingested foods or brushed their teeth after 22:00 p.m. the night before sample collection or were currently smokers or had consumed alcohol within 2 months prior to the examination.

The guidelines (20) for the diagnosis and treatment of pulmonary aspergillosis recommend at least 6 months of voriconazole therapy (200 mg every 12 h) for CPA. As the plasma concentration of voriconazole was detected to maintain the recommended effective concentration range (1~5.5 mg/L), four time points were scheduled for follow-up during the antifungal treatment. The patients were followed up for 9 months (before treatment and at 3, 6, and 9 months after treatment).

VOC Analysis

TD-SPI-MS was performed to obtain qualitative and quantitative data. See **Supplementary Material** for the detailed methods and precautions of exhaled breath collection.

Serum Metabolite Analysis and Metabolic Pathways

Patients fasted for 8–10 h before exhaled gas collection, followed by venipuncture (4 ml) in the morning to collect peripheral blood. The samples were centrifuged at 3,000 rpm for 15 min, and the serum was stored at −80°C for subsequent analysis. For each assay, 100 μl serum plus 300 μl methanol and 20 μl internal standard were added to a centrifuge tube. After vortexing for 30 s, the samples were subjected to ultrasonic treatment in an ice bath for 5 min and kept at −20°C for 2 h. After centrifugation at 13,000 rpm at 4°C for 15 min, 200 μl of the supernatant was transferred to a 2-ml sample vial. All serum metabolites were analyzed using an ultrahigh-performance liquid chromatography-pristine instrument.

Statistical Analysis

Clinical data were analyzed using IBM SPSS Statistics (version 20, SPSS Inc., USA). A *P*-value of 0.05 or less indicated statistical significance. Categorical data are presented as numbers and percentages and continuous data as medians and ranges or interquartile ranges (IQRs). Comparison of continuous data was performed using Student's *t*-test or Mann-Whitney test. Fisher's exact test was applied to compare categorical variables. Partial least squares discrimination analysis (OPLS-DA) with SIMCA software (version 14.1, MKS Umetrics, Sweden) (22) was adopted. High-dimensional data were further processed

TABLE 1 | Baseline characteristics of the study participants.

Characteristics	Group CPA (n = 53)	Group CAP (n = 32)	Group N (n = 48)	*P*-value
Age (year, x ± S)	49.0 ± 15.8	38.0 ± 18.5	26.2 ± 7.0	0.001
Sex, male (No, %)	35 (66.0%)	11 (34.4%)	33 (68.8%)	0.004
Height (cm, x ± S)	162.9 ± 10.0	161.4 ± 9.0	162.2 ± 9.2	0.762
Weight (kg, x ± S)	51.6 ± 10.9	56.3 ± 12.5	59.0 ± 10.6	0.003
Smoking status[a]				
Ex-smoker (No, %)	13 (24.5%)	5 (15.6%)	3 (6.3%)	0.010
Never-smoker (No, %)	40 (75.5%)	27 (84.4%)	45 (93.8%)	
Drinking status[a]				
Ex-drinker (No, %)	3 (5.8%)	1 (3.1%)	0	0.121
Never-drinker (No, %)	50 (94.3%)	31 (96.9%)	48 (100.0%)	
Eating habits[a]				
Light diet (No, %)	45 (83.2%)	30 (93.8%)	43 (89.6%)	0.078
Non-light diet (No, %)	8 (16.8%)	2 (6.3%)	5 (10.4%)	

a: Ex-smokers were defined as those who smoked continuously for at least 6 months but had quit smoking for more than 2 months at the time of recruitment; the definitions of ex-drinkers were similar to those of ex-smokers; light diet refers to daily diet habits, including spicy food such as pepper, garlic, and green onion.

through dimensionality reduction, and the variable importance for projection (VIP) in the OPLS-DA model was calculated (23). For VIPs equal to or >1.0, an array of characteristic ions in the CPA group was selected as potential targets. As each substance may have the same germplasm charge ratio, each *m/z* value can correspond to one or more VOCs. The possible ion range can be inferred according to the CAS (Chemical Abstracts Service, USA).

Metabolites were qualitatively evaluated according to the KEGG (Kyoto Encyclopedia of Genes and Genomes) (http://www.genome.jp/kegg/) database and a customized database. Multivariate statistical analysis was performed using the normalized data matrix with PCA, PLS-DA, OPLS-DA and sequencing tests. Multivariate (OPLS-DA) and univariate statistical (Student's *t*-test) analyses were applied to screen and cluster differentially expressed metabolites, perform metabolic pathway KEGG enrichment analysis, and construct a metabolite regulation network. Potential metabolic pathways between exhaled breath and blood were explored by performing Venn analysis and enrichment analysis. The digital matrix composed of the selected characteristic VOCs was imported into MATLAB (version R2017b, MathWorks, Inc., USA) to construct different classification models, and the accuracy, sensitivity and characteristics of the models were verified by binary logistic regression analysis. The optimal model was selected for simulation operation, which further confirmed the value of characteristic VOCs for CPA diagnosis. Pearson's correlation analysis was used to analyze correlations between exhaled breath VOC expression levels and anti-*Aspergillus* IgG titers in the CPA group.

RESULTS

Baseline Characteristics

We included 53 patients in the CPA group and 32 in the CAP group and 48 subjects in group N. The study flow chart is provided in **Supplementary Figure 1**, and the baseline characteristics of the included participants are shown in **Table 1**. Most of the subjects were male (59.4%), and the male subjects were significantly older than the female subjects [median: 54 (range 38–65 years) vs. 39 (range 29–54 years)]. Patients in the CPA group rarely smoked or drank alcohol. Additionally, age and sex differed significantly between the CPA group and group N ($P < 0.01$). Both weight and smoking history ($P < 0.01$), but not height, drinking history or eating habits, differed significantly among the three groups.

Characteristic Exhaled VOCs

To avoid artifacts, the sampling temperature was controlled between 20 and 25°C, and a regular ultraviolet lamp was applied for environmental irradiation to minimize contamination before sample collection. Despite certain differences in demographic characteristics, we recruited study participants without a recent smoking history.

According to the OPLS-DA model of the entire cohort, VOCs in exhaled breath were capable of distinguishing the three groups ($R^2 = 0.954$, $Q^2 = 0.745$, **Figures 1A,B**). Therefore, the original data model explained the differences among the CPA, CAP and N groups. The *m/z* value of the characteristic VOCs was derived based on the VIP value (**Figure 1C**). After incorporating information from Chemical Abstracts Database (Chemical Abstracts Service, CAS), the characteristic VOCs in patients with CPA were found to be ketones, aldehydes, esters, hydrocarbons and benzenes; the detailed characteristics of these compounds are shown in **Table 2**.

Characteristic Serum Metabolites and Metabolic Pathways

At present, existing theories show that the exhaled VOCs are the product of blood metabolism after pathogen infection (5, 6, 24). Therefore, the purpose of our study on serum metabolomics is to preliminarily explore the source of exhaled VOCs. To identify

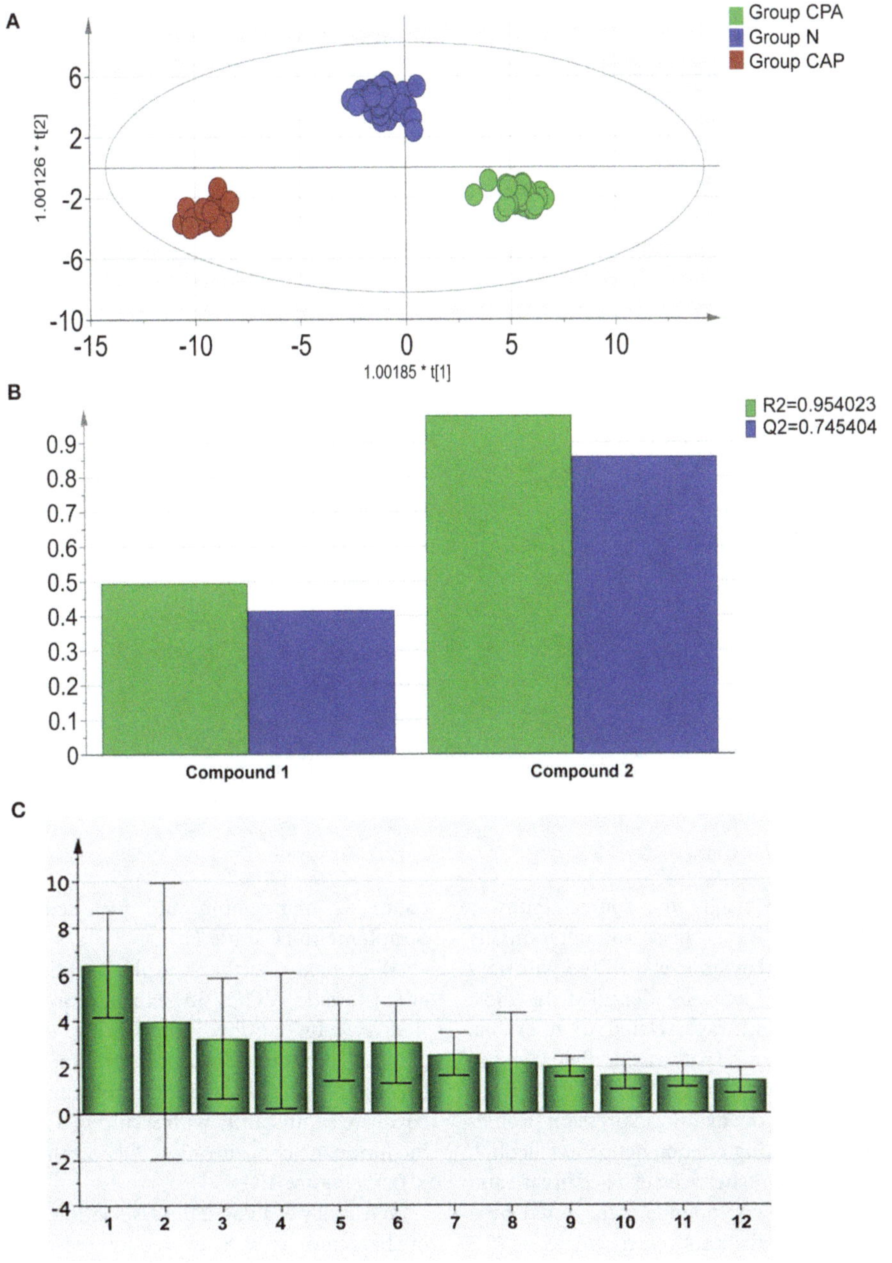

FIGURE 1 | Statistical analysis of characteristic VOCs in exhaled breath of patients with CPA. **(A)** OPLS-DA score plot of characteristic VOCs in exhaled breath samples in group CPA, group CAP and group N. **(B)** Parameters of the OPLS-DA model of characteristic VOCs in exhaled breath samples in group CPA, group CAP and group N. **(C)** VIP value of characteristic VOCs in exhaled breath samples of patients with CPA.

characteristic serum metabolites, we randomly selected samples from subjects with paired serum samples (10 cases in group CPA, 5 in group CAP and 5 in group N). Except for a significant difference in age between group CPA and group N, there were no significant differences in sex, weight or height among the three groups ($P > 0.05$).

The OPLS-DA score chart (**Figure 2A**) showed that the original model was able to explain the differences in serum metabolites among the CPA, CAP and N groups. According to the VIP value of OPLS-DA and between-group comparisons (Student's *t*-test), we identified 24 differentially expressed metabolites between groups CPA and N and 17 differentially expressed metabolites between groups CPA and CAP (**Figure 2B**). A Venn diagram further illustrated 7 metabolites in group CPA that were differentially expressed compared with groups N and CAP (**Figure 2C**).

The same characteristic VOC expressed metabolites between exhaled breath and serum in CPA patients were enriched in

TABLE 2 | Reference compounds of characteristic VOCs of patients in the CPA group.

Number	m/z value	Compound name	CAS number
1	m/z 58	Propanone/Acetone	7-64-1
2	m/z 62	Dimethyl sulfide	75-18-3
		Ethylthiol	75-08-1
3	m/z 68	Isoprene/2-Methyl-1,3-Butadiene	78-79-5
4	m/z 69	1,2-Pentadiene	591-95-7
		Ethyl acetate	141-78-6
5	m/z 88	Neopentyl alcohol	75-84-3
		2-Methyl-2-butanol	75-85-5
6	m/z 92	Toluene	108-88-3
7	m/z 94	Phenol	108-95-2
		Methyl disulfide	624-92-0
8	m/z 106	M-Xylene	108-38-3
		P-Xylene	106-42-3
		Ethylbenzene	100-41-4
9	m/z 134	1-Methyl-2-propylbenzene	1074-17-5
		1-Methyl-4-propylbenzene	1074-55-1
10	m/z 136	2-Methyl-3-propylpyrazine	15986-80-8
		3,7-dimethyl-1,3,7-Octatriene	502-99-8
		2-(sec-Butyl)pyrazine	124070-52
		Dipentene	138-86-3
		Phenyl acetate	122-79-2
11	m/z 281	Diphenyl hydrogen phosphate	838-85-7
12	m/z 282	–	–

different metabolic pathways to clarify the source. Pathway analysis based on the latest KEGG database for differentially expressed metabolites was assigned to six level-1 KEGG pathways (**Figure 3A**). Pathway enrichment analysis identified the most significantly altered metabolic pathways related to microbial metabolism in diverse environments (pathway 1, $P<0.05$) and degradation of aromatic compounds (pathway 2, $P < 0.05$) (**Figure 3B**). In these metabolic pathways, the expression profiles of the characteristic VOCs (including phenol, neopentyl alcohol, toluene, limonene and ethylbenzene) between exhaled breath and serum matched (**Table 3**). These compounds were tested by a logistic regression model, with a sensitivity and specificity of 95.8 and 96.9% for discriminating patients in the CPA group from those in the CAP group and 95.8 and 97.9% for discriminating patients in the CPA group from healthy controls, respectively (**Figures 4A,B**).

Correlation of Characteristic VOCs With Clinical Parameters

In the CAP group, 13 patients (40.6%) had *Mycoplasma* pneumonia, 11 (34.4%) bacterial pneumonia and 8 (25.0%) viral pneumonia. Among CPA patients, the main presenting symptoms were fever, cough, expectoration, hemoptysis and dyspnea. The dominant radiologic characteristics included cavitation, nodules, patchy shadows and ground-glass opacities. There were no significant differences in the neutrophil count or hemoglobin and procalcitonin levels ($P < 0.05$, **Supplementary Table 1**).

We next further explored the association between characteristic VOCs in exhaled breath and anti-*Aspergillus fumigatus* IgG antibody titers in the serum of those in the CPA group. Although the concentration of characteristic VOCs (neopentyl alcohol, phenol, toluene, ethylbenzene) did not correlate significantly with serum IgG antibody titers ($P > 0.05$), the limonene concentration did correlate positively ($r = 0.420$, $P < 0.01$, **Figure 4B**).

We finally evaluated the association between dynamic changes in characteristic VOC expression levels and disease outcomes as well as the efficacy of antifungal treatment. Data were available during longitudinal follow-up four patients (**Figure 4D**). The concentration of VOC *m/z* 136 (limonene) progressively declined after the initiation of antifungal treatment. After anti-fungal treatment for 9 months, the health status of three patients (PA-13, PA-27 and PA-48) improved, as reflected by the alleviation of cough or hemoptysis, decreased anti-*A. fumigatus* IgG antibody titers (negative in one case, positive in two cases), decreased absorption of lesions on chest computed tomography, and a stable blood voriconazole concentration. In support of these clinical signs, the concentration of exhaled breath limonene was also markedly decreased. After 3 months of treatment, PA-27 was readmitted to the hospital due to the recurrence of hemoptysis. Meanwhile, the anti-*Aspergillus* IgG antibody titer decreased compared with the first clinical visit. In contrast, the

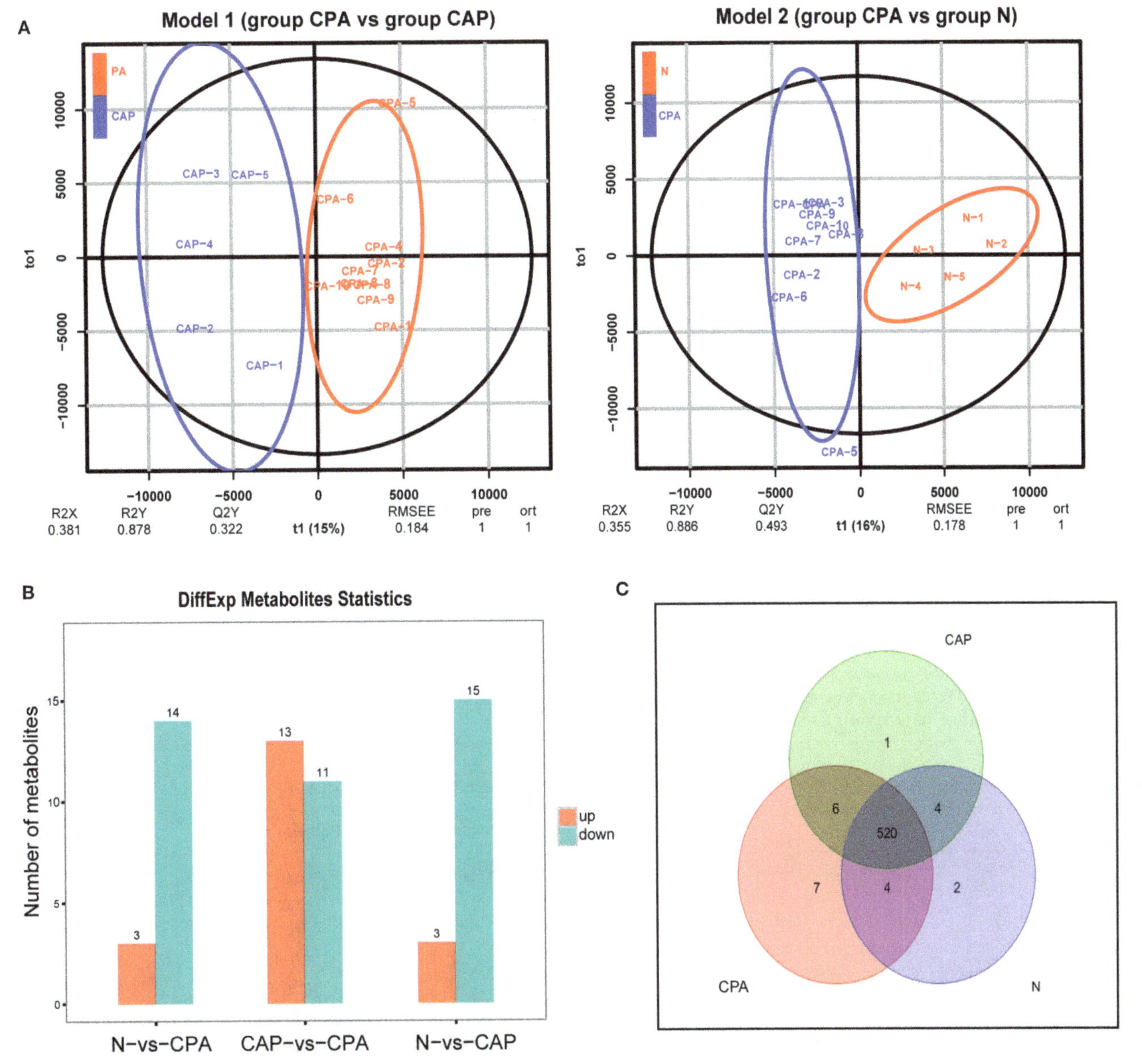

FIGURE 2 | Serum metabolome analysis for distinguishing group CPA from group CAP and group N. **(A)** OPLS-DA score plot of serum characteristic metabolites between the CPA group and the CAP and N groups. **(B)** Quantity change of different serum metabolites among group CPA, group CAP and group N. **(C)** Venn analysis of serum characteristic metabolites in patients with CPA.

concentration of exhaled breath limonene increased significantly and then decreased significantly with improvement of the disease. Patient No. PA-20 exhibited disease progression after 9 months of antifungal treatment, with a recurrence of hemoptysis and an increase in pulmonary infiltration, as revealed by chest computed tomography. Nevertheless, negative conversion was achieved for anti-*Aspergillus* IgG antibodies, with the concentration of limonene remaining relatively stable over the course of follow-up (**Figure 4C**).

DISCUSSION

We identified several characteristic VOCs by performing TD-SPI-MS in the exhaled breath and serum of patients with CPA, revealing biological pathways associated with microbial metabolism in diverse environments and the degradation of aromatic compounds. Detection of these compounds can effectively distinguish patients with CPA; therefore, some characteristic compounds from exhaled breath or serum VOCs might help with the diagnosis of CPA.

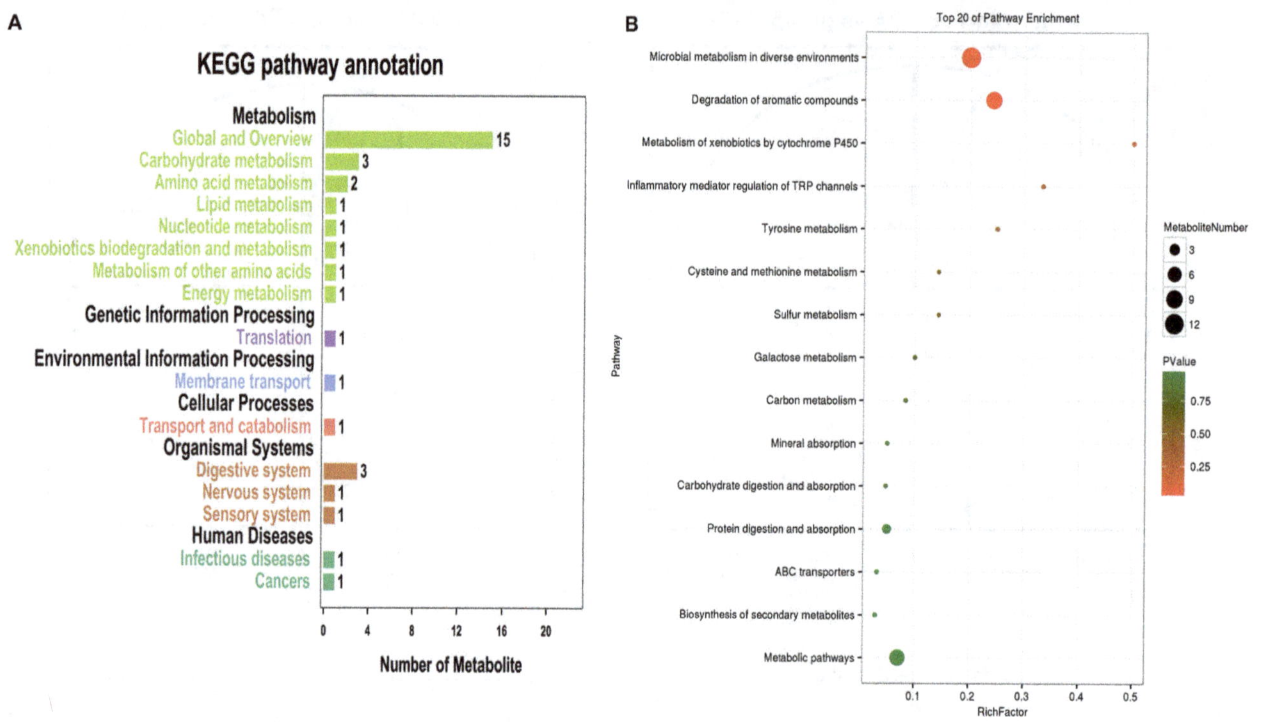

FIGURE 3 | Common metabolic pathways of characteristic VOCs and serum-specific metabolites in patients with CPA. **(A)** Pathway enrichment histogram of candidate metabolites. **(B)** Bubble diagram of pathway enrichment results of candidate metabolites. the *P**value ranges from 0 to 1. The closer to zero, the closer the color is to red, indicating that the enrichment is more significant.

TABLE 3 | Common metabolic pathways of characteristic VOCs in exhaled breath and serum metabolites of patients in the CPA group.

KEGG pathway ID	Pathway	*P*-value	Pathway C-id**	Compound
ko01120	Microbial metabolism in diverse environments	0.0068	C00146	Phenol
			C00556	Neopentyl alcohol*
			C00556	Neopentyl alcohol
			C01455	Toluene
			C06104	Dipentene*
			C07111	Ethylbenzene
ko01220	Degradation of aromatic compounds	0.0140	C00146	Phenol
			C00556	Neopentyl alcohol*
			C01455	Toluene
			C06104	Di pentene*
			C07111	Ethylbenzene

*1. **: ID (C number) of metabolites in the KEGG database; 2. *: serum differential metabolites; 3. Other unmarked metabolites are characteristic VOCs of exhaled breath.*

Exhaled breath analysis is prone to bias by environmental or host factors (25, 26). In our study, we conducted rigorous screening for the inclusion of patients, environmental controls and repeated sample collection to minimize measurement bias. The statistical analysis model consistently indicated a good separation of exhaled breath and serum VOCs among the three groups. Our findings confirmed the results from the study by Koo et al. (12), in which alkenes, ketones and alkanes (including limonene) were detected by GC-MS in the exhaled breath of patients with pulmonary aspergillosis. These findings indicate the value of these compounds as exhaled biomarkers to differentiate pulmonary aspergillosis from other diseases and healthy subjects as well as alkenes and ketones as exhaled breath biomarkers (such as acetone, limonene, isoprene and 1,2-pentadiene). Benzene compounds have not been confirmed as characteristic VOCs of CPA. Our study found that phenol, toluene and ethylbenzene might serve as biomarkers for CPA. The high sensitivity and specificity for differentiating the CPA group might be related to differences in expression levels of benzene, toluene, xylene and chlorobenzene, which are oxidative stress markers of aspergillosis

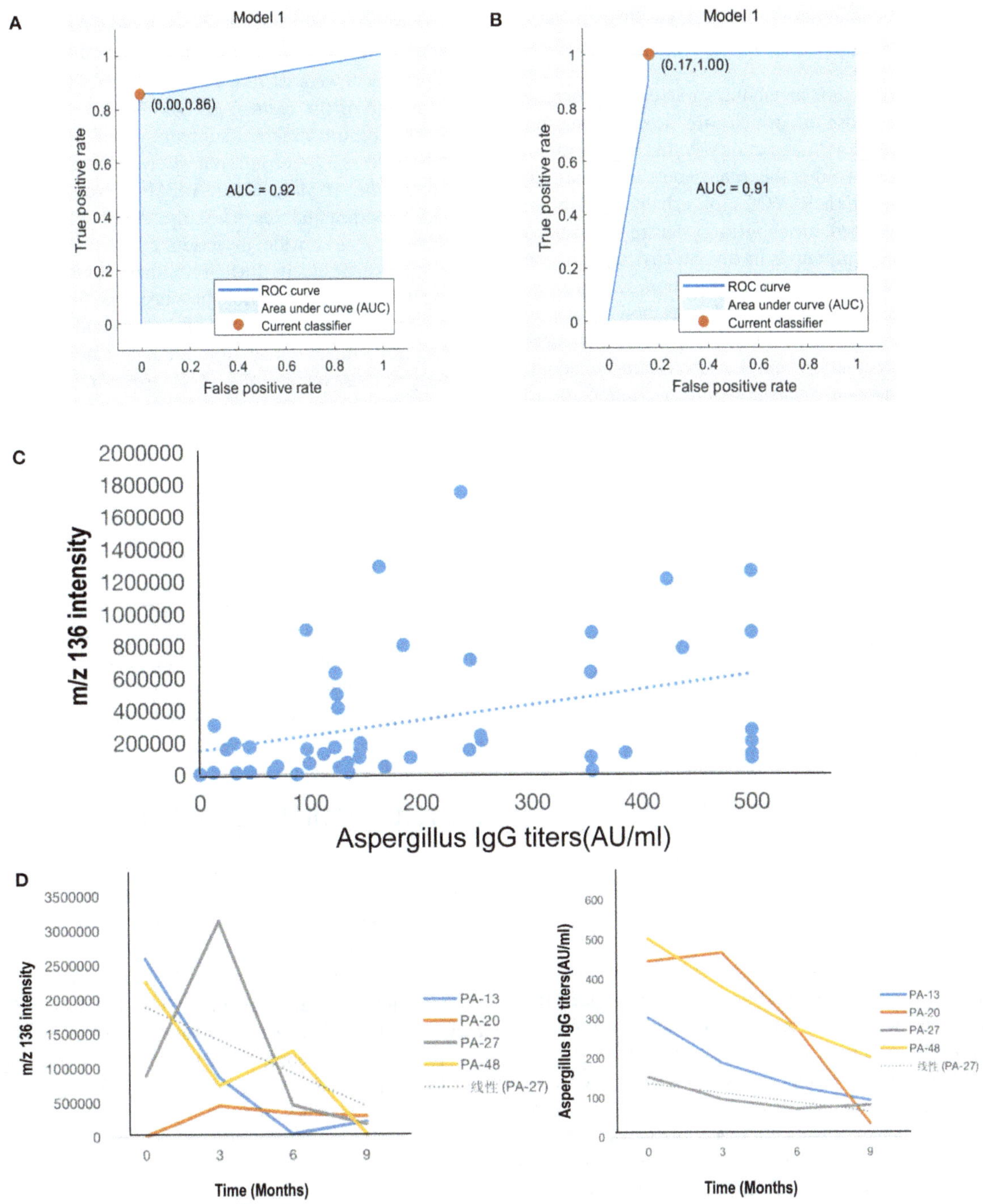

FIGURE 4 | Clinical correlation of characteristic VOCs in exhaled breath of patients with CPA. **(A)** Univariate logistic regression model of the CPA group and CAP group. **(B)** Univariate logistic regression model of group CPA and group N. **(C)** Correlation analysis between characteristic VOCs and serum anti-*Aspergillus fumigatus* IgG antibody titers. **(D)** Dynamic changes in levels of breath characteristic VOCs and serum anti-*Aspergillus fumigatus* IgG antibody titers of 4 patients in the CPA group for baseline and follow-up in the third, sixth, and ninth month after voriconazole treatment.

(27). For example, 2-pentyl furan has been considered an important marker of exhaled breath VOCs of patients with *Aspergillus* infection (11, 28, 29). *Aspergillus spp.* produce 2-PF on blood agar, nutrient agar and other media. In our study, the substance at *m/z* 128 had a VIP value of <1 and was not confirmed as a characteristic VOC of PA. 2-PF might have originated from hemoglobin, which is produced by blood agar culture medium or pulmonary hemorrhage rather than

Aspergillus spp. per se (30). Therefore, it is important to explore the source of these compounds, for instance, by performing metabolomic analysis.

There are more than 200 metabolites related to *Aspergillus sp.* infections (31), most of which are toxins, yet most metabolites produced by interactions with the host are still unknown. In our study, the main metabolic pathways involved in the characteristic VOCs of exhaled breath and the differentially expressed metabolites in serum consisted of microbial metabolism compounds in diverse environments and the products of aromatic compound degradation. Characteristic VOCs in microbial metabolism and metabolic pathways (degradation of aromatic compounds) were shared between the exhaled breath and serum samples. The main metabolites (including phenol, neopentyl alcohol, toluene, limonene and ethylbenzene) suggested that *Aspergillus sp.* infection might result in the production of characteristic metabolites through microbial metabolism and aromatic compound degradation (12, 30). Consistent with this finding, our study also showed limonene to be a potential characteristic compound, thus confirming its value for differential diagnosis based on exhaled breath analysis. It has been reported that aromatic hydrocarbons can regulate inflammatory T cell and dendritic cell (DC) responses (32) and induce oxidative stress and airway tissue injury (33). These compounds in the exhaled breath might also be products of the host's immune response to pathogens (5).

We further confirmed the sensitivity and specificity of the abovementioned characteristic VOCs. According to a previous study, the sensitivity and specificity of exhaled breath VOCs were 95.8 and 96.9% for discriminating patients with CPA from those with CAP and 95.8 and 97.9% for discriminating patients with CPA from healthy controls, respectively. Compared with traditional serologic testing, such as GM tests using serum and bronchoalveolar lavage samples (34), VOC assays *via* TD-SPI-MS might better indicate candidate biomarkers in the exhaled breath of CPA patients. The current international guidelines suggest that IgG antibody detection is the most sensitive laboratory test for the diagnosis of chronic cavitary pulmonary aspergillosis (CCPA) (3). We also showed that changes in serum anti-*A. fumigatus* IgG antibody titers in patients with CPA before and after antifungal treatment may sensitively reveal the occurrence and progression of CPA. Anti-fungal therapy reportedly decreases levels of serum IgG titers in patients with CPA (35). Importantly, during a 9-month follow-up, the intensity of limonene also decreased significantly. In addition, there were two patients who experienced CPA recurrence. Among them, despite an apparent decrease in IgG titer, the limonene concentration remained relatively high, suggesting that exhaled VOCs might be used for evaluating the therapeutic response. Hence, the concentration of characteristic VOCs might indicate the efficacy of antifungal treatment.

Several limitations need to be acknowledged. First, interpretation of the findings (particularly the follow-up investigation) was limited by the small sample size, and only the conformed CPA patients, was taken as the study group. In the future study, we will recruit all suspected CAP patients as many as possible. Thus, there will be enough remaining suspected CAP patients which were excluded from the real CPA patients can be used as one of the control groups. Further investigations that take into account different subtypes of pulmonary aspergillosis are also necessary. Second, our study lacks an *in vitro* analysis of *Aspergillus* strains, which will help validate our findings of cell experimental results. Third, although the TD-SPI-MS instrument has a wide detection range and high sensitivity, the findings should be further validated by GC-MS and other mass spectrometry technologies because there is no unified detection standard for exhaled VOCs and detection results among instruments may differ. Finally, heterogeneity in the underlying diseases of the CAP group might have affected the discriminatory capacity of VOCs, though the inclusion of patients with CAP of different pathogens might have increased the generalizability of our findings.

CONCLUSION

Exhaled breath VOCs (phenol, neopentyl alcohol, toluene, limonene and ethylbenzene), which may help effectively discriminate patients with CPA, are involved in endogenous metabolism. Limonene might be a novel biomarker that reflects the clinical course and treatment response of CPA.

AUTHOR CONTRIBUTIONS

Z-TL, P-YZ, XL, and FY conceived of and designed the study. Z-TL, P-YZ, Z-MC, W-JG, and FY carried out the analyses and wrote the first draft of the manuscript. P-YZ, YL, S-QL, Y-QZ, and M-DW carried out the patient's recruitment, clinical sample collection, and testing. TW, Z-JZ, G-BT, and XL contributed to detection and analysis of VOCs. P-YZ, Z-MC, and YL contributed to the collection of data from the electronic medical records. All authors contributed to data acquisition, data analysis, or data interpretation and reviewed and approved the final version of the manuscript.

ACKNOWLEDGMENTS

We thank the patient; the nurses and clinical staff who are providing care for the patient; staff at the respiratory medicine department of hospital; staff at the clinical lab of hospital; technical staff of the department of State Key Laboratory of Respiratory Disease for excellent assistance. Furthermore, we would also like to thank AJE team for polishing the English language of this manuscript.

REFERENCES

Kosmidis C, Denning DW. The clinical spectrum of pulmonary aspergillosis. *Thorax*. (2015) 70: 270–7. doi: 10.1136/thoraxjnl-2014-206291

Bongomin F, Gago S, Oladele RO, Denning DW. Global and multi-national prevalence of fungal diseases-estimate precision. *J Fungi*. (2017) 3:5247. doi: 10.3390/jof3040057

Patterson TF, Thompson GR, Denning DW, Fishman JA, Hadley S, Herbrecht R, et al. Practice guidelines for the diagnosis and management of aspergillosis: 2016 update by the infectious diseases society of America. *Clin Infect Dis*. (2016) 63:e1–e60. doi: 10.1093/cid/ciw326

Bernal-Martinez L, Alastruey-Izquierdo A, Cuenca-Estrella M. Diagnostics and susceptibility testing in Aspergillus. *Future Microbiol*. (2016) 11:315–28. doi: 10.2217/fmb.15.140

van Oort PM, Povoa P, Schnabel R, Dark P, Artigas A, Bergmans D, et al. The potential role of exhaled breath analysis in the diagnostic process of pneumonia-a systematic review. *J Breath Res*. (2018) 12:024001. doi: 10.1088/1752-7163/aaa499

Tang Z, Liu Y, Duan Y. Breath analysis: technical developments and challenges in the monitoring of human exposure to volatile organic compounds. *J Chromatogr B*. (2015) 1002:285–99. doi: 10.1016/j.jchromb.2015.08.041

Boots AW, Bos LD, van der Schee MP, van Schooten FJ, Sterk PJ. Exhaled molecular fingerprinting in diagnosis and monitoring: validating volatile promises. *Trends Mol Med*. (2015) 21:633–44. doi: 10.1016/j.molmed.2015.08.001

Amann A, Costello BL, Miekisch W, Schubert J, Buszewski B, Pleil J, et al. The human volatilome: volatile organic compounds (VOCs) in exhaled breath, skin emanations, urine, feces and saliva. *J Breath Res*. (2014) 8:034001. doi: 10.1088/1752-7155/8/3/034001

Hong Y, Che X, Su H, Mai Z, Huang Z, Huang W, et al. Exhaled breath analysis using on-line preconcentration mass spectrometry for gastric cancer diagnosis. *J Mass Spectrom*. (2021) 56:e4588. doi: 10.1002/jms.4588

Ratiu IA, Ligor T, Bocos-Bintintan V, Mayhew CA, Buszewski B. Volatile organic compounds in exhaled breath as fingerprints of lung cancer, asthma and COPD. *J Clin Med*. (2020) 10:352. doi: 10.3390/jcm10010032

Chambers ST, Bhandari S, Scott-Thomas A, Syhre M. Novel diagnostics: progress toward a breath test for invasiveAspergillus fumigatus. *Med Mycol*. (2011) 49:S54–61. doi: 10.3109/13693786.2010.508187

Koo S, Thomas HR, Daniels SD, Lynch RC, Fortier SM, Shea MM, et al. A breath fungal secondary metabolite signature to diagnose invasive aspergillosis. *Clin Infect Dis*. (2014) 59:1733–40. doi: 10.1093/cid/ciu725

Gerritsen MG, Brinkman P, Escobar N, Bos LD, de Heer K, Meijer M, et al. Profiling of volatile organic compounds produced by clinical Aspergillus isolates using gas chromatography–mass spectrometry. *Med Mycol*. (2018) 56:253–6. doi: 10.1093/mmy/myx035

Huang Y, Li J, Tang B, Zhu L, Hou K, Li H. Development of a portable single photon ionization-photoelectron ionization time-of-flight mass spectrometer. *Int J Anal Chem*. (2015) 2015:581696. doi: 10.1155/2015/581696

Williams JH, Phillips TD, Jolly PE, Stiles JK, Jolly CM, Aggarwal D. Human aflatoxicosis in developing countries: a review of toxicology, exposure, potential health consequences, and interventions. *Am J Clin Nutr*. (2004) 80:1106–22. doi: 10.1093/ajcn/80.5.1106

Shen B, Yi X, Sun Y, Bi X, Du J, Zhang C, et al. Proteomic and metabolomic characterization of COVID-19 patient sera. *Cell*. (2020) 182:59–72. e15. doi: 10.1016/j.cell.2020.05.032

Cho Y, Park Y, Sim B, Kim J, Lee H, Cho SN, et al. Identification of serum biomarkers for active pulmonary tuberculosis using a targeted metabolomics approach. *Sci Rep*. (2020) 10:3825. doi: 10.1038/s41598-020-6 0669-0

Albors-Vaquer A, Rizvi A, Matzapetakis M, Lamosa P, Coelho AV, Patel AB, et al. Active and prospective latent tuberculosis are associated with different metabolomic profiles: clinical potential for the identification of rapid and non-invasive biomarkers. *Emerg Microbes Infect*. (2020) 9:1131–9. doi: 10.1080/22221751.2020.1760734

Cui L, Zheng D, Lee YH, Chan TK, Kumar Y, Ho WE, et al. Metabolomics investigation reveals metabolite mediators associated with acute lung injury and repair in a murine model of influenza pneumonia. *Sci Rep*. (2016) 6:26076. doi: 10.1038/srep26076

Ullmann AJ, Aguado JM, Arikan-Akdagli S, Denning DW, Groll AH, Lagrou K, et al. Diagnosis and management of Aspergillus diseases: executive summary of the 2017 ESCMID-ECMM-ERS guideline. *Clin Microbiol Infect*. (2018) 24 (Suppl 1):e1–e38. doi: 10.1016/j.cmi.2018.01.002

Cao B, Huang Y, She DY, Cheng QJ, Fan H, Tian XL, et al. Diagnosis and treatment of community-acquired pneumonia in adults: 2016 clinical practice guidelines by the Chinese Thoracic Society, Chinese Medical Association. *Clin Respir J*. (2018) 12:1320–60. doi: 10.1111/crj.12674

Jang HJ, Lee JD, Jeon HS, Kim AR, Kim S, Lee HS, et al. Metabolic profiling of eccentric exercise-induced muscle damage in human urine. *Toxicol Res*. (2018) 34:199–210. doi: 10.5487/TR.2018.34.3.199

Wang C, Li P, Lian A, Sun B, Wang X, Guo L, et al. Blood volatile compounds as biomarkers for colorectal cancer. *Cancer Biol Ther*. (2014) 15:200–6. doi: 10.4161/cbt.26723

Turner C. Techniques and issues in breath and clinical sample headspace analysis for disease diagnosis. *Bioanalysis*. (2016) 8:677–90. doi: 10.4155/bio.16.22

Hlastala MP, Anderson JC. Alcohol breath test: gas exchange issues. *J Appl Physiol*. (2016) 121:367–75. doi: 10.1152/japplphysiol.005 48.2015

Gaugg MT, Gomez DG, Barrios-Collado C, Vidal-de-Miguel G, Kohler M, Zenobi R, et al. Expanding metabolite coverage of real-time breath analysis by coupling a universal secondary electrospray ionization source and high resolution mass spectrometry—a pilot study on tobacco smokers. *J Breath Res*. (2016) 10:016010. doi: 10.1088/1752-7155/10/1/016010

Phillips M, Cataneo RN, Condos R, Ring EG, Greenberg J, La Bombardi V, et al. Volatile biomarkers of pulmonary tuberculosis in the breath. *Tuberculosis*. (2007) 87:44–52. doi: 10.1016/j.tube.2006.03.004

Chambers ST, Syhre M, Murdoch DR, McCartin F, Epton MJ. Detection of 2-Pentylfuran in the breath of patients withAspergillus fumigatus. *Med Mycol*. (2009) 47:468–76. doi: 10.1080/13693780802475212

Syhre M, Scotter JM, Chambers ST. Investigation into the production of 2-Pentylfuran by Aspergillus fumigatus and other respiratory pathogens *in vitro* and human breath samples. *Med Mycol*. (2008) 46:209–15. doi: 10.1080/13693780701753800

Ahmed WM, Geranios P, White IR, Lawal O, Nijsen TM, Bromley MJ, et al. Development of an adaptable headspace sampling method for metabolic profiling of the fungal volatome. *Analyst*. (2018) 143:4155–62. doi: 10.1039/C8AN00841H

Frisvad JC, Rank C, Nielsen KF, Larsen TO. Metabolomics of Aspergillus fumigatus. *Med Mycol*. (2009) 47 (Suppl 1):S53–71. doi: 10.1080/13693780802307720

O'Driscoll CA, Gallo ME, Hoffmann EJ, Fechner JH, Schauer JJ, Bradfield CA, et al. Polycyclic aromatic hydrocarbons (PAHs) present in ambient urban dust drive proinflammatory T cell and dendritic cell responses via the aryl hydrocarbon receptor (AHR) *in vitro*. *PLoS ONE*. (2018) 13:e0209690. doi: 10.1371/journal.pone.0209690

Meldrum K, Gant TW, Macchiarulo S, Leonard MO. Bronchial epithelial innate and adaptive immunity signals are induced by polycyclic aromatic hydrocarbons. *Toxicol Res*. (2016) 5:816–27. doi: 10.1039/C5TX00389J

Mennink-Kersten MA, Donnelly JP, Verweij PE. Detection of circulating galactomannan for the diagnosis and management of invasive aspergillosis. *Lancet Infect Dis*. (2004) 4:349–57. doi: 10.1016/S1473-3099(04)01045-X

Li H, Rui Y, Zhou W, Liu L, He B, Shi Y, et al. Role of the Aspergillus- specific IgG and IgM test in the diagnosis and follow-up of chronic pulmonary aspergillosis. *Front Microbiol*. (2019) 10:1438. doi: 10.3389/fmicb.2019.01438

22

The Immune System in Transfusion-Related Acute Lung Injury Prevention and Therapy

Kai Guo and Shuxuan Ma**

Department of Transfusion Medicine, Beijing Children's Hospital, Capital Medical University, National Center for Children's Health, Beijing, China

***Correspondence:**
Kai Guo
guokai223@outlook.com;
285647152@qq.com
Shuxuan Ma
masxfwyy@sina.com

As an initiator of respiratory distress, transfusion-related acute lung injury (TRALI) is regarded as one of the rare complications associated with transfusion medicine. However, to date, the pathogenesis of TRALI is still unclear, and specific therapies are unavailable. Understanding the mechanisms of TRALI may promote the design of preventive and therapeutic strategies. The immune system plays vital roles in reproduction, development and homeostasis. Sterile tissue damage, such as physical trauma, ischemia, or reperfusion injury, induces an inflammatory reaction that results in wound healing and regenerative mechanisms. In other words, in addition to protecting against pathogens, the immune response may be strongly associated with TRALI prevention and treatment through a variety of immunomodulatory strategies to inhibit excessive immune system activation. Immunotherapy based on immune cells or immunological targets may eradicate complications. For example, IL-10 therapy is a promising therapeutic strategy to explore further. This review will focus on ultramodern advances in our understanding of the potential role of the immune system in TRALI prevention and treatment.

Keywords: transfusion-related acute lung injury, immune system, immune molecule, immunotherapy, prevention

INTRODUCTION

Transfusion-related acute lung injury (TRALI) is the onset of respiratory distress and acute lung injury due to blood product transfusion (Semple et al., 2019), and it is a life-threatening complication characterized by the sudden onset of hypoxemic respiratory failure with non-cardiogenic pulmonary edema and bilateral lung infiltration that developed within 6 h of blood transfusion (Toy et al., 2005; Gokhale and Hendrickson, 2019). Although TRALI develops within 6 hrs of blood transfusion, most occurrences take place during transfusion or within the first 1 or 2 h. According to Voelker and Spieth (2019) TRALI is defined as more complex for cases of seeming TRALI, such as transfusion-associated circulatory overload (TACO), and further testing and diagnosis may be required. TRALI pathophysiology has been partially of elucidated. According to the 2004 Canadian Consensus Conference Panel (Kleinman et al., 2004) and TRALI redefinition

(Vlaar et al., 2019), TRALI can be identified and diagnosed, and the terms TRALI I [without an acute respiratory distress syndrome (ARDS)] and TRALI II (accompanied by ARDS) have been proposed. However, there were some potential TRALI cases did not meet standard clinical definitions (Fuller et al., 2021).

Currently, TRALI is the leading cause of transfusion-related fatalities (Clifford et al., 2015), and the case fatality rate is 5–10% (Swanson et al., 2006). The incidence of TRALI in surgical transfusion patients is 1.3–1.4% (Clifford et al., 2015), and as many as 15% of patients with severe transfusions develop TRALI (Benson et al., 2010). A report from the US FDA showed that 34% of fatalities were due to TRALI from 2012 to 2016 (fatalities reported to FDA following blood collection and transfusion: annual summary for fiscal year 2016: US Food and Drug Administration), which constitutes one of the leading serious adverse reactions to transfusion. Lieberman et al. (2014) suggested that the incidence of TRALI in children is similar to that in adults. Although the numbers are low, there are no differences in outcomes or presentation between adults and children with TRALI.

Generally, the risk factors for blood transfusion can be divided into antibody-independent and antibody-dependent in the context of TRALI. The former is caused by the transfusion of aged red blood cells or platelets, which contain proinflammatory mediators, bioactive lipids, etc. (Mangalmurti et al., 2009; Vlaar et al., 2010; Peters et al., 2015a). The latter is caused by antibody infusions, which mainly contain human leukocyte antigen (HLA) I and II or human neutrophil antigen (HNA) antibodies (Peters et al., 2015b), are mainly obtained from female donors and cause human neutrophil activation (Popovsky et al., 1983). Antibody-dependent TRALI is the most prevalent type (Popovsky and Moore, 1985; Curtis and McFarland, 2006).

Currently, the two-hit model is used to describe the underlying mechanism of TRALI pathology (Peters et al., 2015b; Lorello and Alam, 2018). The predisposing factors of the patient are the first hit, and antibody or non-antibody factors are the second hit (Silliman et al., 1997; Silliman, 2006). Some clinical studies have shown that an inflammatory first hit almost always occurs before TRALI onset and have identified ARDS risk factors that may also be TRALI risk factors in transfusion recipients, including liver surgery, shock, increased peak airway pressure, chronic alcohol abuse and current smoking in the context of immune system balance and inflammation (Toy et al., 2012). Namely, the clinical condition of the patient induces the release of a large number of cytokines, which cause neutrophil activation, accumulation and adhesion to pulmonary microvascular endothelial cells. The second hit is mainly due to HLA or HNA antibodies from the blood products that directly or indirectly activate the recipient's immune system. An increasing number of studies have shown that antibody-dependent TRALI is mediated by the activation of neutrophils, which results in the release of oxygen free radicals and proteases, causes endothelial damage, and increases capillary permeability, ultimately causing pulmonary edema, and inducing TRALI (Silliman, 2006).

According to the classic definition, the immune system is comprised of complement molecules, as well as immune cells and their products, including cytokines, chemokines, antibodies, and growth factors. The immune system is considered to be responsible for defending the host from invading pathogenic microorganisms. In fact, the immune system is an integral part of fundamental physiological processes and immune cells function beyond host defense (Sattler, 2017). Researchers in an expanding range of areas are beginning to recognize continuously the implications of the immune system in their respective fields. The immune system plays an essential role in reproduction both before and during pregnancy, and leukocytes are found in male and female reproductive tissues (Oakley et al., 2011; Care et al., 2013). In other words, the effects of the immune system are not limited to host defense but extend to tissue homeostasis, regeneration and the repair of tissues such as the liver (Meijer et al., 2000), kidney (Lin et al., 2010; Zhang et al., 2012), skin (Goren et al., 2009; Mirza et al., 2009), skeletal muscle, heart (Arnold et al., 2007; Nahrendorf et al., 2007; Frantz et al., 2012; Gallego-Colon et al., 2015; Tonkin et al., 2015; Sattler and Rosenthal, 2016), gut (Seno et al., 2009), and brain (Glod et al., 2006; London et al., 2013). Both evolutionary development and functional variety strongly support the idea of the immune system as an all-encompassing system to ensure systemic integrity.

More importantly, the immune response is closely associated with transfusion therapy (Passwater, 2018). Landers et al. (1996) showed the immunomodulatory effects of blood transfusion in 1996. The immune response is an important basis for the occurrence of TRALI (Tung, 2019). Specifically, before and after transfusion, TRALI patients exhibited elevated levels of IL-6 and IL-8, which are the main contributors to the development of TRALI (Roubinian et al., 2015). Fung et al. (2010) also suggested the importance of T cells in reducing the severity of antibody-dependent TRALI in a murine model. Furthermore, it is believed that TRALI is the result of imbalances in the body's inflammatory response. During infectious diseases, a variety of immunomodulatory molecular mechanisms are activated, including the induction of regulatory T cells (Tregs), regulatory B cells, alternatively activated M2 macrophages or the anti-inflammatory cytokines IL-10 and TGF-β (Taylor et al., 2012; Ziegler et al., 2015; Xu et al., 2016; Loevenich et al., 2017; Soares et al., 2017), which affect all facets of the host immune response to ensure host survival. However, some immune factors, such as B cells, were shown to not play a significant role in the onset of murine antibody-mediated TRALI (Kapur et al., 2017a). Accordingly, in this report, we identified potential immunotherapeutic approaches for TRALI based on immune cells, cytokines and complement molecules by analyzing the literature.

REGULATORY T CELLS

Tregs are essential for maintaining immune homeostasis by regulating effector T cell responses, thus facilitating pathogen immune evasion (Velavan and Ojurongbe, 2011) and preventing potential pathogenic host pathogenic effects through a variety of mechanisms (Shevach, 2009; Maruyama et al., 2011; Gao et al., 2012). For example, Tregs express receptor molecules such as CTLA-4, PD-1 and GITR and directly contact target cells to regulate effector cell function, secrete IL-10, TGF-β and other inhibitory cytokines to exert immunosuppressive effects, and allow antigen-presenting cells to enter a non-response state; the expression of enzymes such as CD39 and CD73 indirectly affects the metabolism of target cells, and the secretion of granzymes A and B directly kills target cells and affects immune responses (Shevach, 2009; Josefowicz et al., 2012; Gubser et al., 2016; Rueda et al., 2016). Tregs represent an antigen-specific mechanism to inhibit potentially harmful autoreactive responses.

Although Tregs are defined as T cells with immunosuppressive activity, it has been documented that Treg populations remain diverse (Miyara and Sakaguchi, 2007). Tregs expressing CD25 and Foxp3 are naturally present in the immune system and are considered to be negative regulators of the T cell response. These natural Tregs originate during thymic development (Mold et al., 2008). In addition, other cells, such as IL-10-secreting $CD4^+CD25^-Foxp3^-$ (Tr1) cells and TGF-β-secreting $CD4^+CD25^-Foxp3^+$ T cells, have also been shown to exert regulatory effects (Lan et al., 2005). While $CD4^+CD25^-Foxp3^+$ T cells, which originate from $CD4^+CD25^-$ T cells that develop in the periphery (Wen et al., 2012), $CD4^+CD25^+Foxp3^+$, $CD4^+CD25^-Foxp3^+$, and Tr1 Tregs can be activated in different microenvironments. Moreover, $CD4^-CD8^-$ Tregs (double-negative Tregs, DNTregs) express the αβ TCR but do not express CD4, CD8, NK cell surface markers or Foxp3, and $CD8^+$ Tregs have no specific surface markers (Lan et al., 2005; Sakaguchi et al., 2010; Murphy and Weaver, 2016). In recent years, a new subpopulation of Tregs (iTR_{35} cells) has been shown to mediate immunosuppression via IL-35 but not IL-10 or TGF-β and is independent of Foxp3 (Collison et al., 2010).

Foxp3-expressing Tregs are known to be indispensable for the maintenance of immunological self-tolerance and immune homeostasis (Sakaguchi et al., 2006). IL-10, TGF-β and Foxp3 are functional and phenotypic markers of natural Tregs (nTregs) and are associated with inducible Tregs (iTregs) (Fontenot et al., 2003). Tregs expressing Foxp3 are able to suppress the activation, proliferation and effector functions (such as cytokine production) of $CD4^+$ and $CD8^+$ T cells, natural killer (NK) cells, NKT cells, B cells and antigen-presenting cells (APCs) *in vitro* and *in vivo* (Sakaguchi et al., 2008). Tregs can also be isolated and expanded *in vitro*; thus far, treatment with this cell product seems safe and well tolerated (Salas and Panes, 2015).

Notably, some researchers have shown that lymphocytes, especially Tregs, are recruited to the lung in response to lung injury. Tregs may play a key role in protecting against TRALI. Tregs can relieve inflammation by regulating immune responses, thereby alleviating lung injury *in vivo* and *in vitro* (D'Alessio et al., 2009). Venet et al. (2009) confirmed that Tregs reduced neutrophil recruitment and activation by producing IL-10 in lipopolysaccharide (LPS)-mediated acute lung injury. Furthermore, Kapur et al. (2017a) demonstrated for the first time that $CD4^+$ $CD25^+$ $Foxp3^+$ Tregs are critical effectors that protect against antibody-dependent murine TRALI via IL-10. Two years later, He et al. (2019) showed that IL-2c and IL-2 derived from $CD4^+CD25^+Foxp3^+$ Tregs increased IL-10 and decreased IL-17A, thereby prophylactically preventing antibody-dependent murine TRALI. Subsequently, different subtypes of Tregs, such as Tr1 and iTR_{35} cells, may play important roles in further studies.

DENDRITIC CELLS

In general, dendritic cells (DCs) are highly specialized antigen-presenting cells that are important in not only initiating immune responses but also in tuning the quality of the immune response or inhibiting the response (Moll, 2003). DCs play a crucial role in this regulatory work, as these cells can regulate T cell-mediated effector responses by generating anti-inflammatory cytokines or inducing Tregs (Maldonado and von Andrian, 2010). Tolerogenic DCs, in particular, can regulate immune responses through various mechanisms (Steinman et al., 2003). Cell fate is predominantly controlled by cytokines in the microenvironment, and to some extent, by the strength of the interaction between the T cell receptor (such as CD45, CTLA-4, and PD-1) and the antigen (Boyton and Altmann, 2002). Tight regulation of effector T cell responses is required to effectively control infections and avoid autoimmune and immunopathological diseases. Aberrant T cell responses, especially those of Th1 and Th17 cells, may play key roles in organ-specific autoimmunity (Dardalhon et al., 2008) and immunopathology (Rutitzky et al., 2008) in the lung. Previously, Kapur R demonstrated that $CD11c^+$ DCs protected against antibody-dependent TRALI via IL-10 in mice (Kapur et al., 2017a). The role of DCs may be essential for TRALI immunotherapy.

MACROPHAGES

Currently, macrophage-targeted therapy has been used in patients (Patel and Janjic, 2015). Alveolar macrophages are central effector cells in the production of proinflammatory mediators. These cells are key in the initiation and resolution of lung inflammation in humans. In the future, the polarization of M1 macrophages may be essential in human TRALI. Lei W et al. (Wang et al., 2020) confirmed that α1-antitrypsin expression improved lung injury by regulating IL-6 production in alveolar macrophages and decreased the M1 macrophage polarization. Modulating macrophage polarization may serve as a potential treatment strategy for human TRALI. By establishing an anti-major histocompatibility complex (MHC) class I monoclonal antibody-induced mouse model of TRALI-like disease, Strait et al. (2011) showed that TRALI induction involves monocytes and macrophages in this murine model.

In addition, osteopontin, a recognized proinflammatory molecule that mediates diverse biological functions (Lund et al., 2009), is involved in various pulmonary disorders, such as fibrosis, inflammation, malignancies, and vascular lung disorders (O'Regan, 2003). Osteopontin is also an important protein involved in regulating the migration of immune cells (Lund et al., 2009). The osteopontin-mediated murine TRALI response is dependent on macrophages, which may be possibly the cellular source of osteopontin (Kapur et al., 2019). In summary, targeting macrophage function may be a critical strategy for TRALI treatment or prevention (Zeeuw van der Laan et al., 2020b).

NEUTROPHILS

Neutrophils, which have diameters of 12–14 μm, are derived from hematopoietic stem cells. As the first line of cellular defense against invading pathogens, neutrophils can rapidly move across the blood-endothelial cell barrier and exert effector functions during inflammation. Neutrophils are the first responders and are recruited in large numbers to the inflammatory microenvironment by the accumulation of lipid mediators, cytokines, and chemokines, as well as changes in the vascular endothelium (Sadik and Luster, 2012; Mocsai et al., 2015). Neutrophil recruitment to inflamed tissues involves elements of neutrophil rolling and firm adhesion (Filippi, 2019). To capture extracellular pathogen-associated molecules and other stimuli, neutrophils release decondensed chromatin coated with granular proteins, which form neutrophil extracellular traps (NETs) (Branzk et al., 2014; Storisteanu et al., 2017; Watanabe and Petri, 2019). However, the secretion of NETs can also cause tissue damage at the expense of the host and has been shown to impair wound healing or facilitate lung injury in diabetes (Wong et al., 2015) and ventilator-induced lung injury (Yildiz et al., 2015). NETs play an essential role in TRALI. Caudrillier et al. (2012) demonstrated that platelets triggered NET formation in an LPS- or anti-MHC class I antibody-based TRALI mouse model. Thomas et al. (2012) showed that NET biomarkers were present in the serum of TRALI patients, as well as in the lungs of LPS- and anti-MHC class I antibody-induced TRALI mice. Treatment with DNaseI IV, which disrupts the formation of the extracellular chromatin web (Hakkim et al., 2010), was shown to have beneficial effects in these two studies. Although DNases are associated with cystic fibrosis in the lung (Thornby et al., 2014), and additional studies on NETs are necessary in the context of DNase therapy for human TRALI.

In addition, as the major producers of reactive oxygen species (ROS), neutrophils can damage the endothelium in antibody-dependent TRALI mice (Strait et al., 2011; Bayat et al., 2013) and in human pulmonary microvascular endothelial cells *in vitro* (Silliman et al., 2007). Other studies has shown neutrophil-mediated endothelial cell damage in antibody-independent TRALI (Xie et al., 2015) and antibody-dependent TRALI (Nishimura et al., 2006; Silliman et al., 2007; Khoy et al., 2017). Moreover, neutrophils and ROS were shown to be critical in antibody-mediated murine TRALI, as demonstrated by *in vivo* neutrophil depletion and the use of gp91phox-knockout mice, respectively (Kapur et al., 2017a).

Lipids in blood products also damage endothelial cells via neutrophils in an antibody-independent TRALI model, and in human pulmonary microvascular endothelial cells that were activated by LPS and cocultured with neutrophils (Wyman et al., 2002). Neutrophil-dependent endothelial cell damage also occurred in the presence of soluble CD40L (Khan et al., 2006). The Fcγ receptor on neutrophils can recognize the Fc-tail of IgG, which binds to pathogens via the IgG-Fab region (Vidarsson and van de Winkel, 1998; Hogarth and Pietersz, 2012; Kapur et al., 2014). A study by Looney MR (Looney et al., 2006) showed that neutrophils and their Fcγ receptors were essential in a TRALI mouse model. Moreover, researchers found that neutrophil Fcγ receptors were critically involved in TRALI, as adoptive transfer of wild-type neutrophils into TRALI-resistant Fcγ receptor-knockout mice ameliorated acute lung injury upon challenge with anti-MHC class I antibodies (Looney et al., 2006). Neutrophil depletion can protect against anti-HNA-3a antibody-mediated TRALI in mice, although TRALI was not completely prevented in this context (Bayat et al., 2013).

Neutrophils are key effectors in TRALI pathogenesis (Rebetz et al., 2018). Pulmonary neutrophil infiltration has been shown to occur in multiple murine TRALI models (Looney et al., 2006, 2009; Kelher et al., 2009; Fung et al., 2010; Tung et al., 2011; Semple et al., 2012; Bayat et al., 2013, 2015; McKenzie et al., 2014; Kapur et al., 2015, 2017a, 2018) and human TRALI patients (Dry et al., 1999; Silliman et al., 2005; Akagi et al., 2020). Currently, new evidence clearly points to the plasticity of neutrophils and may present a new strategy for the potential treatment of TRALI.

IL-10

IL-10 is a member of the IL-10 family of cytokines and a non-covalent homodimeric alpha helical cytokine with structural similarities to IFN-γ. The IL-10 receptor (IL-10R) is expressed on the surface of most hematopoietic cells, including T and B cells and macrophages. Genetically, the immunological and physiological functions of IL-10 were found to be non-redundant in engineered mouse models that lack IL-10 or IL-10R. IL-10 inhibits the proliferation of $CD4^+$ T cells and the secretion of many kinds of cytokines (Fiorentino et al., 1989).

IL-10 expression is altered in patients with TRALI relative to that in control patients. Kapur et al. (2017b) showed reduced IL-10 levels in patients with TRALI. In all pulmonary transfusion reactions, the combination of clinical variables and cytokine measurements indicated optimal diagnostic performance, and the model comparing TACO and TRALI correctly classified 92% of cases relative to expert panel diagnoses (Roubinian et al., 2015). Low plasma IL-10 levels were associated with TRALI susceptibility in a mouse model, and IL-10-knockout mice were also hypersensitive to TRALI induction (Kapur et al., 2017a). These results suggested that low IL-10 levels were a risk factor for TRALI in humans (Kapur et al., 2017b). However, despite this beneficial effect, these data were in contrast to the findings in patients who suffered from other inflammatory/transfusion-associated pulmonary disorders, such as sepsis-associated acute lung injury (Kapur et al., 2017b) or transfusion-associated circulatory overload (Roubinian et al., 2015), in which IL-10 levels were often elevated. This finding may indicate that TRALI has a distinct mechanism of injury and may be uniquely characterized by impaired IL-10 production. However, two reports demonstrated that IL-10 levels were increased in TRALI patients (Looney et al., 2006, 2014). However, the study showed the changes that may indicate risk factors before blood transfusion (Looney et al., 2014) and may explain this discrepancy.

Regardless, IL-10 infusion may have a therapeutic effect in human TRALI and may completely prevent and protect against the development of antibody-dependent TRALI without any apparent side effects both prophylactically and therapeutically by ameliorating the TRALI reaction in mice (Kapur et al.,

2017a). Furthermore, the administration of IL-10 to healthy volunteers was documented as a safe intervention, and only mild to moderate side effects, such as flu-like symptoms, were observed (Moore et al., 2001). We therefore hypothesize that IL-10 administration may be an attractive approach for alleviating TRALI, and clinical studies in humans are highly warranted within 6 h of transfusion for acute lung reactions. However, IL-10 may impair host immune system resistance to infection in clinical settings.

In summary, low plasma IL-10 levels were associated with TRALI susceptibility in a mouse model, and IL-10-knockout mice were also hypersensitive to TRALI induction (Kapur et al., 2017a). IL-10 levels are low in TRALI patients (Kapur et al., 2017b), and very importantly, IL-10 therapy both prophylactically and therapeutically alleviates TRALI in mice (Kapur et al., 2017a). Therefore, IL-10 therapy is a promising therapeutic strategy to explore further.

IL-8

IL-8 is a CXC chemokine that promotes neutrophil chemotaxis and degranulation downstream of CXC-chemokine receptor (CXCR) 1 and CXCR2, which are G protein–coupled receptors (Holmes et al., 1991; Hammond et al., 1995; Waugh and Wilson, 2008). A study by Roubinian NH demonstrated that IL-6 and IL-8 were elevated in patients with TRALI before and after transfusion relative to those in the control group (Roubinian et al., 2015). In H-2Kd/H-2Dd antibody-based severe combined immunodeficient TRALI models, it was demonstrated that the binding of H-2Kd/H-2Dd antibodies to monocytes increased the levels of macrophage inflammatory protein 2 (MIP-2), causing increased pulmonary neutrophil infiltration and subsequently inducing TRALI (McKenzie et al., 2014).

In vivo, peripheral blood monocyte depletion or chemokine blockade completely stopped TRALI induction using an MIP-2 receptor antagonist in severe combined immunodeficiency (SCID) mice (McKenzie et al., 2014). Roubinian et al. (2015) showed that IL-8 is a known risk factor for TRALI, and blocking the IL-8 receptor may also be sufficient to suppress neutrophil chemotaxis and degranulation, thereby counteracting TRALI induction. Moreover, in clinical trials, CXCR2 antagonists were evaluated in other pulmonary disorders, such as cystic fibrosis, asthma and chronic obstructive pulmonary disease (Chapman et al., 2009; O'Byrne et al., 2016), and may have potential efficacy in TRALI as well.

COMPLEMENT CASCADE

One hundred years ago, the complement system was defined based on its ability to "complement" the antibody-dependent and cell-dependent immune responses against pathogens in blood-based antimicrobial system to compared that of global regulators of immunity and tissue homeostasis. Today, many studies have focused on understanding the biology of complement and its mechanisms of action. Our understanding of innate immunity has substantially changed. Complement plays an essential role in modulating innate and adaptive immunity, supports innate immune responses and the initiation of general inflammatory reactions, contributes to tissue and organ development and promotes tissue repair after injury. In cooperation with other immune and physiological systems, the complement system is key in the recognition and elimination of invading pathogens and mediates the clearance of apoptotic cells, cellular debris and immune complexes to remove self-derived danger signals by integrating innate and adaptive immunity (Ricklin et al., 2010; Arbore et al., 2017).

Distinct mechanisms of the complement cascade are triggered by classic, lectin or alternative signals that converge at the third component (C) and lead to the generation of effectors that make up or supplement the ability of antibodies and phagocytes to clear microbial intruders via the opsonization of C3b, which promotes inflammation via anaphylatoxins C3a and C5a and lyses susceptible pathogens via the C5b-9 membrane attack complex (Ricklin et al., 2010). Complement C5a was shown to play an important role in an anti-MHC class I antibody–based TRALI model in BALB/c mice (Strait et al., 2011). Strait et al. (2011) confirmed that the anti-MHC class I antibody-induced murine TRALI model involved complement activation and C5a production (Strait et al., 2011). However, Looney et al. (2006) described the induction of TRALI 2 h after anti-MHC class I antibody injection in C5a receptor-deficient mice (Looney et al., 2006), and additional validation is needed on the role of C5a as a possible TRALI therapy before the use of C5 inhibitors (Nunn et al., 2005). This further research will shed light on the relevance of the complement system in TRALI, which may open up new therapeutic avenues to explore in combatting TRALI. Cleary SJ demonstrated that complement depletion protected the lungs in endothelial MHC I-deficient mice, and targeting complement cascade activation may be useful for TRALI treatment or prevention (Cleary et al., 2020). Zeeuw van der Laan et al. (2020a) further confirmed that TRALI-inducing murine antibodies have increased abilities to activate the complement system, especially Fc-mediated complement activation, compared to those of antibodies that do not cause TRALI. Complement activation by the endothelium initiates antibody-dependent acute lung injury. Neutrophil responses, including NET release, were intact in endothelial MHC I-deficient mice, whereas complement depletion reduced lung injury (Cleary et al., 2020).

In summary, the complement cascade eradicates invading microorganisms, apoptotic cells, and immune complexes. This evidence should significantly increase our understanding of the role of complement in TRALI and thereby potentially result in promising new treatment strategies. Additional systematic studies are needed to elucidate the role of complement in TRALI (Jongerius et al., 2019).

OTHER FACTORS

McKenzie et al. (2014) demonstrated that intact antibody-induced TRALI was abrogated after the depletion of peripheral blood monocytes. However, TRALI was restored upon purified monocyte restoration. Looney et al. (2009) showed that platelet depletion and aspirin treatment protected mice in an antibody-dependent TRALI model. Cognasse et al. (2020) further showed that although platelet depletion did not prevent the occurrence of TRALI in a mouse model, it did reduce TRALI severity and inhibit TRALI development, and recipient platelets are likely involved in TRALI (Semple and Kapur, 2020). The blockade of sphingomyelinase, extracellular vesicle elimination, or supplementation with sphingosine-1-phosphate during platelet storage may present promising new TRALI prevention strategies (McVey et al., 2021).

We should also note that C-reactive protein (CRP) enhances antibody-mediated TRALI induction in mice (Kapur et al., 2015) and that CRP levels are elevated in human TRALI patients (Kapur et al., 2016). Some studies have indicated that targeting the CD40-CD40L interaction could be an important method to prevent or protect against TRALI (Tariket et al., 2019; Hu et al., 2020). The importance of the gut flora in TRALI induction (Kapur et al., 2018) is continuously being studied and explored.

In addition, cytokines connect and interact with each other through a crosstalk network. Cytokines play important roles in regulating the immune response, differentiating and developing immune cells, and mediating the inflammatory response. The TRALI model shows that host inflammation develops, and the disease is the first blow, causing endothelial cells to secrete cytokines, which helps the lung attract neutrophils by increasing the surface expression of cell adhesion molecules. Lung endothelial cells release cytokines and chemokines to activate and induce neutrophils to accumulate in pulmonary capillaries, stimulating neutrophil-mediated endothelial cell interactions and mediating lung injury. Therefore, other than IL-10 and IL-8, other cytokines may be also potential research targets for TRALI prevention and treatment. For example, Qiao et al. (2020) preliminarily confirmed that IL-35 could prevent murine TRALI by inhibiting the activation of endothelial cells. The study of additional immunological factors in combination with previous research findings could shape the field of TRALI research. For example, IL-6, TNF-α, IL-1β and danger-associated molecular patterns (Land, 2013; Tolle and Standiford, 2013; Liu et al., 2017) are factors that induce ARDS.

DISCUSSION

Overall TRALI remains a significant clinical problem. The development of TRALI animal models is highly important in dissecting the disease pathology because factors other than volume appear to play a significant role in TRALI. Based on previously studies, these immune approaches may significantly contribute to combating these life-threatening complications of blood transfusion. Cell-based therapies, such as those based on Treg or DC administration, seem to be safe and well tolerated. Cytokines or secreted factors have increasingly been utilized to validate risk factors for TRALI, and cytokine concentrations are related to the pathogenesis of TRALI. As Semple et al. (2018, 2019) proposed, the most promising therapeutic strategies to explore are interleukin-10 therapy, down-modulating C-reactive

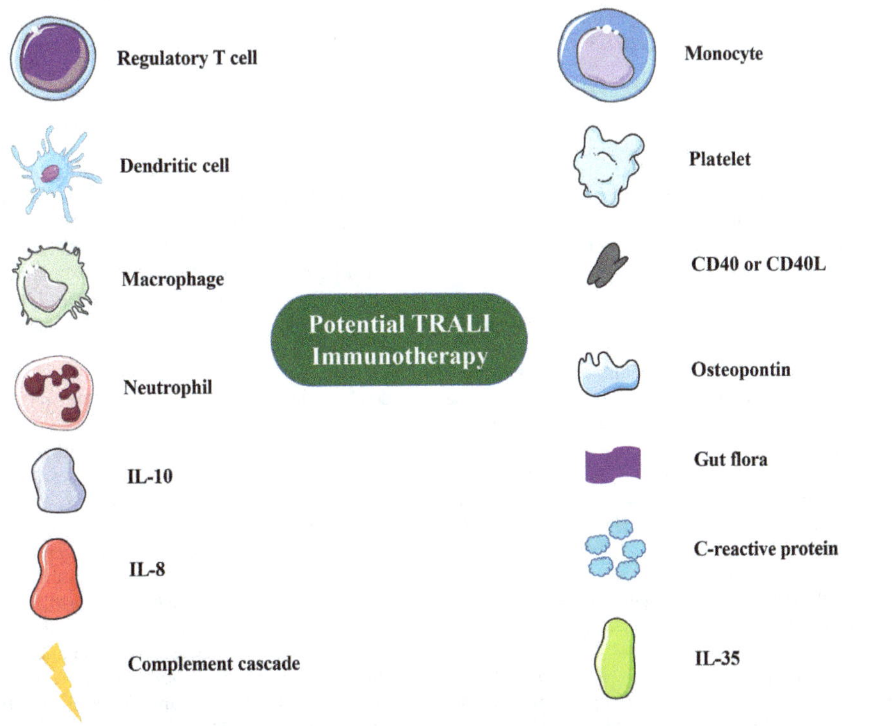

FIGURE 1 | Overview of immune cells or molecules involved in TRALI immunotherapy or prevention. Images of cells and molecules were in part produced or modified using the Smart Servier Medical Art (https://smart.servier.com/), which is licensed under a Creative Commons Attribution 3.0 Unported License (https://screativecommons.org/licenses/by/3.0/).

protein levels, targeting reactive oxygen species, or blocking the interleukin-8 receptor. Innate immune molecules, such as complement, are also important. The immune cells or molecules involvement in TRALI are summarized in **Figure 1**.

These studies focused on the immune system and may provide potential new therapeutic strategies for TRALI. It will be important to expand the investigation of immune-mediated treatments for the clinical diagnosis of and decision making regarding TRALI patients.

AUTHOR CONTRIBUTIONS

KG and SM conceptualized the review. Both authors wrote the review, prepared the figure, and edited and approved the final manuscript.

ACKNOWLEDGMENTS

We thank our colleagues from the Department of Transfusion Medicine, Beijing Children's Hospital, Capital Medical University for all their invaluable efforts.

REFERENCES

Akagi, Y., Murata, S., Yamashita, Y., Tanaka, K., Hiroi, T., Mushino, T., et al. (2020). Two episodes of Transfusion-related Acute Lung Injury (TRALI) occurring within a short period. *Intern. Med.* 59, 2577–2581. doi: 10.2169/internalmedicine.4700-20

Arbore, G., Kemper, C., and Kolev, M. (2017). Intracellular complement - the complosome - in immune cell regulation. *Mol. Immunol.* 89, 2–9. doi: 10.1016/j.molimm.2017.05.012

Arnold, L., Henry, A., Poron, F., Baba-Amer, Y., van Rooijen, N., Plonquet, A., et al. (2007). Inflammatory monocytes recruited after skeletal muscle injury switch into antiinflammatory macrophages to support myogenesis. *J. Exp. Med.* 204, 1057–1069. doi: 10.1084/jem.20070075

Bayat, B., Tjahjono, Y., Berghofer, H., Werth, S., Deckmyn, H., De Meyer, S. F., et al. (2015). Choline transporter-like protein-2: new von willebrand factor-binding partner involved in antibody-mediated neutrophil activation and transfusion-related acute lung injury. *Arterioscler. Thromb. Vasc. Biol.* 35, 1616–1622. doi: 10.1161/ATVBAHA.115.305259

Bayat, B., Tjahjono, Y., Sydykov, A., Werth, S., Hippenstiel, S., Weissmann, N., et al. (2013). Anti-human neutrophil antigen-3a induced transfusion-related acute lung injury in mice by direct disturbance of lung endothelial cells. *Arterioscler. Thromb. Vasc. Biol.* 33, 2538–2548. doi: 10.1161/ATVBAHA.113.301206

Benson, A. B., Austin, G. L., Berg, M., McFann, K. K., Thomas, S., Ramirez, G., et al. (2010). Transfusion-related acute lung injury in ICU patients admitted with gastrointestinal bleeding. *Intens. Care Med.* 36, 1710–1717. doi: 10.1007/s00134-010-1954-x

Boyton, R. J., and Altmann, D. M. (2002). Is selection for TCR affinity a factor in cytokine polarization? *Trends Immunol.* 23, 526–529. doi: 10.1016/s1471-4906(02)02319-0

Branzk, N., Lubojemska, A., Hardison, S. E., Wang, Q., Gutierrez, M. G., Brown, G. D., et al. (2014). Neutrophils sense microbe size and selectively release neutrophil extracellular traps in response to large pathogens. *Nat. Immunol.* 15, 1017–1025. doi: 10.1038/ni.2987

Care, A. S., Diener, K. R., Jasper, M. J., Brown, H. M., Ingman, W. V., and Robertson, S. A. (2013). Macrophages regulate corpus luteum development during embryo implantation in mice. *J. Clin. Invest.* 123, 3472–3487. doi: 10.1172/JCI60561

Caudrillier, A., Kessenbrock, K., Gilliss, B. M., Nguyen, J. X., Marques, M. B., Monestier, M., et al. (2012). Platelets induce neutrophil extracellular traps in transfusion-related acute lung injury. *J. Clin. Invest.* 122, 2661–2671. doi: 10.1172/JCI61303

Chapman, R. W., Phillips, J. E., Hipkin, R. W., Curran, A. K., Lundell, D., and Fine, J. S. (2009). CXCR2 antagonists for the treatment of pulmonary disease. *Pharmacol. Ther.* 121, 55–68. doi: 10.1016/j.pharmthera.2008.10.005

Cleary, S. J., Kwaan, N., Tian, J. J., Calabrese, D. R., Mallavia, B., Magnen, M., et al. (2020). Complement activation on endothelium initiates antibody-mediated acute lung injury. *J. Clin. Invest.* 130, 5909–5923. doi: 10.1172/JCI138136

Clifford, L., Jia, Q., Subramanian, A., Yadav, H., Wilson, G. A., Murphy, S. P., et al. (2015). Characterizing the epidemiology of postoperative transfusion-related acute lung injury. *Anesthesiology* 122, 12–20. doi: 10.1097/ALN.0000000000000514

Cognasse, F., Tariket, S., Hamzeh-Cognasse, H., Arthaud, C. A., Eyraud, M. A., Bourlet, T., et al. (2020). Platelet depletion limits the severity but does not prevent the occurrence of experimental transfusion-related acute lung injury. *Transfusion* 60, 713–723. doi: 10.1111/trf.15738

Collison, L. W., Chaturvedi, V., Henderson, A. L., Giacomin, P. R., Guy, C., Bankoti, J., et al. (2010). IL-35-mediated induction of a potent regulatory T cell population. *Nat. Immunol.* 11, 1093–1101. doi: 10.1038/ni.1952

Curtis, B. R., and McFarland, J. G. (2006). Mechanisms of transfusion-related acute lung injury (TRALI): anti-leukocyte antibodies. *Crit. Care Med.* 34, S118–S123. doi: 10.1097/01.CCM.0000214293.72918.D8

D'Alessio, F. R., Tsushima, K., Aggarwal, N. R., West, E. E., Willett, M. H., Britos, M. F., et al. (2009). CD4+CD25+Foxp3+ Tregs resolve experimental lung injury in mice and are present in humans with acute lung injury. *J. Clin. Invest.* 119, 2898–2913. doi: 10.1172/JCI36498

Dardalhon, V., Korn, T., Kuchroo, V. K., and Anderson, A. C. (2008). Role of Th1 and Th17 cells in organ-specific autoimmunity. *J. Autoimmun.* 31, 252–256. doi: 10.1016/j.jaut.2008.04.017

Dry, S. M., Bechard, K. M., Milford, E. L., Churchill, W. H., and Benjamin, R. J. (1999). The pathology of transfusion-related acute lung injury. *Am. J. Clin. Pathol.* 112, 216–221. doi: 10.1093/ajcp/112.2.216

Filippi, M.-D. (2019). Neutrophil transendothelial migration: updates and new perspectives. *Blood* 133, 2149–2158. doi: 10.1182/blood-2018-12-844605

Fiorentino, D. F., Bond, M. W., and Mosmann, T. R. (1989). Two types of mouse T helper cell. IV. Th2 clones secrete a factor that inhibits cytokine production by Th1 clones. *J. Exp. Med.* 170, 2081–2095.

Fontenot, J. D., Gavin, M. A., and Rudensky, A. Y. (2003). Foxp3 programs the development and function of CD4+CD25+ regulatory T cells. *Nat. Immunol.* 4, 330–336. doi: 10.1038/ni904

Frantz, S., Hofmann, U., Fraccarollo, D., Schäfer, A., Kranepuhl, S., Hagedorn, I., et al. (2012). Monocytes/macrophages prevent healing defects and left ventricular thrombus formation after myocardial infarction. *FASEB J.* 27, 871–881. doi: 10.1096/fj.12-214049

Fuller, C. C., Nambudiri, V. E., Spencer-Smith, C., Curtis, L. H., Shinde, M., Cosgrove, A., et al. (2021). Medical chart validation of inpatient diagnosis codes for transfusion-related acute lung injury 2013-2015. *Transfusion* doi: 10.1111/trf.16251 [Epub ahead of print].

Fung, Y. L., Kim, M., Tabuchi, A., Aslam, R., Speck, E. R., Chow, L., et al. (2010). Recipient T lymphocytes modulate the severity of antibody-mediated transfusion-related acute lung injury. *Blood* 116, 3073–3079. doi: 10.1182/blood-2010-05-284570

Gallego-Colon, E., Sampson, R. D., Sattler, S., Schneider, M. D., Rosenthal, N., and Tonkin, J. (2015). Cardiac-restricted IGF-1Ea overexpression reduces the early accumulation of inflammatory myeloid cells and mediates expression of extracellular matrix remodelling genes after myocardial infarction. *Med. Inflamm.* 2015:484357. doi: 10.1155/2015/484357

Gao, Y., Lin, F., Su, J., Gao, Z., Li, Y., Yang, J., et al. (2012). Molecular mechanisms underlying the regulation and functional plasticity of FOXP3(+) regulatory T cells. *Genes Immun.* 13, 1–13. doi: 10.1038/gene.2011.77

Glod, J., Kobiler, D., Noel, M., Koneru, R., Lehrer, S., Medina, D., et al. (2006). Monocytes form a vascular barrier and participate in vessel repair after brain injury. *Blood* 107, 940–946. doi: 10.1182/blood-2004-11-4403

Gokhale, A., and Hendrickson, J. E. (2019). "*Chapter 66 – Transfusion-Related Acute Lung Injury,*" in *Transfusion Medicine and Hemostasis (Third Edition)*, eds B. H. Shaz, C. D. Hillyer and G. M. Reyes (Elsevier), 405–408. doi: 10.1016/B978-0-12-813726-0.00066-0

Goren, I., Allmann, N., Yogev, N., Schurmann, C., Linke, A., Holdener, M., et al. (2009). A transgenic mouse model of inducible macrophage depletion: effects of diphtheria toxin-driven lysozyme M-specific cell lineage ablation on wound inflammatory, angiogenic, and contractive processes. *Am. J. Pathol.* 175, 132–147. doi: 10.2353/ajpath.2009.081002

Gubser, C., Schmaler, M., Rossi, S. W., and Palmer, E. (2016). Monoclonal regulatory T cells provide insights into T cell suppression. *Sci. Rep.* 6:25758. doi: 10.1038/srep25758

Hakkim, A., Furnrohr, B. G., Amann, K., Laube, B., Abed, U. A., Brinkmann, V., et al. (2010). Impairment of neutrophil extracellular trap degradation is associated with lupus nephritis. *Proc. Natl. Acad. Sci. U.S.A.* 107, 9813–9818. doi: 10.1073/pnas.0909927107

Hammond, M. E., Lapointe, G. R., Feucht, P. H., Hilt, S., Gallegos, C. A., Gordon, C. A., et al. (1995). IL-8 induces neutrophil chemotaxis predominantly via type I IL-8 receptors. *J. Immunol.* 155, 1428–1433.

He, R., Li, L., Kong, Y., Tian, L., Tian, X., Fang, P., et al. (2019). Preventing murine transfusion-related acute lung injury by expansion of CD4(+) CD25(+) FoxP3(+) Tregs using IL-2/anti-IL-2 complexes. *Transfusion* 59, 534–544. doi: 10.1111/trf.15064

Hogarth, P. M., and Pietersz, G. A. (2012). Fc receptor-targeted therapies for the treatment of inflammation, cancer and beyond. *Nat. Rev. Drug Discov.* 11, 311–331. doi: 10.1038/nrd2909

Holmes, W. E., Lee, J., Kuang, W. J., Rice, G. C., and Wood, W. I. (1991). Structure and functional expression of a human interleukin-8 receptor. *Science* 253, 1278–1280. doi: 10.1126/science.1840701

Hu, A., Chen, W., Wu, S., Pan, B., Zhu, A., Yu, X., et al. (2020). An animal model of transfusion-related acute lung injury and the role of soluble CD40 ligand. *Vox Sang.* 115, 303–313. doi: 10.1111/vox.12895

Jongerius, I., Porcelijn, L., van Beek, A. E., Semple, J. W., van der Schoot, C. E., Vlaar, A. P. J., et al. (2019). The role of complement in transfusion-related acute lung injury. *Transfus. Med. Rev.* 33, 236–242. doi: 10.1016/j.tmrv.2019.09.002

Josefowicz, S. Z., Lu, L. F., and Rudensky, A. Y. (2012). Regulatory T cells: mechanisms of differentiation and function. *Annu. Rev. Immunol.* 30, 531–564. doi: 10.1146/annurev.immunol.25.022106.141623

Kapur, R., Einarsdottir, H. K., and Vidarsson, G. (2014). IgG-effector functions: "the good, the bad and the ugly". *Immunol. Lett.* 160, 139–144. doi: 10.1016/j.imlet.2014.01.015

Kapur, R., Kasetty, G., Rebetz, J., Egesten, A., and Semple, J. W. (2019). Osteopontin mediates murine transfusion-related acute lung injury via stimulation of pulmonary neutrophil accumulation. *Blood* 134, 74–84. doi: 10.1182/blood.2019000972

Kapur, R., Kim, M., Aslam, R., McVey, M. J., Tabuchi, A., Luo, A., et al. (2017a). T regulatory cells and dendritic cells protect against transfusion-related acute lung injury via IL-10. *Blood* 129, 2557–2569. doi: 10.1182/blood-2016-12-758185

Kapur, R., Kim, M., Rebetz, J., Rondina, M. T., Porcelijn, L., and Semple, J. W. (2017b). Low levels of interleukin-10 in patients with transfusion-related acute lung injury. *Ann. Transl. Med.* 5:339. doi: 10.21037/atm.2017.04.37

Kapur, R., Kim, M., Rebetz, J., Hallstrom, B., Bjorkman, J. T., Takabe-French, A., et al. (2018). Gastrointestinal microbiota contributes to the development of murine transfusion-related acute lung injury. *Blood Adv.* 2, 1651–1663. doi: 10.1182/bloodadvances.2018018903

Kapur, R., Kim, M., Rondina, M. T., Porcelijn, L., and Semple, J. W. (2016). Elevation of C-reactive protein levels in patients with transfusion-related acute lung injury. *Oncotarget* 7, 78048–78054. doi: 10.18632/oncotarget.12872

Kapur, R., Kim, M., Shanmugabhavananthan, S., Liu, J., Li, Y., and Semple, J. W. (2015). C-reactive protein enhances murine antibody-mediated transfusion-related acute lung injury. *Blood* 126, 2747–2751. doi: 10.1182/blood-2015-09-672592

Kelher, M. R., Masuno, T., Moore, E. E., Damle, S., Meng, X., Song, Y., et al. (2009). Plasma from stored packed red blood cells and MHC class I antibodies causes acute lung injury in a 2-event in vivo rat model. *Blood* 113, 2079–2087. doi: 10.1182/blood-2008-09-177857

Khan, S. Y., Kelher, M. R., Heal, J. M., Blumberg, N., Boshkov, L. K., Phipps, R., et al. (2006). Soluble CD40 ligand accumulates in stored blood components, primes neutrophils through CD40, and is a potential cofactor in the development of transfusion-related acute lung injury. *Blood* 108, 2455–2462. doi: 10.1182/blood-2006-04-017251

Khoy, K., Nguyen, M. V. C., Masson, D., Bardy, B., Drouet, C., and Paclet, M. H. (2017). Transfusion-related acute lung injury: critical neutrophil activation by anti-HLA-A2 antibodies for endothelial permeability. *Transfusion* 57, 1699–1708. doi: 10.1111/trf.14134

Kleinman, S., Caulfield, T., Chan, P., Davenport, R., McFarland, J., McPhedran, S., et al. (2004). Toward an understanding of transfusion-related acute lung injury: statement of a consensus panel. *Transfusion* 44, 1774–1789. doi: 10.1111/j.0041-1132.2004.04347.x

Lan, R. Y., Ansari, A. A., Lian, Z. X., and Gershwin, M. E. (2005). Regulatory T cells: development, function and role in autoimmunity. *Autoimmun. Rev.* 4, 351–363. doi: 10.1016/j.autrev.2005.01.007

Land, W. G. (2013). Transfusion-related acute lung injury: the work of DAMPs. *Transfus. Med. Hemother.* 40, 3–13. doi: 10.1159/000345688

Landers, D. F., Hill, G. E., Wong, K. C., and Fox, I. J. (1996). Blood transfusion-induced immunomodulation. *Anesth. Analg.* 82, 187–204. doi: 10.1097/00000539-199601000-00035

Lieberman, L., Petraszko, T., Yi, Q. L., Hannach, B., and Skeate, R. (2014). Transfusion-related lung injury in children: a case series and review of the literature. *Transfusion* 54, 57–64. doi: 10.1111/trf.12249

Lin, S. L., Li, B., Rao, S., Yeo, E. J., Hudson, T. E., Nowlin, B. T., et al. (2010). Macrophage Wnt7b is critical for kidney repair and regeneration. *Proc. Natl. Acad. Sci. U.S.A.* 107, 4194–4199. doi: 10.1073/pnas.0912228107

Liu, X., Cao, H., Li, J., Wang, B., Zhang, P., Dong Zhang, X., et al. (2017). Autophagy induced by DAMPs facilitates the inflammation response in lungs undergoing ischemia-reperfusion injury through promoting TRAF6 ubiquitination. *Cell Death Differ.* 24, 683–693. doi: 10.1038/cdd.2017.1

Loevenich, K., Ueffing, K., Abel, S., Hose, M., Matuschewski, K., Westendorf, A. M., et al. (2017). DC-Derived IL-10 modulates pro-inflammatory cytokine production and promotes induction of CD4(+)IL-10(+) regulatory t cells during *Plasmodium yoelii* infection. *Front. Immunol.* 8:152. doi: 10.3389/fimmu.2017.00152

London, A., Cohen, M., and Schwartz, M. (2013). Microglia and monocyte-derived macrophages: functionally distinct populations that act in concert in CNS plasticity and repair. *Front. Cell Neurosci.* 7:34. doi: 10.3389/fncel.2013.00034

Looney, M. R., Nguyen, J. X., Hu, Y., Van Ziffle, J. A., Lowell, C. A., and Matthay, M. A. (2009). Platelet depletion and aspirin treatment protect mice in a two-event model of transfusion-related acute lung injury. *J. Clin. Invest.* 119, 3450–3461. doi: 10.1172/JCI38432

Looney, M. R., Roubinian, N., Gajic, O., Gropper, M. A., Hubmayr, R. D., Lowell, C. A., et al. (2014). Prospective study on the clinical course and outcomes in transfusion-related acute lung injury. *Crit. Care Med.* 42, 1676–1687. doi: 10.1097/CCM.0000000000000323

Looney, M. R., Su, X., Van Ziffle, J. A., Lowell, C. A., and Matthay, M. A. (2006). Neutrophils and their Fc gamma receptors are essential in a mouse model of transfusion-related acute lung injury. *J. Clin. Invest.* 116, 1615–1623. doi: 10.1172/JCI27238

Lorello, G. R., and Alam, A. (2018). Perioperative transfusion-related acute lung injury. *Int. Anesthesiol. Clin.* 56, 47–67. doi: 10.1097/AIA.0000000000000178

Lund, S. A., Giachelli, C. M., and Scatena, M. (2009). The role of osteopontin in inflammatory processes. *J. Cell Commun. Signal.* 3, 311–322. doi: 10.1007/s12079-009-0068-0

Maldonado, R. A., and von Andrian, U. H. (2010). How tolerogenic dendritic cells induce regulatory T cells. *Adv Immunol.* 108, 111–165. doi: 10.1016/S0065-2776(10)08004_1

Mangalmurti, N. S., Xiong, Z., Hulver, M., Ranganathan, M., Liu, X. H., Oriss, T., et al. (2009). Loss of red cell chemokine scavenging promotes transfusion-related lung inflammation. *Blood* 113, 1158–1166. doi: 10.1182/blood-2008-07-166264

Maruyama, T., Konkel, J. E., Zamarron, B. F., and Chen, W. (2011). The molecular mechanisms of Foxp3 gene regulation. *Semin. Immunol.* 23, 418–423. doi: 10.1016/j.smim.2011.06.005

McKenzie, C. G., Kim, M., Singh, T. K., Milev, Y., Freedman, J., and Semple, J. W. (2014). Peripheral blood monocyte-derived chemokine blockade prevents murine transfusion-related acute lung injury (TRALI). *Blood* 123, 3496–3503. doi: 10.1182/blood-2013-11-536755

McVey, M. J., Weidenfeld, S., Maishan, M., Spring, C., Kim, M., Tabuchi, A., et al. (2021). Platelet extracellular vesicles mediate transfusion-related acute lung injury by imbalancing the sphingolipid rheostat. *Blood* 137, 690–701. doi: 10.1182/blood.2020005985

Meijer, C., Wiezer, M. J., Diehl, A. M., Schouten, H. J., Schouten, H. J., Meijer, S., et al. (2000). Kupffer cell depletion by CI2MDP-liposomes alters hepatic cytokine expression and delays liver regeneration after partial hepatectomy. *Liver* 20, 66–77. doi: 10.1034/j.1600-0676.2000.020001066.x

Mirza, R., DiPietro, L. A., and Koh, T. J. (2009). Selective and specific macrophage ablation is detrimental to wound healing in mice. *Am. J. Pathol.* 175, 2454–2462. doi: 10.2353/ajpath.2009.090248

Miyara, M., and Sakaguchi, S. (2007). Natural regulatory T cells: mechanisms of suppression. *Trends Mol. Med.* 13, 108–116. doi: 10.1016/j.molmed.2007.01.003

Mocsai, A., Walzog, B., and Lowell, C. A. (2015). Intracellular signalling during neutrophil recruitment. *Cardiovasc. Res.* 107, 373–385. doi: 10.1093/cvr/cvv159

Mold, J. E., Michaelsson, J., Burt, T. D., Muench, M. O., Beckerman, K. P., Busch, M. P., et al. (2008). Maternal alloantigens promote the development of tolerogenic fetal regulatory T cells in utero. *Science* 322, 1562–1565. doi: 10.1126/science.1164511

Moll, H. (2003). Dendritic cells and host resistance to infection. *Cell Microbiol.* 5, 493–500. doi: 10.1046/j.1462-5822.2003.00291.x

Moore, K. W., de Waal Malefyt, R., Coffman, R. L., and O'Garra, A. (2001). Interleukin-10 and the interleukin-10 receptor. *Annu. Rev. Immunol.* 19, 683–765. doi: 10.1146/annurev.immunol.19.1.683

Murphy, K., and Weaver, C. (2016). *Janeway's Immunobiology: Garland Science*, 9th Edn, New York, NY: W.W. Norton & Company.

Nahrendorf, M., Swirski, F. K., Aikawa, E., Stangenberg, L., Wurdinger, T., Figueiredo, J. L., et al. (2007). The healing myocardium sequentially mobilizes two monocyte subsets with divergent and complementary functions. *J. Exp. Med.* 204, 3037–3047. doi: 10.1084/jem.20070885

Nishimura, M., Takanashi, M., Okazaki, H., and Satake, M. (2006). Lung microvascular endothelial cell injury caused by treatment with polymorphonuclear neutrophils and low-IgM serum: a model of transfusion-related acute lung injury. *Lung* 184, 25–32. doi: 10.1007/s00408-005-2559-y

Nunn, M. A., Sharma, A., Paesen, G. C., Adamson, S., Lissina, O., Willis, A. C., et al. (2005). Complement inhibitor of C5 activation from the soft tick *Ornithodoros moubata. J. Immunol.* 174, 2084–2091. doi: 10.4049/jimmunol.174.4.2084

Oakley, O. R., Frazer, M. L., and Ko, C. (2011). Pituitary-ovary-spleen axis in ovulation. *Trends Endocrinol. Metab.* 22, 345–352. doi: 10.1016/j.tem.2011.04.005

O'Byrne, P. M., Metev, H., Puu, M., Richter, K., Keen, C., Uddin, M., et al. (2016). Efficacy and safety of a CXCR2 antagonist, AZD5069, in patients with uncontrolled persistent asthma: a randomised, double-blind, placebo-controlled trial. *Lancet Respir. Med.* 4, 797–806. doi: 10.1016/S2213-2600(16)30227-2

O'Regan, A. (2003). The role of osteopontin in lung disease. *Cytokine Growth Fact. Rev.* 14, 479–488. doi: 10.1016/s1359-6101(03)00055-8

Passwater, M. (2018). Antibody formation in transfusion therapy. *J. Infus. Nurs.* 41, 87–95. doi: 10.1097/NAN.0000000000000264

Patel, S. K., and Janjic, J. M. (2015). Macrophage targeted theranostics as personalized nanomedicine strategies for inflammatory diseases. *Theranostics* 5, 150–172. doi: 10.7150/thno.9476

Peters, A. L., van Hezel, M. E., Juffermans, N. P., and Vlaar, A. P. (2015a). Pathogenesis of non-antibody mediated transfusion-related acute lung injury from bench to bedside. *Blood Rev.* 29, 51–61. doi: 10.1016/j.blre.2014.09.007

Peters, A. L., van Stein, D., and Vlaar, A. P. (2015b). Antibody-mediated transfusion-related acute lung injury; from discovery to prevention. *Br. J. Haematol.* 170, 597–614. doi: 10.1111/bjh.13459

Popovsky, M. A., Abel, M. D., and Moore, S. B. (1983). Transfusion-related acute lung injury associated with passive transfer of antileukocyte antibodies. *Am. Rev. Respir. Dis.* 128, 185–189. doi: 10.1164/arrd.1983.128.1.185

Popovsky, M. A., and Moore, S. B. (1985). Diagnostic and pathogenetic considerations in transfusion-related acute lung injury. *Transfusion* 25, 573–577.

Qiao, J., He, R., Yin, Y., Tian, L., Li, L., Lian, Z., et al. (2020). rIL-35 prevents murine transfusion-related acute lung injury by inhibiting the activation of endothelial cells. *Transfusion* 60, 1434–1442. doi: 10.1111/trf.15805

Rebetz, J., Semple, J. W., and Kapur, R. (2018). The pathogenic involvement of neutrophils in acute respiratory distress syndrome and transfusion-related acute lung injury. *Transfus. Med. Hemother.* 45, 290–298. doi: 10.1159/000492950

Ricklin, D., Hajishengallis, G., Yang, K., and Lambris, J. D. (2010). Complement: a key system for immune surveillance and homeostasis. *Nat. Immunol.* 11, 785–797. doi: 10.1038/ni.1923

Roubinian, N. H., Looney, M. R., Kor, D. J., Lowell, C. A., Gajic, O., Hubmayr, R. D., et al. (2015). Cytokines and clinical predictors in distinguishing pulmonary transfusion reactions. *Transfusion* 55, 1838–1846. doi: 10.1111/trf.13021

Rueda, C. M., Jackson, C. M., and Chougnet, C. A. (2016). Regulatory T-cell-mediated suppression of conventional T-cells and dendritic cells by different cAMP intracellular pathways. *Front. Immunol.* 7:216. doi: 10.3389/fimmu.2016.00216

Rutitzky, L. I., Bazzone, L., Shainheit, M. G., Joyce-Shaikh, B., Cua, D. J., and Stadecker, M. J. (2008). IL-23 is required for the development of severe egg-induced immunopathology in schistosomiasis and for lesional expression of IL-17. *J. Immunol.* 180, 2486–2495.

Sadik, C. D., and Luster, A. D. (2012). Lipid-cytokine-chemokine cascades orchestrate leukocyte recruitment in inflammation. *J. Leukoc. Biol.* 91, 207–215. doi: 10.1189/jlb.0811402

Sakaguchi, S., Miyara, M., Costantino, C. M., and Hafler, D. A. (2010). FOXP3+ regulatory T cells in the human immune system. *Nat. Rev. Immunol.* 10, 490–500. doi: 10.1038/nri2785

Sakaguchi, S., Ono, M., Setoguchi, R., Yagi, H., Hori, S., Fehervari, Z., et al. (2006). Foxp3+ CD25+ CD4+ natural regulatory T cells in dominant self-tolerance and autoimmune disease. *Immunol. Rev.* 212, 8–27. doi: 10.1111/j.0105-2896.2006.00427.x

Sakaguchi, S., Yamaguchi, T., Nomura, T., and Ono, M. (2008). Regulatory T cells and immune tolerance. *Cell* 133, 775–787. doi: 10.1016/j.cell.2008.05.009

Salas, A., and Panes, J. (2015). IBD: regulatory T cells for treatment of Crohn's disease. *Nat. Rev. Gastroenterol. Hepatol.* 12, 315–316. doi: 10.1038/nrgastro.2015.68

Sattler, S. (2017). The role of the immune system beyond the fight against infection. *Adv. Exp. Med. Biol.* 1003, 3–14. doi: 10.1007/978-3-319-57613-8_1

Sattler, S., and Rosenthal, N. (2016). The neonate versus adult mammalian immune system in cardiac repair and regeneration. *Biochim. Biophys. Acta* 1863, 1813–1821. doi: 10.1016/j.bbamcr.2016.01.011

Semple, J. W., and Kapur, R. (2020). The contribution of recipient platelets in TRALI: has the jury reached a verdict? *Transfusion* 60, 886–888. doi: 10.1111/trf.15814

Semple, J. W., Kim, M., Hou, J., McVey, M., Lee, Y. J., Tabuchi, A., et al. (2012). Intravenous immunoglobulin prevents murine antibody-mediated acute lung injury at the level of neutrophil reactive oxygen species (ROS) production. *PLoS One* 7:e31357. doi: 10.1371/journal.pone.0031357

Semple, J. W., McVey, M. J., Kim, M., Rebetz, J., Kuebler, W. M., and Kapur, R. (2018). Targeting transfusion-related acute lung injury: the journey from basic science to novel therapies. *Crit. Care Med.* 46, e452–e458. doi: 10.1097/CCM.0000000000002989

Semple, J. W., Rebetz, J., and Kapur, R. (2019). Transfusion-associated circulatory overload and transfusion-related acute lung injury. *Blood* 133, 1840–1853. doi: 10.1182/blood-2018-10-860809

Seno, H., Miyoshi, H., Brown, S. L., Geske, M. J., Colonna, M., and Stappenbeck, T. S. (2009). Efficient colonic mucosal wound repair requires Trem2 signaling. *Proc. Natl. Acad. Sci. U.S.A.* 106, 256–261. doi: 10.1073/pnas.0803343106

Shevach, E. M. (2009). Mechanisms of foxp3+ T regulatory cell-mediated suppression. *Immunity* 30, 636–645. doi: 10.1016/j.immuni.2009.04.010

Silliman, C. C. (2006). The two-event model of transfusion-related acute lung injury. *Crit. Care Med.* 34, S124–S131. doi: 10.1097/01.CCM.0000214292.62276.8E

Silliman, C. C., Ambruso, D. R., and Boshkov, L. K. (2005). Transfusion-related acute lung injury. *Blood* 105, 2266–2273. doi: 10.1182/blood-2004-07-2929

Silliman, C. C., Curtis, B. R., Kopko, P. M., Khan, S. Y., Kelher, M. R., Schuller, R. M., et al. (2007). Donor antibodies to HNA-3a implicated in TRALI reactions prime neutrophils and cause PMN-mediated damage to human pulmonary microvascular endothelial cells in a two-event in vitro model. *Blood* 109, 1752–1755. doi: 10.1182/blood-2006-05-025106

Silliman, C. C., Paterson, A. J., Dickey, W. O., Stroneck, D. F., Popovsky, M. A., Caldwell, S. A., et al. (1997). The association of biologically active lipids with the development of transfusion-related acute lung injury: a retrospective study. *Transfusion* 37, 719–726. doi: 10.1046/j.1537-2995.1997.37797369448.x

Soares, R. R., Antinarelli, L. M. R., Abramo, C., Macedo, G. C., Coimbra, E. S., and Scopel, K. K. G. (2017). What do we know about the role of regulatory B cells (Breg) during the course of infection of two major parasitic diseases, malaria and leishmaniasis? *Pathog. Glob. Health* 111, 107–115. doi: 10.1080/20477724.2017.1308902

Steinman, R. M., Hawiger, D., and Nussenzweig, M. C. (2003). Tolerogenic dendritic cells. *Annu. Rev. Immunol.* 21, 685–711. doi: 10.1146/annurev.immunol.21.120601.141040

Storisteanu, D. M., Pocock, J. M., Cowburn, A. S., Juss, J. K., Nadesalingam, A., Nizet, V., et al. (2017). Evasion of neutrophil extracellular traps by respiratory pathogens. *Am. J. Respir. Cell Mol. Biol.* 56, 423–431. doi: 10.1165/rcmb.2016-0193PS

Strait, R. T., Hicks, W., Barasa, N., Mahler, A., Khodoun, M., Kohl, J., et al. (2011). MHC class I-specific antibody binding to nonhematopoietic cells drives complement activation to induce transfusion-related acute lung injury in mice. *J. Exp. Med.* 208, 2525–2544. doi: 10.1084/jem.20110159

Swanson, K., Dwyre, D. M., Krochmal, J., and Raife, T. J. (2006). Transfusion-related acute lung injury (TRALI): current clinical and pathophysiologic considerations. *Lung* 184, 177–185. doi: 10.1007/s00408-005-2578-8

Tariket, S., Hamzeh-Cognasse, H., Laradi, S., Arthaud, C. A., Eyraud, M. A., Bourlet, T., et al. (2019). Evidence of CD40L/CD40 pathway involvement in experimental transfusion-related acute lung injury. *Sci. Rep.* 9:12536. doi: 10.1038/s41598-019-49040-0

Taylor, M. D., van der Werf, N., and Maizels, R. M. (2012). T cells in helminth infection: the regulators and the regulated. *Trends Immunol.* 33, 181–189. doi: 10.1016/j.it.2012.01.001

Thomas, G. M., Carbo, C., Curtis, B. R., Martinod, K., Mazo, I. B., Schatzberg, D., et al. (2012). Extracellular DNA traps are associated with the pathogenesis of TRALI in humans and mice. *Blood* 119, 6335–6343. doi: 10.1182/blood-2012-01-405183

Thornby, K. A., Johnson, A., and Axtell, S. (2014). Dornase alfa for non-cystic fibrosis pediatric pulmonary Atelectasis. *Ann. Pharmacother.* 48, 1040–1049. doi: 10.1177/1060028014535199

Tolle, L. B., and Standiford, T. J. (2013). Danger-associated molecular patterns (DAMPs) in acute lung injury. *J. Pathol.* 229, 145–156. doi: 10.1002/path.4124

Tonkin, J., Temmerman, L., Sampson, R. D., Gallego-Colon, E., Barberi, L., Bilbao, D., et al. (2015). Monocyte/macrophage-derived IGF-1 orchestrates murine skeletal muscle regeneration and modulates autocrine polarization. *Mol. Ther.* 23, 1189–1200. doi: 10.1038/mt.2015.66

Toy, P., Gajic, O., Bacchetti, P., Looney, M. R., Gropper, M. A., Hubmayr, R., et al. (2012). Transfusion-related acute lung injury: incidence and risk factors. *Blood* 119, 1757–1767. doi: 10.1182/blood-2011-08-370932

Toy, P., Popovsky, M. A., Abraham, E., Ambruso, D. R., Holness, L. G., Kopko, P. M., et al. (2005). Transfusion-related acute lung injury: definition and review. *Crit. Care Med.* 33, 721–726. doi: 10.1097/01.ccm.0000159849.94750.51

Tung, J.-P. (2019). Transfusion-related acute lung injury (Trali): pathogenesis and diagnosis. *Pathology* 51:S44.

Tung, J. P., Fung, Y. L., Nataatmadja, M., Colebourne, K. I., Esmaeel, H. M., Wilson, K., et al. (2011). A novel in vivo ovine model of transfusion-related acute lung injury (TRALI). *Vox Sang.* 100, 219–230. doi: 10.1111/j.1423-0410.2010.01381.x

Velavan, T. P., and Ojurongbe, O. (2011). Regulatory T cells and parasites. *J. Biomed. Biotechnol.* 2011:520940. doi: 10.1155/2011/520940

Venet, F., Chung, C. S., Huang, X., Lomas-Neira, J., Chen, Y., and Ayala, A. (2009). Lymphocytes in the development of lung inflammation: a role for regulatory CD4+ T cells in indirect pulmonary lung injury. *J. Immunol.* 183, 3472–3480. doi: 10.4049/jimmunol.0804119

Vidarsson, G., and van de Winkel, J. G. (1998). Fc receptor and complement receptor-mediated phagocytosis in host defence. *Curr. Opin. Infect. Dis.* 11, 271–278. doi: 10.1097/00001432-199806000-00002

Vlaar, A. P., Hofstra, J. J., Kulik, W., van Lenthe, H., Nieuwland, R., Schultz, M. J., et al. (2010). Supernatant of stored platelets causes lung inflammation and coagulopathy in a novel in vivo transfusion model. *Blood* 116, 1360–1368. doi: 10.1182/blood-2009-10-248732

Vlaar, A. P. J., Toy, P., Fung, M., Looney, M. R., Juffermans, N. P., Bux, J., et al. (2019). A consensus redefinition of transfusion-related acute lung injury. *Transfusion* 59, 2465–2476. doi: 10.1111/trf.15311

Voelker, M. T., and Spieth, P. (2019). Blood transfusion associated lung injury. *J. Thorac. Dis.* 11, 3609–3615. doi: 10.21037/jtd.2019.06.61

Wang, L., Wu, T., Yan, S., Wang, Y., An, J., Wu, C., et al. (2020). M1-polarized alveolar macrophages are crucial in a mouse model of transfusion-related acute lung injury. *Transfusion* 60, 303–316. doi: 10.1111/trf.15609

Watanabe, K., and Petri, W. A. (2019). Learning from the research on amebiasis and gut microbiome: is stimulation by gut flora essential for effective neutrophil mediated protection from external pathogens? *Gut Microb.* 10, 100–104. doi: 10.1080/19490976.2018.1479626

Waugh, D. J., and Wilson, C. (2008). The interleukin-8 pathway in cancer. *Clin. Cancer Res.* 14, 6735–6741. doi: 10.1158/1078-0432.CCR-07-4843

Wen, K., Li, G., Yang, X., Bui, T., Bai, M., Liu, F., et al. (2012). CD4+ CD25-FoxP3+ regulatory cells are the predominant responding regulatory T cells after human rotavirus infection or vaccination in gnotobiotic pigs. *Immunology* 137, 160–171. doi: 10.1111/j.1365-2567.2012.03617.x

Wong, S. L., Demers, M., Martinod, K., Gallant, M., Wang, Y., Goldfine, A. B., et al. (2015). Diabetes primes neutrophils to undergo NETosis, which impairs wound healing. *Nat. Med.* 21, 815–819. doi: 10.1038/nm.3887

Wyman, T. H., Bjornsen, A. J., Elzi, D. J., Smith, C. W., England, K. M., Kelher, M., et al. (2002). A two-insult in vitro model of PMN-mediated pulmonary endothelial damage: requirements for adherence and chemokine release. *Am. J. Physiol. Cell Physiol.* 283, C1592–C1603. doi: 10.1152/ajpcell.00540.2001

Xie, R. F., Hu, P., Wang, Z. C., Yang, J., Yang, Y. M., Gao, L., et al. (2015). Platelet-derived microparticles induce polymorphonuclear leukocyte-mediated damage of human pulmonary microvascular endothelial cells. *Transfusion* 55, 1051–1057. doi: 10.1111/trf.12952

Xu, A., Liu, Y., Chen, W., Wang, J., Xue, Y., Huang, F., et al. (2016). TGF-beta-induced regulatory T cells directly suppress B cell responses through a noncytotoxic mechanism. *J. Immunol.* 196, 3631–3641. doi: 10.4049/jimmunol.1501740

Yildiz, C., Palaniyar, N., Otulakowski, G., Khan, M. A., Post, M., Kuebler, W. M., et al. (2015). Mechanical ventilation induces neutrophil extracellular trap formation. *Anesthesiology* 122, 864–875. doi: 10.1097/ALN.0000000000000605

Zeeuw van der Laan, E. A. N., van der Velden, S., Bentlage, A. E. H., Larsen, M. D., van Osch, T. L. J., Mok, J. Y., et al. (2020a). Biological and structural characterization of murine TRALI antibody reveals increased Fc-mediated complement activation. *Blood Adv.* 4, 3875–3885. doi: 10.1182/bloodadvances.2020002291

Zeeuw van der Laan, E. A. N., van der Velden, S., Porcelijn, L., Semple, J. W., van der Schoot, C. E., and Kapur, R. (2020b). Update on the pathophysiology of transfusion-related acute lung injury. *Curr. Opin. Hematol.* 27, 386–391. doi: 10.1097/MOH.0000000000000607

Zhang, M. Z., Yao, B., Yang, S., Jiang, L., Wang, S., Fan, X., et al. (2012). CSF-1 signaling mediates recovery from acute kidney injury. *J. Clin. Invest.* 122, 4519–4532. doi: 10.1172/JCI60363

Ziegler, T., Rausch, S., Steinfelder, S., Klotz, C., Hepworth, M. R., Kuhl, A. A., et al. (2015). A novel regulatory macrophage induced by a helminth molecule instructs IL-10 in CD4+ T cells and protects against mucosal inflammation. *J. Immunol.* 194, 1555–1564. doi: 10.4049/jimmunol.1401217

Permissions

 Every chapter published in this book has been scrutinized by our experts. Their significance has been extensively debated. The topics covered herein carry significant findings which will fuel the growth of the discipline. They may even be implemented as practical applications or may be referred to as a beginning point for another development.

The contributors of this book come from diverse backgrounds, making this book a truly international effort. This book will bring forth new frontiers with its revolutionizing research information and detailed analysis of the nascent developments around the world.

We would like to thank all the contributing authors for lending their expertise to make the book truly unique. They have played a crucial role in the development of this book. Without their invaluable contributions this book wouldn't have been possible. They have made vital efforts to compile up to date information on the varied aspects of this subject to make this book a valuable addition to the collection of many professionals and students.

This book was conceptualized with the vision of imparting up-to-date information and advanced data in this field. To ensure the same, a matchless editorial board was set up. Every individual on the board went through rigorous rounds of assessment to prove their worth. After which they invested a large part of their time researching and compiling the most relevant data for our readers.

The editorial board has been involved in producing this book since its inception. They have spent rigorous hours researching and exploring the diverse topics which have resulted in the successful publishing of this book. They have passed on their knowledge of decades through this book. To expedite this challenging task, the publisher supported the team at every step. A small team of assistant editors was also appointed to further simplify the editing procedure and attain best results for the readers.

Apart from the editorial board, the designing team has also invested a significant amount of their time in understanding the subject and creating the most relevant covers. They scrutinized every image to scout for the most suitable representation of the subject and create an appropriate cover for the book.

The publishing team has been an ardent support to the editorial, designing and production team. Their endless efforts to recruit the best for this project, has resulted in the accomplishment of this book. They are a veteran in the field of academics and their pool of knowledge is as vast as their experience in printing. Their expertise and guidance has proved useful at every step. Their uncompromising quality standards have made this book an exceptional effort. Their encouragement from time to time has been an inspiration for everyone.

The publisher and the editorial board hope that this book will prove to be a valuable piece of knowledge for researchers, students, practitioners and scholars across the globe.

List of Contributors

Caleb N. Muefong and Jayne S. Sutherland
Vaccines and Immunity Theme, Medical Research Council Unit, The Gambia at the London School of Hygiene and Tropical Medicine, Fajara, The Gambia

Zirui Meng, Minjin Wang, Zhenzhen Zhao, Shuo Guo, Mengjiao Li, Yanbing Zhou, Shuyu Yang and Binwu Ying
Department of Laboratory Medicine, West China Hospital, Sichuan University, Chengdu, China

Yongzhao Zhou, Ying Wu and Weimin Li
Department of Respiratory and Critical Care Medicine, West China Hospital, Sichuan University, Chengdu, China

Jianjuan Ma
Department of Pathophysiology, School of Basic Medical Sciences, Guizhou Medical University, Guiyang, China
Pulmonary and Critical Care Medicine, Guangzhou Institute of Respiratory Health, National Clinical Research Center for Respiratory Disease, National Center for Respiratory Medicine, State Key Laboratory of Respiratory Diseases, The First Affiliated Hospital of Guangzhou Medical University, Guangzhou, China
Department of Pediatric Hematology, Affiliated Hospital of Guizhou Medical University, Guiyang, China

Cong Dong, Shushan Wei, Minzhi Qiu, Penghui Wu, Changxing Ou, Bomeng Zhang and Qingling Zhang
Pulmonary and Critical Care Medicine, Guangzhou Institute of Respiratory Health, National Clinical Research Center for Respiratory Disease, National Center for Respiratory Medicine, State Key Laboratory

Xueyan Zhang
School of Basic Medical Sciences, The Second Affiliated Hospital, State Key Laboratory of Respiratory Disease, Guangdong Provincial Key Laboratory of Allergy & Clinical Immunology, Guangzhou Medical University, Guangzhou, China

Jie Yan
The Second Affiliated Hospital, State Key Laboratory of Respiratory Disease, Guangdong Provincial Key Laboratory of Allergy & Clinical Immunology, Guangzhou Medical University, Guangzhou, China

Nanshan Zhong
Department of Pathophysiology, School of Basic Medical Sciences, Guizhou Medical University, Guiyang, China
Pulmonary and Critical Care Medicine, Guangzhou Institute of Respiratory Health, National Clinical Research Center for Respiratory Disease, National Center for Respiratory Medicine, State Key Laboratory of Respiratory Diseases, The First Affiliated Hospital of Guangzhou Medical University, Guangzhou, China

Arjun Mohan, Nicole Neequaye, Anagha Malur, Matthew McPeek, Nancy Leffler, David Ogburn Barbara P. Barna and Mary Jane Thomassen
Division of Pulmonary, Critical Care and Sleep Medicine, Department of Medicine, Brody School of Medicine- East Carolina University, Greenville, NC, United States

Eman Soliman
Division of Pulmonary, Critical Care and Sleep Medicine, Department of Medicine, Brody School of Medicine- East Carolina University, Greenville, NC, United States
Department of Pharmacology and Toxicology, Faculty of Pharmacy, Zagazig University, Zagazig, Egypt

Debra A. Tokarz
Department of Population Health and Pathobiology, College of Veterinary Medicine, North Carolina State University, Raleigh, NC, United States

Warren Knudson
Department of Anatomy and Cell Biology, Brody School of Medicine- East Carolina University, Greenville, NC, United States

Sina A. Gharib
Division of Pulmonary, Critical Care and Sleep Medicine, Computational Medicine Core, Center for Lung Biology, Department of Medicine, University of Washington, Seattle, WA, United States

Lynn M. Schnapp
Allergy, Pulmonary and Critical Care Medicine, Department of Medicine, University of Wisconsin Madison School of Medicine and Public Health, Madison, WI, United States

Yuan Cao and Lulu Zheng
Department of Pulmonary and Critical Care Medicine, The Second Affiliated Hospital of Xi'an Jiaotong University (Xibei Hospital), Xi'an, China

Hua Zhang
Department of Respiratory Medicine, Zhangjiakou First Hospital, Zhangjiakou, China

Qiao Li
Clinical Laboratory, The Affiliated Children Hospital of Xi'an Jiaotong University, Xi'an, China

Vanessa Santos, David Araújo and Adriana Magalhães
Pulmonology Department, Centro Hospitalar Universitário São João, Porto, Portugal

David Barros Coelho and Henrique Queiroga
Pulmonology Department, Centro Hospitalar Universitário São João, Porto, Portugal
Faculdade de Medicina, University of Porto, Porto, Portugal

Hélder Novais Bastos, Venceslau Hespanhol and Maria Gabriela O. Fernandes
Pulmonology Department, Centro Hospitalar Universitário São João, Porto, Portugal
Faculdade de Medicina, University of Porto, Porto, Portugal
Institute for Research and Innovation in Health (i3S), University of Porto, Porto, Portugal

Natália Cruz-Martins
Faculdade de Medicina, University of Porto, Porto, Portugal
Institute for Research and Innovation in Health (i3S), University of Porto, Porto, Portugal
Laboratory of Neuropsychophysiology, Faculty of Psychology and Education Sciences, University of Porto, Porto, Portugal

Sarah A. Greaves and Shaikh M. Atif
Department of Medicine, University of Colorado Anschutz Medical Campus, Aurora, CO, United States

Andrew P. Fontenot
Department of Medicine, University of Colorado Anschutz Medical Campus, Aurora, CO, United States
Department of Immunology and Microbiology, University of Colorado Anschutz Medical Campus, mAurora, CO, United States

Xie Xiaohong, Wang Liqiang, Lin Xinqing, Qin Yinyin, Liu Ming, Ouyang Ming, Han Qian, Luo Qun, Li Shiyue and Zhou Chengzhi
State Key Laboratory of Respiratory Disease, National Clinical Research Center of Respiratory Disease, The First Affiliated Hospital of Guangzhou Medical University, Guangzhou Institute of the Respiratory Health, Guangzhou Medical University, Guangzhou, China

Li Na, Yang Shuanying, Huang Wei and Liu Mei
Department of Respiratory and Critical Care Medicine, The Second Affiliated Hospital of Xi'an Jiaotong University, Xi'an, China

Li Chunyan and Wang Xiaoqian
Department of Respiratory and Critical Care Medicine, The First Medical Center of PLA General Hospital, Beijing, China

Wang Ping
Department of Respiratory and Critical Care Medicine, The Eighth Medical Center of PLA General Hospital, Beijing, China

Wenzhe Yang Wei Yang, Pinhua Pan, Chengping Hu, Rongli Lu, Yimin Fang and Yuanyuan Li
Department of Respiratory Medicine (Department of Respiratory and Critical Care Medicine), Xiangya Hospital, Central South University, Changsha, China

Rongjun Wan
Department of Respiratory Medicine (Department of Respiratory and Critical Care Medicine), Xiangya Hospital, Central South University, Changsha, China
National Clinical Research Center for Geriatric Disorders, Xiangya Hospital, Central South University, Changsha, China

Qiong Chen
National Clinical Research Center for Geriatric Disorders, Xiangya Hospital, Central South University, Changsha, China

Xinhua Ma
Department of Critical Care Medicine, Xiangya Hospital, Central South University, Changsha, China

Yaou Zhou
Department of Rheumatology and Immunology, Xiangya Hospital, Central South University, Changsha, China

Raisa Kraaijvanger, Montse Janssen Bonás and Adriane D. M. Vorselaars
Department of Pulmonology, ILD Center of Excellence, St. Antonius Hospital, Nieuwegein, Netherlands

Marcel Veltkamp
Department of Pulmonology, ILD Center of Excellence, St. Antonius Hospital, Nieuwegein, Netherlands
Department of Pulmonology, University Medical Center, Utrecht, Netherlands

Shuangyue Pan
The Second Clinical Medical College, Zhejiang Chinese Medical University, Hangzhou, China
Center of Oncology, Department of Medical Oncology, Zhejiang Provincial People's Hospital, People's Hospital of Hangzhou Medical College, Hangzhou, China

Jiahong Jiang, Zheling Chen and Liu Yang
Center of Oncology, Department of Medical Oncology, Zhejiang Provincial People's Hospital, People's Hospital of Hangzhou Medical College, Hangzhou, China

Zheyi Wang and Yaqian Liu
Dongzhimen Hospital Affiliated to Beijing University of Chinese Medicine, Beijing, China

Yufeng Meng
Department of TCM, Peking University People's Hospital, Beijing, China

Guishu Wang
Department of TCM, Peking University People's Hospital, Beijing, China
Dongzhimen Hospital Affiliated to Beijing University of Chinese Medicine, Beijing, China

Bo Zhou
Xiyuan Hospital Affiliated to China Academy of Chinese Medical Sciences, Beijing, China

Xiaoqin Yao
Department of TCM, Peking University International Hospital, Beijing, China
Department of Integration of Chinese and Western Medicine, School of Basic Medical Sciences, Peking University, Beijing, China

Cuiling Feng
Department of TCM, Peking University People's Hospital, Beijing, China
Department of Integration of Chinese and Western Medicine, School of Basic Medical Sciences, Peking University, Beijing, China

Kerry Maryse Hena
Division of Pulmonary, Critical Care, and Sleep Medicine, Department of Medicine, New York University, New York, NY, United States

Lucy Revercomb
Department of BioSciences, Rice University, Houston, TX, United States
Department of Biochemistry and Molecular Biology, McGovern Medical School, University of Texas Health Science Center at Houston, Houston, TX, United States

Ankit Hanmandlu and Nancy Wareing
Department of Biochemistry and Molecular Biology, McGovern Medical School, University of Texas Health Science Center at Houston, Houston, TX, United States

Bindu Akkanti
Divisions of Critical Care, Pulmonary and Sleep Medicine, McGovern Medical School, University of Texas Health Science Center at Houston, Houston, TX, United States

Harry Karmouty-Quintana
Department of Biochemistry and Molecular Biology, McGovern Medical School, University of Texas Health Science Center at Houston, Houston, TX, United States
Divisions of Critical Care, Pulmonary and Sleep Medicine, McGovern Medical School, University of Texas Health Science Center at Houston, Houston, TX, United States

Pan Li
Department of Cardiology, Changhai Hospital, Second Military Medical University, Shanghai, China
Department of Infection Diseases No. 1, The Maternal and Child Health Hospital of Hubei Province, Wuhan, China

Zhengmao Lu
Department of Infection Diseases No. 1, The Maternal and Child Health Hospital of Hubei Province, Wuhan, China
Department of Gastrointestinal Surgery, Changhai Hospital, Second Military Medical University, Shanghai, China

Qiang Li
Department of Infection Diseases No. 1, The Maternal and Child Health Hospital of Hubei Province, Wuhan, China
Department of Neurosurgery, Changhai Hospital, Second Military Medical University, Shanghai, China

Zhenmeng Wang
Department of Infection Diseases No. 1, The Maternal and Child Health Hospital of Hubei Province, Wuhan, China
Department of Anesthesia, Third Affiliated Hospital, Second Military Medical University, Shanghai, China

Yan Guo
Department of Infection Diseases No. 1, The Maternal and Child Health Hospital of Hubei Province, Wuhan, China
Department of Endocrinology, Changhai Hospital, Second Military Medical University, Shanghai, China

Chen Cai
Department of Infection Diseases No. 1, The Maternal and Child Health Hospital of Hubei Province, Wuhan, China
Department of Special Clinic, Changhai Hospital, Second Military Medical University, Shanghai, China

Shengyun Wang
Department of Infection Diseases No. 1, The Maternal and Child Health Hospital of Hubei Province, Wuhan, China
Department of Emergency and Critical Care Medicine, Changzheng Hospital, Second Military Medical University, Shanghai, China

Peng Liu
Department of Infection Diseases No. 1, The Maternal and Child Health Hospital of Hubei Province, Wuhan, China
Department of Colorectal Surgery, Changhai Hospital, Second Military Medical University, Shanghai, China

Xiaoping Su
School of Basic Medicine, Wenzhou Medical University, Wenzhou, China

Yi Huang, Yuchao Dong and Chong Bai
Department of Respiratory and Critical Care Medicine, Changhai Hospital, Second Military Medical University, Shanghai, China

Wei Zhang
Department of Infection Diseases No. 1, The Maternal and Child Health Hospital of Hubei Province, Wuhan, China
Department of Respiratory and Critical Care Medicine, Changhai Hospital, Second Military Medical University, Shanghai, China

Wenjuan Qiu
Department of Infection Diseases No. 1, The Maternal and Child Health Hospital of Hubei Province, Wuhan, China
Department of Cardiovascular ICU, Changhai Hospital, Second Military Medical University, Shanghai, China

Yueming Ling
Department of Infection Diseases No. 1, The Maternal and Child Health Hospital of Hubei Province, Wuhan, China
Department of Clinical Laboratory Science of No. 910 Hospital of PLA Joint Support Force, Quanzhou, China

Lonny Yarmus
Department of Infection Diseases No. 1, The Maternal and Child Health Hospital of Hubei Province, Wuhan, China
Division of Pulmonary and Critical Care, Johns Hopkins University School of Medicine, Baltimore, MD, United States

Fengming Luo
Department of Infection Diseases No. 1, The Maternal and Child Health Hospital of Hubei Province, Wuhan, China
Department of Pulmonary and Critical Care Medicine, West China Hospital, Sichuan University, Chengdu, China

Li Zeng
Department of Infection Diseases No. 1, The Maternal and Child Health Hospital of Hubei Province, Wuhan, China
Department of Organ Transplantation, Changhai Hospital, Second Military Medical University, Shanghai, China

Jaya Talreja
Division of Pulmonary, Critical Care and Sleep Medicine, Department of Internal Medicine, School of Medicine and Detroit Medical Center, Wayne State University, Detroit, MI, United States

Christian Bauerfeld
Division of Critical Care, Department of Pediatrics, School of Medicine and Detroit Medical Center, Wayne State University, Detroit, MI, United States

Edward Sendler
Center for Molecular Medicine and Genetics, School of Medicine, Wayne State University, Detroit, MI, United States

Roger Pique-Regi and Francesca Luca
Center for Molecular Medicine and Genetics, School of Medicine, Wayne State University, Detroit, MI, United States
Department of Obstetrics and Gynecology, School of Medicine, Wayne State University, Detroit, MI, United States

Lobelia Samavati
Division of Pulmonary, Critical Care and Sleep Medicine, Department of Internal Medicine, School of Medicine and Detroit Medical Center, Wayne State University, Detroit, MI, United States
Center for Molecular Medicine and Genetics, School of Medicine, Wayne State University, Detroit, MI, United States

Xue Yang, Minglei Zhuo, Meina Wu, Tongtong An, Ziping Wang, Yuyan Wang, Jianjie Li, Jia Zhong, Hanxiao Chen, Bo Jia, Jingjing Wang and Jun Zhao
Key Laboratory of Carcinogenesis and Translational Research (Ministry of Education), Department of Thoracic Medical Oncology, Peking University Cancer Hospital and Institute, Beijing, China

Yang Xia
Key Laboratory of Respiratory Disease of Zhejiang Province, Department of Respiratory and Critical Care Medicine, Second Affiliated Hospital of Zhejiang University School of Medicine, Hangzhou, Zhejiang, China

Liyan Xu
Department of Medical Oncology, Beijing Chest Hospital, Capital Medical University, Beijing, China

Li Liang
Department of Tumor Chemotherapy and Radiation Sickness, Peking University Third Hospital, Beijing, China

Nicholas K. Arger, Siddharth Machiraju, Prescott G. Woodruff and Laura L. Koth
Division of Pulmonary and Critical Care, University of California, San Francisco, San Francisco, CA, United States

Isabel E. Allen
Department of Epidemiology and Biostatistics, University of California, San Francisco, San Francisco, CA, United States

Ling Zhou, Yuanyuan Fang and Huiguo Liu
Department of Respiratory and Critical Care Medicine, Tongji Hospital, Tongji Medical College, Huazhong University of Science and Technology, Wuhan, China

Wei Liu
Department of Respiratory and Critical Care Medicine, Renmin Hospital of Wuhan University, Wuhan, China

Jianchu Zhang
Department of Respiratory and Critical Care Medicine, Union Hospital, Tongji Medical College, Huazhong University of Science and Technology, Wuhan, China

Yingnan Wang
Department of Respiratory and Critical Care Medicine, The People's Hospital of China Three Gorges University, The First People's Hospital of Yichang, Yichang, China

Sheng Xie
Department of Respiratory and Critical Care Medicine, Huangshi Central Hospital, Affiliated Hospital of Hubei Polytechnic University, Huangshi, China

Minhua Zhong
Department of Respiratory and Critical Care Medicine, Xiaogan Hospital Affiliated to Wuhan University of Science and Technology, The Central Hospital of Xiaogan, Xiaogan, China

Zhengyan Wang
Department of Respiratory Medicine, Suizhou Hospital, Hubei University of Medicine, Suizhou, China

Guangcai Li
Department of Respiratory and Critical Care Medicine, The Central Hospital of Enshi Tujia and Miao Autonmous Prefecture, Enshi Clinical College of Wuhan University, Enshi Tujia and Miao Autonomous Prefecture, Hubei, China

Hongyan Ai
Department of Respiratory and Critical Care Medicine, Hanyang Hospital Affiliated to Wuhan University of Science and Technology, Wuhan, China

Hongrong Guo
Department of Respiratory and Critical Care Medicine, Wuhan Third Hospital, Tongren Hospital of Wuhan University, Wuhan, China

Fanjun Zeng
Department of Respiratory and Critical Care Medicine, The First College of Clinical Medicine Science, China Three Gorges University, Yichang Central People's Hospital, Yichang, China

Wei Xiao
Department of Respiratory and Critical Care Medicine, The First People's Hospital of Jingzhou, Jingzhou, China

Chenghong Li
Department of Respiratory and Critical Care Medicine, The Sixth Hospital of Wuhan, Jianghan University, Wuhan, China

Yi Hu
Department of Respiratory and Critical Care Medicine, The Central Hospital of Wuhan, Tongji Medical College, Huazhong University of Science and Technology, Wuhan, China

Yijun Tang
Department of Respiratory and Critical Medical, Taihe Hospital, Affiliated Hospital of Hubei University of Medicine, Shiyan, China

Marc A. Judson
Albany Medical College, Albany, NY, United States

Zheng-Tu Li, Pei-Ying Zeng, Zhao-Ming Chen, Ye Lin, Shao-Qiang Li, Yang-Qing Zhan, Ming-Die Wang and Feng Ye
State Key Laboratory of Respiratory Disease, National Clinical Research Center for Respiratory Disease, National Center for Respiratory Medicine, Guangzhou Institute of Respiratory Health, The First Affiliated Hospital of Guangzhou Medical University, Guangzhou, China

Wei-Jie Guan
State Key Laboratory of Respiratory Disease, National Clinical Research Center for Respiratory Disease, National Center for Respiratory Medicine, Guangzhou Institute of Respiratory Health, The First Affiliated Hospital of Guangzhou Medical University, Guangzhou, China
Department of Thoracic Surgery, Guangzhou Institute for Respiratory Health, The First Affiliated Hospital of Guangzhou Medical University, Guangzhou, Guangdong, China

Tong Wang
Institute of Mass Spectrometry and Atmospheric Environment, Jinan University, Guangzhou, China
Guangdong Provincial Engineering Research Center for On-Line Source Apportionment System of Air Pollution, Guangzhou, China

Zhi-Juan Zhang
Institute of Mass Spectrometry and Atmospheric Environment, Jinan University, Guangzhou, China
Guangdong Provincial Engineering Research Center for On-Line Source Apportionment System of Air Pollution, Guangzhou, China
College of Pharmacy, Hena University of Chinese Medicine, Zhengzhou, China

Guo-Bin Tan
Institute of Mass Spectrometry and Atmospheric Environment, Jinan University, Guangzhou, China
Guangdong Provincial Engineering Research Center for On-Line Source Apportionment System of Air Pollution, Guangzhou, China
Guangzhou Hexin Instrument Co., Ltd., Guangzhou, China

Xue Li
Institute of Mass Spectrometry and Atmospheric Environment, Jinan University, Guangzhou, China
Guangdong Provincial Engineering Research Center for On-Line Source Apportionment System of Air Pollution, Guangzhou, China

Kai Guo and Shuxuan Ma
Department of Transfusion Medicine, Beijing Children's Hospital, Capital Medical University, National Center for Children's Health, Beijing, China

Index

M

N

O

P

Q

S

T

U

W

www.ingramcontent.com/pod-product-compliance
Lightning Source LLC
LaVergne TN
LVHW082127200926
848484LV00008B/2019